STATISTICAL METHODS IN
MEDICAL RESEARCH

To J. O. Irwin

MENTOR AND FRIEND

Statistical Methods in Medical Research

P. ARMITAGE
MA, PhD
Emeritus Professor of Applied Statistics,
University of Oxford

G. BERRY
MA, PhD
Professor in Epidemiology and Biostatistics,
University of Sydney

THIRD EDITION

b

Blackwell
Science

© 1971, 1987, 1994 by
Blackwell Science Ltd
Editorial Offices:
Osney Mead, Oxford OX2 0EL
25 John Street, London WC1N 2BL
23 Ainslie Place, Edinburgh EH3 6AJ
238 Main Street, Cambridge
  Massachusetts 02142, USA
54 University Street, Carlton
  Victoria 3053, Australia

Other Editorial Offices:
Arnette Blackwell SA
  224, Boulevard Saint Germain
  75007 Paris, France

Blackwell Wissenschafts-Verlag GmbH
  Kurfürstendamm 57
  10707 Berlin, Germany

  Zehetnergasse 6
  A-1140 Wien
  Austria

First published 1971
Reprinted 1973, 1974, 1977, 1980, 1983, 1985
Italian editions 1975, 1977, 1979, 1981
Polish edition 1978
Second edition 1987
Reprinted 1988 (twice), 1990, 1991, 1993
Spanish edition 1992
Third edition 1994
Reprinted 1995, 1996

Set by Macmillan India Ltd
Printed and bound in Great Britain
at the University Press, Cambridge

DISTRIBUTORS

  Marston Book Services Ltd
  PO Box 269
  Abingdon
  Oxon OX14 4YN
  (*Orders*: Tel: 01235 465500
             Fax: 01235 465555)

USA
  Blackwell Science, Inc.
  238 Main Street
  Cambridge, MA 02142
  (*Orders*: Tel: 800 215-1000
                   617 876-7000
             Fax: 617 492-5263)

Canada
  Copp Clark, Ltd
  2775 Matheson Blvd East
  Mississauga, Ontario
  Canada, L4W 4P7
  (*Orders*: Tel: 800 263-4374
                   905 238-6074)

Australia
  Blackwell Science Pty Ltd
  54 University Street
  Carlton, Victoria 3053
  (*Orders*: Tel: 03 9347 0300
             Fax: 03 9349 3016)

A catalogue record for this title
is available from the British Library

ISBN 0-632-03695-8

Library of Congress
Cataloging-in-Publication Data

Armitage, P.
  Statistical methods in medical research/
  P. Armitage and G. Berry.—3rd ed.
       p.   cm.
  Includes bibliographical references
  and index.
  ISBN 0-632-03695-8
  1. Medicine—Research
  Statistical methods
  I. Berry, G. (Geoffrey)
  II. Title.
  [DNLM: 1. Biometry.
  2. Research—methods.
  WA 950 A733s 1994]
  R853.S7A743 1994
  610´.72—dc20
  DNLM/DLC
  for Library of Congress

Contents

Preface to the Third Edition ix

1 The Scope of Statistics 1
  1.1 General, 1
  1.2 Diagrams, 4
  1.3 Tabulation and data processing, 7
  1.4 Summarizing numerical data, 14
  1.5 Means and other measures of location, 26
  1.6 Measures of variation, 31

2 Probability 41
  2.1 The meaning of probability, 41
  2.2 Probability calculations, 44
  2.3 Probability distributions, 48
  2.4 Expectation, 52
  2.5 The binomial distribution, 55
  2.6 The Poisson distribution, 59
  2.7 The normal (or Gaussian) distribution, 66
  2.8 Bayes' theorem, 71
  2.9 Subjective probability, 76

3 Sampling 78
  3.1 Population and sample, 78
  3.2 The sampling error of a mean, 80
  3.3 The sampling error of a proportion, 84
  3.4 The sampling error of a variance, 85
  3.5 The sampling error of a difference, 88
  3.6 Some other variance formulae, 90

4 Statistical Inference 93
  4.1 General, 93
  4.2 Significance tests and confidence intervals, 94
  4.3 Inferences from means, 99
  4.4 Comparison of two means, 106
  4.5 Inferences from variances, 114
  4.6 Comparison of two variances, 115
  4.7 Inferences from proportions, 118
  4.8 Comparison of two proportions, 125
  4.9 2×2 Tables and χ^2 tests, 132

    4.10 Inferences from counts, 141
    4.11 Comparison of two counts, 144
    4.12 Likelihood and Bayesian methods, 146
    4.13 Some further Bayesian methods, 149

5   **Regression and Correlation** 154
    5.1 Association, 154
    5.2 Linear regression, 156
    5.3 Correlation, 163
    5.4 Sampling errors in regression and correlation, 165
    5.5 Regression to the mean, 172

6   **The Planning of Statistical Investigations** 175
    6.1 General, 175
    6.2 The planning of surveys: estimation of population parameters, 176
    6.3 Surveys to investigate associations, 183
    6.4 The design of experiments, 187
    6.5 Clinical trials, 189
    6.6 The size of a statistical investigation, 195

7   **Comparison of Several Groups** 207
    7.1 One-way analysis of variance, 207
    7.2 The method of weighting, 215
    7.3 Components of variance, 219
    7.4 Multiple comparisons, 224
    7.5 Comparison of several proportions: the $2 \times k$ contingency table, 228
    7.6 General contingency tables, 232
    7.7 Comparison of several variances, 234
    7.8 Comparison of several counts: the Poisson heterogeneity test, 234

8   **Further Experimental Designs** 237
    8.1 Two-way analysis of variance: randomized blocks, 237
    8.2 The simple crossover design, 245
    8.3 Factorial designs, 249
    8.4 Latin squares, 259
    8.5 Other incomplete designs, 264
    8.6 Split-unit designs, 268
    8.7 Intraclass correlation, 273
    8.8 Non-orthogonal two-way tables: some simple cases, 276

9   **Further Analysis of Straight-Line Data** 283
    9.1 Analysis of variance applied to regression, 283
    9.2 Errors in both variables, 288
    9.3 Straight lines through the origin, 291
    9.4 Regression in groups, 292
    9.5 The analysis of covariance, 301

10   Multiple Measurements 312
   10.1   Multiple regression, 312
   10.2   Multiple regression in groups, 334
   10.3   Polynomial and other curvilinear regressions, 341
   10.4   Multiple regression in the analysis of non-orthogonal data, 348
   10.5   Multivariate methods, 350
   10.6   Time series, 375
   10.7   Repeated measurements and growth curves, 380

11   Data Editing 386
   11.1   Preliminary remarks, 386
   11.2   Transformations in general, 386
   11.3   Logarithmic and power transformations, 389
   11.4   Transformations for proportions, 392
   11.5   Goodness of fit of frequency distributions, 394
   11.6   Outlying observations, 399

12   Further Analysis of Categorical Data 402
   12.1   Introduction, 402
   12.2   Trends in proportions, 403
   12.3   Trends in larger contingency tables, 408
   12.4   Trends in counts, 410
   12.5   Other components of χ^2, 411
   12.6   Combination of 2×2 tables, 415
   12.7   Combination of larger tables, 420
   12.8   Generalized linear models, 422
   12.9   Standardization, 436
   12.10 Kappa measure of agreement, 443

13   Distribution-Free Methods 448
   13.1   Introduction, 448
   13.2   One-sample tests for location, 449
   13.3   Comparison of two independent groups, 453
   13.4   Comparison of several groups, 461
   13.5   Rank correlation, 464
   13.6   General comments, 467

14   Survival Analysis 469
   14.1   Introduction, 469
   14.2   Life tables, 470
   14.3   Follow-up studies, 472
   14.4   Sampling errors in the life table, 475
   14.5   The product-limit estimate of survival, 476
   14.6   The logrank test, 477
   14.7   Parametric models, 482
   14.8   Regression and proportional-hazards models, 483
   14.9   Subject-years methods, 489

15 Sequential Methods 493
15.1 General, 493
15.2 Sequential tests for binary data, 495
15.3 Normal approximations, 500
15.4 Group sequential plans, 502
15.5 Concluding remarks, 505

16 Statistical Methods in Epidemiology 507
16.1 Introduction, 507
16.2 Relative risk, 508
16.3 Attributable risk, 519
16.4 Diagnostic tests and screening procedures, 522
16.5 Disease clustering, 530

17 Biological Assay 535
17.1 Introduction, 535
17.2 Parallel-line assays, 537
17.3 Slope-ratio assays, 544
17.4 Quantal-response assays, 547

18 Statistical Computation 551
18.1 Introduction, 551
18.2 Data processing, 552
18.3 Statistical analysis, 553
18.4 Statistical packages, 554
18.5 General remarks, 557

Appendix Tables 559
A1   Areas in tail of the normal distribution, 560
A2   Percentage points of the χ^2 distribution, 562
A3   Percentage points of the t distribution, 564
A4   Percentage points of the F distribution: $P = 0.05, 0.025, 0.01, 0.005$, 566
A5   Percentage points of the distribution of studentized range: $\alpha = 0.05, 0.01$, 570
A6   Random sampling numbers, 572
A7   Percentage points for the Wilcoxon signed rank sum test, 577
A8   Percentage points for the Wilcoxon two-sample rank sum test, 578
A9   Sample size for comparing two proportions, 579
A10 Sample size table for detecting relative risk in case–control study, 580

References 581

Author Index 595

Subject Index 601

Preface to the Third Edition

There are many excellent introductory books on medical statistics, providing simple expositions of basic statistical techniques and describing some of the problems that beset the statistician practising his or her art in medical applications. The aim of the present book, as of its earlier editions, is a little more ambitious. We have tried to gather together the majority of statistical techniques that are used at all frequently in medical research, and to describe them in terms accessible to the non-mathematician. Our scope clearly overlaps that of a number of other, more general, books on applied statistics. We hope, though, that the present book, explicitly directed towards medical applications, will have two special assets. First, the use of examples selected almost entirely from medical research projects will, we believe, help the reader to understand the underlying concepts. Second, the choice of statistical topics reflects the extent of their usage in medical research; some of these would not appear in a general book on applied statistics but find a natural place here.

The book is intended to be useful both for the medical research worker with no particular mathematical expertise but with the ability to follow straightforward formulae, and for the professional statistician interested in medical applications. The emphasis throughout is on the general concepts underlying statistical techniques, the purposes for which they are designed, and the form of calculations required for their implementation. Proofs are regarded as of secondary importance and are usually omitted or (when they involve relatively simple mathematics) relegated to small type. The level of mathematics is in the main that of simple algebraic manipulation, and the symbolism (such as the use of the summation sign) can be mastered quite easily. Calculus and matrix operations are used very occasionally, but the reader unfamiliar with these techniques will be able to skip judiciously without loss of continuity. We have dealt in a fairly leisurely way with some of the basic concepts, which are often found to be difficult at first encounter, but readers who are already familiar with these (from introductory courses, for instance) will be able to skip the early chapters and make immediate use of the later material. Medical research is gradually becoming more statistical in character, and research workers are increasingly called upon to design their studies and analyse their data with no more than occasional consultations with specialist statisticians. This book may help them to extend the range of statistical methods that they can confidently apply without recourse to expert advice.

The present edition follows the same general approach as its predecessors. We have preserved the original order of the chapters, although some of the sections have been rearranged, renumbered or retitled, and a small amount of material has been transferred between chapters. The last few years have seen a substantial output of papers developing new statistical methods specifically for medical research, with several thousand pages each year in the three or four principal journals. We have tried to take account of some of these developments, particularly in the sections on Bayesian methods (Chapters 2 and 4), clinical trials (Chapter 6) and survival analysis (Chapter 14). We have also rewritten or enlarged some of the more general sections, especially in Chapter 6 on sample size determination, Chapter 10 on regression diagnostics, Chapter 12 on categorical data and Chapter 13 on distribution-free methods.

Two changes have been made which affect the reporting of significance levels. First, it is now unnecessary always to refer P values to a few standard levels such as 0·05 and 0·01. Most statistical packages for computers quote precise P values for standard tests, and we recommend that these values are used. The second change is more fundamental and applies to the calculation of P values for discrete distributions, such as those occurring in the analysis of binary data. We advocate the 'mid-P' significance value, which was originally suggested over 40 years ago and has recently received a good deal of attention in the statistical literature. Associated with this is the concept of mid-P confidence intervals, which we also recommend.

We noted in the Preface to the Second Edition the impact on statistical practice of the widespread use of computers and the availability of powerful statistical packages. Since that date (1987) the influence of the computer has grown apace. Few scientists, whether statisticians, clinicians or laboratory workers, would nowadays conduct any but the most trivial statistical analysis without a computer. Indeed, we strongly urge any reader intending to make serious use of the methods described in this book to gain access to a computer equipped with one of the standard statistical packages (such as those outlined in Chapter 18). This trend has enabled us to remove or reduce descriptions of some of the methods designed for hand calculation. We have, though, deliberately retained full descriptions of the intermediate steps of many of the calculations to enable the reader to gain understanding of the logical steps involved, even though, in practice, few if any of our readers will need to carry out the calculations other than with a statistical package. We aim, in short, to explain the concepts and detailed methods more fully than is possible in a computer manual. Statistical packages are developing so rapidly that it seemed unwise to try to provide comprehensive descriptions of individual systems. Chapter 18 provides short notes on some of these, which may be amplified by reference to the relevant manuals. We have occasionally referred to particular programs in the text, where this seemed appropriate—usually because they offer special facilities.

Statisticians engaged in medical work or interested in medical applications will, we hope, find many points of interest in this review of the subject. In particular, the book may provide a useful framework for the teaching of courses for students trained in medical or biological science. Much of the exposition and many of the examples are based on material used in courses for postgraduate students in the medical sciences. The book as a whole is more extensive than would be required for a single course, but the statistics teacher would have little difficulty in making appropriate selections for particular groups of students.

For much of the material included in the book, both illustrative and general, we owe our thanks to our present and former colleagues. We have not attempted systematically to give attributions for all quoted data, some of which are hidden in the mists of time, and must apologize to any authors who find their data put to unsuspected purposes in these pages. Nor have we identified all the computer programs used for computations. However, for the calculation of precise P values, referred to earlier, we have found it particularly convenient to use a small package, Arcus Pro-II developed by Iain E. Buchan, to cover many of the methods described in this book.

In preparing each of these editions for the press we have had much secretarial and other help from many people, to all of whom we express our thanks.

P. Armitage
G. Berry

1: The Scope of Statistics

1.1 General

In one sense medical statistics are merely numerical statements about medical matters: how many people die from a certain cause each year, how many hospital beds are available in a certain area, how much money is spent on a certain medical service. Such facts are clearly of administrative importance. To plan the maternity-bed service for a community we need to know how many women in that community give birth to a child in a given period, and how many of these should be cared for in hospitals or maternity homes. Numerical facts also supply the basis for a great deal of medical research; examples will be found throughout this book. It is no purpose of the book to list or even to summarize numerical information of this sort. Such facts may be found in official publications of national or international health departments, in the published reports of research investigations and in textbooks and monographs on medical subjects. The book is concerned with the general rather than the particular, with methodology rather than with factual information, with the general principles of statistical investigations rather than with the results of particular studies.

Statistics may be defined as the discipline concerned with the treatment of numerical data derived from groups of individuals. These individuals will often be people—for instance, those suffering from a certain disease or those living in a certain area. They may be animals or other organisms. They may be different administrative units, as when we measure the case-fatality rate in each of a number of hospitals. They may be merely different occasions on which a particular measurement has been made.

Why should we be interested in the numerical properties of groups of people or objects? Sometimes, for administrative reasons like those mentioned earlier, statistical facts are needed: these may be contained in official publications; they may be derivable from established systems of data collection such as cancer registries or systems for the notification of congenital malformations; they may, however, require specially designed statistical investigations.

This book is concerned particularly with the use of statistics in medical research, and here—in contrast to its administrative uses—the case for statistics is not free from controversy. The argument is occasionally heard that statistical information contributes little or nothing to the progress of medicine, because the physician is concerned at any one time with the treatment of a single patient, and

1

every patient differs in important respects from every other patient. An eminent psychiatrist wrote, in a letter to the *Lancet*, 'One must go on repeating the fact that if, in the past 30 years, one had ever paid very much attention to statistics, especially when they were not supported by clinical bedside findings, treatment progress in psychiatry in this country would not have got very far.' Two points may be made at this stage. First, the variability of disease is an argument *for* statistical information, not *against* it. If the bedside physician finds that on one occasion a patient with migraine feels better after drinking plum juice, it does not follow, from this single observation, that plum juice is a useful therapy for migraine. The doctor needs statistical information showing, for example, whether in a group of patients improvement is reported more frequently after the administration of plum juice than after the use of some alternative treatment. Secondly, the 'bedside findings' referred to in the quotation above are likely to be essentially statistical comparisons derived from a lifetime of clinical practice. The argument, then, is whether such information should be stored in a rather informal way in the physician's mind or whether it should be collected and reported in a systematic way. Very few doctors acquire, by personal experience, factual information over the whole range of medicine, and it is partly by the collection, analysis and reporting of statistical information that a common body of knowledge is built and solidified.

The difficulty of arguing from a single instance is equally apparent in studies of the aetiology of disease. The fact that a particular person was alive and well at the age of 95 and that he smoked 50 cigarettes a day and drank heavily would not convince one that such habits are conducive to good health and longevity. Individuals vary greatly in their susceptibility to disease. Many abstemious non-smokers die young. To study these questions one should look at the morbidity and mortality experience of groups of people with different habits; that is, one should do a statistical study.

The first chapter in this book is concerned mainly with some of the basic tools for collecting and presenting numerical data, a part of the subject usually called *descriptive statistics*.

The statistician needs to go beyond this descriptive task, in two important respects. First, it may be possible to improve the quality of the information by careful planning of the data collection. Secondly, the methods of *statistical inference* provide a largely objective means of drawing conclusions from the data about the issues under research. Both these developments, of planning and inference, owe much to the work of R. A. (later Sir Ronald) Fisher (1890–1962), whose influence is apparent throughout modern statistical practice.

Almost all the techniques described in this book can be used in a wide variety of branches of medical research, and indeed frequently in the non-medical sciences also. To set the scene it may be useful to mention five quite different investigations in which statistical methods played an essential part.

1 Smith *et al.* (1962) described a study of antibody titres after vaccination against yellow fever. The investigators had records of blood samples from 100 or so vaccinated subjects, and wanted to know whether the level of antibody production depended on the level before vaccination; whether it depended on the presence of antibodies against certain other viruses related to yellow fever; whether the antibody level against the other viruses was also affected; and so on. The investigation of all these possible associations was clearly a substantial task. Moreover, the determination of antibody level from each blood sample required an animal experiment in which groups of animals were inoculated with mixtures of serum and varying dilutions of virus, the results of which had to be interpreted statistically.

2 MacKie *et al.* (1992) studied the trend in the incidence of primary cutaneous malignant melanoma in Scotland during the period 1979–89. In assessing trends of this sort it is important to take account of such factors as changes in standards of diagnosis and in definitions of disease categories, changes in the pattern of referrals of patients in and out of the area under study, and changes in the age structure of the population. The study group was set up with these points in mind, and dealt with almost 4000 patients. The investigators found that the annual incidence rate increased during the period from 3·4 to 7·1 per 100 000 for men, and from 6·6 to 10·4 for women. These findings suggest that the disease, which is known to be affected by high levels of ultraviolet radiation, may be becoming more common even in areas where these levels are relatively low.

3 Women who have had a pregnancy with a neural tube defect (NTD) are known to be at higher than average risk of having a similar occurrence in a future pregnancy. During the early 1980s two studies were published which suggested that vitamin supplementation around the time of conception might reduce this risk. In one study, women who agreed to participate were given a mixture of vitamins including folic acid, and they showed a much lower incidence of NTD in their subsequent pregnancies than women who were already pregnant or who declined to participate. It was possible, however, that some systematic difference in the characteristics of those who participated and those who did not might explain the results. The second study attempted to overcome this ambiguity by allocating women randomly to receive folic acid supplementation or a placebo, but it was too small to give clear-cut results. The MRC Vitamin Study Research Group (1991) reported a much larger randomized trial, in which the separate effects could be studied both of folic acid and of other vitamins. The outcome was clear. Of 593 women receiving folic acid and becoming pregnant, six had NTD; of 602 not receiving folic acid, 21 had NTD. No effect of other vitamins was apparent. Statistical methods confirmed the immediate impression that the contrast between the folic acid and control groups is very unlikely to be due to chance and can safely be ascribed to the treatment used.

4 The World Health Organization carried out a collaborative case–control study at 12 participating centres in 10 countries to investigate the possible association between breast cancer and the use of oral contraceptives (WHO Collaborative Study of Neoplasia and Steroid Contraceptives, 1990). In each hospital, women with breast cancer and meeting specified age and residential criteria were taken as cases. Controls were selected from among women who were admitted to the same hospital, who satisfied the same age and residential criteria as the cases, and who were not suffering from a condition considered as possibly influencing contraceptive practices. The study included 2116 cases and 13 072 controls. The analysis of the association between breast cancer and use of oral contraceptives had to consider a number of other variables that are associated with breast cancer and which might differ between users and non-users of oral contraceptives. These variables included age, age at first live birth (2·7-fold effect between age 30 or older and less than 20 years), a socio-economic index (two-fold effect), year of marriage and family history of breast cancer (three-fold effect). After making allowances for these possible confounding variables as necessary, the risk of breast cancer for users of oral contraceptives was estimated as 1·15 times the risk for non-users, a weak association in comparison with the size of the associations of some of the other variables that had to be considered.

5   A final example of the use of statistical arguments is a study to quantify illness in babies under 6 months of age reported by Cole *et al.* (1991). It is important that parents and general practitioners have an appropriate method for identifying severe illness requiring referral to a specialist paediatrician. Whether this is possible can only be determined by the study of a large number of babies for whom possible signs and symptoms are recorded, and for whom the severity of illness is also determined. In this study the authors considered 28 symptoms and 47 physical signs. The analysis showed that it was sufficient to use seven of the symptoms and 12 of the signs, and each symptom or sign was assigned an integer score proportional to its importance. A baby's illness score was then derived by adding the scores for any signs or symptoms that were present. The score was then considered in three categories, 0–7, 8–12 and 13 or more, indicating well or mildly ill, moderate illness and serious illness respectively. It was predicted that the use of this score would correctly classify 98% of the babies who were well or mildly ill and correctly identify 92% of the seriously ill.

1.2 Diagrams

One of the principal methods of displaying statistical information is the use of diagrams. Trends and contrasts are often more readily apprehended, and perhaps retained longer in the memory, by casual observation of a well-proportioned diagram than by scrutiny of the corresponding numerical data presented in tabular form. Diagrams must, however, be simple. If too much information is presented in one diagram it becomes too difficult to unravel and the reader is unlikely even to make the effort. Furthermore, details will usually be lost when data are shown in diagrammatic form. For any critical analysis of the data, therefore, reference must be made to the relevant numerical quantities.

Statistical diagrams serve two main purposes. The first is the presentation of statistical information in articles and other reports, when it may be felt that the reader will appreciate a simple, evocative display. Official statistics of trade, finance and medical and demographic data are often illustrated by diagrams in newspaper articles and in annual reports of government departments. The powerful impact of diagrams makes them also a potential means of misrepresentation by the unscrupulous. The reader should pay little attention to a diagram unless the definition of the quantities represented and the scales on which they are shown are all clearly explained. In research papers it is inadvisable to present basic data solely in diagrams because of the loss of detail referred to above. The use of diagrams here should be restricted to the emphasis of important points, the detailed evidence being presented separately in tabular form.

The second main use is as a private aid to statistical analysis. The statistician will often have recourse to diagrams to gain insight into the structure of the data and to check assumptions which might be made in an analysis. This informal use of diagrams will often reveal new aspects of the data or suggest hypotheses which may be further investigated.

Various types of diagrams are discussed at appropriate points in this book. It will suffice here to mention a few of the main uses to which statistical diagrams are put, illustrating these from official publications.

1 *To compare two or more numbers.* The comparison is often by bars of different lengths (Fig. 1.1), but another common method (the *pictogram*) is to use rows of repeated symbols; for example, the populations of different countries may be depicted by rows of 'people', each 'person' representing 1 000 000 people. Care should be taken not to use symbols of the same shape but different sizes because of ambiguity in interpretation; for example, if exports of different countries are represented by money bags of different sizes the reader is uncertain whether the numerical quantities are represented by the linear or the areal dimensions of the bags.

2 *To express the distribution of individual objects or measurements into different categories.* The frequency distribution of different values of a numerical measurement is usually depicted by a histogram, a method discussed more fully in § 1.4 (see Figs 1.6–1.8). The distribution of individuals into non-numerical categories can be shown as a *bar diagram* as in **1**, the length of each bar representing the number of observations (or *frequency*) in each category. If the frequencies are expressed as percentages, totalling 100%, a convenient device is the *pie chart* (Fig. 1.2).

3 *To express the change in some quantity over a period of time.* The natural method here is a graph in which points, representing the values of the quantity at

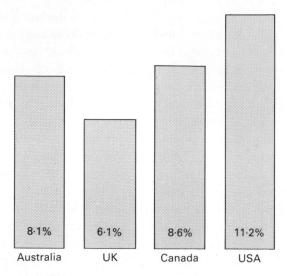

Fig. 1.1 A 'bar diagram' showing the percentages of gross domestic product spent on health care in four countries in 1987 (reproduced with permission from Macklin, 1990).

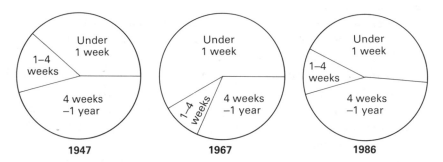

Fig. 1.2 A 'pie chart' showing for three different years the proportions of infant deaths in England and Wales that occur in different parts of the first year of life. The amount for each category is proportional to the angle subtended at the centre of the circle and hence to the area of the sector.

successive times, are joined by a series of straight-line segments (Fig. 1.3). If the time intervals are very short the graph will become a smooth curve. If the variation in the measurement is over a small range centred some distance from zero it will be undesirable to start the scale (usually shown vertically) at zero for this will leave too much of the diagram completely blank. A non-zero origin should be indicated by a break in the axis at the lower end of the scale, to attract the readers' attention (Fig. 1.3). A slight trend can, of course, be made to appear much more dramatic than it really is by the judicious choice of a non-zero

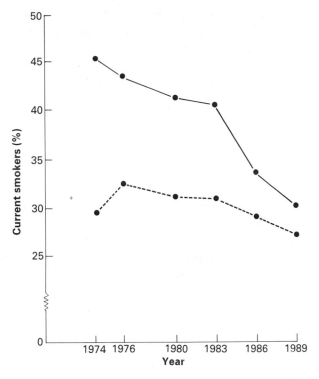

Fig. 1.3 A 'line diagram' showing the changes between six surveys in the proportion of men (solid line) and women (dashed line) in Australia who were current smokers (adapted from Hill *et al.* 1991).

origin, and it is unfortunately only too easy for the unscrupulous to support a chosen interpretation of a time trend by a careful choice of origin. A sudden change of scale over part of the range of variation is even more misleading and should almost always be avoided. Special scales based on logarithmic and other transformations are discussed in Chapter 11.

4   *To express the relationship between two measurements, in a situation where they occur in pairs.* The usual device is the *scatter diagram* (see Fig. 5.1), which is described in detail in Chapter 5 and will not be discussed further here. Time trends, discussed in **3**, are of course a particular form of relationship, but they called for special comment because the data often consist of one measurement at each point of time (these times being often equally spaced). In general, data on relationships are not restricted in this way and the continuous graph is not generally appropriate.

1.3 Tabulation and data processing

Another way of summarizing and presenting some of the important features of a set of data is in the form of a table. There are many variants, but the essential features are that the structure and meaning of a table are indicated by headings or labels and the statistical summary is provided by numbers in the body of the table. Frequently the table is two-dimensional, in that the headings for the horizontal rows and vertical columns define two different ways of categorizing the data. Each portion of the table defined by a combination of row and column is called a *cell*. The numerical information may be counts of numbers of individuals in different cells, mean values of some measurements (see §1.5) or more complex indices.

Some useful guidelines in the presentation of tables for publication are given by Ehrenberg (1975, 1977). Points to note are the avoidance of an unnecessarily large number of digits (since shorter, rounded-off numbers convey their message to the eye more effectively) and care that the layout allows the eye easily to compare numbers that need to be compared.

Table 1.1, taken from a report on assisted conception (AIH National Perinatal Statistics Unit, 1991), is an example of a table summarizing counts. It summarizes information on 5116 women who conceived following *in vitro* fertilization (IVF), and shows that the proportion of women whose pregnancy resulted in a live birth was related to age. How is such a table constructed? With a small number of data a table of this type could be formed by manual sorting and counting of the original records, but if there were many observations (as in Table 1.1) or if many tables had to be produced the labour would obviously be immense.

We may distinguish first between the problems of preparing the data in a form suitable for tabulation, and the mechanical (or electronic) problems of getting the

Table 1.1 Outcome of pregnancies according to maternal age (adapted from AIH National Perinatal Statistics Unit, 1991)

Age		Live birth	Spontaneous abortion	Ectopic pregnancy	Stillbirth	Termination of pregnancy	Total
< 25	No.	94	21	10	2	0	127
	%	74·0	16·5	7·9	1·6	0·0	100·0
25–29	No.	962	272	96	36	2	1368
	%	70·3	19·9	7·0	2·6	0·1	99·9
30–34	No.	1615	430	143	58	8	2254
	%	71·7	19·1	6·3	2·6	0·4	100·1
35–39	No.	789	338	66	27	6	1226
	%	64·4	27·6	5·4	2·2	0·5	100·1
40 +	No.	69	60	6	1	5	141
	%	48·9	42·6	4·3	0·7	3·5	100·0
Total	No.	3529	1121	321	124	21	5116
	%	69·0	21·9	6·3	2·4	0·4	100·0

computations done. Some studies, particularly small laboratory experiments, give rise to relatively few observations, and the problems of data preparation are correspondingly simple. Indeed, tabulations of the type under discussion may not be required, and the statistician may be concerned solely with more complex forms of analysis.

Data preparation is, in contrast, a problem of serious proportions in many large-scale investigations, whether with complex automated laboratory measurements or in clinical or other studies on a 'human' scale. In large-scale therapeutic and prophylactic trials, in prognostic investigations, in studies in epidemiology and social medicine and in many other fields, a large number of people may be included as subjects, and very many observations may be made on each subject. Furthermore, much of the information may be difficult to obtain in unambiguous form and the precise definition of the variables may require careful thought.

In most investigations of this type it will be necessary to collect the information on specially designed record forms or questionnaires. The design of forms and questionnaires is considered in some detail by Babbie (1989). The following points may be noted briefly here.

1   There is a temptation to attempt to collect more information than is clearly required, in case it turns out to be useful in either the present or some future study. While there is obviously a case for this course of action it carries serious disadvantages. The collection of data costs money and, although the cost of collecting extra information from an individual who is in any case providing some information may be relatively low, it must always be considered. The most serious disadvantage, though, is that the collection of marginally useful information may detract from the value of the essential data. The interviewer faced with 50 items for each subject may take appreciably less care than if only 20 items were required. If there is a serious risk of non-cooperation of the subject, as perhaps in postal surveys using questionnaires which are self-administered, the length of a questionnaire may be a strong disincentive and the list of items must be severely pruned. Similarly, if the data are collected by telephone interview, cooperation may be reduced if the respondent expects the call to take more than a few minutes.

2   Care should be taken over the wording of questions to ensure that their interpretation is unambiguous and in keeping with the purpose of the investigation. Whenever possible the various categories of response that are of interest should be enumerated on the form. This helps to prevent meaningless or ambiguous replies and saves time in the later classification of results. For example,

What is your working status? (circle number)

1   Domestic duties with no paid job outside home.
2   In part-time employment (less than 25 hours per week).
3   In full-time employment.
4   Unemployed seeking work.

5   Retired due to disability or illness (please specify cause) ....
6   Retired for other reasons.
7   Other (please specify)..

If the answer to a question is a numerical quantity the units required should be specified. For example,

Your weight:........ kg.

In some cases more than one set of units may be in common use and both should be allowed for. For example,

Your height:........ cm.
             Or........ feet .... inches.

In other cases it may be sufficient to specify a number of categories. For example,

How many years have you lived in this town? (circle number)

1   Less than 5.
2   5–9.
3   10–19.
4   20–29.
5   30–39.
6   40 or more.

When the answer is qualitative but may nevertheless be regarded as a gradation of a single dimensional scale, a number of ordered choices may be given. For example,

How much stress or worry have you had in the last month with:

		None	A little	Some	Much	Very much
1	Your spouse?	1	2	3	4	5
2	Other members of your family?	1	2	3	4	5
3	Friends?	1	2	3	4	5
4	Money or finance?	1	2	3	4	5
5	Your job?	1	2	3	4	5
6	Your health?	1	2	3	4	5

The next step is to transfer the relevant information from the records into a form suitable for analysis. Formerly this would have involved transferring the data to 80-column punch cards but now the data are entered directly from a visual display unit (VDU) through a computer on to disk, either the computer's own hard disk or a floppy disk or both. Editing facilities allow amendments to be made directly on the stored data. As it is no longer necessary to keep a 'hard' copy of the data in computer-readable form, it is essential to maintain back-up copies of data files to guard against computer malfunctions that may result in a particular file becoming unreadable. Back-up copies may be kept on floppy disks or magnetic tape.

The initial entry of data may be through a personal computer, and editing and analysis may sometimes be completed on this computer. For other sets of data it is necessary to transfer the analysis to a larger computer, either because of the size of the data set or to obtain access to a wider range of software.

There are two strategies for the entry of data. In the first the data are regarded as a row of characters, and no interpretation occurs until a data file has been created. The second method is much more powerful and involves using the computer interactively as the data are entered. Thus logical errors and unlikely values (see §11.6) can be reported to the operator immediately. If such an error is due to a mistake by the operator, it can be corrected immediately; otherwise it would be necessary to refer it to the investigator. Questionnaires often contain items that are only applicable if a particular answer has been given to an earlier item. For example, if a detailed smoking history is required, the first question might be 'Have you smoked?' If the answer was 'yes', there would follow several questions on the number of years smoked, the amount smoked, the brands of cigarettes, etc. On the other hand, if the answer was 'no', these questions would not be applicable and should be skipped. With screen-based data entry the controlling program would automatically display the next applicable item on the VDU screen.

Whilst screen-based data entry is usually carried out working from a completed questionnaire, for telephone interviews it may be possible to dispense with the paper record and for the interviewer to read a question on the VDU screen, enter the response on the keyboard, and so on, with any branching to different parts of the questionnaire or skipping of questions controlled by the computer. In this case any logical errors detected can be queried immediately with the respondent.

There are various ways in which information from a form or questionnaire can be represented in a computer record. In the simplest method the reply to each question is given in one or more specific columns and each column contains a digit from 0 to 9. This means that non-numerical information must be 'coded'. For example, the coding of the first few questions might be as in Fig. 1.4. In some systems leading zeros must be punched, e.g. if three digits were allowed for a variable like diastolic blood pressure, a reading of 88 mmHg would be recorded

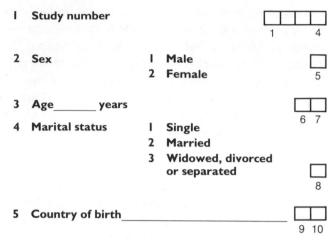

Fig. 1.4 An example of part of a questionnaire with coding indicated.

as 088, whereas other systems allow blanks instead. For the subject with study number 122 who was a married woman aged 49, the first eight columns of the record given in Fig. 1.4 would be punched as the following codes:

Column	1	2	3	4	5	6	7	8
Code	0	1	2	2	2	4	9	2

Clearly the person entering the data must know which code to enter for any particular column. Two different approaches are possible. The information may be transferred from the original record to a 'coding sheet' which will show for each column of each record precisely which code is to be punched. This may be a sheet of paper, ruled as a grid, in which the rows represent the different individuals and the vertical columns represent the columns of the record. Such coding sheets are available commercially. Except for small jobs it will usually be preferable to design a special coding form showing clearly the different items; this will reduce the frequency of transcription errors. Alternatively, the coding may be included on the basic record form so that the punching may be done direct from this form and the need for an intermediate coding sheet is removed. If sufficient care is given to the design of the record form, this second method is preferable, as it removes a potential source of copying errors. This is the approach shown in Fig. 1.4, where the boxes on the right are used for coding. For the first four items the codes are shown and an interviewer could fill in the coding boxes immediately. For item 5 there are so many possibilities that all the codes cannot be shown. Instead the response would be recorded in open form, e.g. 'Greece', and the code looked up later in a detailed set of coding instructions.

It was stated above that it is preferable to use the record form or questionnaire also for the coding. One reservation must, however, be made. The purpose of the questionnaire is to obtain accurate information, and anything that detracts from this should be removed. Particularly with self-administered questionnaires the presence of coding boxes, even though the respondent is not asked to use them, may reduce the cooperation a subject would otherwise give. This may be because of an abhorrence of what may be regarded as looking like an 'official' form, or it may be simply that the boxes have made the form appear cramped and less interesting. This should not be a problem where a few interviewers are being used but if there is any doubt separate coding sheets should be used.

With screen-based data entry the use of coding boxes is not necessary but care is still essential in the questionnaire design to ensure that the information required by the operator is easy to find.

The statistician or investigator wishing to tabulate the data in various ways using a computer must have access to a suitable program. It would probably not be necessary to write a special program since statistical packages are widely available for standard statistical tasks such as tabulation.

It is essential that the data and the instructions for the particular analysis required be punched in the form specified by the package. The investigator should therefore study the specification of the program before arranging for the data to be punched. In a large-scale study involving a record form and questionnaire these matters should be considered at an early stage before the design of the record form is finally decided.

Most of the methods of analysis described later in this book may be carried out using standard statistical packages or languages. Widely available packages include SAS, BMDP, SPSS and Minitab. A discussion of these and some other packages or programs is contained in Chapter 18.

Although computers are increasingly used for analysis, with smaller sets of data it is often convenient to use a calculator, the most convenient form of which is the pocket calculator. These machines perform at high speed all the basic arithmetic operations, and have a range of mathematical functions such as the square, square root, exponential, logarithm, etc. An additional feature particularly useful in statistical work is the automatic calculation and accumulation of sums of squares of numbers. Some machines have a special range of extended facilities for statistical analyses. It is particularly common for the automatic calculation of the mean and standard deviation to be available. Programmable calculators are available and these facilitate repeated use of statistical formulae.

The user of a calculator often finds it difficult to know how much rounding off is permissible in the data and in the intermediate or final steps of the computations. Some guidance will be derived from the examples in this book, but the following general points may be noted.

1 Different values of any one measurement should normally be expressed to the same degree of precision. If a series of children's heights are generally given to the nearest inch, but a few are expressed to the nearest 0·25 in, this extra precision will be wasted in any calculations done on the series as a whole. All the measurements should therefore be rounded to the nearest inch for convenience of calculation.

2   A useful rule in rounding midpoint values (such as a height of 127·5 cm when rounding to whole numbers) is to round to the nearest even number. Thus 127·5 would be rounded to 128. This rule prevents a slight bias which would otherwise occur if the figures were always rounded up or always rounded down.

3   It may occasionally be justifiable to quote the results of calculations to a little more accuracy than the original data. For example, if a large series of heights is measured to the nearest centimetre the mean may sometimes be quoted to one decimal point. The reason for this is that, as we shall see, the effect of the rounding errors is reduced by the process of averaging.

4   If any quantity calculated during an intermediate stage of the calculations is quoted to, say, n significant digits, the result of any multiplication or division of this quantity will be valid to, at the most, n digits. The significant digits are those from the first non-zero digit to the last meaningful digit, irrespective of the position of the decimal point. Thus, 1·002, 10·02, 100 200 (if this number is expressed to the nearest 100) all have four significant digits. Cumulative inaccuracy arises with successive operations of multiplication or division.

5   The result of an addition or subtraction is valid to at most the number of decimal digits of the least accurate figure. Thus the result of adding 101 (accurate to the nearest integer) and 4·39 (accurate to two decimal points) is 105 (to the nearest integer). The last digit may be in error by one unit; for example, the exact figure corresponding to 101 may have been 101·42, in which case the result of the addition now should have been 105·81, or 106 to the nearest integer. These considerations are particularly important in subtraction. Very frequently in statistical calculations one number is subtracted from another of very similar size. The result of the subtraction may then be accurate to many fewer significant digits than either of the original numbers. For example, 3212·78 − 3208·44 = 4·34; three digits have been lost by the subtraction. For this reason it is essential in some early parts of a computation to keep more significant digits than will be required in the final result.

A final general point about computation is the importance of keeping a tidy layout on paper, with adequate labelling and vertical and horizontal alignment of figures and without undue crowding. Paper ruled in two directions at intervals of about 0·25 in or 0·5 cm is often found convenient.

1.4 Summarizing numerical data

The raw material of all statistical investigations consists of individual observations, and these almost always have to be summarized in some way before any use can be made of them. We have discussed in the last two sections the use of diagrams and tables to present some of the main features of a set of data. We must now examine some particular forms of table, and the associated diagrams, in more detail. As we have seen, the aim of statistical methods goes beyond the mere presentation of data to include the drawing of inferences from them. These two aspects—description and inference—cannot be entirely separated. We cannot discuss the descriptive tools without some consideration of the purpose for which they are needed. In the next few sections, we shall occasionally have to anticipate questions of inference which will be discussed in more detail later in the book.

Any class of measurement or classification on which individual observations are made is called a *variable* or *variate*. For instance, in one problem the variable might be a particular measure of respiratory function in schoolboys, in another it might be the number of bacteria found in samples of water. In most problems many variables are involved. In a study of the natural history of a certain disease, for example, observations are likely to be made, for each patient, on a number of variables measuring the clinical state of the patient at various times throughout the illness, and also on certain variables, such as age, not directly relating to the patient's health.

It is useful first to distinguish between two types of variable, *qualitative* (or *categorical*) and *quantitative*. Qualitative observations are those that are not characterized by a numerical quantity, but whose possible values consist of a number of categories, with any individual recorded as belonging to just one of these categories. Typical examples are sex, hair colour, death or survival in a certain period of time, and occupation. Qualitative variables may be subdivided into *nominal* and *ordinal* observations. An ordinal variable is one where the categories have an unambiguous natural order. For example, the stage of a cancer at a certain site may be categorized as stage A, B, C or D, where previous observations have indicated that there is a progression through these stages in sequence from A to D. Sometimes the fact that the stages are ordered may be indicated by referring to them in terms of a number, stage 1, 2, 3 or 4, but the use of a number here is as a label and does not indicate that the variable is quantitative. A nominal variable is one for which there is no natural order of the categories. For example, certified cause of death might be classified as infectious disease, cancer, heart disease, etc. Again, the fact that cause of death is often referred to as a number (the International Classification of Diseases, or ICD, code) does not obscure the fact that the variable is nominal, with the codes serving only as shorthand labels.

The problem of summarizing qualitative nominal data is relatively simple. The main task is to count the number of observations in various categories, and perhaps to express them as proportions or percentages of appropriate totals. These counts are often called *frequencies* or *relative frequencies*. Examples are shown in Tables 1.1 and 1.2. If relative frequencies in certain subgroups are shown, it is useful to add them to give 1·00, or 100%, so that the reader can easily see which total frequencies have been subdivided. (Slight discrepancies in these

Table 1.2 Result of sputum examination 3 months after operation in group of patients treated with streptomycin and control group treated without streptomycin

	Streptomycin		Control	
	Frequency	%	Frequency	%
Smear negative, culture negative	141	45·0	117	41·8
Smear negative, not cultured	90	28·8	67	23·9
Smear or culture positive	82	26·2	96	34·3
Total with known sputum result	313	100·0	280	100·0
Results not known	12		17	
Total	325		297	

totals, due to rounding the relative frequencies (for examples, see Tables 1.1 and 1.3), may be ignored.)

Ordinal variables may be summarized in the same way as nominal variables. One difference is that the order of the categories in any table or figure is predetermined, whereas it is arbitrary for a nominal variable. The order also allows the calculation of *cumulative relative frequencies*, which are the sums of all relative frequencies up to each category.

A particularly important type of qualitative observation is that in which a certain characteristic is either present or absent, so that the observations fall into one of two categories. Examples are sex, and survival or death. Such variables are variously called *quantal*, *binary* or *dichotomous*.

Quantitative variables are those for which the individual observations are numerical quantities, usually either measurements or counts. It is useful to subdivide quantitative observations into *discrete* and *continuous* variables. Discrete measurements are those for which the possible values are quite distinct and separated. Often they are counts such as the number of times an individual has been admitted to hospital in the last five years.

Continuous variables are those which can assume a continuous uninterrupted range of values. Examples are height, weight, age and blood pressure. Continuous measurements usually have an upper and a lower limit. For instance, height cannot be less than zero, and there is presumably some lower limit above zero and some upper limit, but it would be difficult to say exactly what these limits are. The distinction between discrete and continuous variables is not always clear, because all continuous measurements are in practice rounded off; for instance, a series of heights might be recorded to the nearest centimetre and so appear discrete. Any ambiguity rarely matters, since the same statistical methods can often be safely applied to both continuous and discrete variables, particularly if the scale used for the latter is fairly finely subdivided. On the other hand, there are some special methods applicable to counts, which as we have seen must be positive whole numbers. The problems of summarizing quantitative data are much more complex than those for qualitative data, and the remainder of this chapter will be devoted almost entirely to them.

Sometimes a continuous or a discrete quantitative variable may be summarized by dividing the range of values into a number of categories, or *grouping intervals*, and producing a table of frequencies. For example, for age a number of age groups could be created and each individual put into one of the groups. The variable, age, has then been transformed into a new variable, age group, which has all the characteristics of an ordered categorical variable. Such a variable may be called an *interval* variable.

A useful first step in summarizing a fairly large collection of quantitative data is the formation of a *frequency distribution*. This is a table showing the number of observations, or frequency, at different values or within certain ranges of values of the variable. For a discrete variable with a few categories the frequency may be tabulated at each value, but if there is a wide range of possible values, it will be convenient to subdivide the range into categories. An example is shown in Table 1.3. (In this example the reader should note the distinction between two types of count—the variable, which is the number of lesions on an individual chorioallantoic membrane, and the frequency, which is the number of membranes on which the variable falls within a specified range.) With continuous measurements one *must* form grouping intervals (Table 1.4). In Table 1.4 the cumulative relative frequencies are also tabulated. These give the percentages of the total who are younger than the lower limit of the following interval, that is, 9.8% of the subjects are in the age groups 25–34 and 35–44 and so are younger than 45.

Table 1.3 Frequency distribution of number of lesions caused by smallpox virus in egg membranes

Number of lesions	Frequency (number of membranes)	Relative frequency (%)
0–	1	1
10–	6	8
20–	14	18
30–	14	18
40–	17	21
50–	8	10
60–	9	11
70–	3	4
80–	6	8
90–	1	1
100–	0	0
110–119	1	1
Total	80	101

Table 1.4 Frequency distribution of age for 1357 male patients with lung cancer

Age (years)	Frequency (number of patients)	Relative frequency (%)	Cumulative relative frequency (%)
25–	17	1·3	1·3
35–	116	8·5	9·8
45–	493	36·3	46·1
55–	545	40·2	86·3
65–74	186	13·7	100·0
Total	1357	100·0	

The advantages in presenting numerical data in the form of a frequency distribution rather than a long list of individual observations are too obvious to need stressing. On the other hand, if there are only a few observations, a frequency distribution will be of little value since the number of readings falling into each group will be too small to permit any meaningful pattern to emerge.

We now consider in more detail the practical task of forming a frequency distribution. If the variable is to be grouped, a decision will have to be taken about the end-points of the groups. For convenience these should be chosen, as far as possible, to be 'round' numbers. For distributions of age, for example, it is customary to use multiples of 5 or 10 as the boundaries of the groups. Care should be taken in deciding in which group to place an observation falling on one of the group boundaries, and the decision must be made clear to the reader. Usually such an observation is placed in the group of which the observation is the lower limit. For example, in Table 1.3 a count of 20 lesions would be placed in the group 20–, which includes all counts between 20 and 29, and this convention is indicated by the notation used for the groups.

How many groups should there be? No clear-cut rule can be given. To provide a useful, concise indication of the nature of the distribution, fewer than five groups will usually be too few and more than 20 will usually be too many. Again, if too large a number of groups is chosen, the investigator may find that many of the groups contain frequencies which are too small to provide any regularity in the shape of the distribution. For a given size of grouping interval this difficulty will become more acute as the total number of observations is reduced, and the choice of grouping interval may, therefore, depend on this number. If in doubt, the grouping interval may be chosen smaller than that to be finally used, and groups may be amalgamated in the most appropriate way after the distribution has been formed.

The count should be made by going systematically through the list of measurements and making a mark in the appropriate group. This process, called *tallying*, is illustrated in Table 1.5. It is convenient to form groups of five marks to

Table 1.5 The formation of a frequency distribution by tallying

Counts of trypanosomes in the tail blood of a rat, each count being from a different cell of a haemocytometer

4	6	2	2	2	1	3	5	1	2	2	3	2	4	1	1
5	3	2	6	4	3	3	1	2	6	7	3	5	5	2	2
5	5	6	2	5	1	3	1	9	1	1	2	2	4	1	1
4	4	4	6	1	2	2	1	2	1	0	3	3	4	3	1
4	2	6	2	3	3	7	4	2	6	1	5	2	2	1	9
3	4	4	1	4	6	4	2	5	4	5	4	5	5	6	2
3	1	0	1	5	5	2	2	6	1	3	1	1	1	5	3
1	0	1	5	3	3	6	8	2	0	1	3	6	2	3	5

Steps in the formation of a frequency distribution

Count	First tally mark	First five tally marks (reading along first row)	Final tally	Frequency
0			IIII	4
1			ЖЖ ЖЖ ЖЖ ЖЖ ЖЖ II	27
2		III	ЖЖ ЖЖ ЖЖ ЖЖ ЖЖ II	27
3			ЖЖ ЖЖ ЖЖ ЖЖ	20
4	I	I	ЖЖ ЖЖ ЖЖ I	16
5			ЖЖ ЖЖ ЖЖ II	17
6		I	ЖЖ ЖЖ II	12
7			II	2
8			I	1
9			II	2
				128

facilitate counting. The whole process should be repeated as a check. The alternative method of taking each group in turn and counting the observations falling into that group is not to be recommended, as it requires the scanning of the list of observations once for each group (or more than once if a check is required) and thus encourages mistakes.

If the number of observations is not too great (say, fewer than about 50), a frequency distribution can be depicted graphically by a diagram such as Fig. 1.5. Here each individual observation is represented by a dot or some other mark opposite the appropriate point on a scale. The general shape of the distribution can be seen at a glance, and it is easy to compare visually two or more distributions of the same variable (Fig. 1.5). With larger numbers of observations this method is unsuitable because the marks tend to become congested, and a *box-and-whisker* plot is more suitable (see p. 34).

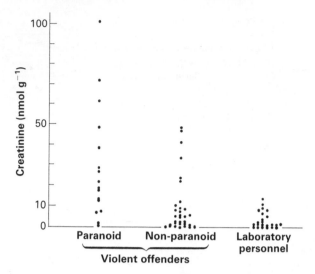

Fig. 1.5 Dot diagram showing the distribution of urinary excretion of bufotenin in three groups of subjects (reprinted from Räisänen *et al.*, 1984, by permission of the authors and the editor of *The Lancet*).

When the number of observations is large the original data may be grouped into a frequency distribution table and the appropriate form of diagram is then the *histogram*. Here the values of the variable are by convention represented on the horizontal scale, and the vertical scale represents the frequency, or relative frequency, at each value or in each group. If the variable is discrete and un-grouped (Fig. 1.6), the frequencies may be represented by vertical lines. The more general method, which must be applied if the variable is grouped, is to draw rectangles based on the different groups (Figs 1.7 and 1.8). It may happen that the grouping intervals are not of constant length. In Table 1.3, for example, suppose we decided to pool the groups 60–, 70– and 80–. The total frequency in these groups is 18, but it would clearly be misleading to represent this frequency by a rectangle on a base extending from 60 to 90 and with a height of 18. The correct procedure would be to make the height of the rectangle 6, the average frequency in the three groups (as indicated by the dotted line in Fig. 1.7). One way of interpreting this rule is to say that the height of the rectangle in a histogram is the frequency per standard grouping of the variable (in this example the standard grouping is 10 lesions). Another way is to say that the frequency for a group is proportional to the *area* rather than the height of the rectangle (in this example the area of any of the original rectangles, or of the composite rectangle formed by the dotted line, is 10 times the frequency for the group). If there is no variation in length of grouping interval, areas are of course proportional to heights, and frequencies are represented by either heights or areas.

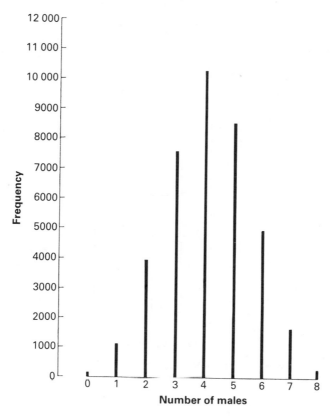

Fig. 1.6 Histogram representing the frequency distribution for an ungrouped discrete variable (number of males in sibships of eight children).

The cumulative relative frequency may be represented by a line diagram (Fig. 1.9). The positioning of the points on the age axis needs special care, since in the frequency distribution (Table 1.4) the cumulative relative frequencies in the final column are plotted against the start of the age group in the next line. That is, since none of the men are younger than 25, zero is plotted on the vertical axis at age 25, 1·3% are younger than 35 so 1·3% is plotted at age 35, 9·8% at age 45, and so on to 100% at age 75.

The *stem-and-leaf display*, illustrated in Table 1.6, is a useful way of tabulating the original data and, at the same time, depicting the general shape of the frequency distribution. In Table 1.6, the first column lists the initial digit in the count, and in each row (or 'stem') the numbers to the right (the 'leaves') are the values of the second digit for the various observations in that group. Thus, the single observation in the first group is 7, and the observations in the second group are 10, 12, 14, 17, 17 and 19. The leaves have been ordered on each stem. The similarity in the shape of the stem-and-leaf display and the histogram in Fig. 1.7 is apparent.

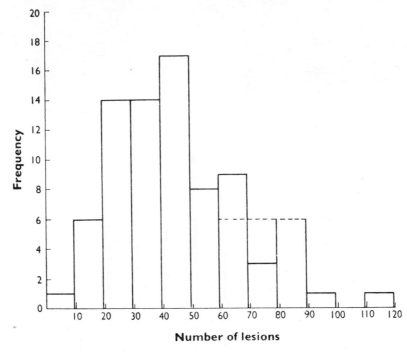

Fig. 1.7 Histogram representing the frequency distribution for a grouped discrete variable (Table 1.3).

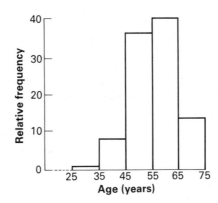

Fig. 1.8 Histogram representing the relative frequency distribution for a continuous variable (age of 1357 men with lung cancer, Table 1.4). Note that the variable shown here is exact age. The age at last birthday is a discrete variable and would be represented by groups displaced half a year to the left from those shown here; see p. 29.

The number of asterisks * indicates how many digits are required for each leaf. Thus, in Table 1.6, one asterisk is shown because the observations require only one digit from the leaf in addition to the row heading. Suppose that, in the distribution shown in Table 1.6, there had been four outlying values over 100: say, 112,

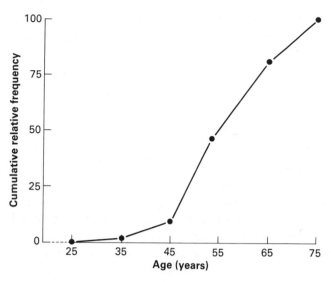

Fig. 1.9 Cumulative frequency plot for age of 1357 men with lung cancer (Table 1.4 and Fig. 1.8).

Table 1.6 Stem-and-leaf display for distribution of number of lesions caused by smallpox virus in egg membranes (see Table 1.3)

Number of lesions	
0*	7
1	024779
2	11122266678999
3	00223456788999
4	01233346677888999
5	11234478
6	014567779
7	057
8	023447
9	8
10	
11	2

187, 191 and 248. Rather than having a large number of stems with no leaves and a few with only one leaf, it would be better to use a wider group interval for these high readings. The observations over 100 could be shown as:

1**	12, 87, 91
2	48

Sometimes it might be acceptable to drop some of the less significant digits. Thus, if such high counts were needed only to the nearest 10 units, they could be displayed as:

$$1** \quad 199$$

$$2 \qquad 5$$

representing 110, 190, 190 and 250.

For other variants on stem-and-leaf displays, see Tukey (1977).

If the main purpose of a visual display is to compare two or more distributions, the histogram is a clumsy tool. Superimposed histograms are usually confusing, and spatially separated histograms are often too distant to provide a means of comparison. The dot diagram of Fig. 1.5 or the box-and-whisker plot of Fig. 1.12 (p. 34) is preferable for this purpose.

Alternatively, use may be made of the representations of three-dimensional figures now available in some computer programs; an example is shown in Fig. 1.10 of a bar diagram plotted against two variables simultaneously. With this representation care must be taken not to mislead because of the effects of perspective.

The frequency in a distribution or in a histogram is often expressed not as an absolute count but as a relative frequency, i.e. as a proportion or percentage of the total frequency. If the standard grouping of the variable in terms of which the

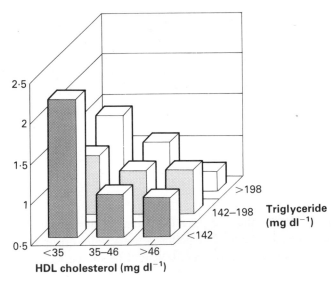

Fig. 1.10 A 'three-dimensional' bar diagram showing the relative risk of coronary heart disease according to high density lipoprotein (HDL) cholesterol concentration and triglyceride (reproduced with permission from Simons *et al.*, 1991).

frequencies are expressed is a single unit, the total area under the histogram will be 1 (or 100% if percentage frequencies are used), and the area between any two points will be the relative frequency in this range.

Suppose we had a frequency distribution of heights of 100 men, in 1 cm groups. The relative frequencies would be rather irregular, especially near the extremes of the distribution, owing to the small frequencies in some of the groups. If the number of observations were increased to, say, 1000, the trend of the frequencies would become smoother and we might then reduce the grouping to 0.5 cm, still making the vertical scale in the histogram represent the relative frequency per cm. We could imagine continuing this process indefinitely, if there were no limit to the fineness of the measurement of length or to the number of observations we could make. In this imaginary situation the histogram would approach closer and closer to a smooth curve, the *frequency curve*, which can be thought of as an idealized form of histogram (Fig. 1.11). The area between the ordinates erected at any two values of the variable will represent the relative frequency of observations between these two points. These frequency curves are useful as models on which statistical theory is based, and should be regarded as idealized approximations to the histograms which might be obtained in practice with a large number of observations on a variable which can be measured extremely accurately.

We now consider various features which may characterize frequency distributions. Any value of the variable at which the frequency curve reaches a peak is called a *mode*. Most frequency distributions encountered in practice have one peak and are described as *unimodal*. For example, the distribution in Fig. 1.6 has a mode at four males, and that in Table 1.3 at 40–49 lesions. Usually, as in these two

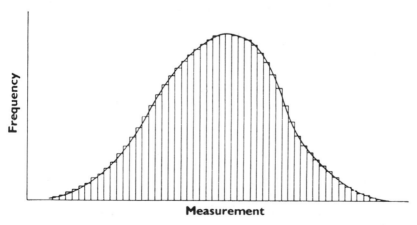

Fig. 1.11 Histogram representing the frequency distribution for a very large number of measurements finely subdivided, with an approximating frequency curve.

examples, the curve is 'bell-shaped'; that is, the mode occurs somewhere between the two extremes of the distribution. These extreme portions, where the frequency becomes low, are called *tails*. Some unimodal distributions have the mode at one end of the range. For instance, if the emission of γ-particles by some radioactive material is being studied, the frequency distribution of the time interval between successive emissions is shaped like a letter J (or rather its mirror image), with a mode at zero. Similarly, if we take families with four children and record the numbers of families in which there have been 0, 1, 2, 3 or 4 cases of poliomyelitis, we shall find a very pronounced mode at zero.

Some distributions will appear to have more than one mode owing to the inevitable random fluctuations of small numbers. In Table 1.3, for example, the observed frequencies show subsidiary modes at 60–69, 80–89 and 110–119, although we should be inclined to pay no great attention to these. Occasionally, even with very large numbers of observations, distributions with more than one mode are found. There has been a great deal of discussion as to whether the distribution of casual blood pressure in a large population free from known circulatory diseases is *bimodal*, i.e. has two modes, because the presence of a second mode at blood pressures higher than the principal mode might indicate that a substantial proportion of the population suffered from essential hypertension.

Another characteristic of some interest is the symmetry or lack of symmetry of the distribution. An asymmetric distribution is called *skew*. The distribution in Fig. 1.6 is fairly symmetrical about the mode. That in Table 1.3 and Fig. 1.7, in which the upper tail is longer than the lower, would be called *positively* skew. The distribution in Table 1.4 and Fig. 1.8 has a slight negative skewness.

Two other characteristics of distributions are of such importance that separate sections will be devoted to them. They are the general location of the distribution on the scale of the variable, and the degree of variation of the observations about the centre of the distribution. Indeed, measures of location and variation are of such general importance that we shall discuss them first without reference to frequency distributions.

1.5 Means and other measures of location

It is often important to give, in a single figure, some indication of the general level of a series of measurements. Such a figure may be called a *measure of location*, a *measure of central tendency*, a *mean* or an *average*. The most familiar of these measures is the *arithmetic* mean, and is customarily referred to as the 'average'. In statistics the term is often abbreviated to 'mean'.

The mean is the sum of the observations divided by the number of observations. It is awkward to have to express rules of calculation verbally in this way, and we shall therefore digress a little to discuss a convenient notation. A single algebraic symbol, like x or y, will often be used to denote a particular variable. For each variable there may be one or more observations. If there are n observations of variable x they will be denoted by

$$x_1, x_2, x_3, \ldots, x_{n-1}, x_n.$$

The various xs are not necessarily or even usually arranged in order of magnitude. They may be thought of as arranged in the order in which they were calculated or observed. It is often useful to refer to a typical member of the group in order to show some calculation which is to be performed on each member. This is done by introducing a 'dummy' suffix which will often be i or j. Thus, if x is the height of a schoolchild and $x_1, x_2, \ldots, x_n$ are n values of x, a typical value may be denoted by x_i.

The arithmetic mean of the xs will be denoted by $\bar{x}$ (spoken 'x bar'). Thus,

$$\bar{x} = \frac{x_1 + x_2 + \ldots + x_n}{n}.$$

The summation occurring in the numerator can be denoted by use of the *summation sign* $\sum$ (the capital Greek letter 'sigma'), which means 'the sum of'. The range of values taken by the dummy suffix is indicated above and below the summation sign. Thus,

$$\sum_{i=1}^{n} x_i = x_1 + x_2 + \ldots + x_n$$

and

$$\bar{x} = \frac{\sum_{i=1}^{n} x_i}{n}.$$

If, as in this instance, it is clear which values the dummy suffix assumes throughout the summation, the range of the summation, and even occasionally the dummy suffix, may be omitted. Thus,

$$\sum_{i=1}^{n} x_i$$

may be abbreviated to $\sum x_i$ or to $\sum x$. Sometimes the capital letter S is used instead of $\sum$. It is important to realize that $\sum$ stands for an operation (that of obtaining the sum of quantities which follow), rather than a quantity itself.

Some simplification in the calculation of the mean may occasionally be achieved by the introduction of *working units*. Some simple examples are shown in Table 1.7. In (1), the xs are close to each other, relative to their mean, and a convenient working unit is $u = x - 100$, involving a change of origin. We find $\bar{u} = 5$ and convert back by taking $\bar{x} = 100 + \bar{u} = 105$. In (2) the factor of 1000 is superfluous to the calculation. We therefore make a change of scale, taking as

Table 1.7 The use of working units in the calculation of a mean

(1)		(2)		(3)	
x	$u = x - 100$	x	$u = x/1000$	x	$u = (x - 1000)/10$
102	2	2000	2	1020	2
104	4	4000	4	1040	4
105	5	5000	5	1050	5
109	9	9000	9	1090	9
	20		20		20

$\bar{u} = 20/4 = 5$ $\qquad\qquad$ $\bar{u} = 20/4 = 5$ $\qquad\qquad$ $\bar{u} = 20/4 = 5$

$\bar{x} = 100 + \bar{u} = 105$ $\qquad$ $\bar{x} = 1000\,\bar{u} = 5000$ $\qquad$ $\bar{x} = 1000 + 10\,\bar{u} = 1050$

working unit $u = x/1000$. We find $\bar{u} = 5$ and convert back by the formula $\bar{x} = \bar{u} \times 1000$. A change of both origin and scale is illustrated in (3).

Working units would be particularly useful if all calculations had to be done by hand. In practice, with a calculator it is usually preferable to do rather more calculation than necessary to save writing down working units and perhaps introducing errors in doing so. Nevertheless, the principle underlying working units is important and the reader should become familiar with their use.

It is sometimes required to obtain the mean of a series of measurements which have already been formed into a frequency distribution, without having recourse to the original list. Indeed, if the number of observations is very large and computational aids are lacking, the preliminary formation of a distribution may be undertaken to save computational labour, although if a calculator is available it is usually preferable to work from the original observations.

If the distribution is expressed in terms of a grouping of the original variable, no further calculations will yield the exact value of the mean (except by a fluke), for the mean depends on the precise value of each observation, and these values are lost once a grouping system is adopted. The best we can hope to do, therefore, is to get an approximation to the mean. The calculations are illustrated in Table 1.8. Some definite value must be attached to the observations in each group, and the simplest rule is to suppose them all to be located at the midpoint of the group. In Table 1.8, therefore, we suppose there are 17 observations at age 30, 116 observations at age 40, and so on. To obtain the mean age we could form a sum by adding in 30 seventeen times, 40 one hundred and sixteen times, and so on, and finally dividing by 1357. Column (1) shows the contribution made by each group to the sum of the ages. The mean age is calculated as 55·7 years.

The determination of the midpoint of each group requires a knowledge of the extent, if any, to which the original readings have been rounded off. In the above example the ages of individuals included in the group 25– would range from 25

Table 1.8 Calculation of mean from frequency distribution (data of Table 1.4)

Age (years)	Frequency f	Midpoint x (years)	(1) fx
25–	17	30	510
35–	116	40	4 640
45–	493	50	24 650
55–	545	60	32 700
65–74	186	70	13 020
	1357		75 520

$$\bar{x} = \frac{75\,520}{1357} = 55 \cdot 7 \text{ years}$$

years 0 days to 34 years 364 days, and the midpoint would be 30 years. If, on the other hand, the variable was length in metres, rounded off to the nearest half-metre, the group would include lengths from 24·75 to 34·75 m, and the midpoint would be 29·75 m. If the original readings were integers, or were rounded off to the nearest integer, the midpoint would be 29·5. Age is an unusual variable in that by convention it is rounded downwards. In many research investigations ages are recorded only as 'age last birthday'. The mean of a series of 'ages last birthday' will be approximately half a year below the mean of the exact ages, and it is quite common practice to quote the former rather than to add half a year to provide an estimate of the mean exact age. In the example in Table 1.8, we have assumed that the mean exact age was required. If we had required the mean 'age last birthday', the midpoint would have been 29·5 (the midpoint of 25, 26, . . ., 34), 39·5, etc., and the calculated mean age last birthday would have been 55·2 instead of 55·7.

Another useful measure of location is the *median*. If the observations are arranged in increasing or decreasing order, the median is the middle observation. If the number of observations, n, is odd, there will be a unique median—the $\frac{1}{2}(n + 1)$th observation from either end. If n is even, there is strictly no middle observation, but the median is defined by convention as the mean of the two middle observations—the $\frac{1}{2}n$th and the $(\frac{1}{2}n + 1)$th from either end.

The median has several disadvantages in comparison with the mean.

1   It takes no account of the precise magnitude of most of the observations, and is therefore usually less efficient than the mean because it wastes information.

2   If two groups of observations are pooled, the median of the combined group cannot be expressed in terms of the medians of the two component groups. This is not so with the mean. If groups containing n_1 and n_2 observations have means of $\bar{x}_1$ and $\bar{x}_2$ respectively, the mean of the combined group is

$$(n_1 \bar{x}_1 + n_2 \bar{x}_2)/(n_1 + n_2).$$

3   The median is much less amenable than the mean to mathematical treatment, and is not much used in the more elaborate statistical techniques.

For descriptive work, however, the median is occasionally useful. Consider the following series of durations (in days) of absence from work owing to sickness.

1, 1, 2, 2, 3, 3, 4, 4, 4, 4, 5, 6, 6, 6, 6, 7, 8, 10, 10, 38, 80.

From a purely descriptive point of view the mean might be said to be misleading. Owing to the highly skew nature of the distribution the mean of 10 days is not really typical of the series as a whole, and the median of 5 days might be a more useful index. Another point is that in skew distributions of this type the mean is very much influenced by the presence of isolated high values. The median is therefore more stable than the mean in the sense that it is likely to fluctuate less from one series of readings to another.

The calculation of a median from a grouped frequency distribution is illustrated using Table 1.4. We require the value of age below which it is estimated that 50% of the observations lie. We have that

46·1% of the patients have an age less than 55 years,

86·3% of the patients have an age less than 65 years.

The median clearly lies between 55 and 65 years, and is estimated by linear interpolation as

$$55 + \left(\frac{50 \cdot 0 - 46 \cdot 1}{86 \cdot 3 - 46 \cdot 1} \times 10 \right) = 56 \cdot 0 \text{ years,}$$

very slightly higher than the mean of 55·7 years. This method corresponds to the cumulative frequency plot (Fig. 1.9). The median may be read off this plot by finding the point on the age axis corresponding to 50% on the cumulative relative frequency axis.

The median and mean are equal if the series of observations is symmetrically distributed about their common value (as is nearly the case in Table 1.8). For a positively skew distribution (as in Table 1.3) the mean will be greater than the median, while if the distribution is negatively skew the median will be the greater.

A third measure of location, the mode, was introduced in §1.4. It is not widely used in analytical statistics, mainly because of the ambiguity in its definition as the fluctuations of small frequencies are apt to produce spurious modes.

Finally, reference must be made to the *geometric mean*, which is used extensively in microbiological and serological research. Observations are sometimes expressed as *titres*, which are the dilutions of certain suspensions or reagents at which a specified phenomenon, like agglutination of red cells, first takes place. If repeated observations are made during the same investigation, the possible values of a titre will usually be multiples of the same dilution factor: for example, 2, 4, 8,

16, etc., for twofold dilutions. It is commonly found that a series of titres, obtained, for example, from different sera, is distributed with marked positive skewness on account of the increasingly wide intervals between possible values. Now, if a series of numbers increases by a constant multiplying factor, their logarithms must increase by a constant difference, which is the logarithm of the multiplying factor. The series of titres 2, 4, 8, 16, etc., for example, has logarithms very nearly equal to 0·3, 0·6, 0·9, 1·2, etc., which increase successively by an increment of 0·3 (= log 2). It is often found, empirically, that the use of log titres rather than titres gives a series of observations which is more symmetrically distributed and for which, therefore, the use of the arithmetic mean is more appropriate. Denote the titre by x and the log titre by $u(= \log x)$. The arithmetic mean of u is, like the individual values of u, measured on a logarithmic scale, and to get back to the original scale of titres we take $\bar{x}_g = $ antilog $\bar{u}$. This is called the geometric mean of x. It can never be greater than the arithmetic mean, and the two means will be equal only if all the xs are the same.

The geometric mean cannot be used if any of the original observations are negative, since a negative number has no logarithm. Its use with series of dilutions is particularly appropriate because of the underlying equally spaced logarithmic series, but it may occasionally be used more generally whenever a series of positive readings shows a degree of positive skewness which is largely removed by taking logarithms. The conditions under which its use is appropriate are thus rather similar to those for which the median is often used, and indeed for this type of data the median and the geometric mean will often have similar values. As an example, consider the following set of antibody titres: 4, 8, 16, 16, 64. Their logarithms are 0·60, 0·90, 1·20, 1·20, 1·81, the mean logarithm is 1·142 and the geometric mean is antilog 1·142 = 13·9. In contrast, the arithmetic mean of the titres is 21·6 and the median is 16.

Another measure, the *harmonic mean*, which is much more rarely used, is described in §11.3.

1.6 Measures of variation

When the mean value of a series of measurements has been obtained it is usually a matter of considerable interest to express the degree of variation or scatter around this mean. Are the readings all rather close to the mean or are some of them scattered widely in each direction? This question is important for purely descriptive reasons, as we shall emphasize below. It is important also since the measurement of variation plays a central part in the methods of statistical inference which are described in this book. To take a simple example, the reliability of the mean of 100 values of some variable depends on the extent to which the 100 readings differ among themselves; if they show little variation the mean value is more reliable, more precisely determined, than if the 100 readings vary widely. The role of variation in statistical inference will be clarified in later chapters of this book. At present we are concerned more with the descriptive aspects.

In works of reference it is common to find a single figure quoted for the value of some biological quantity and the reader may not always realize that the stated figure is some sort of average. In a textbook on nutrition, for example, we find the vitamin A content of 'cheese—Cheddar-type' given as 2000 international units per 100 g. Clearly, not all specimens of 'cheese—Cheddar-type' contain precisely 2000 i.u. per 100 g; how much variation, then, is there from one piece of cheese to another? To take another example from nutrition, the daily calorie requirement for a man of 25 years is given as 3200. This requirement must vary from one person to another; how large is the variation?

There is unlikely to be a single answer to questions of this sort, because the amount of variation to be found in a series of measurements will usually depend on the circumstances in which they are made, and in particular on the way in which these circumstances change from one reading to another. Specimens of Cheddar cheese are likely to vary in their vitamin A content for a number of reasons: major differences in the place and method of manufacture; variation in composition from one specimen to another even within the same batch of manufacture; the age of the cheese, and so on. Variation in the recorded measurement may be partly due to measurement error—in the method of assay, for example, or because of observer errors. Similarly, if reference is made to the variation in systolic blood pressure it must be made clear what sort of comparison is envisaged. Are we considering differences between various types of individual (for example, groups defined by age or by clinical state); differences between individuals classified in the same group; or variation from one occasion to another in the same individual? And are the instrument and the observer kept constant throughout the series?

We now consider some methods of measuring the variation or scatter of a series of continuous measurements.

This scatter is, of course, one of the features of the data which is elucidated by a frequency distribution. It is, however, convenient to use some single quantity to measure this feature of the data, first for economy of presentation, secondly because the statistical methods to be described later require such an index, and thirdly because the data may be too sparse to enable a distribution to be formed. We therefore require what is variously termed a measure of *variation*, *scatter*, *spread* or *dispersion*.

An obvious candidate is the *range*, which is defined as the difference between the maximum value and the minimum value. (Note that the range is a definite quantity, measured in the same units as the original observations; if the highest and lowest of a series of diastolic blood pressures are 95 and 65 mmHg, we may say not only (as in conversation) that the readings range from 65 to 95 mmHg, but also that the range *is* 30 mmHg.) There are three main difficulties about the use of the range as a measure of variation. The first is that the numerical value assumed by the range is determined by only two of the original observations. It is true that, if we say that the minimum and maximum readings have the values 65 and 95, we are saying something about the other readings—that they are between these extremes—but apart from this their exact values have no effect on the range. In this example, the range would be 30 whether (i) all the other readings were concentrated between 75 and 80, or (ii) they were spread rather evenly between 65 and 95. A desirable measure of the variation of the whole set of readings should be greater in case (ii) than in case (i). Secondly, the interpretation of the range depends on the number of observations. If observations are selected serially from a large group (for example, by taking the blood pressures of one individual after another), the range cannot possibly decrease; it will increase whenever a new reading falls outside the interval between the two previous extremes. The interpretation of the range as a measure of variation of the group as a whole must therefore depend on a knowledge of the number of observations on which it is based. This is an undesirable feature; no such allowance is required, for instance, in the interpretation of a mean value as a measure of location. Thirdly, calculations based on extreme values are rather unreliable because big differences in these extremes are liable to occur between two similar investigations.

If the number of observations is not too small a modification may be introduced which avoids the use of the absolute extreme values. If the readings are arranged in ascending or descending order two values may be ascertained which cut off a small fraction of the observations at each end, just as the median breaks the distribution into two equal parts. The value below which a quarter of the observations fall is called the *lower quartile*, that which is exceeded by a quarter of the observations is called the *upper quartile*, and the distance between them is called the *interquartile range*. This measure is not subject to the second disadvantage of the range and is less subject to the other disadvantages.

The evaluation of the quartiles for a set of n values is achieved by first calculating the corresponding ranks by

$$r_l = \tfrac{1}{4}n + \tfrac{1}{2}$$

and

$$r_u = \tfrac{3}{4}n + \tfrac{1}{2}$$

and then calculating the quartiles as the corresponding values in the ordered set of values, using interpolation if necessary. For example, in the data on duration of absence from work (p. 30) where n is 21, $r_l = 5\tfrac{3}{4}$ and $r_u = 16\tfrac{1}{4}$. The lower quartile is then obtained by interpolation between the 5th and 6th values; these are both 3 days, so the lower quartile is also 3 days. The upper quartile is obtained by interpolation between the 16th and 17th values, 7 and 8 days. The interpolation involves moving $\tfrac{1}{4}$ of the way from the 16th value towards the 17th value, to give

$7 + \frac{1}{4}(8 - 7) = 7\frac{1}{4}$ days. It should be noted that there is not a single standard convention for calculating the quartiles. Some authors define the quartiles in terms of the ranks $r_l = \frac{1}{4}(n + 1)$ and $r_u = \frac{3}{4}(n + 1)$. It is also common to round $\frac{1}{4}$ and $\frac{3}{4}$ to the nearest integer and only use interpolation when this involves calculation of the midpoint between two values. Differences between the results using the different conventions are usually small and unimportant in practice.

The quartiles are particular examples of the more general quantity, the *percentile*. The value below which $P\%$ of the values fall is called the Pth percentile. Thus the lower and upper quartiles are the 25th and 75th percentiles respectively. The quartiles or any other percentiles could be read off a plot of cumulative relative frequency such as Fig. 1.9.

A convenient method of displaying the location and variability of a set of data is the box-and-whisker plot. The basic form of this plot shows a box defined by the lower and upper quartiles and with the median marked by a subdivision of the box. The whiskers extend from both ends of the box to the minimum and maximum values. Elaborations of this plot show possible outlying values (§11.6) separately beyond the ends of the whiskers by redefining the whiskers to have a maximum length in terms of the interquartile range. Box-and-whisker plots facilitate a visual comparison of groups. Figure 1.12 shows a comparison of birth

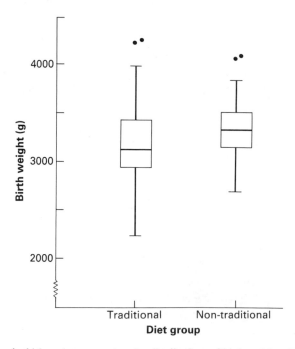

Fig. 1.12 Box-and-whisker plot comparing the distributions of birth weight of babies between two groups of Vietnamese mothers (data of J. Mitchell).

weight between two groups of migrant Vietnamese mothers, one group following a traditional diet and the other a non-traditional diet. In this plot the whiskers extend to the most extreme observations within ± 1.5 interquartile ranges of the quartiles and more extreme points are plotted individually. The higher median and quartiles for the group with the non-traditional diet show clearly, as also does the lower variability associated with this diet.

An alternative approach is to make some use of all the deviations from the mean, $x_i - \bar{x}$. Clearly, the greater the scatter of the observations the greater will the magnitude of these deviations tend to be. It would be of no use to take the mean of the deviations $x_i - \bar{x}$, since some of these will be negative and some positive. In fact,

$$\sum (x_i - \bar{x}) = \sum x_i - \sum \bar{x}$$

$$= \sum x_i - n\bar{x}$$

$$= 0 \quad \text{since } \bar{x} = \sum x_i / n.$$

Therefore the mean of the deviations $x_i - \bar{x}$ will always be zero. We could, however, take the mean of the deviations ignoring their sign, i.e. counting them all as positive. These quantities are called the absolute values of the deviations and are denoted by $|x_i - \bar{x}|$. Their mean, $\sum |x_i - \bar{x}|/n$, is called the *mean deviation*. This measure has the drawback of being difficult to handle mathematically, and we shall not consider it any further in this book.

Another way of getting over the difficulty caused by the positive and negative signs is to square them. The mean value of the squared deviations is called the *variance* and is a most important measure in statistics. Its formula is

$$\text{Variance} = \frac{\sum (x_i - \bar{x})^2}{n}. \tag{1.1}$$

The numerator is often called the *sum of squares about the mean*. The variance is measured in the square of the units in which x is measured. For example, if x is height in cm, the variance will be measured in cm^2. This might seem not to matter, because these units are often used for the measurement of area. On the other hand, if x was a time measurement in seconds, it would be undesirable to have variation measured in square seconds. It is convenient, therefore, to have a measure of variation expressed in the original units of x, and this can be easily done by taking the square root of the variance. This quantity is known as the *standard deviation*, and its formula is

$$\text{Standard deviation} = \sqrt{\left[\frac{\sum (x_i - \bar{x})^2}{n}\right]}. \tag{1.1a}$$

In practice, in calculating variances and standard deviations, the n in the denominator is almost always replaced by $n - 1$. The reason for this is that in applying the methods of statistical inference, developed later in this book, it is useful to regard the collection of observations as being a *sample* drawn from a much larger group of possible readings. The large group is often called a *population*. When we calculate a variance or a standard deviation we may wish not merely to describe the variation in the sample with which we are dealing, but also to estimate as best we can the variation in the population from which the sample is supposed to have been drawn. In a certain respect (see §3.4) a better estimate of the population variance is obtained by using a divisor $n - 1$ instead of n. Thus, we shall almost always use the formula for the *estimated variance* or *sample variance*:

$$\text{Estimated variance, } s^2 = \frac{\sum (x_i - \bar{x})^2}{n - 1}, \tag{1.2}$$

and, similarly,

$$\text{Estimated standard deviation, } s = \sqrt{\left[\frac{\sum (x_i - \bar{x})^2}{n - 1} \right]}. \tag{1.2a}$$

Having established the convention we shall very often omit the word 'estimated' and refer to s^2 and s as 'variance' and 'standard deviation', respectively.

The modification of the divisor from n to $n - 1$ is clearly not very important when n is large. It is more important for small values of n. Although the theoretical justification will be discussed more fully in §3.4, two heuristic arguments may be used now which may make the divisor $n - 1$ appear more plausible. First, consider the case when $n = 1$; that is, there is a single observation. Formula (1.1) with a divisor n gives a variance $0/1 = 0$. Now, this is a reasonable expression of the complete absence of variation in the available observation: it cannot differ from itself. On the other hand, a single observation provides no information at all about the variation in the population from which it is drawn, and this fact is reflected in the calculation of the estimated variance, s^2, from (1.2), which becomes $0/0$, an indeterminate quantity.

Secondly, in the general case when n takes any value, we have already seen that $\sum (x_i - \bar{x}) = 0$. This means that if $n - 1$ of these deviations $x_i - \bar{x}$ are chosen arbitrarily, the nth is determined automatically. (It is the sum of the $n - 1$ chosen values of $x_i - \bar{x}$ with the sign changed.) In other words, only $n - 1$ of the n deviations which are squared in the numerator of (1.1) or (1.2) are *independent*. The divisor $n - 1$ in (1.2) may be regarded as the number of independent quantities amongst the sum of squared deviations in the numerator. The divisor $n - 1$ is, in fact, a particular case of a far-reaching concept known as the *degrees of freedom* of an estimate of variance, which will be developed in §3.4.

Table 1.9 Calculation of estimated variance and standard deviation: direct formula

x_i	$x_i - \bar{x}$	$(x_i - \bar{x})^2$
8	0	0
5	-3	9
4	-4	16
12	4	16
15	7	49
5	-3	9
7	-1	1
$\sum x_i = 56$		$\sum (x_i - \bar{x})^2 = 100$

$$n = 7$$
$$\bar{x} = 56/7 = 8$$
$$s^2 = 100/6 = 16{\cdot}67$$
$$s = \sqrt{16{\cdot}67} = 4{\cdot}08$$

The direct calculation of the estimated variance is illustrated in Table 1.9. In this particular example the calculation is fairly straightforward. In general, two features of the method are likely to cause trouble. Errors can easily arise in the subtraction of the mean from each reading. Further, if the mean is not a 'round' number, as it was in this example, it will need to be rounded off. The deviations $x_i - \bar{x}$ will then need to be written with several significant digits and doubt will arise as to whether an adequate number of significant digits was retained for $\bar{x}$. These difficulties have led to the widespread use of an alternative method of calculating the sum of squares about the mean, $\sum (x_i - \bar{x})^2$. It is based on the following algebraic identity:

$$\sum (x_i - \bar{x})^2 = \sum (x_i^2 - 2x_i\bar{x} + \bar{x}^2)$$

$$= \sum x_i^2 - 2\bar{x}\sum x_i + n\bar{x}^2$$

$$= \sum x_i^2 - 2\frac{(\sum x_i)^2}{n} + \frac{(\sum x_i)^2}{n}$$

$$= \sum x_i^2 - \frac{(\sum x_i)^2}{n}. \tag{1.3}$$

This is called the short-cut formula for the sum of squares about the mean. The derivation of (1.3) uses the fact that $\sum x_i = n\bar{x}$.

The important point about (1.3) is that the computation is performed without the need to calculate individual deviations from the mean, $x_i - \bar{x}$. The sum of squares of the original observations, x_i, is corrected by subtraction of a quantity

Table 1.10 Calculation of estimated variance and standard deviation: short-cut formula (same data as in Table 1.9)

x_i	x_i^2
8	64
5	25
4	16
12	144
15	225
5	25
7	49
56	548

$$\sum(x_i - \bar{x})^2 = \sum x_i^2 - (\sum x_i)^2/n$$
$$= 548 - 56^2/7$$
$$= 548 - 448$$
$$= 100$$

Subsequent steps as in Table 1.9

dependent only on the mean (or, equivalently, the total) of the x_i. This second term is therefore often called the *correction term*, and the whole expression a *corrected* sum of squares.

The previous example is reworked in Table 1.10. We again have the result $\sum(x_i - \bar{x})^2 = 100$, and the subsequent calculations follow as in Table 1.9.

The short-cut formula avoids the need to square individual deviations with many significant digits, but involves the squares of the x_i, which may be large numbers. This rarely causes trouble using a calculator, although care must be taken to carry sufficient digits in the correction term to give the required number of digits in the difference between the two terms. (For example, if $\sum x_i^2 = 2025$ and $(\sum x_i)^2/n = 2019 \cdot 3825$, the retention of all these decimals will give $\sum(x_i - \bar{x})^2 = 5 \cdot 6175$; if the correction term had been rounded off to the nearest whole number it would have given $\sum(x_i - \bar{x})^2 = 6$—an accuracy of only 1 significant digit.) Indeed, this rounding error can cause problems in high-speed computing, and computer programs should use the direct rather than the short-cut formula for the sum of squares about the mean.

Most scientific calculators have a summation key which accumulates n, $\sum x$ and $\sum x^2$ in stores and then the mean and standard deviation are each calculated by successive key strokes, the latter invoking calculation of (1.3). Calculators usually have separate keys for (1.1a) and (1.2a), often called σ_n and σ_{n-1} respectively.

If the observations are presented in the form of a frequency distribution, the standard deviation may be obtained by a method analogous to that used for the mean. If the original variable is grouped, only an approximate estimate of the standard deviation may be obtained. The calculations are illustrated in

Table 1.11 Calculation of standard deviation from frequency distribution (same data as in Table 1.8)

Age (years)	Frequency f	(1) Midpoint x (years)	(2) fx	(1) × (2) fx^2
25–	17	30	510	15 300
35–	116	40	4 640	185 600
45–	493	50	24 650	1232 500
55–	545	60	32 700	1962 000
65–74	186	70	13 020	911 400
	1357		75 520	4306 800
	n		$\sum x$	$\sum x^2$

$$\sum (x - \bar{x})^2 = 4\,306\,800 - \frac{75\,520^2}{1357} = 103\,948$$

$$s^2 = 103\,948/1356 = 76\cdot66$$

$$s = \sqrt{76\cdot66} = 8\cdot76 \text{ years}$$

Note that $\sum x$ denotes the sum over all $n\,(=1357)$ observations. It is calculated as $\sum fx$, where the summation now refers to the five age groups. Similarly $\sum x^2$ over all observations is calculated as $\sum fx^2$ over the five groups.

Table 1.11, which shows the same data as in the corresponding calculations for the mean (Table 1.8). The standard deviation of x is 8·76 years.

The assumption that all the values of x within a group can safely be replaced by the midpoint of the interval, although reasonable for the calculation of the mean, is slightly suspect for the calculation of the standard deviation, for the following reason. When the distribution is unimodal, as in Table 1.11, the observations within each group will tend to be pulled towards the middle of the distribution instead of being distributed evenly throughout the interval. That is, the mean values of the observations in the intervals 25–, 35– are likely to be rather greater than 30 and 40; those in the intervals 55–, 65– rather less than 60 and 70, respectively. These biases will tend to even out in the calculation of the mean age, and may safely be ignored. The calculated standard deviation will, however, tend to be exaggerated. An appropriate correction for this effect, called *Sheppard's correction*, is to subtract $\frac{1}{12}h^2$ from the calculated variance, h being the size of the grouping interval. (If the grouping interval is not constant an average value may be used.) In the present example, h is 10, and the corrected variance would be

$$76\cdot66 - \frac{1}{12}(10^2) = 68\cdot33$$

giving

$$\text{SD}(x) = 8\cdot27 \text{ years,}$$

where SD( ) denotes the standard deviation of the variable in question. The correction is thus rather small unless the grouping is quite crude, and for this reason is often ignored.

The standard deviation of a set of measurements is expressed in the same units as the measurements and hence in the same units as the mean. It is occasionally useful to describe the variability by expressing the standard deviation as a proportion, or a percentage, of the mean. The resulting measure, called the *coefficient of variation*, is thus a dimensionless quantity—a pure number. In symbols,

$$CV(x) = \frac{s}{\bar{x}} \times 100\%. \tag{1.4}$$

The coefficient of variation is most useful as a descriptive tool in situations in which a change in the conditions under which measurements are made alters the standard deviation in the same proportion as it alters the mean. The coefficient of variation then remains unchanged and is a useful single measure of variability. It is mentioned again in a more substantive context in §3.6.

2: Probability

2.1 The meaning of probability

A clinical trial shows that 50 patients receiving treatment A for a certain disease fare better, on the average, than 50 similar patients receiving treatment B. Is it safe to assume that treatment A is really better than treatment B for this condition? Should the investigator use A rather than B for future patients? These are questions typical of those arising from any statistical investigation. The first is one of inference: what conclusions can reasonably be drawn from this investigation? The second question is one of decision: what is the rational choice of future treatment, taking into account the information provided by the trial and the known or unknown consequences of using an inferior treatment? The point to be emphasized here is that the answers to both questions, and indeed those to almost all questions asked about statistical data, are in some degree couched in uncertainty. There may be a very strong suggestion indeed that A is better than B, but can we be entirely sure that the patients receiving B were not more severely affected than those on A and that this variability between the patients was not a sufficient reason for their different responses to treatment? This possibility may, in any particular instance, seem unlikely, but it can rarely, if ever, be completely ruled out. The questions that have to be asked, therefore, must receive an answer phrased in terms of uncertainty. If the uncertainty is low, the conclusion will be firm, the decision will be safe. If the uncertainty is high the investigation must be regarded as inconclusive. It is thus important to consider the measurement of uncertainty, and the appropriate tool for this purpose is the *theory of probability*. Initially the approach will be rather formal; later chapters are concerned with the application of probability theory to statistical problems of various types.

If a coin is tossed a very large number of times and the result of each toss written down, the results may be something like the following (*H* standing for heads and *T* for tails):

$$TTHTHHTHTTTHTHHTHHHHHTTH...$$

Such a sequence will be called a *random sequence* or *random series*, each place in the sequence will be called a *trial*, and each result will often be called an *event* or *outcome*. A random sequence of binary outcomes, such as *H* and *T* in this example, is sometimes called a *Bernoulli sequence* (James Bernoulli, 1654–1705).

41

A random sequence is characterized by a complete lack of pattern or of predicta-
bility. In coin tossing the chance of finding *H* at any one stage is just the same as
at any other stage, and is quite uninfluenced by the outcomes of the previous
tosses. (Contrary to some people's intuition, the chance of getting a head would be
neither raised nor lowered by a knowledge that there had just occurred a run of,
say, six tails.)

In such a sequence it will be found that as the sequence gets larger and larger
the proportion of trials resulting in a particular outcome becomes less and less
variable and settles down closer to some limiting value. This long-run proportion
is called the *probability* of the particular outcome. Figure 2.1 shows the proportion of heads after various numbers of tosses, in an actual experiment. Clearly the
proportion is settling down close to $\frac{1}{2}$, and it would be reasonable to say that the
probability of a head is about $\frac{1}{2}$. Considerations of symmetry would of course
have led us to this conclusion before seeing the experimental results. The slight
differences between the indentations on the two sides of a coin, possibly variations
in density, and even some minor imbalance in the tossing method, might make the
probability very slightly different from $\frac{1}{2}$, but we should be unlikely ever to do
a tossing experiment sufficiently long to distinguish between a probability of 0·5
and one of, say, 0·5001.

The reader will observe that this definition of probability is rather heuristic.
We can never observe a sequence of trials and say unambiguously 'This is

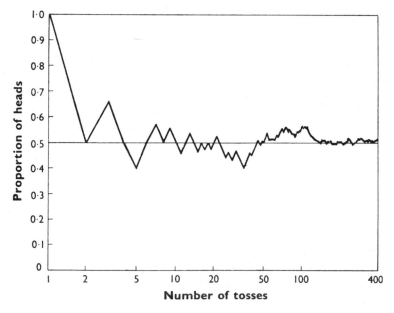

Fig. 2.1 Proportion of heads in a sequence of tosses of a coin with a logarithmic scale for the number
of tosses (reprinted from Cramér, 1946, by permission of the author and publishers).

a random sequence'; we observe only a finite portion of the sequence and there may be underlying patterns in the outcomes which cannot readily be discerned. Nor can we observe a sequence and state precisely the probability of a certain outcome; the probability is a long-run property and again an insufficient portion of the sequence is observed. Nevertheless, there are many phenomena which apparently behave in this way, and the concept of a random sequence should be regarded as an idealistic concept which apparently describes these phenomena very faithfully indeed. Here are some other examples of empirical 'random' (Bernoulli) sequences.

1 *The throws of a die* (*commonly, but incorrectly, called a 'dice'*). If the die is well made the probability of each outcome, 1–6, will be very close to $\frac{1}{6}$.

2 *The sex of successive live births occurring in a large human population.* The probability of a male is known to vary from population to population (for example, it depends on the stillbirth rate) but it is usually a little over $\frac{1}{2}$. In England and Wales it is currently about 0·515; the probability of a female birth is correspondingly about $1 - 0·515 = 0·485$.

3 *A sequence of outcomes of antenatal screening examinations, each classified by whether or not a specific fetal abnormality is present.* Thus, the probability that open spina bifida is present might be about 0·0012.

A consequence of this definition of probability is that it is measured by a number between 0 and 1. If an event never occurs in any of the trials in a random sequence, its probability is zero. If it occurs in every trial, its probability is unity.

A further consequence is that probability is not defined for sequences in which the succession of events follows a manifestly non-random pattern. If a machine were invented which tossed heads and tails in strict alternation (*H, T, H, T, H, T, . . .* , etc.), the long-run proportions of heads and tails would both be $\frac{1}{2}$, but it would be incorrect to say that the probabilities of these events were $\frac{1}{2}$. The sequence is non-random because the behaviour of the odd-numbered trials is different from that of the even-numbered trials. It would be better to think of the series as a mixture of two separate series: the odd-numbered trials, in which the probability of *H* is 1, and the even-numbered trials, in which this probability is 0.

This concept of probability provides a measure of uncertainty for certain types of phenomena which occur in nature. There is a fairly high degree of certainty that any one future birth will not exhibit spina bifida because the probability for that event is low. There is considerable uncertainty about the sex of a future birth because the probabilities of both outcomes are about $\frac{1}{2}$. The definition is, however, much more restrictive than might be wished. What is the probability that smoking is a contributory cause of lung cancer? This question uses the word 'probability' in a perfectly natural conversational way. It does not, however, accord with our technical definition, for it is impossible to think of a random sequence of trials, in some of which smoking is a contributory cause of lung cancer and in some of which it is not.

It will appear in due course that the so-called 'frequency' definition of probability, which has been put forward above, can be used as the basis of statistical inference, and often some rewording of the question can shed some light on the plausibility of hypotheses such as 'Smoking is a contributory cause of lung cancer'. However, many theoretical statisticians, probabilists and logicians advocate a much wider interpretation of the concept of probability than is permitted in the frequency definition outlined above. On this broader view, one should interpret probability as a measure of one's degree of belief in a proposition, and direct statements about the probability that a certain scientific hypothesis is true are quite in order. We return to this point of view in §2.9, but until that section is reached we shall restrict our attention to the frequency definition.

2.2 Probability calculations

The main purpose of allotting numerical values to probabilities is to allow calculations to be performed on these numbers. The two basic operations which concern us here are *addition* and *multiplication*, and we consider first the addition of probabilities.

Consider a random sequence of trials with more than one possible outcome for each trial. In a series of throws of a die, for example, we might ask for the probability of *either* a 1 *or* a 3 being thrown. The answer is fairly clear. If the die is perfectly formed, the probability of a 1 is $\frac{1}{6}$, and the probability of a 3 is $\frac{1}{6}$. That is, a 1 will appear in $\frac{1}{6}$ of trials in the long run, and a 3 will appear in the same proportion of a long series of trials. In no trial will a 1 *and* a 3 appear together. Therefore the compound event 'either a 1 or a 3' will occur in $\frac{1}{6} + \frac{1}{6}$, or $\frac{1}{3}$, of the trials in the long run. The probabilities for the two separate events have been added together.

Note the importance of the observation that a 1 and a 3 cannot both occur together; they are, in other words, *mutually exclusive*. Without this condition the simple form of the addition rule could not be valid. For example, if a doctor's name is chosen haphazardly from the *British Medical Register*, the probability that the doctor is male is about 0·8. The probability that the doctor qualified at an English medical school is about 0·6. What is the probability that the doctor either is male or qualified in England, or both? If the two separate probabilities are added the result is 0·8 + 0·6 = 1·4, clearly a wrong answer since probabilities cannot be greater than 1. The trouble is that the probability of the double event—male and qualified in England—has been counted twice, once as part of the probability of being male and once as part of the probability of being qualified in England. To obtain the right answer, the probability of the double event must be subtracted. Thus, denoting the two events by *A* and *B*, we have the more general form of the *addition rule*.

Probability of A or B or both = (Probability of A)

+ (Probability of B)

− (Probability of A and B).

It will be convenient to write this as

$$P(A \text{ or } B \text{ or both}) = P(A) + P(B) - P(A \text{ and } B). \qquad (2.1)$$

In this particular example the probability of the double event has not been given, but it must clearly be greater than 0·4, to ensure that the right side of the equation (2.1) is less than 1.

If the two events are mutually exclusive, the last term on the right of (2.1) is zero, and we have the *simple form of the addition rule*:

$$P(A \text{ or } B) = P(A) + P(B).$$

Suppose now that two random sequences of trials are proceeding simultaneously; for example, at each stage a coin may be tossed and a die thrown. What is the *joint probability* of a particular combination of results, for example a head (H) on the coin and a 5 on the die? The result is given by the *multiplication rule*:

$$P(H \text{ and } 5) = P(H) \times P(5, \text{ given } H). \qquad (2.2)$$

That is, the long-run proportion of pairs of trials in which both H and 5 occur is equal to the long-run proportion of trials in which H occurs on the coin, multiplied by the long-run proportion of those trials which occur with 5 on the die. The second term on the right of (2.2) is an example of a *conditional probability*, the first event, 5, being 'conditional' on the second, H.

In this particular example, there would be no reason to suppose that the probability of 5 on the die was in the least affected by whether or not H occurred on the coin. In other words,

$$P(5, \text{ given } H) = P(5).$$

A common notation is to replace 'given' by a vertical line, that is $P(5 \mid H)$. The conditional probability is equal to the unconditional probability. The two events are now said to be *independent*, and we have the *simple form of the multiplication rule*:

$$P(H \text{ and } 5) = P(H) \times P(5)$$
$$= \tfrac{1}{2} \times \tfrac{1}{6}$$
$$= \tfrac{1}{12}.$$

Effectively, in this example, there are 12 combinations which occur equally often in the long run: $H1, H2, \ldots, H6, T1, T2, \ldots, T6$.

In general, pairs of events need not be independent, and the general form of the multiplication rule (2.2) must be used. In the earlier example we referred to the probability of a doctor being male and having qualified in England. If these events were independent, we could calculate this as

$$0.8 \times 0.6 = 0.48,$$

and, denoting the events by A and B, (2.1) would give

$$P(A \text{ or } B \text{ or both}) = 0.80 + 0.60 - 0.48$$
$$= 0.92.$$

These events may not be independent, however, since some medical schools are more likely to accept women than others. The correct value for $P(A \text{ and } B)$ could only be ascertained by direct investigation.

As another example of the lack of independence, suppose that in a certain large community 30% of individuals have blue eyes. Then

$$P(\text{blue right eye}) = 0.3$$
$$P(\text{blue left eye}) = 0.3.$$

$P(\text{blue right eye and blue left eye})$ is not given by

$$P(\text{blue right eye}) \times P(\text{blue left eye}) = 0.09.$$

It is obtained by the general formula (2.2) as

$$P(\text{blue right eye}) \times P(\text{blue left eye, given blue right eye})$$
$$= 0.3 \times 1.0$$
$$= 0.3.$$

Addition and multiplication may be combined in the same calculation. In the double sequence with a coin and a die, what is the probability of getting either heads and 2 *or* tails and 4? Each of these combinations has probability $\frac{1}{12}$ (by the multiplication rule for independent events). Each combination is a possible outcome in the double sequence and the outcomes are mutually exclusive. The two probabilities of $\frac{1}{12}$ may therefore be added to give a final probability of $\frac{1}{6}$ that either one or the other combination occurs.

As a slightly more complicated example, consider the sex composition of families of four children. As an approximation, let us assume that the proportion of males at birth is 0·51, that all the children in the families may be considered as independent random selections from a sequence in which the probability of a boy is 0·51, and that the question relates to all liveborn infants so that differential survival does not concern us. The question is, what are the probabilities that a family of four contains no boys, one boy, two boys, three boys and four boys?

The probability that there will be no boys is the probability that each of the four children will be a girl. The probability that the first child is a girl is

$1 - 0\cdot51 = 0\cdot49$. By successive applications of the multiplication rule for independent events, the probability that the first two are girls is $(0\cdot49)^2$; the probability that the first three are girls is $(0\cdot49)^3$; and the probability that all four are girls is $(0\cdot49)^4 = 0\cdot0576$. About 1 in 17 of all families of four will consist of four girls. Write this

$$P(GGGG) = 0\cdot0576.$$

A family with one boy and three girls might arise in any of the following ways, $BGGG$, $GBGG$, $GGBG$, $GGGB$, according to which of the four children is the boy. Each of these ways has a probability of $(0\cdot49)^3 (0\cdot51) = 0\cdot0600$. The total probability of one boy is therefore, by the addition rule,

$$0\cdot0600 + 0\cdot0600 + 0\cdot0600 + 0\cdot0600$$

$$= 4(0\cdot0600)$$

$$= 0\cdot2400.$$

A family with two boys and two girls might arise in any of the following ways: $BBGG$, $BGBG$, $BGGB$, $GBBG$, $GBGB$, $GGBB$. Each of these has a probability of $(0\cdot49)^2 (0\cdot51)^2$, and the total probability of two boys is

$$6(0\cdot49)^2 (0\cdot51)^2 = 0\cdot3747.$$

Similarly for the other family composition types. The complete results are shown in Table 2.1.

Note that the five probabilities total to 1, as they should since this total is the probability that one or other of the five family composition types arises (these being mutually exclusive). Since these five types exhaust all the possibilities, the total probability must be unity. If one examined the records of a very large number of families experiencing four live births, would the proportions of the five types be close to the values shown in the last column? Rather close, perhaps, but it would not be surprising to find some slight but systematic discrepancies because

Table 2.1 Calculation of probabilities of families with various sex compositions

Composition		Probability
Boys	Girls	
0	4	$(0\cdot49)^4 = 0\cdot0576$
1	3	$4(0\cdot49)^3 (0\cdot51) = 0\cdot2400$
2	2	$6(0\cdot49)^2 (0\cdot51)^2 = 0\cdot3747$
3	1	$4(0\cdot49)(0\cdot51)^3 = 0\cdot2600$
4	0	$(0\cdot51)^4 = 0\cdot0677$
		$1\cdot0000$

the formal assumptions underlying our argument may not be strictly correct. For one thing, the probability of a male birth may vary slightly from family to family (as pointed out in §2.1). More importantly, families that start in an unbalanced way, with several births of the same sex, are more likely to be continued than those that are better balanced. The first two births in families that are continued to the third stage will then not be representative of all two-birth families. A similar bias may exist in the progression from three births to four. The extent of these biases would be expected to differ from one community to another, and this seems to be borne out by actual data, some of which agree more closely than others with the theoretical probabilities.

It is sometimes convenient to express a probability in terms of the *odds*, which equal the probability that the event occurs divided by the probability that it does not occur. Thus the odds of throwing a 6 with a die are $\frac{1}{5}$.

2.3 Probability distributions

Table 2.1 provides our first example of a *probability distribution*. That is, it shows how the total probability, equal to 1, is distributed among the different types of family. A variable whose different values follow a probability distribution is known as a *random variable*. In Table 2.1 the number of boys in a family is a random variable. So is the number of girls.

If a random variable can be associated with different points on a scale, the probability distribution can be represented visually by a histogram, just as for frequency distributions. We shall consider first some examples of ungrouped discrete random variables. Here the vertical scale of the histogram measures the probability for each value of the random variable, and each probability is represented by a vertical line.

Example 2.1

In repeated tosses of an unbiased coin, the outcome is a random variable with two values, H and T. Each value has a probability $\frac{1}{2}$. The distribution is shown in Fig. 2.2, where the two outcomes, H and T, are allotted to arbitrary points on the horizontal axis.

Example 2.2

In a genetic experiment we may cross two heterozygotes with genotypes Aa (that is, at a particular gene locus, each parent has one gene of type A and one of type a). The progeny will be homozygotes (aa or AA) or heterozygotes (Aa), with the probabilities shown below.

Genotype	No. of A genes	Probability
aa	0	$\frac{1}{4}$
Aa	1	$\frac{1}{2}$
AA	2	$\frac{1}{4}$
		$\overline{1}$

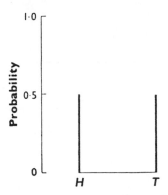

Fig. 2.2 Probability distribution for random variable with two values: the results of tossing a coin with equal probabilities of heads and tails.

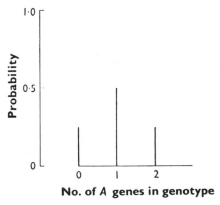

No. of A genes in genotype

Fig. 2.3 Probability distribution for random variable with three values: the number of A genes in the genotype of progeny of an $Aa \times Aa$ cross.

The three genotypes may be allotted to points on a scale by using as a random variable the number of A genes in the genotype. This random variable takes the values 0, 1 and 2, and the probability distribution is depicted in Fig. 2.3.

Example 2.3

A third example is provided by the characterization of families of four children by the number of boys. The probabilities, in the particular numerical case considered in §2.2, are given in Table 2.1, and they are depicted in Fig. 2.4.

When the random variable is continuous it is of little use to refer to the probabilities of particular values of the variable, because these probabilities are in general zero. For example, the probability that the exact height of a male adult is 70 in is zero, because in the virtually infinite population of exact heights of adult males a negligible proportion will be exactly 70 in. If, however, we consider

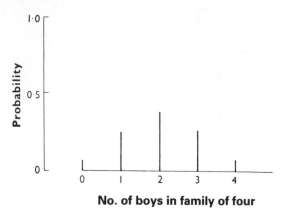

No. of boys in family of four

Fig. 2.4 Probability distribution of number of boys in family of four children if male births occur independently with probability 0·51 (Table 2.1).

a small interval centred at 70 in, say 70 − h to 70 + h, where h is very small, there will be a small non-zero probability associated with this interval. Furthermore, the probability will be very nearly proportional to h. Thus, the probability of a height between 69·98 and 70·02 in will be very nearly double the probability for the interval 69·99 to 70·01. It is therefore a reasonable representation of the situation to suppose that there is a *probability density* characteristic of the value 70 in, which can be denoted by $f(70)$, such that the probability for a small interval 70 − h to 70 + h is very close to

$$2hf(70).$$

The probability distribution for a continuous random variable, x, can therefore be depicted by a graph of the probability density $f(x)$ against x, as in Fig. 2.5. This is, in fact, the frequency curve discussed in §1.4. The reader familiar with the calculus will recognize $f(x)$ as the derivative with respect to x of the probability $F(x)$ that the random variable assumes a value less than or equal to x. $F(x)$ is called the *distribution function* and is represented by the area underneath the curve in Fig. 2.5 from the left end of the distribution (which may be at minus infinity) up to the value x. The distribution function corresponding to the density function of Fig. 2.5 is shown in Fig. 2.6. Note that the height of the density function is proportional to the slope of the distribution function; in the present example both these quantities are zero at the lower and upper extremes of the variables and attain a maximum at an intermediate point.

The shape of a probability distribution may be characterized by the features already used for frequency distributions. In particular, we may be concerned with the number and position of the modes, the values of the random variable at which the probability, or (for continuous variables) the probability density, reaches

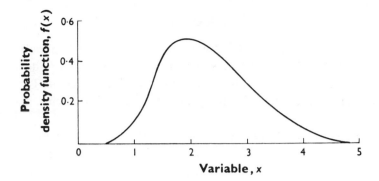

Fig. 2.5 Probability density function for a continuous random variable.

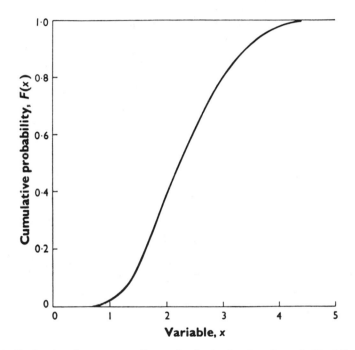

Fig. 2.6 Distribution function corresponding to the density function shown in Fig. 2.5.

a maximum. We may be interested too in the skewness of a probability distribution.

By analogy with §1.5 and §1.6 we are particularly interested in the mean and standard deviation of a random variable, and these concepts are discussed in the next section.

2.4 Expectation

There is some difficulty in deciding what is meant by the phrase 'mean of a random variable'. The mean has been defined earlier only for a finite number, n, of observations. With a probability distribution such as that in Table 2.1 the number of observations must be thought of as infinite. How, then, is the mean to be calculated?

Suppose n is very large—so large that the relative frequencies of the different values of a discrete random variable like that in Table 2.1 can be taken to be very nearly equal to the probabilities. If they were exactly equal to the probabilities, the frequency distribution of the number of boys would be as follows:

x No. of boys	Frequency
0	$0.0576n$
1	$0.2400n$
2	$0.3747n$
3	$0.2600n$
4	$0.0677n$
	n

The mean value of x would be

$$\frac{(0 \times 0.0576n) + (1 \times 0.2400n) + (2 \times 0.3747n) + (3 \times 0.2600n) + (4 \times 0.0677n)}{n}.$$

The factor n may be cancelled from the numerator and denominator of the expression, to give the numerical result 2.04. The arbitrary sample size, n, does not appear.

If the probabilities of 0, 1, ..., 4 boys are denoted by $P_0, P_1, \ldots, P_4$, the formula for the mean is clearly

$$(0 \times P_0) + (1 \times P_1) + (2 \times P_2) + (3 \times P_3) + (4 \times P_4).$$

In general, if x is a discrete random variable taking values $x_0, x_1, x_2, \ldots$, with probabilities $P_0, P_1, P_2, \ldots$, the mean value of x is calculated as

$$\sum_i x_i P_i. \tag{2.3}$$

The mean value of a random variable, calculated in this way, is often called the *expected value*, the *mathematical expectation* or simply the *expectation* of x, and the operation involved (multiplying each value of x by its probability, and then adding) is denoted by $E(x)$. The expectation of a random variable is often allotted a Greek symbol like μ (lower case Greek letter 'mu'), to distinguish it from a mean value calculated from a finite number of observations (denoted usually by symbols such as $\bar{x}$ or $\bar{y}$).

As a second example, consider the probability distribution of x, the number of A genes in the genotypes shown in Example 2.2. Here,

$$E(x) = (0 \times 0.25) + (1 \times 0.50) + (2 \times 0.25)$$

$$= 1.$$

If x follows a continuous distribution, the formula given above for $E(x)$ cannot be used. However, one could consider a discrete distribution in which possible values of x differed by a small interval $2h$. To any value X_0 we could allot the probability given by the continuous distribution for values of x between $X_0 - h$ and $X_0 + h$ (which, as we have seen, will be close to $2hf(X_0)$ if h is small enough). The expectation of x in this discrete distribution can be calculated by the general rule. As the interval h gets smaller and smaller, the discrete distribution will approach more and more closely the continuous distribution, and in general the expectation will approach a quantity which formally is given by the expression

$$\mu = \int_{-\infty}^{\infty} x f(x) \, dx.$$

This provides a definition of the expectation of x for a continuous distribution.

The *variance* of a random variable is defined as

$$\text{var}(x) = E(x - \mu)^2;$$

that is, as the expectation of the squared difference from the mean. This is an obvious development from the previous formula $\sum (x_i - \bar{x})^2 / n$ for the variance of a finite number, n, of observations, since this quantity is the mean value of the squared difference from the sample mean, $\bar{x}$. The distinction between the divisor of n and that of $n - 1$ becomes of no importance when we are dealing with probability distributions since n is effectively infinite.

The variance of a random variable is customarily given the symbol σ^2 (σ being the lower case Greek letter 'sigma'). The standard deviation is again defined as σ, the square root of the variance.

By analogy with the short-cut formula for the sample variance (§1.6), we shall find it convenient to use the following relationship:

$$\sigma^2 = E(x^2) - \mu^2.$$

The proof* is as follows:

$$\sigma^2 = E(x - \mu)^2$$
$$= E(x^2 - 2x\mu + \mu^2)$$
$$= E(x^2) - 2\mu E(x) + \mu^2$$
$$= E(x^2) - 2\mu^2 + \mu^2$$
$$= E(x^2) - \mu^2. \tag{2.4}$$

The two formulae for the variance may be illustrated by the distribution in Example 2.2, for which we have already obtained $\mu = 1$. With the direct formula, we proceed as follows:

x	P	$x - \mu$	$(x - \mu)^2$
0	0·25	−1	1
1	0·50	0	0
2	0·25	1	1

$$\sigma^2 = E(x - \mu)^2$$
$$= (1 \times 0·25) + (0 \times 0·50) + (1 \times 0·25)$$
$$= 0·5.$$

With the short-cut formula,

x	P	x^2
0	0·25	0
1	0·50	1
2	0·25	4

$$E(x^2) = (0 \times 0·25) + (1 \times 0·50) + (4 \times 0·25)$$
$$= 1·5;$$
$$\sigma^2 = E(x^2) - \mu^2$$
$$= 1·5 - 1^2$$
$$= 0·5,$$

as before.

We have so far discussed probability distributions in rather general terms. In the next three sections we consider three specific forms of distribution which play a very important role in statistical theory and practice.

---

*Note that in this proof we make use of some properties of the expectation which are intuitively acceptable, but which we shall not attempt to prove rigorously: (i) in going from the second to the third line, the expectation of a sum (or difference) of two random variables is the sum (or difference) of their expectations; (ii) in treating the middle term on the third line, the expectation of a constant times a random variable is equal to the constant times the expectation.

2.5 The binomial distribution

We have already met a particular case of this form of distribution in the example of §2.2 on the sex distribution in families of four.

In general, suppose we have a random sequence in which the outcome of each individual trial is of one of two types, A or B, these outcomes occurring with probabilities π and $1 - \pi$, respectively. (The symbol π, the lower case Greek letter 'pi', is used merely as a convenient Greek letter and has no connection at all with the mathematical constant $\pi = 3\cdot14159\ldots\ldots$) In the previous example, A and B were boys and girls, and π was $0\cdot51$.

Consider now a group of n observations from this random sequence (in the example $n = 4$). It will be convenient to refer to each such group as a 'sample' of n observations. What is the probability distribution of the number of As in the sample? This number we shall call r, and clearly r must be one of the numbers 0, 1, 2, $\ldots$, $n - 1$, n. Define also $p = r/n$, the *proportion* of As in the sample, and $q = (n - r)/n = 1 - p$, the proportion of Bs.

As in the example, we argue that the probability of r As and $n - r$ Bs is

$$\pi^r(1 - \pi)^{n-r}$$

multiplied by the number of ways in which one can choose r out of the n sample members to receive a label 'A'. This multiplying factor is called a *binomial coefficient*. In the example the binomial coefficients were worked out by simple enumeration, but clearly this could be tedious with large values of n and r. The binomial coefficient is usually denoted by

$$\binom{n}{r}$$

(referred to in speaking as 'n binomial r'), or

$$^nC_r.$$

Tables of binomial coefficients are provided in most books of mathematical tables. For moderate values of n and r they can be calculated directly from:

$$\binom{n}{r} = \frac{n(n - 1)(n - 2)\ldots(n - r + 1)}{1\,.\,2\,.\,3\ldots r} \tag{2.5}$$

(where the single dots are multiplication signs and the rows mean that all the intervening integers are used). The quantity $1\,.\,2\,.\,3\ldots r$ is called 'factorial r' or 'r factorial' and is usually written $r!$. Since the expression $n(n - 1)\ldots(n - r + 1)$, which occurs in the numerator of

$$\binom{n}{r},$$

can be written as

$$\frac{n!}{(n-r)!},$$

it follows that

$$\binom{n}{r} = \frac{n!}{r!(n-r)!}. \tag{2.6}$$

This formula involves unnecessarily heavy multiplication, but it draws attention to the symmetry of the binomial coefficients:

$$\binom{n}{r} = \binom{n}{n-r}. \tag{2.7}$$

This is, indeed, obvious from the definition. Any selection of r objects out of n is automatically a selection of the $n-r$ objects which remain.

If we put $r = 0$ in (2.5), both the numerator and the denominator are meaningless. Putting $r = n$ would give

$$\binom{n}{n} = \frac{n!}{n!} = 1,$$

and it would accord with the symmetry result to put

$$\binom{n}{0} = 1. \tag{2.8}$$

This is clearly the correct result, since there is precisely one way of selecting 0 objects out of n to be labelled as As: namely to select all the n objects to be labelled as Bs. Note that (2.8) accords with (2.6) if we agree to call $0! = 1$; this is merely a convention since 0! is strictly not covered by our previous definition of the factorial, but it provides a useful extension of the definition which is used generally in mathematics.

The binomial coefficients required in the example of §2.2 could have been obtained from (2.5) as follows:

$$\binom{4}{0} = 1$$

$$\binom{4}{1} = \frac{4}{1} = 4$$

$$\binom{4}{2} = \frac{4 \cdot 3}{1 \cdot 2} = 6$$

$$\binom{4}{3} = \frac{4 \cdot 3 \cdot 2}{1 \cdot 2 \cdot 3} = 4$$

$$\binom{4}{4} = \frac{4 \cdot 3 \cdot 2 \cdot 1}{1 \cdot 2 \cdot 3 \cdot 4} = 1.$$

A useful way to obtain binomial coefficients for small values of n, without any multiplication, is by means of Pascal's triangle:

$$
\begin{array}{cccccccccccc}
n & & & & & & 1 & & & & & \\
1 & & & & & 1 & & 1 & & & & \\
2 & & & & 1 & & 2 & & 1 & & & \\
3 & & & 1 & & 3 & & 3 & & 1 & & \\
4 & & 1 & & 4 & & 6 & & 4 & & 1 & \\
5 & 1 & & 5 & & 10 & & 10 & & 5 & & 1 \\
\text{etc.} & & & & & & \text{etc.} & & & & &
\end{array}
$$

In this triangle of numbers, which can be extended downwards indefinitely, each entry is obtained as the sum of the two adjacent numbers on the line above. Thus, in the fifth row (for $n = 4$),

$$4 = 1 + 3, \quad 6 = 3 + 3, \quad \text{etc.}$$

Along each row are the binomial coefficients

$$\binom{n}{0}, \ \binom{n}{1}, \ \ldots \ \text{up to} \ \binom{n}{n-1}, \ \binom{n}{n}.$$

The probability that the sample of n individuals contains r As and $n - r$ Bs, then, is

$$\binom{n}{r} \pi^r (1 - \pi)^{n-r}. \tag{2.9}$$

If this expression is evaluated for each value of r from 0 to n, the sum of these $n + 1$ values will represent the probability of obtaining 0 As or 1 A or 2 As, etc., up to n As. These are the only possible results from the whole sequence and they are mutually exclusive; the sum of the probabilities is, therefore, 1. That this is so follows algebraically from the classical binomial theorem, for

$$\binom{n}{0} \pi^0 (1 - \pi)^n + \binom{n}{1} \pi^1 (1 - \pi)^{n-1} + \ldots + \binom{n}{n} \pi^n (1 - \pi)^0$$

$$= [\pi + (1 - \pi)]^n$$

$$= 1^n$$

$$= 1.$$

This result was verified in the particular example of Table 2.1.

The expectation and variance of r can now be obtained by applying the general formulae (2.3) and (2.4) to the probability distribution (2.9) and using standard algebraic results on the summation of series. We shall defer a proof until we can apply some general results given in Chapter 3, and merely give the results here:

$$E(r) = n\pi \qquad\qquad\qquad (2.10)$$

and

$$\text{var}(r) = n\pi(1 - \pi). \qquad\qquad\qquad (2.11)$$

The formula for the expectation is intuitively acceptable. The mean number of As is equal to the number of observations multiplied by the probability that an individual result is an A. The expectation of the number of boys out of four, in our previous example, was shown in §2.4 to be 2·04. We now see that this result could have been obtained from (2.10):

$$E(r) = 4 \times 0.51 = 2.04.$$

The formula (2.11) for the variance is less obvious. For a given value of n, var(r) reaches a maximum value when $\pi = 1 - \pi = \frac{1}{2}$ (when var$(r) = \frac{1}{4}n$), and falls off markedly as π approaches 0 or 1. If π is very small the factor $1 - \pi$ in (2.11) is very close to 1, and var(r) becomes very close to $n\pi$, the value of E(r).

We shall often be interested in the probability distribution of p, the *proportion* of As in the sample. Now $p = r \times (1/n)$, and the multiplying factor $1/n$ is constant from one sample to another. It follows that

$$E(p) = E(r) \times (1/n) = \pi \qquad\qquad\qquad (2.12)$$

and

$$\text{var}(p) = \text{var}(r) \times (1/n)^2 = \frac{\pi(1 - \pi)}{n}. \qquad\qquad\qquad (2.13)$$

The square in the multiplying factor for the variance arises because the units in which the variance is measured are the squares of the units of the random variable.

It will sometimes be convenient to refer to the standard deviations of r or of p. These are the square roots of the corresponding variances:

$$\text{SD}(r) = \sqrt{[n\pi(1 - \pi)]}$$

and

$$\text{SD}(p) = \sqrt{\left[\frac{\pi(1 - \pi)}{n}\right]}.$$

Some further properties of the binomial distribution are given in §3.3. A brief table of the probabilities for various values of π and n is in Pearson and Hartley (1966, Table 37). Fuller tables for $n \leqslant 25$ are given by Owen (1962, Table 9.5); for $n < 50$ by National Bureau of Standards (1950); and for $50 \leqslant n \leqslant 100$ by Romig (1947).

Example 2.4

Table 2.2 is given by Lancaster (1965) from data published by Roberts *et al.* (1939). These authors observed 551 crosses between rats, with one parent heterozygous for each of five factors and the other parent homozygous recessive for each. The distribution is that of the number of dominant genes out of five, for each offspring. The theoretical distribution is the binomial with $n = 5$ and $\pi = \frac{1}{2}$, and the 'expected' frequencies, obtained by multiplying the binomial probabilities by 551, are shown in the table. The agreement between observed and expected frequencies is satisfactory.

Table 2.2 Distribution of number of dominant genes at five loci, in crosses between parents heterozygous for each factor and those homozygous recessive for each (Lancaster, 1965)

Number of dominant genes	Number of offspring	
	Observed	Expected
0	17	17·2
1	81	86·1
2	152	172·2
3	180	172·2
4	104	86·1
5	17	17·2
	551	551·0

The binomial distribution is characterized by the mathematical variables π and n. Variables such as these which partly or wholly characterize a probability distribution are known as *parameters*. They are of course entirely distinct from random variables. Figure 2.7 illustrates the shape of the distribution for various combinations of π and n. Note that, for a particular value of n, the distribution is symmetrical for $\pi = \frac{1}{2}$ and asymmetrical for $\pi < \frac{1}{2}$ or $\pi > \frac{1}{2}$; and that for a particular value of π the asymmetry decreases as n increases.

Statistical methods based on the binomial distribution are described in detail in §§4.7, 4.8, 4.9 and 7.5.

2.6 The Poisson distribution

This distribution is named after S. D. Poisson (1781–1840), a French mathematician. It is sometimes useful as a limiting form of the binomial, but it is important also in its own right as a distribution arising when events of some sort occur randomly in time, or when small particles are distributed randomly in space.

We shall first consider random events in time. Suppose that a certain type of event occurs repeatedly, with an average rate of λ per unit time but in an entirely random fashion. To make the idea of randomness rather more precise we can

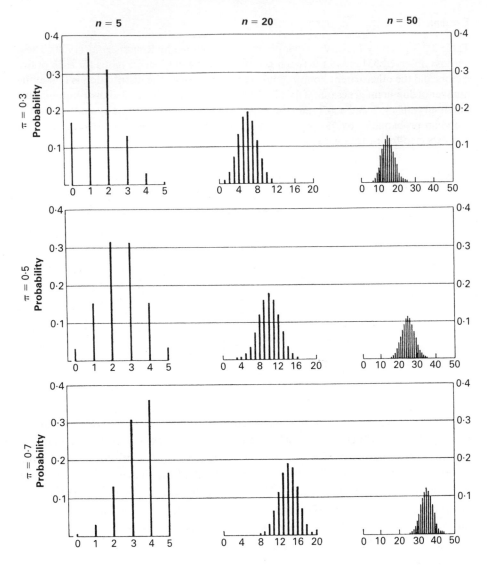

Fig. 2.7 Binomial distribution for various values of π and n. The horizontal scale in each diagram shows values of r.

postulate that in any very small interval of time of length h (say 1 ms) the probability that an event occurs is approximately proportional to h, say λh. (For example, if h is doubled the very small probability that the interval contains an event is also doubled.) The probability that the interval contains more than one event is supposed to be proportionately smaller and smaller as h gets smaller, and can therefore be ignored. Furthermore, we suppose that what happens in any small interval is independent of what happens in any other small interval which does not overlap the first.

A very good instance of this probability model is that of the emission of radioactive particles from some radioactive material. The rate of emission, λ, will be constant, but the particles will be emitted in a purely random way, each successive small interval of time being on exactly the same footing, rather than in a regular pattern. The model is the analogy, in continuous time, of the random sequence of independent trials discussed in §2.1, and is called the *Poisson process*.

Suppose that we observe repeated stretches of time, of length T time units, from a Poisson process with a rate λ. The number, x, of events occurring in an interval of length T will vary from one interval to another. In fact, it is a random variable, the possible values of which are 0, 1, 2, . . . etc. What is the probability of a particular value x?

A natural guess at the value of x would be λT, the rate of occurrence multiplied by the time interval. We shall see later that λT is the mean of the distribution of x, and it will be convenient to denote λT by the single symbol μ.

Let us split any one interval of length T into a large number n of subintervals each of length T/n (Fig. 2.8). Then, if n is sufficiently large, the number of events in

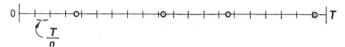

Fig. 2.8 The occurrence of events in a Poisson process, with the time-scale subdivided into small intervals.

the subinterval will almost always be 0, will occasionally be 1 and will hardly ever be more than 1. The situation is therefore almost exactly the same as a sequence of n binomial trials (a trial being the observation of a subinterval), in each of which there is a probability $\lambda(T/n) = \mu/n$ of there being an event and $1 - \mu/n$ of there being no event. The probability that the whole series of n trials provides exactly x events is, in this approximation, given by the binomial distribution:

$$\frac{n(n-1)\ldots(n-x+1)}{x!}\left(\frac{\mu}{n}\right)^x\left(1-\frac{\mu}{n}\right)^{n-x}. \tag{2.14}$$

Now, this binomial approximation will get better and better as n increases. What happens to (2.14) as n increases indefinitely? We can replace

$$n(n-1)\ldots(n-x+1)$$

by n^x since x will be negligible in comparison with n. Similarly we can replace $(1 - \mu/n)^{n-x}$ by $(1 - \mu/n)^n$ since $(1 - \mu/n)^x$ will approach 1 as n increases. It is a standard mathematical result that, as n increases indefinitely, $(1 - \mu/n)^n$ approaches $e^{-\mu}$, where e is the base of natural (or Napierian) logarithms (e = 2·718. . .).

Finally, then, in the limit as n increases indefinitely, the probability of x events approaches

$$P_x = \frac{n^x}{x!}\left(\frac{\mu}{n}\right)^x e^{-\mu} = \frac{\mu^x e^{-\mu}}{x!}. \tag{2.15}$$

The expression (2.15) defines the Poisson probability distribution. The random variable x takes the values $0, 1, 2, \ldots$ with the successive probabilities obtained by putting these values of x in (2.15). Thus,

$$P_0 = e^{-\mu}$$
$$P_1 = \mu e^{-\mu}$$
$$P_2 = \tfrac{1}{2}\mu^2 e^{-\mu}, \text{ etc.}$$

Note that, for $x = 0$, we replace $x!$ in (2.15) by the value 1, as was found to be appropriate for the binomial distribution. To verify that the sum of the probabilities is 1,

$$P_0 + P_1 + P_2 + \ldots = e^{-\mu}(1 + \mu + \tfrac{1}{2}\mu^2 + \ldots)$$
$$= e^{-\mu} \times e^{\mu}$$
$$= 1,$$

the replacement of the infinite series on the right-hand side by e^{μ} being a standard mathematical result.

Before proceeding to further consideration of the properties of the Poisson distribution, we may note that a similar derivation may be applied to the situation in which particles are randomly distributed in space. If the space is one-dimensional (for instance the length of a cotton thread along which flaws may occur with constant probability at all points), the analogy is immediate. With two-dimensional space (for instance a microscopic slide over which bacteria are distributed at random with perfect mixing technique) the total area of size A may be divided into a large number n of subdivisions each of area A/n; the argument then carries through with A replacing T. Similarly, with three-dimensional space (bacteria well mixed in a fluid suspension), the total volume V is divided into n small volumes of size V/n. In all these situations the model envisages particles distributed at random with density λ per unit length (area or volume). The number of particles found in a length (area or volume) of size l (A or V) will follow the Poisson distribution (2.15) where the parameter $\mu = \lambda l$ (λA or λV).

The shapes of the distribution for $\mu = 1, 4$ and 15 are shown in Fig. 2.9. Note that for $\mu = 1$ the distribution is very skew, for $\mu = 4$ the skewness is much less and for $\mu = 15$ it is almost absent.

The distribution (2.15) is determined entirely by the one parameter, μ. It follows that all the features of the distribution in which one might be interested

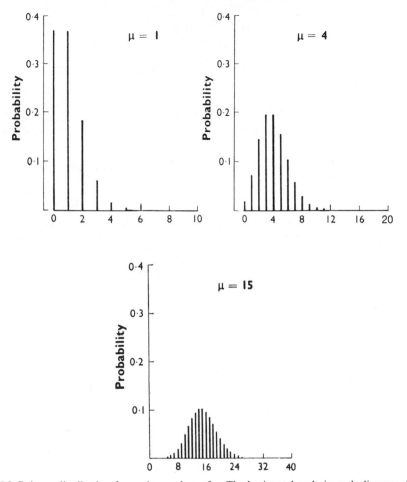

Fig. 2.9 Poisson distribution for various values of μ. The horizontal scale in each diagram shows values of x.

are functions only of μ. In particular the mean and variance must be functions of μ. The mean is

$$E(x) = \sum_{x=0}^{\infty} x P_x$$

$$= \sum_{x=0}^{\infty} \frac{x \mu^x e^{-\mu}}{x!}$$

$$= \sum_{x=1}^{\infty} \frac{\mu^x e^{-\mu}}{(x-1)!} \quad \text{since} \quad \frac{x}{x!} = \frac{1}{(x-1)!}$$

and the term in the summation corresponding to $x = 0$ is zero.

$$E(x) = \mu \sum_{x=1}^{\infty} \frac{\mu^{x-1}e^{-\mu}}{(x-1)!}$$

$$= \mu \sum_{i=0}^{\infty} \frac{\mu^{i}e^{-\mu}}{i!}, \quad \text{putting } i = x - 1$$

$$= \mu,$$

since the summation contains all the terms of the Poisson distribution, which sum to 1.

To find the variance, which by the short-cut formula is $E(x^2) - \mu^2$, we first find $E[x(x-1)] = E(x^2) - E(x)$.

$$E[x(x-1)] = \sum_{x=0}^{\infty} x(x-1)P_x$$

$$= \mu^2 \sum_{x=2}^{\infty} \frac{\mu^{x-2}e^{-\mu}}{(x-2)!}$$

$$= \mu^2$$

by the same sort of argument as before. Thus,

$$E(x^2) - E(x) = \mu^2,$$

$$E(x^2) = \mu^2 + E(x)$$

$$= \mu^2 + \mu$$

and

$$var(x) = E(x^2) - \mu^2$$

$$= (\mu^2 + \mu) - \mu^2$$

$$= \mu. \tag{2.16}$$

Thus, the variance of x, like the mean, is equal to μ. The standard deviation is therefore $\sqrt{\mu}$.

Much use is made of the Poisson distribution in bacteriology. To estimate the density of live organisms in a suspension the bacteriologist may dilute the suspension by a factor of, say, 10^{-5}, take samples of, say, 1 cm^3 in a pipette and drop the contents of the pipette on to a plate containing a nutrient medium on which the bacteria grow. After some time each organism dropped on to the plate will have formed a colony and these colonies can be counted. If the original suspension was well mixed, the volumes sampled are accurately determined and the medium is uniformly adequate to sustain growth, the number of colonies in a large series of plates could be expected to follow a Poisson distribution. The mean colony count per plate, $\bar{x}$, is an estimate of the mean number of bacteria per 10^{-5} cm^3 of the original suspension, and a knowledge of the theoretical properties of the Poisson distribution permits one to measure the precision of this estimate (see §4.10).

Similarly, for total counts of live and dead organisms, repeated samples of constant volume may be examined under the microscope and the organisms counted directly.

Example 2.5

As an example, Table 2.3 shows a distribution observed during a count of the root nodule bacterium (*Rhizobium trifolii*) in a Petroff–Hausser counting chamber. The 'expected' frequencies are obtained by calculating the mean number of organisms per square, $\bar{x}$, from the frequency distribution (giving $\bar{x} = 2\cdot50$) and calculating the probabilities P_x of the Poisson distribution with μ replaced by $\bar{x}$. The expected frequencies are then given by $400\,P_x$. The observed and expected frequencies agree quite well. This organism normally produces gum and therefore clumps readily. Under these circumstances one would not expect a Poisson distribution, but the data in Table 2.3 were collected to show the effectiveness of a method of overcoming the clumping.

Table 2.3 Distribution of counts of root nodule bacterium (*Rhizobium trifolii*) in a Petroff–Hausser counting chamber (data from Wilson and Kullman, 1931)

Number of bacteria per square	Number of squares	
	Observed	Expected
0	34	32·8
1	68	82·1
2	112	102·6
3	94	85·5
4	55	53·4
5	21	26·7
6	12	11·1
7–	4	5·7
	400	399·9

In the derivation of the Poisson distribution use was made of the fact that the binomial distribution with a large n and small π is an approximation to the Poisson with mean $\mu = n\pi$.

Conversely, when the correct distribution is a binomial with large n and small π, one can approximate this by a Poisson with mean $n\pi$. For example, the number of deaths from a certain disease, in a large population of n individuals subject to a probability of death π, is really binomially distributed but may be taken as approximately a Poisson variable with mean $\mu = n\pi$. Note that the standard deviation on the binomial assumption is $\sqrt{[n\pi(1-\pi)]}$, whereas the Poisson standard deviation is $\sqrt{(n\pi)}$. When π is very small these two expressions are almost

Table 2.4 Binomial and Poisson distributions with $\mu = 5$

r	π n	0·5 10	0·10 50	0·05 100	Poisson
0		0·0010	0·0052	0·0059	0·0067
1		0·0098	0·0286	0·0312	0·0337
2		0·0439	0·0779	0·0812	0·0842
3		0·1172	0·1386	0·1396	0·1404
4		0·2051	0·1809	0·1781	0·1755
5		0·2461	0·1849	0·1800	0·1755
6		0·2051	0·1541	0·1500	0·1462
7		0·1172	0·1076	0·1060	0·1044
8		0·0439	0·0643	0·0649	0·0653
9		0·0098	0·0333	0·0349	0·0363
10		0·0010	0·0152	0·0167	0·0181
> 10		0	0·0094	0·0115	0·0137
		1·0000	1·0000	1·0000	1·0000

equal. Table 2.4 shows the probabilities for the Poisson distribution with $\mu = 5$, and those for various binomial distributions with $n\pi = 5$. The similarity between the binomial and the Poisson improves with increases in n (and corresponding decreases in π).

Probabilities for the Poisson distribution are tabulated in Tables 7 and 39 of Pearson and Hartley (1966).

2.7 The normal (or Gaussian) distribution

The binomial and Poisson distributions both relate to a discrete random variable. The most important continuous probability distribution is the *Gaussian* (C. F. Gauss, 1777–1855, German mathematician) or, as it is frequently called, the *normal* distribution. Figures 2.10 and 2.11 show two frequency distributions, of height and of blood pressure, which are similar in shape. They are both approximately symmetrical about the middle and exhibit a shape rather like a bell, with a pronounced peak in the middle and a gradual falling off of the frequency in the two tails. The observed frequencies have been approximated by a smooth curve, which is in each case the probability density of a normal distribution.

Frequency distributions resembling the normal probability distribution in shape are often observed, but this form should not be taken as the norm, as the name 'normal' might lead one to suppose. Many observed distributions are undeniably far from 'normal' in shape and yet cannot be said to be abnormal in the ordinary sense of the word. The importance of the normal distribution lies not so much in any claim to represent a wide range of observed frequency distributions but in the central place it occupies in sampling theory, as we shall see

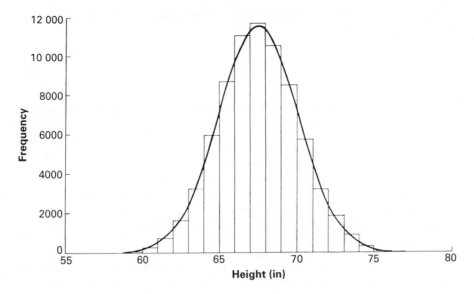

Fig. 2.10 A distribution of heights of young adult males, with an approximating normal distribution (Martin, 1949, Table 17 (Grade 1)).

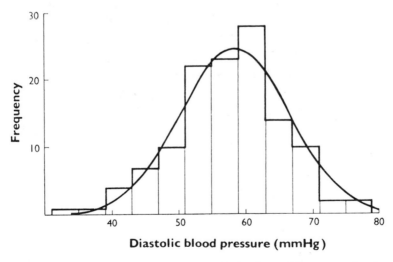

Fig. 2.11 A distribution of diastolic blood pressures of schoolboys with an approximating normal distribution (Rose, 1962, Table 1).

in Chapter 3. For the purposes of the present discussion we shall regard the normal distribution as one of a number of theoretical forms for a continuous random variable, and proceed to describe some of its properties.

The probability density, $f(x)$, of a normally distributed random variable, x, is given by the expression

$$f(x) = \frac{1}{\sigma \sqrt{(2\pi)}} \exp\left[-\frac{(x - \mu)^2}{2\sigma^2} \right], \qquad (2.17)$$

where $\exp(z)$ is a convenient way of writing the exponential function e^z (e being the base of natural logarithms), μ is the expectation or mean value of x and σ is the standard deviation of x. (Note that π is the mathematical constant $3\cdot14159\ldots$, not, as in §2.5, the parameter of a binomial distribution.)

The curve (2.17) is shown in Fig. 2.12, on the horizontal axis of which are marked the positions of the mean, μ, and the values of x which differ from μ by $\pm\sigma$, $\pm2\sigma$ and $\pm3\sigma$. The symmetry of the distribution about μ may be inferred from (2.17), since changing the sign but not the magnitude of $x - \mu$ leaves $f(x)$ unchanged.

Figure 2.12 shows that a relatively small proportion of the area under the curve lies outside the pair of values $x = \mu + 2\sigma$ and $x = \mu - 2\sigma$. The area under the curve between two values of x represents the probability that the random variable x takes values within this range (see §2.3). In fact the probability that x lies within $\mu \pm 2\sigma$ is very nearly $0\cdot95$, and the probability that x lies outside this range is, correspondingly, $0\cdot05$.

It is important for the statistician to be able to find the area under any part of a normal distribution. Now, the density function (2.17) depends on two parameters, μ and σ. It might be thought, therefore, that any relevant probabilities would have to be worked out separately for every pair of values of μ and σ. Fortunately this is not so. In the previous paragraph we made a statement about

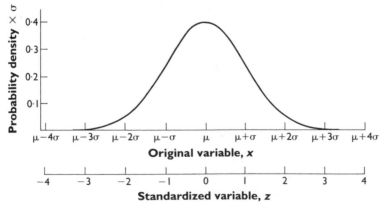

Fig. 2.12 The probability density function of a normal distribution showing the scales of the original variable and the standardized variable.

the probabilities inside and outside the range $\mu \pm 2\sigma$, without any assumption about the particular values taken by μ and σ. In fact the probabilities depend on an expression of the departure of x from μ as a multiple of σ. For example, the points marked on the axis of Fig. 2.12 are characterized by the multiples ± 1, ± 2, and ± 3, as shown on the lower scale. The probabilities under various parts of any normal distribution can therefore be expressed in terms of the *standardized deviate* (or *z-value*)

$$z = \frac{x - \mu}{\sigma}.$$

A few important results are given in Table 2.5. More detailed results are given in Appendix Table A1.

Table 2.5 Some probabilities associated with the normal distribution

Standardized deviate $z = (x - \mu)/\sigma$	Probability of greater deviation	
	In either direction	In one direction
0·0	1·000	0·500
1·0	0·317	0·159
2·0	0·046	0·023
3·0	0·0027	0·0013
1·645	0·10	0·05
1·960	0·05	0·025
2·576	0·01	0·005

The use of tables of the normal distribution may be illustrated by the next example.

Example 2.6

The heights of a large population of men are found to follow closely a normal distribution with a mean of 172·5 cm and a standard deviation of 6·25 cm. We shall use Table A1 to find the proportions of the population corresponding to various ranges of height.

1 *Above 180 cm.* If $x = 180$, the standardized deviate $z = (180 - 172·5)/6·25 = 1·20$. The required proportion is the probability that z exceeds 1·20, which is found from Table A1 to be 0·115.

2 *Below 170 cm.* $z = (170 - 172·5)/6·25 = -0·40$. The probability that z falls below $-0·40$ is the same as that of exceeding $+0·40$, namely 0·345.

3 *Below 185 cm.* $z = (185 - 172·5)/6·25 = 2·00$. The probability that z falls below 2·00 is one minus the probability of exceeding 2·00, namely $1 - 0·023 = 0·977$.

4 *Between 165 and 175 cm.* For $x = 165$, $z = -1\cdot20$; for $x = 175$, $z = 0\cdot40$. The probability that z falls between $-1\cdot20$ and $0\cdot40$ is one minus the probability of (i) falling below $-1\cdot20$ or (ii) exceeding $0\cdot40$, namely

$$1 - (0\cdot115 + 0\cdot345) = 1 - 0\cdot460 = 0\cdot540.$$

The normal distribution is often useful as an approximation to the binomial and Poisson distributions. The binomial distribution for any particular value of π approaches the shape of a normal distribution as the other parameter n increases indefinitely (see Fig. 2.7); the approach to normality is more rapid for values of π near $\frac{1}{2}$ than for values near 0 or 1, since all binomial distributions with $\pi = \frac{1}{2}$ have the advantage of symmetry. Thus, provided n is large enough, a binomial variable r (in the notation of §2.5) may be regarded as approximately normally distributed with mean $n\pi$ and standard deviation $\sqrt{[n\pi(1 - \pi)]}$.

The Poisson distribution with mean μ approaches normality as μ increases indefinitely (see Fig. 2.9). A Poisson variable x may, therefore, be regarded as approximately normal with mean μ and standard deviation $\sqrt{\mu}$.

If tables of the normal distribution are to be used to provide approximations to the binomial and Poisson distributions, account must be taken of the fact that these two distributions are discrete whereas the normal distribution is continuous. It is useful to introduce what is known as a *continuity correction*, whereby the exact probability for, say, the binomial variable r (taking integral values) is approximated by the probability of a normal variable between $r - \frac{1}{2}$ and $r + \frac{1}{2}$. Thus, the probability that a binomial variable took values greater than or equal to r when $r > n\pi$ (or less than or equal to r when $r < n\pi$) would be approximated

Table 2.6 Examples of the approximation to the binomial distribution by the normal distribution with continuity correction

π	n	Mean $n\pi$	Standard deviation $\sqrt{[n\pi(1 - \pi)]}$	Values of r	Exact probability	Normal approximation with continuity correction	
						z	Probability
0·5	10	5	1·581	$\leqslant 2$	0·0547	1·581	0·0579
				$\geqslant 8$	0·0547		
0·1	50	5	2·121	$\leqslant 2$	0·1117	1·179	0·1192
				$\geqslant 8$	0·1221		
0·5	40	20	3·162	$\leqslant 14$	0·0403	1·739	0·0410
				$\geqslant 26$	0·0403		
0·2	100	20	4·000	$\leqslant 14$	0·0804	1·375	0·0846
				$\geqslant 26$	0·0875		

by the normal tail area beyond a standardized normal deviate

$$z = \frac{|r - n\pi| - \frac{1}{2}}{\sqrt{[n\pi(1 - \pi)]}},$$

the vertical lines indicating that the 'absolute value', or the numerical value ignoring the sign, is to be used.

Tables 2.6 and 2.7 illustrate the normal approximations to some probabilities for binomial and Poisson variables.

Table 2.7 Examples of the approximation to the Poisson distribution by the normal distribution with continuity correction

Mean μ	Standard deviation $\sqrt{\mu}$	Values of x	Exact probability	Normal approximation with continuity correction	
				$z = \dfrac{\lvert x - \mu\rvert - \frac{1}{2}}{\sqrt{\mu}}$	Probability
5	2·236	0	0·0067	2·013	0·0221
		≤ 2	0·1246	1·118	0·1318
		≥ 8	0·1334	1·118	0·1318
		≥ 10	0·0318	2·013	0·0221
20	4·472	≤ 10	0·0108	2·214	0·0168
		≤ 15	0·1565	1·006	0·1572
		≥ 25	0·1568	1·006	0·1572
		≥ 30	0·0218	2·124	0·0168
100	10·000	≤ 80	0·0226	1·950	0·0256
		≤ 90	0·1714	0·950	0·1711
		≥ 110	0·1706	0·950	0·1711
		≥ 120	0·0282	1·950	0·0256

2.8 Bayes' theorem

It was pointed out in §2.1 that the frequency definition of probability does not normally permit one to allot a numerical value to the probability that a certain proposition or hypothesis is true. There are, however, some situations in which the relevant alternative hypotheses can be thought of as presenting themselves in a random sequence so that numerical probabilities can be associated with them. For instance, a doctor in charge of a clinic may be interested in the hypothesis: 'This patient has disease A.' By regarding this patient as a random member of a large collection of patients presenting themselves at the clinic he may be able to associate with the hypothesis a certain probability, namely the long-run proportion of patients with disease A. This may be regarded as a *prior probability*, since it can be ascertained (or at least estimated roughly) from retrospective observations.

Suppose the doctor now makes certain new observations, after which he again considers the probability of the hypothesis: 'This patient has disease A.' The new value may be called a *posterior probability* because it refers to the situation after the new observations have been made. Intuitively one would expect the posterior probability to exceed the prior probability if the new observations were particularly common on the hypothesis in question and relatively uncommon on any alternative hypothesis. Conversely, the posterior probability would be expected to be less than the prior probability if the observations were not often observed in disease A but were common in other situations.

Consider a simple example in which there are only three possible diseases (A, B and C), with prior probabilities π_A, π_B and π_C (with $\pi_A + \pi_B + \pi_C = 1$). Suppose that the doctor's observations fall conveniently into one of four categories 1, 2, 3, 4, and that the probability distributions of the various outcomes for each disease are as follows:

	Outcome				
Disease	1	2	3	4	Total
A	l_{A1}	l_{A2}	l_{A3}	l_{A4}	1
B	l_{B1}	l_{B2}	l_{B3}	l_{B4}	1
C	l_{C1}	l_{C2}	l_{C3}	l_{C4}	1

Suppose the doctor observes outcome 2. The total probability of this outcome is

$$\pi_A l_{A2} + \pi_B l_{B2} + \pi_C l_{C2}.$$

The three terms in this expression are in fact the probabilities of disease A and outcome 2, disease B and outcome 2, disease C and outcome 2. Once the doctor has observed outcome 2, therefore, the posterior probabilities of A, B and C, $\pi_{A|2}$, $\pi_{B|2}$ and $\pi_{C|2}$, are

$$\frac{\pi_A l_{A2}}{\pi_A l_{A2} + \pi_B l_{B2} + \pi_C l_{C2}}, \frac{\pi_B l_{B2}}{\pi_A l_{A2} + \pi_B l_{B2} + \pi_C l_{C2}}, \frac{\pi_C l_{C2}}{\pi_A l_{A2} + \pi_B l_{B2} + \pi_C l_{C2}}.$$

The prior probabilities have been multiplied by factors proportional to l_{A2}, l_{B2} and l_{C2}. Although these three quantities are straightforward probabilities, they do not form part of the same distribution, being entries in a column rather than a row of the table above. Probabilities of a particular outcome on different hypotheses are often called *likelihoods* of these hypotheses.

This is an example of the use of Bayes' theorem (named after an English clergyman, Thomas Bayes, 1702–61). More generally, if the hypothesis H_i has a prior probability π_i and outcome j has a probability l_{ij} when H_i is true, the posterior probability of H_i after outcome j has been observed is

$$\pi_{i|j} = \frac{\pi_i l_{ij}}{\sum_h \pi_h l_{hj}}. \tag{2.18}$$

An alternative form of this equation is in terms of the odds

$$\frac{\pi_{i|j}}{1 - \pi_{i|j}} = \frac{\pi_i}{1 - \pi_i} \times \frac{l_{ij}}{l_{(\text{not } i)j}} \tag{2.19}$$

where $l_{(\text{not } i)j}$ is the probability of outcome j if the hypothesis is not i. The left-hand side is the posterior odds, and the terms on the right-hand side are the prior odds and the likelihood ratio for outcome j.

In some examples, the outcomes will be continuous random variables, in which case the l_{ij} terms will be probability densities rather than probabilities. The hypothesis H_i may form a continuous set (for example H_i may specify that the mean μ of a normal distribution is equal to i, which can therefore take any negative or positive value); in this case the summation in the denominator of (2.18) must be replaced by an integral. But Bayes' theorem always takes the same basic form: prior probabilities are converted to posterior probabilities by multiplication in proportion to likelihoods.

The example provides an indication of the way in which Bayes' theorem may be used as an aid to diagnosis. In practice there are severe problems in estimating the probabilities appropriate for the population of patients under treatment; for example, the distribution of diseases observed in a particular centre is likely to vary with time. The determination of the likelihoods will involve extensive and carefully planned surveys and the definition of the outcome categories may be difficult.

One of the earliest applications of Bayes' theorem to medical diagnosis was that of Warner *et al.* (1961). They examined data from a large number of patients with congenital heart disease. For each of 33 different diagnoses they estimated the prior probability, π_i, and the probabilities l_{ij} of various combinations of symptoms. Altogether 50 symptoms, signs and other variables were measured on each individual. Even if all these had been dichotomies there would have been 2^{50} possible values of j, and it would clearly be impossible to get reliable estimates of all the l_{ij}. Warner *et al.* overcame this problem by making an assumption which has often been made by later workers in this field, namely that the symptoms and other variables are statistically independent. The probability of any particular combination of symptoms, j, can then be obtained by multiplying together the separate, or *marginal*, probabilities of each. In this study firm diagnoses for certain patients could be made by intensive investigation and these were compared with the diagnoses given by Bayes' theorem and also with those made by experienced cardiologists using the same information. Bayes' theorem seems to emerge well from the comparison. Nevertheless the assumption of independence of symptoms is potentially dangerous and should not be made without careful thought.

A number of papers illustrating the use of Bayesian methods and related techniques of decision theory to problems in medical diagnosis, prognosis and decision-making are to be found in the journal *Medical Decision Making*. For a recent review of decision analysis see Glasziou and Schwartz (1991). The aim here is to provide rules for the choice amongst decisions to be made during the course of medical treatment. These may involve such questions as whether to proceed immediately with an operation or whether to delay the decision while the patient is kept under observation or until the results of laboratory tests become available. Such choices depend not only on assessments of the probabilities of life-treatening diseases, based on the evidence currently available, but also on assessments of the expected gain (or *utility*) to be derived from various outcomes. Bayesian methods are central to the calculation of probabilities, but the assignment of utilities may be difficult and indeed highly subjective.

For further discussion see Bailey (1977, §4.7), Spiegelhalter and Knill-Jones (1984), Pauker and Kassirer (1992) and Weinstein and Fineberg (1980).

Example 2.7

Fraser and Franklin (1974) studied 700 case records of patients with liver disease. The initial set of over 300 symptoms, signs and test results was reduced to 97 variables for purposes of analysis. In particular, groups of symptoms and signs recognized to be clinically interdependent were amalgamated so as to minimize the danger inherent in the independence assumption discussed above. Patients with rare diagnoses (those represented by less than 12 patients) or multiple diagnoses were omitted, as were those with incomplete records. There remained 480 cases. Prior probabilities were estimated from the relative frequencies of the various diagnoses, and likelihoods for particular combinations of symptoms, signs and test results were obtained by multiplication of marginal frequencies.

Application of Bayes' theorem to each of the patient records gave posterior probabilities. For example, the posterior probabilities for one patient were:

Acute infective hepatitis	0·952,
Cholestatic infective hepatitis	0·048,
All other diagnoses	0·000.

In a large number of cases the first or first two diagnoses accounted for a high probability, as in this instance.

This first analysis led to some revisions of the case records, and the exercise was repeated on a reduced set of 419 patients and the predicted diagnoses compared with the true diagnoses. A result was categorized as 'equivocal' if the highest posterior probability was less than three times as great as the second highest. Similar predictions were done on the basis of the likelihoods alone (i.e. ignoring the prior probabilities). The results were:

	Correct	Equivocal	Incorrect
Likelihood	316 (75%)	51 (12%)	52 (12%)
Bayesian	325 (78%)	48 (11%)	46 (11%)

It seems likely that the Bayesian results would have shown a greater improvement over the likelihood results if the rare diseases had not been excluded (because the priors would then have been relatively more important).

There is a danger in validating such a diagnostic procedure on the data set from which the method has been derived, because the estimates of probability are 'best' for this particular set and less appropriate for other sets. Fraser and Franklin therefore checked the method on 70 new cases with diagnoses falling into the group previously considered. The Bayesian method gave 44 (63%) correct, 12 (17%) equivocal and 14 (20%) incorrect results, with the likelihood method again slightly worse.

The following example illustrates the application of Bayes' theorem to genetic counselling.

Example 2.8

From genetic theory it is known that a woman with a haemophiliac brother has a probability of $\frac{1}{2}$ of being a carrier of a haemophiliac gene. A recombinant DNA diagnostic probe test provides information that contributes towards discriminating between carriers and non-carriers of a haemophiliac gene. It has been observed that 90% of women known to be carriers give a positive test result, whilst 20% of non-carriers have a positive result. The woman has the test. What is the probability that she is a carrier if the result is negative?

The probability may be evaluated using (2.18). Let H_1 be the hypothesis that the woman is a carrier and H_2 that she is not. Then $\pi_1 = \pi_2 = 0.5$. If outcome j represents a negative test then l_{1j}, the probability of a negative test result if the woman is a carrier, equals $1 - 0.9 = 0.1$, and l_{2j}, the probability of a negative test result if the woman is not a carrier, equals 0.8. Therefore

$$P \text{ (carrier given } -\text{ve test)} = \frac{0.5 \times 0.1}{0.5 \times 0.1 + 0.5 \times 0.8}$$

$$= 0.11.$$

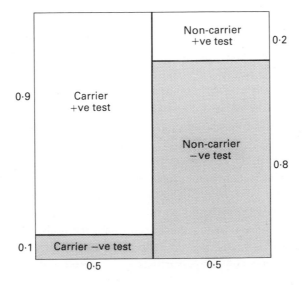

Thus the posterior probability is less than the prior probability, as would be expected, since the extra information, a negative test, is more probable if the woman is not a carrier.

A diagrammatic representation of the calculation is as follows. A square with sides of length 1 unit is divided vertically according to the prior probabilities of each hypothesis, and then horizontally within each column according to the probabilities of outcome. Then by the multiplication rule (2.2) each of the four rectangles has an area equal to the probability of the corresponding hypothesis and outcome.

Once it is known that the outcome is negative then only the shaded area is relevant and the probability that the woman is a carrier is the proportion of the shaded area that is in the carrier column, leading to the same numerical answer as direct application of (2.18).

2.9 Subjective probability

The use of Bayes' theorem described in §2.8 is restricted to situations in which the hypothesis can be regarded as having prior and posterior probabilities in the usual sense of long-run frequencies. It would be attractive if one could allot probabilities to hypotheses like the following: 'The use of tetanus antitoxin in cases of clinical tetanus reduces the fatality of the disease by more than 20%', for which no frequency interpretation is possible.

Suppose we interpret the probability of a hypothesis as a measure of our degree of belief in its truth. A probability of zero would correspond to complete disbelief, a value of one representing complete certainty. Such numerical values could now be manipulated by Bayes' theorem, measures of prior belief being modified in the light of observations on random variables by multiplication by likelihoods, resulting in measures of posterior belief. Many writers (Jeffreys, 1961; Good, 1950; Savage, 1954; Lindley, 1965) have advocated this method as the basis of statistical inference, and the so-called Bayesian approach is at present very influential.

The main problem is how to determine prior probabilities in situations in which frequency interpretations are meaningless. One approach is to accept arbitrary 'indifference' rules for distributing probability amongst the alternative hypotheses when one is in a state of ignorance about their relative plausibilities. Another approach is to ask oneself what odds one would be prepared to accept for a bet on the truth or falsehood of a particular proposition. If the acceptable odds were judged to be 4 to 1 against, the proposition could be regarded as having a probability of $\frac{1}{5}$ or 0·2.

The main body of statistical methods described in this book was built on the basis of a frequency view of probability, and we shall adhere mainly to this approach. Bayesian methods based on suitable indifference rules (Lindley, 1965) often correspond precisely to the more traditional methods, when appropriate changes of wording are made. We shall indicate many of these points of correspondence (for example in §4.12). Nevertheless, there are points at which conflicts between the viewpoints necessarily arise, and it is wrong to suggest that they are merely different ways of saying the same thing.

In our view both Bayesian and non-Bayesian methods have their proper place in statistical methodology. If the purpose of an analysis is to express the way in which a set of initial beliefs is modified by the evidence provided by the data, then Bayesian methods are clearly appropriate. If the emphasis is on the evidence provided by the data, without the need to formulate prior and posterior beliefs, the statistician has two options: either to use frequency-based methods such as those described later in this book, or to keep within the Bayesian framework by calculating likelihoods (for direct presentation or for possible future use in Bayes' theorem). The two approaches can and should coexist.

Bayesian methods are discussed further in §§4.12 and 4.13. Fuller accounts are to be found in books such as Lee (1989) and, at a rather more advanced level, Box and Tiao (1973).

3: Sampling

3.1 Population and sample

Statistics as a subject is very much concerned with the properties of large collections of individual items. Such large collections are usually called *populations*. The word 'population' is commonly used in conversation to refer to a large collection of human beings or other living organisms. The statistician refers also to collections of inanimate objects, such as birth certificates or parishes. He or she will also often refer to a population of observations—for example, the population of heights of adult males resident in England at a certain moment, or the population of outcomes (death or survival) for all patients suffering from a particular illness during some period.

To study the properties of some populations we often have recourse to a *sample* drawn from that population. This is a subgroup of the individuals in the population, usually proportionately few in number, selected so as to be, to some degree, representative of the population. In most situations the sample will not be fully representative. Something is lost by the process of sampling. Any one sample is likely to differ in some respect from any other sample which might have been chosen and there will be some risk in taking any sample as representing the population. However, much may be gained by having to make relatively few observations. If a national census is conducted by interviewing, say, only 1 in 100 rather than the whole of the population, it may be possible to devote more resources to training the interviewers, who will be fewer in number, and thereby to obtain more accurate records.

The most familiar example of a sampling enquiry is perhaps the public opinion poll, in which a very small proportion of the population is interviewed for some specific purpose. Many sampling enquiries are concerned with topics in medicine and health. In the United States National Health Interview Survey, over 2000 people are interviewed each week to provide a continuous picture of the nation's health. In Great Britain similar questions are included as part of the General Household Survey, which covers over 10 000 households annually. Apart from these continuous surveys, many *ad hoc* surveys are carried out for specific purposes. Current examples in the UK include surveys on dental health, children's smoking, health and nutrition, infant feeding, and health and activity.

Techniques for the design of sample surveys are discussed in §6.2. In the present section we are concerned with only the simplest sort of sampling procedure, *random sampling*, and in the remainder of the present chapter we shall consider the consequences of following this procedure in various circumstances.

The first step is usually to define the *sampling frame*, which is essentially a list tor form of identification of the individuals in the population to be sampled. For example, if the aim is to sample adults resident in England, one useful way is to define the sampling frame as the individuals listed in the current electoral registers (lists of people entitled to vote at elections). If the intention is to sample small areas of a country, the sampling frame may be defined by marking a map into appropriate subdivisions by a grid. Once the individuals to be sampled have been defined they can be numbered, and the problem will now be to decide which numbers to select for the sample.

How is the sample to be chosen? If some characteristics of the population are known, perhaps as a result of previous surveys, it is sometimes suggested that the sample should be chosen by *purposive selection*, whereby certain features of the sample are made to agree exactly or almost exactly with those of the population. For example, in sampling for market research or opinion polls, some organizations use *quota sampling*, a method by which each interviewer is given instructions about certain characteristics (such as age, sex and social status of the individuals to be selected), the proportions in various subgroups being chosen to agree with the corresponding proportions in the population. The difficulty with this method is that serious discrepancies between the sample and the population may arise in respect of characteristics which have not been taken into account. There is nothing in the sampling procedure to give any general confidence about the representativeness of the sample.

In general it is preferable to use some form of random sampling. In *simple random sampling*, every possible sample of a given size from the population has an equal probability of being chosen. A particular sample may, purely by chance, happen to be dissimilar from the population in some serious respect, but the theory of probability enables us to calculate how large these discrepancies are likely to be. Much of statistical analysis is concerned with the estimation of the likely magnitude of these *sampling errors*, and in this chapter we consider some of the most important results.

To draw a simple random sample from a population we could imagine some physical method of randomization. For instance, if 10 people were to be selected at random from a population of 100, a card could be produced for each member of the population, the cards thoroughly shuffled, and 10 cards selected. Such a method would be tedious, particularly with large population sizes, and it is convenient to make use of tables of *random sampling numbers*, which effectively give the results of very extensive random selections made in the past by various reliable methods. A set of random numbers is given in Table A6, and instructions on the use of the table will be found on p. 576.

3.2 The sampling error of a mean

Suppose that x is a quantitative random variable with mean μ and variance σ^2, and that $\bar{x}$ is the mean of a random sample of n values of x. For example x may be the systolic blood pressure of men aged 30–34 employed in a certain industrial occupation, and $\bar{x}$ the mean of a random sample of n men from this very large population. We may think of $\bar{x}$ as itself a random variable, for each sample will have its own value of $\bar{x}$, and if the random sampling procedure is repeated indefinitely the values of $\bar{x}$ can be regarded as following a probability distribution (Fig. 3.1). The nature of this distribution of $\bar{x}$ is of considerable importance, for it determines how much uncertainty is conferred upon $\bar{x}$ by the very process of sampling.

Two features of the variability of $\bar{x}$ seem intuitively clear. First, it must depend on σ: the more variable is the blood pressure in the industrial population, the more variable will be the means of different samples of size n. Secondly, the variability of $\bar{x}$ must depend on n: the larger the size of each random sample, the closer together the values of $\bar{x}$ will be expected to lie.

Mathematical theory provides three basic results concerning the distribution of $\bar{x}$, which are of great importance in applied statistics. The first two results are

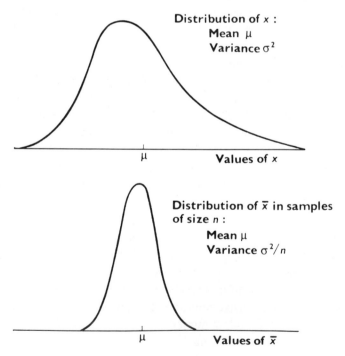

Fig. 3.1 The distribution of a random variable and the sampling distribution of means in random samples of size n.

proved at the end of this section, but a proof of the third result is beyond the scope of this book.

1 $E(\bar{x}) = \mu$; that is, the mean of the distribution of the sample mean is the same as the mean of the individual measurements.

2 $\text{var}(\bar{x}) = \sigma^2/n$. The variance of the sample mean is equal to the variance of the individual measurements divided by the sample size. This provides a formal expression of the intuitive feeling, mentioned above, that the variability of $\bar{x}$ should depend on both σ and n; the precise way in which this dependence acts would perhaps not have been easy to guess. The standard deviation of $\bar{x}$ is

$$\sqrt{\left(\frac{\sigma^2}{n}\right)} = \frac{\sigma}{\sqrt{n}}. \tag{3.1}$$

This quantity is often called the *standard error* of the mean and written $\text{SE}(\bar{x})$. It is quite convenient to use this nomenclature as it helps to avoid confusion between the standard deviation of x and the standard deviation of $\bar{x}$, but it should be remembered that a standard error is not really a new concept: it is merely the standard deviation of some quantity calculated from a sample (in this case, the mean) in an indefinitely long series of repeated samplings.

3   If the distribution of x is normal, so will be the distribution of $\bar{x}$. Much more importantly, even if the distribution of x is not normal, that of $\bar{x}$ will become closer and closer to the normal distribution with mean μ and variance σ^2/n as n gets larger. This is a consequence of a mathematical result known as the *central limit theorem*, and it accounts for the central importance of the normal distribution in statistics.

The normal distribution is strictly only the limiting form of the sampling distribution of $\bar{x}$ as n increases to infinity, but it provides a remarkably good approximation to the sampling distribution even when n is small and the distribution of x is far from normal. Table 3.1 shows the results of taking random samples of five digits from tables of random numbers. These tables may be thought of as forming a probability distribution for a discrete random variable x, taking the values $0, 1, 2, \ldots, 9$ with equal probabilities of 0.1. This is clearly far from normal in shape. The mean and variance may be found by the methods of §2.4.

$$\mu = E(x) = 0.1(1 + 2 + \ldots + 9) = 4.5,$$

$$\sigma^2 = E(x^2) - \mu^2$$

$$= 0.1(1^2 + 2^2 + \ldots + 9^2) - (4.5)^2$$

$$= 8.25,$$

$$\sigma = \sqrt{8.25} = 2.87,$$

$$\text{SE}(\bar{x}) = \sqrt{(8.25/5)} = \sqrt{1.65} = 1.28.$$

Table 3.1   Distribution of means of 2000 samples of five random numbers

Mean, $\bar{x}$	Frequency
0.4–	1
0.8–	4
1.2–	11
1.6–	22
2.0–	43
2.4–	88
2.8–	104
3.2–	178
3.6–	196
4.0–	210
4.4–	272
4.8–	200
5.2–	193
5.6–	154
6.0–	129
6.4–	92
6.8–	52
7.2–	30
7.6–	13
8.0–	7
8.4–	1
	2000

Two thousand samples of size 5 were taken (actually, by generating the random numbers on a computer rather than reading from printed tables), the mean $\bar{x}$ was calculated for each sample, and the 2000 values of $\bar{x}$ formed into the frequency distribution shown in Table 3.1. The distribution can be seen to be similar in shape to the normal distribution. The closeness of the approximation may be seen from Fig. 3.2, which shows the histogram corresponding to Table 3.1, together with a curve the height of which is proportional to the density of a normal distribution with mean 4·5 and standard deviation 1·28.

The theory outlined above applies strictly to random sampling from an infinite population or for successive independent observations on a random variable. Suppose a sample of size n has to be taken from a population of finite size N. Sampling is usually *without replacement*, which means that if an individual member of the population is selected as one member of a sample it cannot again be chosen in that sample. The expectation of $\bar{x}$ is still equal to μ, the population mean. The formula (3.1) must, however, be modified by a 'finite population correction', to become

$$\text{SE}(\bar{x}) = \frac{\sigma}{\sqrt{n}} \sqrt{(1 - f)}, \tag{3.2}$$

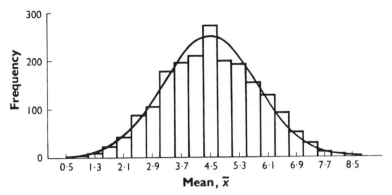

Fig. 3.2 The distribution of means from 2000 samples of five random digits (Table 3.1), with the approximating normal distribution.

where $f = n/N$, the *sampling fraction*. In (3.2), σ is defined as the standard deviation of x in the population, using a divisor $N - 1$. Thus

$$\mu = \frac{\sum_{i=1}^{N} x_i}{N}$$

and

$$\sigma^2 = \frac{\sum_{i=1}^{N} (x_i - \mu)^2}{N - 1}.$$

The effect of the finite population correction, $1 - f$, is to reduce the sampling variance substantially as f approaches 1, i.e. as the sample size approaches the population size. Clearly, when $n = N$, $f = 1$ and $SE(\bar{x}) = 0$: there is only one possible random sample, consisting of all the members of the population, and for this sample $\bar{x} = \mu$.

The sampling error of the sample median has no simple general expression. In random samples from a normal distribution however, the standard error of the median for large n is approximately $1{\cdot}253\sigma/\sqrt{n}$. The fact that this exceeds $\sigma/\sqrt{n}$ shows that the median is more variable than the sample mean (or, technically, it is less *efficient* as an estimator of μ). This comparison depends on the assumption of normality for the distribution of x, however, and for certain other distributional forms the median provides the more efficient estimator.

Proofs of results 1 and 2

1 $E(\bar{x}) = \mu$.
Denote the individual observations in the sample by $x_1, x_2, \ldots, x_n$. Then

$$\bar{x} = (x_1 + x_2 + \ldots + x_n)/n$$
$$= (1/n)x_1 + (1/n)x_2 + \ldots + (1/n)x_n.$$

Using the intuitive steps referred to in the footnote on p. 54,

$$E(\bar{x}) = (1/n)E(x_1) + (1/n)E(x_2) + \ldots + (1/n)E(x_n).$$

But

$$E(x_1) = E(x_2) = \ldots = E(x_n) = \mu.$$

Hence

$$E(\bar{x}) = (1/n)\mu + (1/n)\mu + \ldots + (1/n)\mu$$
$$= \mu,$$

since there are n identical terms to be added.

2 $\text{var}(\bar{x}) = \sigma^2/n.$

$$\text{var}(\bar{x}) = E(\bar{x} - \mu)^2$$

$$= E\left(\frac{x_1 + x_2 + \ldots + x_n}{n} - \mu\right)^2$$

$$= E\left[\frac{(x_1 - \mu) + (x_2 - \mu) + \ldots + (x_n - \mu)}{n}\right]^2$$

$$= (1/n^2)E[(x_1 - \mu)^2 + (x_2 - \mu)^2 + \ldots + 2(x_1 - \mu)(x_2 - \mu) + \ldots],$$

where the square brackets include all squared terms like $(x_i - \mu)^2$ and twice each product of terms like $(x_i - \mu)(x_j - \mu)$. The expectation of each term $(x_i - \mu)^2$ is σ^2. The expectation of each term $(x_i - \mu)(x_j - \mu)$ is zero since, for any value of x_i, x_j independently ranges over all possible values so that $E(x_j - \mu) = 0$. Hence

$$\text{var}(\bar{x}) = (1/n^2)(\sigma^2 + \sigma^2 + \ldots \text{(to } n \text{ terms)} \ldots + 0)$$
$$= (1/n^2)(n\sigma^2)$$
$$= \sigma^2/n.$$

3.3   The sampling error of a proportion

This has already been fully discussed in §2.5. If individuals in an infinitely large population are classified into two types A and B, with probabilities π and $1 - \pi$, the number r of individuals of type A in a random sample of size n follows a binomial distribution. We shall now apply the results of §3.2 to prove the formulae previously given for the mean and variance of r.

Suppose we define a quantitative variable x, which takes the value 1 for each A individual and 0 for each B. We may think of x as a score attached to each member of the population. The point of doing this is that, in a sample of n consisting of r As and $n - r$ Bs,

$$\sum x = (r \times 1) + [(n - r) \times 0]$$
$$= r$$

and

$$\bar{x} = r/n, \; = p \quad \text{in the notation of §2.5.}$$

The sample proportion p may therefore be identified with the sample mean of x, and to study the sampling variation of p we can apply the general results established in §3.2. We shall need to know the population mean and standard deviation of x. From first principles these are

$$E(x) = (\pi \times 1) + [(1 - \pi) \times 0]$$
$$= \pi, \tag{3.3}$$

and

$$\text{var}(x) = E(x^2) - [E(x)]^2$$
$$= (\pi \times 1^2) + [(1 - \pi) \times 0^2] - \pi^2$$
$$= \pi(1 - \pi).$$

From (3.1),

$$\text{var}(\bar{x}) = \frac{\pi(1 - \pi)}{n}. \tag{3.4}$$

Writing (3.3) and (3.4) in terms of p rather than x and $\bar{x}$, we have

$$E(p) = \pi$$

and

$$\text{var}(p) = \frac{\pi(1 - \pi)}{n},$$

as in (2.12) and (2.13). Since $r = np$,

$$E(r) = n\pi$$

and

$$\text{var}(r) = n\pi(1 - \pi),$$

as in (2.10) and (2.11).

One more result may be taken from §3.2. As n approaches infinity, the distribution of $\bar{x}$ (that is, of p) approaches the normal distribution with the corresponding mean and variance. The increasing symmetry has already been noted in §2.5.

3.4 The sampling error of a variance

Suppose that a quantitative random variable x follows a distribution with mean μ and variance σ^2. In a sample of size n, the estimated variance is

$$s^2 = \frac{\sum (x_i - \bar{x})^2}{n - 1}.$$

In repeated random sampling from the distribution, s^2 will vary from one sample to another; it will itself be a random variable. We now consider the nature of the variation in s^2.

The expectation of s^2 can be derived as follows:

$$E(s^2) = \frac{1}{n-1} E\left[\sum (x_i - \bar{x})^2\right]$$

$$= \frac{1}{n-1} E\left\{\sum [(x_i - \mu) - (\bar{x} - \mu)]^2\right\}$$

$$= \frac{1}{n-1} E\left[\sum (x_i - \mu)^2 - 2\sum (x_i - \mu)(\bar{x} - \mu) + \sum (\bar{x} - \mu)^2\right]$$

$$= \frac{1}{n-1} E\left[\sum (x_i - \mu)^2 - n(\bar{x} - \mu)^2\right],$$

since

$$\sum (x_i - \mu)(\bar{x} - \mu) = \sum (\bar{x} - \mu)^2 = n(\bar{x} - \mu)^2.$$

Now, $E(x_i - \mu)^2 = \sigma^2$ by definition, and $E(\bar{x} - \mu)^2 = \text{var}(\bar{x}) = \sigma^2/n$. Hence

$$E(s^2) = \frac{1}{n-1}\left[n\sigma^2 - n\left(\frac{\sigma^2}{n}\right)\right],$$

$$= \frac{1}{n-1}(n-1)\sigma^2$$

$$= \sigma^2. \tag{3.5}$$

Another way of stating the result (3.5) is that s^2 is an *unbiased* estimator of σ^2. It is this property which makes s^2, with its divisor of $n-1$, a satisfactory estimator of the population variance: the statistic (1.1), with a divisor of n, has an expectation $(n-1)\sigma^2/n$, which is less than σ^2. Note that $E(s)$ is not equal to σ; it is in fact less than σ. The reason for paying so much attention to $E(s^2)$ rather than $E(s)$ will appear in Chapters 7 and 8.

What else can be said about the sampling distribution of s^2? Let us, for the moment, tighten our requirements about the distribution of x by assuming that it is strictly normal. In this particular instance, the distribution of s^2 is closely related to one of a family of distributions called the χ^2 distributions ('chi-square' or 'chi-squared'), which are of very great importance in statistical work, and it will be useful to introduce these distributions by a short discussion before returning to the distribution of s^2 which is the main concern of this section.

Denote by X_1 the standardized deviate corresponding to the variable x. That is, $X_1 = (x - \mu)/\sigma$. X_1^2 is a random variable, whose value must be non-negative. The distribution of X_1^2 is called the χ^2 *distribution on one degree of freedom* (1 DF), and is often called

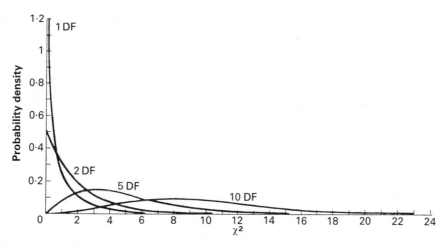

Fig. 3.3 Probability density functions for χ^2 distributions with various numbers of degrees of freedom.

the $\chi^2_{(1)}$ distribution. It is depicted as the first curve in Fig. 3.3. The *percentage points* of the χ^2 distribution are tabulated in Table A2. The values exceeded with probability P are often called the $100(1-P)$th *percentiles*; thus, the column headed $P = 0.050$ gives the 95th percentile. Two points may be noted at this stage.

1 $E(X_1^2) = E(x-\mu)^2/\sigma^2 = \sigma^2/\sigma^2 = 1$. The mean value of the distribution is 1.

2 The percentiles may be obtained from those of the normal distribution. From Table A1 we know, for instance, that there is a probability 0.05 that $(x-\mu)/\sigma$ exceeds $+1.960$ or falls below -1.960. Whenever either of these events happens, $(x-\mu)^2/\sigma^2$ exceeds $(1.960)^2 = 3.84$. Thus, the 0.05 level of the $\chi^2_{(1)}$ distribution is 3.84. A similar relationship holds for all the other percentiles.

Now let x_1 and x_2 be two independent observations on x, and define

$$X_2^2 = \frac{(x_1-\mu)^2}{\sigma^2} + \frac{(x_2-\mu)^2}{\sigma^2}.$$

X_2^2 follows what is known as the χ^2 *distribution on two degrees of freedom* ($\chi^2_{(2)}$). The variable X_2^2, like X_1^2, is necessarily non-negative. Its distribution is shown as the second curve in Fig. 3.3, and is tabulated along the second line of Table A2. Note that X_2^2 is the sum of two independent observations on X_1^2. Hence

$$E(X_2^2) = 2E(X_1^2) = 2.$$

Similarly, in a sample of n independent observations x_i, define

$$X_n^2 = \sum_{i=1}^{n} \frac{(x_i-\mu)^2}{\sigma^2} = \frac{\sum (x_i-\mu)^2}{\sigma^2}. \tag{3.6}$$

This follows the χ^2 *distribution on n degrees of freedom* ($\chi^2_{(n)}$), and $E(X_n^2) = n$.

Figure 3.3 and Table A2 show that, as the degrees of freedom increase, the χ^2 distribution becomes more and more symmetric. Indeed, since it is the sum of n

independent $\chi^2_{(1)}$ variables, the central limit theorem (which applies to sums as well as to means) shows that $\chi^2_{(n)}$ tends to normality as n increases. The variance of the $\chi^2_{(n)}$ distribution is $2n$.

The result (3.6) enables us to find the distribution of the sum of squared deviations about the population mean μ. In the formula for s^2, we use the sum of squares about the sample mean $\bar{x}$, and it can be shown that

$$\sum (x_i - \bar{x})^2 \leqslant \sum (x_i - \mu)^2.$$

In fact, $\sum (x_i - \bar{x})^2/\sigma^2$ follows the $\chi^2_{(n-1)}$ distribution. The fact that differences are taken from the sample mean rather than the population mean is compensated for by the subtraction of 1 from the degrees of freedom. Now

$$s^2 = \frac{\sum (x_i - \bar{x})^2}{n - 1} = \frac{\sigma^2}{n - 1} \frac{\sum (x_i - \bar{x})^2}{\sigma^2}$$

$$= \frac{\sigma^2}{n - 1} \chi^2_{(n-1)}.$$

That is, s^2 behaves as $\sigma^2/(n - 1)$ times a $\chi^2_{(n-1)}$ variable. It follows that

$$E(s^2) = \frac{\sigma^2}{n - 1} E(\chi^2_{(n-1)}) = \frac{\sigma^2}{n - 1} (n - 1) = \sigma^2,$$

as we proved directly at (3.5), and

$$\text{var}(s^2) = \frac{\sigma^4}{(n - 1)^2} \text{var}(\chi^2_{(n-1)}) = \frac{\sigma^4}{(n - 1)^2} 2(n - 1)$$

$$= \frac{2\sigma^4}{n - 1}. \tag{3.7}$$

The formula (3.7) for $\text{var}(s^2)$ is true only for samples from a normal distribution; indeed, the whole sampling theory for s^2 is more sensitive to non-normality than that for the mean.

3.5 The sampling error of a difference

Many statistical investigations lead to a consideration of a difference between two quantities—the difference between the mean weight gain in two groups of animals receiving different diets, for example; or the difference between the proportions of 10-year-old children in two different areas who show a certain serum antibody level.

We shall therefore be much concerned with the sampling error to be attached to the difference between two quantities, such as means or proportions calculated from two independently drawn random samples. It will be useful to consider a rather general situation first, and to consider cases of particular interest later. Suppose, then, that we have two random variables y_1 and y_2, that y_1 is distributed with mean m_1 and variance v_1, and y_2 with mean m_2 and variance v_2. We take an observation at random on y_1 and an *independent* random observation on y_2. What can be said about the distribution of $y_1 - y_2$ in an indefinite series of repetitions of this procedure?

$$E(y_1 - y_2) = E(y_1) - E(y_2) = m_1 - m_2. \tag{3.8}$$

$$var(y_1 - y_2) = E[(y_1 - y_2) - (m_1 - m_2)]^2$$

$$= E[(y_1 - m_1) - (y_2 - m_2)]^2$$

$$= E[(y_1 - m_1)^2 - 2(y_1 - m_1)(y_2 - m_2) + (y_2 - m_2)^2]$$

$$= v_1 + v_2, \tag{3.9}$$

the middle term on the previous line being zero, because, for any given value of y_1, $E(y_2 - m_2) = 0$, and consequently when y_1 is allowed to vary $E(y_1 - m_1)(y_2 - m_2)$ is also zero. This term could not be equated to zero if y_1 and y_2 were not drawn independently.

We now apply the general results (3.8) and (3.9) to the particular case in which $y_1 = \bar{x}_1$, the mean of a random sample of size n_1 from a population with mean μ_1 and variance σ_1^2; and $y_2 = \bar{x}_2$, the mean of an independent random sample of size n_2 from a population with mean μ_2 and variance σ_2^2. Here, from the results of §3.2,

$$m_1 = \mu_1 \text{ and } v_1 = \sigma_1^2/n_1;$$

$$m_2 = \mu_2 \text{ and } v_2 = \sigma_2^2/n_2.$$

Therefore, from (3.8) and (3.9),

and

$$\left. \begin{array}{c} E(\bar{x}_1 - \bar{x}_2) = \mu_1 - \mu_2 \\ \\ var(\bar{x}_1 - \bar{x}_2) = \dfrac{\sigma_1^2}{n_1} + \dfrac{\sigma_2^2}{n_2}. \end{array} \right\} \tag{3.10}$$

Similarly, suppose $y_1 = p_1$, the proportion of individuals showing some characteristic in a random sample of size n_1 from a population in which this characteristic occurs with probability π_1; and $y_2 = p_2$, the proportion in an independent sample of size n_2 from a population with parameter π_2. From §3.3,

$$m_1 = \pi_1 \text{ and } v_1 = \pi_1(1 - \pi_1)/n_1;$$

$$m_2 = \pi_2 \text{ and } v_2 = \pi_2(1 - \pi_2)/n_2.$$

From (3.8) and (3.9),

$$E(p_1 - p_2) = \pi_1 - \pi_2$$

and   (3.11)

$$\text{var}(p_1 - p_2) = \frac{\pi_1(1 - \pi_1)}{n_1} + \frac{\pi_2(1 - \pi_2)}{n_2}.$$

The results (3.10) and (3.11) are of great importance in the statistical methods to be described in the next chapter. It is important here to emphasize the condition of independence. If the two samples are not independent, for example because of some constraint in the design of the investigation, the expectation formulae in (3.10) and (3.11) will still hold, but the variance formulae will be invalid.

3.6 Some other variance formulae

In §3.5 we derived a general formula for the variance of a difference between two random variables, and applied it to two different sampling problems. It is convenient to mention here one or two other useful formulae for the variances of various functions of independent random variables. Two random variables are said to be *independent* if the distribution of one is unaffected by the value taken by the other. One important consequence of independence is that mean values can be multiplied. That is, if $y = x_1 x_2$, where x_1 and x_2 are independent, then

$$E(y) = E(x_1)E(x_2).$$ (3.12)

Linear function

Suppose $x_1, x_2, \ldots, x_k$ are independent random variables, and

$$y = a_1 x_1 + a_2 x_2 + \ldots + a_k x_k,$$

the as being constants. Then,

$$\text{var}(y) = a_1^2 \text{var}(x_1) + a_2^2 \text{var}(x_2) + \ldots + a_k^2 \text{var}(x_k).$$ (3.13)

The result (3.9) is a particular case of (3.13) when $k = 2$, $a_1 = 1$ and $a_2 = -1$.
The independence condition is important. If the xs are not independent, there must be added to the right-hand side of (3.13) a series of terms like

$$2a_i a_i \text{cov}(x_i, x_j),$$ (3.14)

where 'cov' stands for the *covariance* of x_i and x_j, which is defined by

$$\text{cov}(x_i, x_j) = E\{[x_i - E(x_i)][(x_j - E(x_j)]\}.$$

The covariance is the expectation of the product of deviations of two random variables from their means. When the variables are independent, the covariance is zero (see the proof of (3.9)). When all k variables are independent, all the covariance terms vanish and we are left with (3.13).

Ratio

Let $y = x_1/x_2$, where again x_1 and x_2 are independent. No general formula can be given for the variance of y. Indeed, it may be infinite. However, if x_2 has a small coefficient of variation, the distribution of y will be rather similar to a distribution with a variance given by the following formula:

$$\text{var}(y) = \frac{\text{var}(x_1)}{[E(x_2)]^2} + \frac{[E(x_1)]^2}{[E(x_2)]^4}\text{var}(x_2). \tag{3.15}$$

Note that if x_2 has no variability at all, (3.15) reduces to

$$\text{var}(y) = \frac{\text{var}(x_1)}{x_2^2},$$

which is an exact result when x_2 is a constant.

Product

Let $y = x_1 x_2$, where x_1 and x_2 are independent. Denote the means of x_1 and x_2 by μ_1 and μ_2, and their variances by σ_1^2 and σ_2^2. Then

$$\text{var}(y) = E(y^2) - [E(y)]^2$$

$$= E(x_1^2)E(x_2^2) - [E(x_1)E(x_2)]^2$$

$$= (\mu_1^2 + \sigma_1^2)(\mu_2^2 + \sigma_2^2) - \mu_1^2\mu_2^2$$

$$= \mu_1^2\sigma_2^2 + \mu_2^2\sigma_1^2 + \sigma_1^2\sigma_2^2. \tag{3.16}$$

Note that the step from the first to the second line of this proof uses the assumption that x_1 and x_2 are independent. For example, if x_1 and x_2 were not independent it would not necessarily be true that $E(y) = E(x_1)E(x_2)$.

General function

Suppose we know the mean and variance of the random variable x. Can we calculate the mean and variance of any general function of x such as $3x^3$ or $\sqrt{(\log x)}$? There is no simple formula, but again a useful approximation is available when the coefficient of variation of x is small. We have to assume some knowledge of calculus at this point. Denote the function of x by y. Then

$$\text{var}(y) \simeq \left(\frac{dy}{dx}\right)^2_{x=E(x)} \text{var}(x), \tag{3.17}$$

the symbol $\simeq$ standing for 'approximately equal to'. In (3.17), dy/dx is the differential coefficient (or derivative) of y with respect to x, evaluated at the mean value of x.

If y is a function of two variables, x_1 and x_2,

$$\text{var}(y) \simeq \left(\frac{\partial y}{\partial x_1}\right)^2 \text{var}(x_1) + 2\left(\frac{\partial y}{\partial x_1}\right)\left(\frac{\partial y}{\partial x_2}\right)\text{cov}(x_1, x_2) + \left(\frac{\partial y}{\partial x_2}\right)^2 \text{var}(x_2),$$

$$\tag{3.18}$$

where $\partial y/\partial x_1$ and $\partial y/\partial x_2$ are the *partial* derivatives of y with respect to x_1 and x_2, and these are again evaluated at the mean values. The reader with some knowledge of calculus will be able to derive (3.9) as a particular case of (3.18) when $\text{cov}(x_1, x_2) = 0$. An obvious extension of (3.18) to k variables gives (3.13) as a special case. Equation (3.16) is another special case of (3.18), when $\text{cov}(x_1, x_2) = 0$. In (3.16), the last term becomes negligible if the coefficients of variation of x_1 and x_2 are very small; the first two terms agree with (3.18).

4: Statistical Inference

4.1 General

The argument in Chapter 3 has been essentially from the population to the sample. Given the distribution of a variable in a population we obtained results about the distributions of various quantities, such as the mean and variance, calculated from sample observations. Such a quantity is called a *statistic*. These results are of direct interest in the planning of sampling enquiries, as they enable the investigator to estimate the precision attainable with a sample of a given size, and hence help to decide how large a sample should be taken. This question will be discussed again in §6.6.

We have not yet, however, come to grips with another problem that interests the investigator. When the sample has been taken, what sort of inferences can be drawn about the population on the basis of the sample? The argument here must be in the opposite direction to that previously used. We do not know the characteristics of the population. We have taken one random sample and wish to use our knowledge of sampling theory to make whatever inference can be made about the population. One fundamental difficulty usually arises. The expressions of sampling variation given by the various formulae for standard errors or variances in the last chapter usually involve some parameters of the population. For instance the standard error of the sample mean is $\sigma/\sqrt{n}$. If we are attempting to make an inference about a normal distribution on the basis of one random sample, we shall know the sample size, n, but not the population standard deviation, σ. We cannot, therefore, calculate the standard error exactly. A similar point arises in other situations, and the discussion of methods to overcome the difficulty will be a constant theme in this chapter.

We shall continue to suppose that the data at our disposal form a random sample from some population. In some sampling enquiries this is known to be true by virtue of the design of the investigation. In other studies a more complex form of sampling may have been used; consideration of some more complex designs is deferred until Chapter 6. A more serious conceptual difficulty is that in many statistical investigations there is no formal process of sampling from a well-defined population. For instance the prevalence of a certain disease may be calculated for all the inhabitants of a village and compared with that for another village. A clinical trial may be conducted in a clinic, with the participation of all the patients seen at the clinic during a given period. A doctor may report the mean duration of symptoms amongst a consecutive series of 50 patients with a certain form of illness. Individual readings vary haphazardly whether they form a random sample or whether they are collected in a less formal way, and it will often be desirable to assess the effect which this basic variability has on any statistical calculations that are performed. How can this be done if there is no infinite population and no strictly random sample?

It can be done by arguing that the observations are subject to random, unsystematic variation, which makes them appear very much like observations on random variables. The population formed by the whole distribution is not a real, well-defined entity, but it may be helpful to think of it as a hypothetical population which would be generated if an indefinitely large number of observations showing the same sort of random variation as those at our disposal could be made. This concept seems satisfactory when the observations vary in a patternless way. We are putting forward a 'model', or conceptual framework, for the random variation, and propose to make whatever statements we can about the relevant features of this model, just as we wish to make statements about the relevant features of a population in a strict sampling situation. Sometimes, of course, the supposition that the data behave like a random sample is blatantly unrealistic. There may, for instance, be a systematic tendency for the earliest observations to be greater in magnitude than those made later. Such trends, and other systematic features, can be allowed for by increasing the complexity of the model. When such modifications have been made, there will still remain some degree of apparently random variation, the underlying probability distribution of which is a legitimate object of study.

In §6.4 and §6.5 we shall discuss comparative experiments in which experimental units are allocated at random to various groups which are to receive different treatments. It will be of considerable importance to compare two or more groups of observations made on units receiving different treatments, and to assess the extent to which such contrasts are affected by random variation. In most experiments the whole collection of units is not selected by strictly random sampling; the clinical trial mentioned earlier provides an example. Nevertheless, because of random allocation the differences between groups behave like differences between random samples—from the same population if all treatments are alike, from different populations if the treatments differ in their effects. The sampling theory of differences is therefore directly relevant.

4.2 Significance tests and confidence intervals

Significance tests

Data are often collected in order to answer specified questions, such as: (i) do workers in a particular industry have reduced lung function compared with a control group? or (ii) is a new treatment beneficial to those suffering from a certain disease compared with the existing treatment? Such questions may be answered by setting up a hypothesis and then using the data to test this hypothesis. It is generally agreed that some caution should be exercised before claiming that some effect, such as a reduced lung function or an improved cure rate, has been established. The way of proceeding is to set up a *'null' hypothesis*, that there is no effect. So in (ii) above the null hypothesis is that the new treatment and the existing treatment were equally beneficial. Then an effect is claimed only if the data are inconsistent with this null hypothesis, that is, unlikely to have occurred if it were true.

The formal way of proceeding is one of the most important methods of statistical inference, and is called the *significance test*. Suppose a series of observations is selected randomly from a population and we are interested in a certain null hypothesis that specifies values for one or more of the parameters of the population. The question then arises: do the observations in the sample throw any light on the plausibility of the hypothesis? Some samples will be, in some sense, reasonably typical of those which might be expected by sampling theory if the null hypothesis were true. Other samples will have certain features which would be unlikely to arise if the null hypothesis were true; if such a sample were observed, there would be reason to suspect that the null hypothesis was untrue.

The significance test is a rule for deciding whether any particular sample is in the 'likely' or 'unlikely' class, or, more usefully, for assessing the strength of the conflict between what is found in the sample and what is predicted by the null hypothesis. The dividing line between the 'likely' and 'unlikely' classes is clearly arbitrary but is usually defined in terms of a probability, P, which is referred to as the *significance level*. Thus a result would be declared as *significant at the 5% level*, if the sample was in the class containing those samples most removed from the null hypothesis and that class contained no more than 5% of all possible samples. An alternative and common way of expressing this is to state that the result was statistically significant ($P < 0.05$).

The 5% level, and to a lesser extent the 1% level, have become widely accepted as convenient yardsticks for assessing the significance of departures from a null hypothesis. This is unfortunate in a way, because there should be no rigid distinction between a departure which is just beyond the 5% significance level and one which just fails to reach it. It is perhaps preferable to avoid the dichotomy—'significant' and 'not significant'—by attempting to measure *how* significant the departure is. A convenient way of measuring this is to measure the probability, P, of obtaining, if the null hypothesis were true, a sample as extreme as, or more extreme than, the sample obtained. One reason for the origin of the use of the dichotomy, significant or not significant, is that significance levels had to be looked up in tables, such as Appendix Tables A2, A3 and A4, and this restricted the evaluation of P to a range. Nowadays significance tests are often carried out on a computer and many statistical computing packages give the calculated P value. It is preferable to quote this value and we will follow this practice. However, when analyses are carried out by hand, or the calculated P value is not given in computer output, then a range of values could be stated. This should be done as precisely as possible, particularly when a result is 'almost significant'; thus '$0.05 < P < 0.1$' is far preferable to 'not significant ($P > 0.05$)'.

The test to be used in any situation will depend on what alternatives to the null hypothesis are contemplated. If the null hypothesis specifies the mean and standard deviation of a normal distribution as μ_0 and σ_0, a significance test which is particularly designed to detect departures of the population mean from μ_0 could reasonably be based on an examination of the sample mean, $\bar{x}$. A test designed to detect departures of the standard deviation from σ_0 should be based on some measure of variation in the sample, such as the sample standard deviation, s.

Although a 'significant' departure provides some degree of evidence against a null hypothesis, it is important to realize that a 'non-significant' departure does not provide positive evidence in favour of that hypothesis. The situation is rather that we have failed to find strong evidence against the null hypothesis.

It is important also to grasp the distinction between statistical significance and clinical significance or practical importance. The analysis of a large body of data might produce evidence of a departure from a null hypothesis which is highly significant, and yet the difference may be of no practical importance—either because the effect is clinically irrelevant or because it is too small. Conversely, another investigation may fail to show a significant effect—perhaps because the study is too small or because of excessive random variation—and yet an effect large enough to be important may be present: the investigation may have been too insensitive to reveal it.

The significance test is generally *two-sided*, in the sense that sufficiently large departures from the null hypothesis, in either direction, will be judged significant. If, for some reason, we decided that we were interested in possible departures only in one particular direction, say that a new treatment was superior to an old treatment, it would be reasonable to count as significant only those samples that differed sufficiently from the null hypothesis in that direction. Such a test is called *one-sided*. For a one-sided test at, say, the 5% level, sensitive to positive deviations from the null hypothesis, a sample would be significant if it was in the class of samples deviating most from the null hypothesis in the positive direction and this class contained at most 5% of possible samples.

A one-sided test at level P is therefore the same as a two-sided test at level $2P$, except that departures from the null hypothesis are only counted in one direction. In a sense the distinction is semantic. On the other hand, there may be a temptation to use one-sided tests rather than two-sided tests because the probability level is lower, and therefore the *apparent* significance is greater. A decision to use a one-sided test should *never* be made after looking at the data and observing the direction of the departure. Before the data are examined one should decide to use a one-sided test only if it is quite certain that departures in one direction will always be ascribed to chance, and therefore regarded as non-significant however large they are. This situation rarely arises in practice, and it will be safe to assume that significance tests should almost always be two-sided. We shall make this assumption in this book unless otherwise stated.

No null hypothesis is likely to be exactly true. Why, then, should we bother to test it, rather than immediately rejecting it as implausible? There are several rather different situations in which the use of significance tests can be justified.

1 *To test a simplifying hypothesis.* Sometimes the null hypothesis specifies a simple model for a situation which is really likely to be more complex than the model admits. For instance, in studying the relationship between two variables, as in Chapter 5, it will be useful to assume for simplicity that a trend is linear (i.e. follows a straight line) if there is no evidence to the contrary, even though common sense tells us that the true trend is highly unlikely to be precisely linear.

2 *To test a null hypothesis which may be approximately true.* In a clinical trial to test a new drug against a placebo, it may be that the drug will either be very nearly inert or will have a marked effect. The null hypothesis that the drug is completely inert (and therefore has exactly the same effect as a placebo) is then a close approximation to a possible state of affairs.

3 *To test the direction of a difference from a critical value.* Suppose we are interested in whether a certain parameter, θ, has a value greater or less than some value θ_0. We could test the null hypothesis that θ is precisely θ_0. It may be quite clear that this will not be true. Nevertheless we give ourselves the opportunity to assert in which direction the difference lies. If the null hypothesis is significantly contradicted, we shall have good evidence either that $\theta > \theta_0$ or that $\theta < \theta_0$.

Confidence intervals

Questions of the type considered in the context of hypothesis testing can be looked at from a different point of view, leading to another very important concept of statistical inference. Instead of asking 'is a new treatment beneficial to those suffering from a certain disease compared with the existing treatment?', we might ask 'how large is the benefit of a new treatment compared with the existing treatment to those suffering from a certain disease?'. The question could be answered by quoting a single figure and this is termed the *point estimate*. But additionally we should like some indication of how accurate this estimate is. This is provided by the *confidence interval* which has a specified probability (the *confidence coefficient*) of containing the population value. The most commonly used probability is 95%. The interval is then called the 95% confidence interval, and the ends of this intervals the 95% *confidence limits*; less frequently 90% or

99% confidence limits may be used. The confidence interval provides a formal expression of the uncertainty which must be attached to the point estimate on account of sampling errors alone.

Two slightly different ways of interpreting a confidence interval may be useful.
1   The values of the parameter inside the 95% confidence interval are precisely those which would not be contradicted by a significance test at the 5% level, because there is only a probability of 5% that the interval does not contain the population value. Values outside the interval, on the other hand, would all be contradicted by a two-sided test at the 5% level.
2   We have said that the confidence interval contains the population value with probability 0.95. This is not quite the same thing as saying that the population value has a probability of 0.95 of being within the interval, because the population value is not a random variable. In any particular case the population value either is or is not in the interval. What we are doing is to imagine a series of repeated random samples from a population with a fixed parameter value. In the long run, 95% of the confidence intervals will include the parameter value and the confidence statement will then be true. Five per cent of the time the interval will not include the parameter value and the confidence statement is then untrue. If, in any particular problem, we calculate a confidence interval, we may happen to be unlucky in that this may be one of the 5% of cases in which the interval does not contain the population parameter; but we are applying a procedure that will work 95% of the time. For a somewhat different approach, see §4.12.

It follows from **1** above that a confidence interval may be regarded as equivalent to performing a significance test for all values of a parameter, not just the single value corresponding to the null hypothesis. Thus the confidence interval contains more information than the corresponding significance test and, for this reason, it is sometimes argued that significance tests could be dispensed with and all results expressed in terms of an estimate together with the confidence interval of that estimate. On the other hand quoting the value of the significance level, and not just whether the result is or is not significant at the 5% level, does provide information additional to that provided by the 95% confidence interval. In the last decade or so there has been an increasing tendency to put more emphasis on expressing results using confidence intervals and less on significance testing (Rothman, 1978; Gardner and Altman, 1989). In general we recommend that where possible results should be expressed using a confidence interval, and that possibly the significance level is quoted as well.

The use of confidence intervals facilitates the distinction between statistical significance and clinical significance or practical importance. Five possible interpretations of a significance test are illustrated in terms of the confidence interval of a difference between two groups in Fig. 4.1, adapted from Berry (1986, 1988): (a) the difference is significant and certainly large enough to be of practical importance; (b) the difference is significant but it is unclear whether it is large enough to

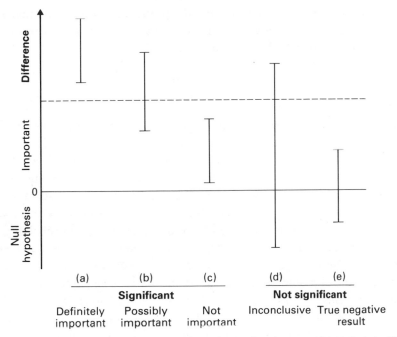

Fig. 4.1 Confidence intervals showing five possible interpretations in terms of statistical significance and practical importance.

be important; (c) the difference is significant but too small to be important; (d) the difference is not significant but may be large enough to be important; and (e) the difference is not significant and also not large enough to be important. One of the tasks in planning investigations is to ensure that a difference large enough to be important is likely, if it really exists, to be statistically significant and thus to be detected (cf. §6.6), and possibly to ensure that it is clear whether or not the difference is large enough to be important.

In the following sections these two methods of statistical inference will be applied to a number of different situations and the detailed methodology set out.

4.3 Inferences from means

We consider first the situation in which the population standard deviation, σ, is known; later we consider what to do when σ is unknown.

Known σ

Let us consider in some detail the problem of testing the null hypothesis (which we shall denote by H_0) that the parameters of a normal distribution are $\mu = \mu_0$ and $\sigma = \sigma_0$, using the mean, $\bar{x}$, of a random sample of size n.

If H_0 is true, we know from §3.2 that the probability is only 0·05 that $\bar{x}$ falls outside the interval $\mu_0 - 1·96\sigma_0/\sqrt{n}$ to $\mu_0 + 1·96\sigma_0/\sqrt{n}$. For a value of $\bar{x}$ outside this range, the standardized normal deviate

$$z = \frac{\bar{x} - \mu_0}{\sigma_0/\sqrt{n}} \qquad (4.1)$$

would be less than $-1·96$ or greater than $1·96$. Such a value of $\bar{x}$ could be regarded as sufficiently far from μ_0 to cast doubt on the null hypothesis. Certainly, H_0 *might* be true, but if so an unusually large deviation would have arisen—one of a class that would arise by chance only once in 20 times. On the other hand such a value of $\bar{x}$ would be quite likely to occur if μ had some value other than μ_0, closer, in fact, to the observed $\bar{x}$. The particular critical values adopted here for z, $\pm 1·96$, corresponds to the quite arbitrary probability level of 0·05. If z is numerically greater than $1·96$ the difference between μ_0 and $\bar{x}$ is said to be *significant at the 5% level*. Similarly, an even more extreme difference yielding a value of z numerically greater than $2·58$ is *significant at the 1% level*. Rather than using arbitrary levels, such as 5% or 1%, we might enquire how far into the tails of the expected sampling distribution the observed value of $\bar{x}$ falls. A convenient way of measuring this tendency is to measure the probability, P, of obtaining, if the null hypothesis were true, a value of $\bar{x}$ as extreme as, or more extreme than, the value observed. If $\bar{x}$ is just significant at the 5% level, $z = \pm 1·96$ and $P = 0·05$ (the probability being that in both tails of the distribution). If $\bar{x}$ is beyond the 5% significance level, $z > 1·96$ or $< -1·96$ and $P < 0·05$. If $\bar{x}$ is not significant at the 5% level, $P > 0·05$ (see Fig. 4.2). If the observed value of z were, say, 2·20, one could either give the exact value of P as 0·028 (from Table A1), or, by comparison with the percentage points of the normal distribution, write $0·02 < P < 0·05$.

Example 4.1

A large number of patients with cancer at a particular site, and of a particular clinical stage, are found to have a mean survival time from diagnosis of 38·3 months with a standard deviation of 43·3 months. One hundred patients are treated by a new technique and their mean survival time is 46·9 months. Is this apparent increase in mean survival explicable as a random fluctuation?

We test the null hypothesis that the 100 recent results are effectively a random sample from a population with mean $\mu_0 = 38·3$ and standard deviation $\sigma_0 = 43·3$. Note that this distribution must be extremely skew, since a deviation of even one standard deviation below the mean gives a negative value ($38·3 - 43·3 = -5·0$), and no survival times can be negative. However, 100 is a reasonably large sample size, and it would be safe to use the normal theory for the distribution of the sample mean. Putting $n = 100$ and $\bar{x} = 46·9$, we have a standardized normal deviate

$$\frac{46 \cdot 9 - 38 \cdot 3}{(43 \cdot 3/\sqrt{100})} = \frac{8 \cdot 6}{4 \cdot 33} = 1.99.$$

This value just exceeds the 5% value of 1·96, and the difference is therefore just significant at the 5% level ($P < 0.05$). Referring to Appendix Table A1 the actual value of P is $2 \times 0.0233 = 0.047$.

This significant difference suggests that the increase in mean survival time is rather unlikely to be due to chance. It would not be safe to assume that the new treatment has improved survival, as certain characteristics of the patients may have changed since the earlier data were collected; for example, the disease may be diagnosed earlier. All we can say is that the difference is not very likely to be a chance phenomenon.

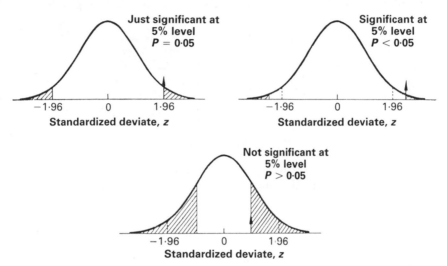

Fig. 4.2 Significance tests at the 5% level based on a standardized normal deviate. The observed deviate is marked by an arrow.

Suppose we wish to draw inferences about the population mean, μ, without concentrating on a single possible value μ_0. In a rough sense, μ is more likely to be near $\bar{x}$ than very far from $\bar{x}$. Can this idea be made more precise by asserting something about the probability that μ lies within a given interval around $\bar{x}$? This is the confidence interval approach. Suppose that the distribution of x is normal with known standard deviation, σ. From the general sampling theory (§3.2), the probability is 0·95 that $\bar{x} - \mu$ lies between $-1.96\sigma/\sqrt{n}$ and $+1.96\sigma/\sqrt{n}$, i.e. that

$$-1.96\sigma/\sqrt{n} < \bar{x} - \mu < 1.96\sigma/\sqrt{n}. \tag{4.2}$$

Rearrangement of the left part of (4.2), namely $-1.96\sigma/\sqrt{n} < \bar{x} - \mu$, gives $\mu < \bar{x} + 1.96\sigma/\sqrt{n}$; similarly the right part gives $\bar{x} - 1.96\sigma/\sqrt{n} < \mu$. Therefore (4.2) is equivalent to the statement that

$$\bar{x} - 1.96\sigma/\sqrt{n} < \mu < \bar{x} + 1.96\sigma/\sqrt{n}. \tag{4.3}$$

The statement (4.3), which as we have seen, is true with probability 0·95, asserts that μ lies in a certain interval called the 95% *confidence interval*. The ends of this interval, which are called the 95% *confidence limits*, are symmetrical about $\bar{x}$ and (since σ and n are known) can be calculated from the sample data. The confidence interval provides a formal expression of the uncertainty which must be attached to $\bar{x}$ on account of sampling errors alone.

Interpretation **2** of a confidence interval is illustrated in Fig. 4.3. An imaginary series of repeated random samples from a population with a fixed value of μ will give different values of $\bar{x}$ and therefore different confidence intervals but, in the long run, 95% of these intervals will include μ, whilst in 5% $\bar{x}$ will be more than 1·96 standard errors away from μ (as in the fourth sample in Fig. 4.3) and the interval will not include μ.

Example 4.1, continued

In this example, the 95% confidence limits are

$$46·9 \pm (1·96)(4·33)$$

$$= 38·4 \text{ and } 55·4.$$

The fact that this interval just excludes the possible value 38·3, which was tested previously, corresponds to the fact that this value was just contradicted by a significance test at the 5% level.

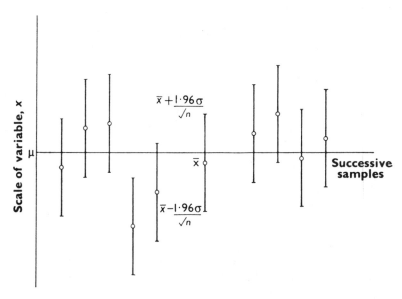

Fig. 4.3 Confidence limits (95%) for the mean of a normal distribution with known standard deviation, from a series of random samples of size n.

The assumption of normality is not crucial if n is reasonably large, because of the near-normality of the distribution of $\bar{x}$ in samples from almost any population.

For a higher degree of confidence than 95% we may use some other percentile of the normal distribution. The 99% limits, for instance, are

$$\bar{x} \pm 2 \cdot 58\sigma/\sqrt{n}.$$

In general, the $1 - 2\alpha$ confidence limits are

$$\bar{x} \pm z_{2\alpha}\sigma/\sqrt{n},$$

where $z_{2\alpha}$ is the standardized normal deviate exceeded (in either direction) with probability 2α.

Unknown σ—the t distribution

Suppose now that we wish to test a null hypothesis which specifies the mean value of a normal distribution ($\mu = \mu_0$) but does not specify the variance σ^2, and that we have no evidence about σ^2 besides that contained in our sample. The procedure outlined above cannot be followed because the standard error of the mean, $\sigma/\sqrt{n}$, cannot be calculated. It seems reasonable to replace σ by the estimated standard deviation in the sample, s, giving a standardized deviate

$$t = \frac{\bar{x} - \mu_0}{s/\sqrt{n}} \tag{4.4}$$

instead of the normal deviate z given by (4.1). The statistic t would be expected to follow a sampling distribution close to that of z (i.e. close to a standard normal distribution with mean 0 and variance 1) when n is large, because then s will be a good approximation to σ. When n is small, s may differ considerably from σ, purely by chance, and this will cause t to have substantially greater random variability than z.

In fact, t follows what is known as the t *distribution on $n - 1$ degrees of freedom.* The t distributions form a family, distinguished (rather like the χ^2 distributions) by an index, the 'degrees of freedom', which in the present application is one less than the sample size. As the degrees of freedom increase, the t distribution tends towards the standard normal distribution (Fig. 4.4). Appendix Table A3 shows the percentiles of t, i.e. the values exceeded with specified probabilities, for different values of the degrees of freedom, ν. For $\nu = \infty$, the tabulated values agree with those of the standard normal distribution. The 5% point, which always exceeds the normal value of 1·960, is nevertheless close to 2·0 for all except quite small values of ν. The t distribution was derived by

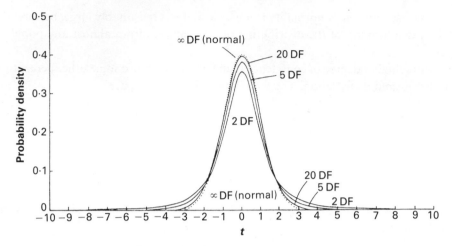

Fig. 4.4 Probability density function for t distributions on 2, 5, 20 and infinite degrees of freedom; the last is the standard normal distribution.

W. S. Gosset (1876–1937) and published under the pseudonym of 'Student' in 1908; the distribution is frequently referred to as Student's t distribution.

The t distribution is strictly valid only if the distribution of x is normal. Nevertheless, it is reasonably '*robust*' in the sense that it is approximately valid for quite marked departures from normality.

Calculation of the confidence interval proceeds as before, but using the t distribution instead of the normal distribution. If

$$t = \frac{\bar{x} - \mu}{s/\sqrt{n}},$$

the probability is 0·95 that t lies between $\pm t_{v, 0 \cdot 05}$, the tabulated 5% point of the t distribution on $v = n - 1$ degrees of freedom. A little rearrangement gives an equivalent statement: the probability is 0·95 that

$$\bar{x} - t_{v, 0 \cdot 05}(s/\sqrt{n}) < \mu < \bar{x} + t_{v, 0 \cdot 05}(s/\sqrt{n}). \tag{4.5}$$

This is the 95% confidence interval. It differs from (4.3) in the replacement of the percentage point of the normal distribution by that of the t distribution, which as we have seen is a somewhat large number. The necessity to estimate the standard error from the sample has led to an interval based on a somewhat larger multiple of the standard error.

As in significance tests, normality of the distribution of x is necessary for the strict validity of (4.5), but moderate departures from normality will have little effect on the validity.

Example 4.2

The following data are the uterine weights (in mg) of each of 20 rats drawn at random from a large stock. Is it likely that the mean weight for the whole stock could be 24 mg, a value observed in some previous work?

9	18	21	26
14	18	22	27
15	19	22	29
15	19	24	30
16	20	24	32

Here $n = 20$, $\sum x = 420$ and $\bar{x} = 420/20 = 21\cdot0$. For t, we need the estimated standard error of the mean, $s/\sqrt{n}$, which it is convenient to calculate as $\sqrt{(s^2/n)}$, to avoid taking two separate square roots. From the usual short-cut formula,

$$\sum (x - \bar{x})^2 = \sum x^2 - \left(\sum x\right)^2 / n$$

$$= 9484 - 8820$$

$$= 664,$$

$$s^2 = 664/19 = 34\cdot947,$$

$$s^2/n = 34\cdot947/20 = 1\cdot7474,$$

$$\sqrt{(s^2/n)} = 1\cdot3219$$

and

$$t = \frac{21\cdot0 - 24\cdot0}{1\cdot3219} = -2\cdot27.$$

The degrees of freedom are $v = 20 - 1 = 19$, and Table A3 shows the relevant percentage points as

P	0·05	0·02
t	2·093	2·539

Thus, the observed value is significant at between 2% and 5% ($0\cdot02 < P < 0\cdot05$). If these calculations had been done on a computer which gave the precise significance level we should have had $P = 0\cdot035$. There is a rather strong suggestion that the mean weight of the stock is different from 24 mg (and, indeed, *less* than this value).

The 95% confidence limits for μ are

$$21\cdot00 \pm (2\cdot093)(1\cdot3219)$$

$$= 18\cdot23 \text{ and } 23\cdot77.$$

The exclusion of the value 24 corresponds to the significant result of testing this value at the 5% level. The 99% limits are

$$21\cdot00 \pm (2\cdot861)(1\cdot3219)$$

$$= 17\cdot22 \text{ and } 24\cdot78,$$

now including 24, since this value for μ was not significantly contradicted at the 1% level.

The limits calculated here are sometimes called *fiducial limits*, this being the term used by R. A. Fisher in his approach to the problem of interval estimation. Fisher's approach was more akin to interpretation **1** (p. 98) rather than **2**, the latter being particularly stressed by J. Neyman (1894–1981), who was responsible for the concept of confidence limits. In most situations, fiducial and confidence limits are (as here) numerically the same, and the interpretation is a matter of choice. In a few situations minor differences arise, a circumstance which has given rise to some controversy.

4.4 Comparison of two means

The sampling error of the difference between two means has been considered in §3.5, where the importance of the independence or dependence of the two samples was stressed. We shall accordingly distinguish between two situations: the paired case, in which the two samples are of equal size and the individual members of one sample are paired with particular members of the other sample; and the unpaired case, in which the samples are quite independent.

Paired case

Suppose we have two samples of size n:

$$x_{11}, x_{12}, \ldots, x_{1i}, \ldots x_{1n}$$

drawn at random from a distribution with mean μ_1 and variance σ_1^2, and

$$x_{21}, x_{22}, \ldots, x_{2i}, \ldots, x_{2n}$$

drawn at random from a distribution with mean μ_2 and variance σ_2^2. If there is some sense in which x_{1i} is paired with x_{2i}, it will usually be true that high values of x_{1i} tend to be associated with high values of x_{2i}, and low with low. For example, x_{1i} and x_{2i} might be blood pressure readings on the ith individual in a group of n, on each of two occasions. Some individuals would tend to give high values on both occasions, and some would tend to give low values. In such situations,

$$E(x_{1i} - x_{2i}) = \mu_1 - \mu_2,$$

but $\text{var}(x_{1i} - x_{2i})$ is (by application of (3.13) and (3.14)) less than the value $\sigma_1^2 + \sigma_2^2$ which would be appropriate for independent observations. Now, $\bar{x}_1 - \bar{x}_2$, the difference between the two means, is the mean of the n individual differences $x_{1i} - x_{2i}$, and these differences are independent of each other. The sampling error of $\bar{x}_1 - \bar{x}_2$ can therefore be obtained by analysing the n individual differences. This automatically ensures that, whatever the nature of the relationship between the paired readings, the appropriate sampling error is calculated. If the differences are normally distributed then the methods of §4.3 can be applied.

Table 4.1 Anxiety scores recorded for 10 patients receiving a new drug and a placebo in random order

| Patient | Anxiety score | | Difference d_i |
	Drug	Placebo	(drug − placebo)
1	19	22	−3
2	11	18	−7
3	14	17	−3
4	17	19	−2
5	23	22	1
6	11	12	−1
7	15	14	1
8	19	11	8
9	11	19	−8
10	8	7	1
			−13

Example 4.3

In a small clinical trial to assess the value of a new tranquillizer on psychoneurotic patients, each patient was given a week's treatment with the drug and a week's treatment with a placebo, the order in which the two sets of treatments were given being determined at random. At the end of each week the patient had to complete a questionnaire, on the basis of which he was given an 'anxiety score' (with possible values from 0 to 30), high scores corresponding to states of anxiety. The results are shown in Table 4.1.

The last column of Table 4.1 shows the difference, d_i, between the anxiety score for the ith subject on the drug and on the placebo. A t test on the 10 values of d_i gives

$$\sum d_i = -13,$$
$$\sum d_i^2 = 203,$$
$$\sum (d_i - \bar{d})^2 = 186 \cdot 1.$$

Therefore,

$$\bar{d} = -1 \cdot 30.$$
$$s^2 = 186 \cdot 1/9 = 20 \cdot 68,$$
$$\sqrt{(s^2/n)} = \sqrt{(20 \cdot 68/10)} = \sqrt{2 \cdot 068} = 1 \cdot 438,$$

and, to test the null hypothesis that $E(d_i) = 0$,

$$t = \frac{-1 \cdot 30}{1 \cdot 438} = -0 \cdot 90 \text{ on 9 DF.}$$

The difference is clearly not significant ($P = 0 \cdot 39$).

The 95% confidence limits for the mean difference are

$$-1 \cdot 30 \pm (2 \cdot 262)(1 \cdot 438)$$
$$= -4 \cdot 55 \text{ and } 1 \cdot 95.$$

To conclude, this trial provided no convincing evidence that the new tranquillizer reduced anxiety when compared with a placebo ($P = 0\cdot39$). The 95% confidence interval for the reduction in anxiety was from 4·6 points on a 30-point scale in the tranquillizer's favour to 2·0 units in favour of the placebo.

In Table 4.1, some subjects, like Nos. 6 and 10, tend to give consistently low scores, whereas others, like Nos. 1 and 5, score highly on both treatments. These systematic differences between subjects are irrelevant to the comparison between treatments, and it is therefore appropriate that the method of differencing removes their effect.

Unpaired case

Suppose $x_{11}, x_{12}, \ldots, x_{1n_1}$ are drawn at random from a distribution with mean μ_1 and variance σ_1^2, and $x_{21}, x_{22}, \ldots, x_{2n_2}$ from a distribution with mean μ_2 and variance σ_2^2. Let $\bar{x}_1$ and $\bar{x}_2$ be the sample means. If the two samples are independent, we have, from (3.10),

and
$$\left. \begin{aligned} \mathrm{E}\,(\bar{x}_1 - \bar{x}_2) &= \mu_1 - \mu_2 \\[2mm] \mathrm{var}\,(\bar{x}_1 - \bar{x}_2) &= \frac{\sigma_1^2}{n_1} + \frac{\sigma_2^2}{n_2}. \end{aligned} \right\} \tag{4.6}$$

If the distributions of the xs are normal, and σ_1^2 and σ_2^2 are known, (4.6) can be used immediately for inferences about $\mu_1 - \mu_2$. To test the null hypothesis that $\mu_1 = \mu_2$, the standardized normal deviate

$$z = \frac{\bar{x}_1 - \bar{x}_2}{\sqrt{\left(\dfrac{\sigma_1^2}{n_1} + \dfrac{\sigma_2^2}{n_2}\right)}}$$

is used. For confidence limits for $\mu_1 - \mu_2$, the appropriate multiple of the standard error (i.e. of the denominator of z) is measured on either side of $\bar{x}_1 - \bar{x}_2$.

The normality of the xs is not a serious restriction if the sample sizes are not too small, because $\bar{x}_1 - \bar{x}_2$, like $\bar{x}_1$ and $\bar{x}_2$ separately, will be almost normally distributed. The lack of knowledge of σ_1^2 and σ_2^2 is more serious. These variances have to be estimated in some way, and we shall distinguish between two situations, in the first of which σ_1^2 and σ_2^2 are assumed to be equal and a common estimate is used for both parameters, and in the second of which no such assumption is made.

Equal variances: the two-sample t test

There are many instances in which it is reasonable to assume $\sigma_1^2 = \sigma_2^2$.

1 In testing a null hypothesis that the two samples are from distributions with the same mean and variance. For example, if the two samples are observations made on patients treated with a possibly active drug and on other patients treated with a pharmacologically inert placebo, the null hypothesis might specify that the drug was completely inert. In that case equality of variance is as much a part of the null hypothesis as equality of means, although we want a test based on $\bar{x}_1 - x_2$ so that we can hope to detect drugs which particularly affect the mean value of x.

2 It may be known from general experience that the sort of changes which distinguish sample 1 from sample 2 may affect the mean but are not likely to affect the variance appreciably. The sample estimates of variance, s_1^2 and s_2^2, may differ considerably, but in these situations we should, on general grounds, be prepared to regard most of the difference as due to sampling fluctuations in s_1^2 and s_2^2 rather than to a corresponding difference in σ_1^2 and σ_2^2.

If σ_1^2 and σ_2^2 are equal, their common value may be denoted by σ^2 without a subscript. How should σ^2 be estimated? From the first sample we have the estimator

$$s_1^2 = \frac{\sum_{(1)} (x - \bar{x}_1)^2}{n_1 - 1},$$

the subscript (1) after $\sum$ denoting a summation over the first sample. From the second sample, similarly, σ^2 is estimated by

$$s_2^2 = \frac{\sum_{(2)} (x - \bar{x}_2)^2}{n_2 - 1}.$$

A common estimate could be got by a straightforward mean of s_1^2 and s_2^2, but it is better to take a weighted mean, giving more weight to the estimate from the larger sample. It can be shown to be appropriate to take

$$s^2 = \frac{(n_1 - 1)s_1^2 + (n_2 - 1)s_2^2}{(n_1 - 1) + (n_2 - 1)}$$

$$= \frac{\sum_{(1)} (x - \bar{x}_1)^2 + \sum_{(2)} (x - \bar{x}_2)^2}{n_1 + n_2 - 2}.$$

This step enables us to use the t distribution on $n_1 + n_2 - 2$ degrees of freedom, as an exact solution to the problem if the xs are exactly normally distributed and as an approximate solution if the distribution of the xs is not grossly non-normal.

The standard error of $\bar{x}_1 - \bar{x}_2$ is now estimated by

$$\text{SE}(\bar{x}_1 - \bar{x}_2) = \sqrt{\left[s^2 \left(\frac{1}{n_1} + \frac{1}{n_2} \right) \right]}.$$

To test the null hypothesis that $\mu_1 = \mu_2$, we take

$$t = \frac{\bar{x}_1 - \bar{x}_2}{\text{SE}(\bar{x}_1 - \bar{x}_2)}$$

as following the t distribution on $n_1 + n_2 - 2$ DF.

Confidence limits are given by

$$\bar{x}_1 - \bar{x}_2 \pm t_{v,0\cdot05}\, \text{SE}(\bar{x}_1 - \bar{x}_2),$$

with $v = n_1 + n_2 - 2$.

Example 4.4

Two groups of female rats were placed on diets with high and low protein content, and the gain in weight between the 28th and 84th days of age was measured for each rat. The results are given in Table 4.2.

The calculations proceed as follows

$\sum_{(1)} x =$	1440		$\sum_{(2)} x =$	707
$n_1 =$	12		$n_2 =$	7
$\bar{x}_1 =$	120·0		$\bar{x}_2 =$	101·0
$\sum_{(1)} x^2 =$	177832		$\sum_{(2)} x^2 =$	73959
$(\sum_{(1)} x)^2 / n_1 =$	172800·00		$(\sum_{(2)} x)^2 / n_2 =$	71407·00
$\sum_{(1)} (x - \bar{x}_1)^2 =$	5032·00		$\sum_{(2)} (x - \bar{x}_2)^2 =$	2552·00

$$s^2 = \frac{5032 + 2552}{17} = 446\cdot12.$$

$$\begin{aligned}
\text{SE}(\bar{x}_1 - \bar{x}_2) &= \sqrt{[(446\cdot12)\,(\tfrac{1}{12} + \tfrac{1}{7})]} \\
&= \sqrt{[(446\cdot12)\,(0\cdot22619)]} \\
&= \sqrt{100\cdot9} \\
&= 10\cdot04.
\end{aligned}$$

To test the null hypothesis that $\mu_1 = \mu_2$,

$$t = \frac{120\cdot0 - 101\cdot0}{10\cdot04} = \frac{19\cdot0}{10\cdot04} = 1\cdot89 \text{ on 17 DF } (P = 0\cdot076).$$

The difference is not quite significant at the 5% level, and would provide merely suggestive evidence for a dietary effect.

Table 4.2 Gain in weight (g) between 28th and 84th days of age of rats receiving diets with high and low protein content

High protein	Low protein
134	70
146	118
104	101
119	85
124	107
161	132
107	94
83	
113	
129	
97	
123	
Total 1440	707

The 95% confidence limits for $\mu_1 - \mu_2$ are

$$19{\cdot}0 \pm (2{\cdot}110)\,(10{\cdot}04)$$

$$= 19{\cdot}0 \pm 21{\cdot}2$$

$$= -2{\cdot}2 \text{ and } 40{\cdot}2.$$

The range of likely values for $\mu_1 - \mu_2$ is large. If the experimenter feels dissatisfied with this range of uncertainty, the easiest remedy is to repeat the experiment with more observations. Higher values of n_1 and n_2 will tend to decrease the standard error of $\bar{x}_1 - \bar{x}_2$ and hence increase the precision of the comparison.

It might be tempting to apply the unpaired method to paired data. This would be incorrect because systematic differences between pairs would not be eliminated but would form part of the variance used in the denominator of the t statistic. Thus, using the unpaired method for paired data would lead to a less sensitive analysis except in cases where the pairing proved ineffective.

Unequal variances

In other situations it may be either clear that the variances differ considerably or prudent to assume that they may do so. One possible approach, in the first case, is to work with a transformed scale of measurement (Chapter 11). If the means, as well as the variances, differ, it may be possible to find a transformed scale, such as the logarithm of the original measurement, on which the means differ but the variances are similar. On the other hand, if the original means are not too different, it will usually be difficult to find a transformation that substantially reduces the disparity between the variances.

In these situations the main defect in the methods based on the t distribution is the use of a pooled estimate of variance. It is better to estimate the standard error of the difference between the two means as

$$\text{SE}(\bar{x}_1 - \bar{x}_2) = \sqrt{\left(\frac{s_1^2}{n_1} + \frac{s_2^2}{n_2}\right)}.$$

A significance test of the null hypothesis may be based on the statistic

$$d = \frac{\bar{x}_1 - \bar{x}_2}{\sqrt{\left(\frac{s_1^2}{n_1} + \frac{s_2^2}{n_2}\right)}},$$

which is approximately a standardized normal deviate if n_1 and n_2 are reasonably large. Similarly, approximate confidence limits are given by

$$\bar{x}_1 - \bar{x}_2 \pm z_{2\alpha} \, \text{SE}(\bar{x}_1 - \bar{x}_2),$$

where $z_{2\alpha}$ is the appropriate standardized normal deviate corresponding to the two-sided probability 2α.

However, this method is no more exact for finite values of n_1 and n_2 than would be the use of the normal approximation to the t distribution in the case of equal variances. The appropriate analogue of the t distribution is both more complex than the t distribution and more contentious. One solution, due to B. L. Welch, is to use a distribution for d (tabulated, for example, in Pearson and Hartley, 1966, Table 11). The critical value for any particular probability level depends on s_1^2/s_2^2, n_1 and n_2. Another solution, similarly dependent on s_1^2/s_2^2, n_1 and n_2, is that of W. V. Behrens, tabulated as Table VI in Fisher and Yates (1963). The distinction between these two approaches is due to different approaches to the logic of statistical inference. Underlying Welch's test is an interpretation of probability levels, either in significance tests or confidence intervals, as long-term frequencies in repeated samples from the same populations. The Behrens test was advocated by R. A. Fisher as an example of the use of fiducial inference, and it arises also from the Bayesian approach (§4.12).

A feature of Welch's approach is that the critical value for d may be less than the critical value for a t distribution with $n_1 + n_2 - 2$ DF, and this is unsatisfactory. A simpler approximate solution which does not have this disadvantage is to test d against the t distribution with degrees of freedom, v, dependent on s_1^2/s_2^2, n_1 and n_2 according to the following formula:

$$\frac{(s_1^2/n_1 + s_2^2/n_2)^2}{v} = \frac{(s_1^2/n_1)^2}{n_1 - 1} + \frac{(s_2^2/n_2)^2}{n_2 - 1}. \tag{4.7}$$

This formula, originally due to Satterthwaite (1946), can be derived using (3.7) and (3.18). Although this test uses the t distribution it should not be confused with the more usual two-sample t test based on equal variances. This approximate test is included in some statistical software packages.

Example 4.5

A suspension of virus particles is prepared at two dilutions. If the experimental techniques are perfect, preparation B should have 10 times as high a concentration of virus particles as preparation A. Equal volumes from each suspension are inoculated on to the chorioallantoic membrane of chick embroys. After an appropriate incubation period the membranes are removed and the number of pocks on each membrane is counted. The numbers are as follows:

Preparation	A	B
Counts	0	10
	0	13
	1	13
	1	14
	1	19
	1	20
	2	21
	2	26
	3	29

Are these results consistent with the hypothesis that, in a large enough series of counts, the mean for preparation B will be 10 times that for preparation A? If the counts on B are divided by 10 and denoted by x_2, the counts on A being denoted by x_1, an equivalent question is whether the means of x_1 and x_2 differ significantly.

Preparation	A	B
Counts	x_1	x_2
	0	1·0
	0	1·3
	1	1·3
	1	1·4
	1	1·9
	1	2·0
	2	2·1
	2	2·6
	3	2·9

$$n_1 = 9 \qquad n_2 = 9$$
$$\bar{x}_1 = 1{\cdot}2222 \qquad \bar{x}_2 = 1{\cdot}8333$$
$$s_1^2 = 0{\cdot}9444 \qquad s_2^2 = 0{\cdot}4100.$$

The estimates of variance are perhaps not sufficiently different here to cause great disquiet, but it is known from experience with this type of data that estimates of variance of pock counts, standardized for dilution as we did for x_2, tend to decrease as the original counts increase. The excess of s_1^2 over s_2^2 is therefore probably not due to sampling error. We have

$$d = \frac{1 \cdot 2222 - 1 \cdot 8333}{\sqrt{\left(\dfrac{0 \cdot 9444}{9} + \dfrac{0 \cdot 4100}{9}\right)}} = \frac{-0 \cdot 6111}{0 \cdot 3879} = -1 \cdot 58.$$

Note that, when, as here, $n_1 = n_2$, d turns out to have exactly the same numerical value as t, because the expression inside the square root can be written either as

$$\frac{s_1^2}{n} + \frac{s_2^2}{n}$$

or as

$$\frac{1}{2}(s_1^2 + s_2^2)\left(\frac{1}{n} + \frac{1}{n}\right).$$

Using Satterthwaite's approximation the test statistic of $1 \cdot 58$ can be referred to the t distribution with DF given by

$$v = \frac{0 \cdot 1504^2}{0 \cdot 1049^2/8 + 0 \cdot 0455^2/8} = 13 \cdot 8.$$

Using 14 DF the significance level is $0 \cdot 14$. The 95% confidence limits for the difference between the two means are

$$-0 \cdot 6111 \pm 2 \cdot 145 \times 0 \cdot 3879$$

$$= -1 \cdot 4 \text{ and } 0 \cdot 2.$$

4.5 Inferences from variances

For normally distributed variables the methods follow immediately from the results of §3.4.

Suppose s^2 is the usual estimate of variance in a random sample of size n from a normal distribution with variance σ^2; the population mean need not be specified. For a test of the null hypothesis that $\sigma^2 = \sigma_0^2$, calculate

$$X^2 = \frac{(n-1)s^2}{\sigma_0^2}, \quad \text{or equivalently} \quad \frac{\sum(x - \bar{x})^2}{\sigma_0^2}, \tag{4.8}$$

and refer this to the $\chi_{(n-1)}^2$ distribution. For a two-sided test at a significance level α, the critical values for X^2 will be those corresponding to tabulated probabilities of $1 - \frac{1}{2}\alpha$ and $\frac{1}{2}\alpha$. For a two-sided 5% level, for example, the entries under the headings 0·975 and 0·025 must be used. We may denote these by $\chi_{n-1, 0 \cdot 975}^2$ and $\chi_{n-1, 0 \cdot 025}^2$.

For confidence limits for σ^2 we can argue that the probability is, say, 0·95 that

$$\chi_{n-1, 0 \cdot 975}^2 < \frac{\sum(x - \bar{x})^2}{\sigma^2} < \chi_{n-1, 0 \cdot 025}^2$$

and hence that

$$\frac{\sum(x-\bar{x})^2}{\chi^2_{n-1,0\cdot025}} < \sigma^2 < \frac{\sum(x-\bar{x})^2}{\chi^2_{n-1,0\cdot975}} .$$

These are the required confidence limits.

As pointed out in §3.4, the sampling theory for s^2 is particularly sensitive to non-normality, and the results in the present section should be interpreted cautiously if serious departures from normality are present.

4.6 Comparison of two variances

Suppose that two independent samples provide observations on a variable x, the first sample of n_1 observations giving an estimated variance s_1^2, and the second sample of n_2 observations giving an estimated variance s_2^2. If each sample is from a normal distribution the two estimates of variance can be compared by considering the *ratio* of the two variance estimates,

$$F = s_1^2/s_2^2.$$

If the null hypothesis is true, the distribution of F, in repeated pairs of samples of size n_1 and n_2 from normal distributions, is known exactly. It depends on n_1 and n_2 (or, equivalently, on the degrees of freedom, $v_1 = n_1 - 1$ and $v_2 = n_2 - 1$) but not on the common population variance σ^2. A tabulation of the F distributions as complete as that provided in Table A2 for the χ^2 distributions is impracticable because of the dependence on both v_1 and v_2. The standard books of tables (Fisher and Yates, 1963; Pearson and Hartley, 1966; Geigy Scientific Tables, 1982) provide a table of critical values of F at each of a number of significance levels. An abbreviated version is shown in Table A4.

For particular values of v_1 and v_2, F can clearly assume values on either side of 1, and significant departures from the null hypothesis may be marked either by very small or by very large values of F. The tabulated critical values are, however, all greater than 1 and refer only to the upper tail of the F distribution. This is not a serious restriction because the labelling of the two samples by the numbers 1 and 2 is arbitrary, and a mere reversal of the labels will convert a ratio less than 1 into a value greater than 1.

To use Table A4 we denote by s_1^2 the *larger* of the two variance estimates; v_1 is the corresponding number of degrees of freedom (which, of course, is not necessarily the larger of v_1 and v_2). For a two-sided test care should be taken to set P in Table A4 equal to half the two-sided significance level. For a two-sided test at the 5% level, for instance, the entries for $P = 0\cdot025$ are used.

The tables of the F distribution may be used to provide confidence limits for σ_1^2/σ_2^2. The ratio

$$F' = \frac{s_1^2/\sigma_1^2}{s_2^2/\sigma_2^2}$$

follows the F distribution on v_1 and v_2 degrees of freedom (on the null hypothesis $\sigma_1^2 = \sigma_2^2$ and $F' = F$). We no longer require $s_1^2 > s_2^2$. Denote by F_{α,v_1,v_2} the tabulated critical value of F for v_1 and v_2 degrees of freedom and a one-sided significance level α; and by F_{α,v_2,v_1}, the corresponding entry with v_1 and v_2 interchanged. Then the probability is α that

$$F' > F_{\alpha,v_1,v_2},$$

i.e. that

$$F > F_{\alpha,v_1,v_2}(\sigma_1^2/\sigma_2^2);$$

and also α that

$$1/F' > F_{\alpha,v_2,v_1},$$

i.e. that

$$F < (1/F_{\alpha,v_2,v_1})(\sigma_1^2/\sigma_2^2).$$

Consequently, the probability is $1 - 2\alpha$ that

$$(1/F_{\alpha,v_2,v_1})(\sigma_1^2/\sigma_2^2) < F < F_{\alpha,v_1,v_2}(\sigma_1^2/\sigma_2^2)$$

or that

$$F/F_{\alpha,v_1,v_2} < \sigma_1^2/\sigma_2^2 < F \times F_{\alpha,v_2,v_1}.$$

For a 95% confidence interval, therefore, the observed value of F must be divided by the tabulated value $F_{0.025,v_1,v_2}$ and multiplied by the value $F_{0.025,v_2,v_1}$.

Example 4.6

Two different microscopic methods, A and B, are available for the measurement of very small dimensions. Repeated observations on the same standard object give estimates of variance as follows:

Method	A	B
Number of observations	$n_1 = 10$	$n_2 = 20$
Estimated variance (square micrometres)	$s_1^2 = 1{\cdot}232$	$s_2^2 = 0{\cdot}304$

For a significance test we calculate

$$F = s_1^2/s_2^2 = 4{\cdot}05.$$

The tabulated value for $v_1 = 9$ and $v_2 = 19$ for $P = 0.025$ is 2·88 and for $P = 0.005$ is 4·04. (Interpolation in Table A4 is needed.) The observed ratio is thus just significant at the two-sided 1% level, that is $P = 0.010$.

For 95% confidence limits we need the tabulated values

$$F_{0.025, 9, 19} = 2.88$$

and

$$F_{0.025, 19, 9} = 3.69$$

(interpolating in the table where necessary). The confidence limits for the ratio of population variances, σ_1^2/σ_2^2, are therefore

$$\frac{4.05}{2.88} = 1.24$$

and

$$(4.05)(3.69) = 14.9.$$

Two connections may be noted between the F distributions and other distributions already met.

1 When $v_1 = 1$, the F distribution is that of the square of a quantity following the t distribution on v_2 DF. For example, for a one-sided significance level 0·05, the tabulated value of F for $v_1 = 1$, $v_2 = 10$ is 4·96; the two-sided value for t on 10 DF is 2·228; $(2·228)^2 = 4·96$.

This relationship follows because a t statistic is essentially the ratio of a normal variable with zero mean to an independent estimate of its standard deviation. Squaring the numerator gives a χ^2 variable (equivalent to an estimate of variance on 1 DF), and squaring the denominator similarly gives an estimate of variance on the appropriate number of degrees of freedom. Both the positive and negative tails of the t distribution have to be included because, after squaring, they both give values in the upper tail of the F distribution.

2 When $v_2 = \infty$, the F distribution is the same as that of a $\chi^2_{(v_1)}$ variable divided by v_1. Thus, for $v_1 = 10$, $v_2 = \infty$, the tabulated F for a one-sided level 0·05 is 1·83; that for $\chi^2_{(10)}$ is 18·31; $18·31/10 = 1·83$.

The reason here is similar to that advanced above. An estimate of variance s_2^2 on $v_2 = \infty$ DF must be exactly equal to the population variance σ^2. Thus, F may be written as $s_1^2/\sigma^2 = \chi^2_{(v_1)}/v_1$ (see §3.4).

The F test and the associated confidence limits provide an exact treatment of the comparison of two variance estimates from two independent *normal* samples. Unfortunately the methods are rather sensitive to the assumption of normality—much more so than in the corresponding uses of the t distribution to compare two means. This defect is called a lack of *robustness*.

The methods described in this section are appropriate only for the comparison of two *independent* estimates of variances. Sometimes this condition fails because the observations in the two samples are paired, as in the first situation considered in §4.4. The appropriate method for this case makes use of a technique described in Chapter 5, and is therefore postponed until p. 171.

4.7 Inferences from proportions

Consider now the binomial situtation discussed in §2.5 and §3.3. Individuals drawn at random from a large population have a probability π of being of type A. In a random sample of n individuals, a proportion $p(=r/n)$ are of type A. What can be said about π?

Suppose first that we wish to test a null hypothesis specifying that π is equal to some value π_0. On this hypothesis, the number of type A individuals, r, found in repeated random samples of size n would follow a binomial distribution. To express the departure of any observed value, r, from its expected value, $n\pi_0$, we could state the extent to which r falls into either of the tails of its sampling distribution. As in §4.2 this extent could be measured by calculating the probability in the tail area. The situation is a little different here because of the discreteness of the distribution of r. Do we calculate the probability of obtaining a larger deviation than that observed, $r - n\pi_0$, or the probability of a deviation at least as great? Since we are saying something about the degree of surprise elicited by a certain observed result, it seems reasonable to include the probability of this result in the summation. Thus, if $r > n\pi_0$ and the probabilities in the binomial distribution with parameters π_0 and n are $P_0, P_1, \ldots, P_n$, the P value for a one-sided test will be

$$P_+ = P_r + P_{r+1} + \ldots + P_n.$$

For a two-sided test we could add the probabilities of deviations at least as large as that observed, in the other direction. The P value for the other tail is

$$P_- = P_{r'} + P_{r'-1} + \ldots + P_0,$$

where r' is equal to $2n\pi_0 - r$ if this is an integer, and the highest integer less than this quantity otherwise. The P value for the two-sided test is then $P = P_- + P_+$.

For example, if $r = 8$, $n = 10$ and $\pi_0 = \frac{1}{2}$,

$$P_+ = P_8 + P_9 + P_{10}$$

and

$$P_- = P_2 + P_1 + P_0.$$

If $r = 17$, $n = 20$ and $\pi_0 = \frac{1}{3}$,

$$P_+ = P_{17} + P_{18} + P_{19} + P_{20}$$

$$P_- = 0.$$

If $r = 15$, $n = 20$ and $\pi_0 = 0.42$,

$$P_+ = P_{15} + P_{16} + P_{17} + P_{18} + P_{19} + P_{20}$$
$$P_- = P_1 + P_0.$$

An alternative, and perhaps preferable, approach is to obtain the two-sided P value by doubling the one-sided value (see p. 139).

Considerable simplification is achieved by approximating to the binomial distribution by the normal (§2.7). On the null hypothesis

$$\frac{r - n\pi_0}{\sqrt{[n\pi_0(1 - \pi_0)]}}$$

is approximately a standardized normal deviate. Using the continuity correction, the tail area required in the significance test is approximated by the area beyond a standardized normal deviate

$$z = \frac{|r - n\pi_0| - \frac{1}{2}}{\sqrt{[n\pi_0(1 - \pi_0)]}}, \tag{4.9}$$

and the result will be significant at, say, the 5% level if this probability is less than 0.05.

Example 4.7

In a clinical trial to compare the effectiveness of two analgesic drugs, X and Y, each of 100 patients receives X for a period of 1 week and Y for another week, the order of administration being determined randomly. Each patient then states a preference for one of the two drugs. Sixty-five patients prefer X and 35 prefer Y. Is this strong evidence for the view that, in the long run, more patients prefer X than Y?

Test the null hypothesis that the preferences form a random series in which the probability of an X preference is $\frac{1}{2}$. This would be true if X and Y were equally effective in all respects affecting the patients' judgements. The standard error of r is

$$\sqrt{(100 \times \tfrac{1}{2} \times \tfrac{1}{2})} = \sqrt{25} = 5.$$

The observed deviation, $r - n\pi_0$, is

$$65 - 50 = 15.$$

With continuity correction, the standardized normal deviate is $(15 - \frac{1}{2})/5 = 2.90$. Without continuity correction, the value would have been $15/5 = 3.00$, a rather trivial difference. In this case the continuity correction could have been ignored. The normal tail area for $z = 2.90$ is 0.0037; the departure from the null hypothesis is highly significant, and the evidence in favour of X is strong. The exact value of P, from the binomial distribution, is 0.0035, very close to the normal approximation.

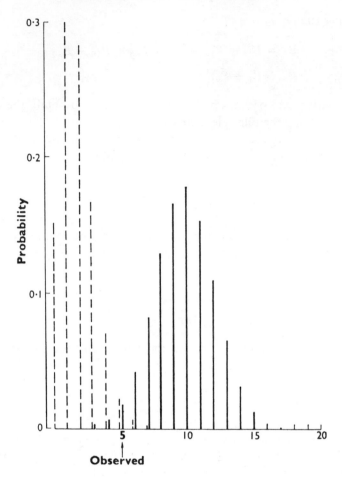

Fig. 4.5 Binomial distributions illustrating the 95% confidence limits for the parameter π based on a sample with five individuals of a certain type out of 20. For $\pi = \pi_L = 0.09$ the probability of 5 or more is 0.025; for $\pi = \pi_U = 0.49$ the probability of 5 or less is 0.025. (— —) $\pi_L = 0.09$; (——) $\pi_U = 0.49$.

The 95% confidence limits for π are the two values, π_L and π_U, for which the observed value of r is just significant on a one-sided test at the $2\frac{1}{2}$% level (Fig. 4.5). These values may be obtained fairly readily from tables of the binomial distribution, and are tabulated in the Geigy Scientific Tables (1982, Vol. 2, pp. 89–102). They may be obtained also from Fisher and Yates (1963, Table VIII1).

The normal approximation may be used in a number of ways.

1 The tail areas could be estimated from (4.9). Thus, for 95% confidence limits, approximations to π_L and π_U are given by the formulae

$$\frac{r - n\pi_L - \frac{1}{2}}{\sqrt{[n\pi_L(1 - \pi_L)]}} = 1.96$$

and

$$\frac{r - n\pi_U + \frac{1}{2}}{\sqrt{[n\pi_U(1 - \pi_U)]}} = -1.96.$$

2 In method **1**, if n is large, the continuity correction of $\frac{1}{2}$ may be omitted.

Method **1** involves the solution of a quadratic equation for each of π_L and π_U; method **2** involves a single quadratic equation. A further simplification is as follows.

3 Replace $\pi_L(1 - \pi_L)$ and $\pi_U(1 - \pi_U)$ by $p(1 - p)$. This is not too drastic a step, as $p(1 - p)$ changes rather slowly with changes in p, particularly for values of p near $\frac{1}{2}$. Ignoring the continuity correction, as in **2**, we have the most frequently used approximation to the 95% confidence limits:

$$p \pm 1.96\sqrt{(pq/n)},$$

where, as usual, $q = 1 - p$. The simplification here is due to the replacement of the standard error of p, which involves the unknown value π, by the approximate form $\sqrt{(pq/n)}$, which can be calculated entirely from known quantities.

The exact limits may be obtained using tables of the F distribution. This follows from the mathematical link between the binomial and the F distributions. Although the mathematical property has been known for many years, this method of working has not been widely adopted.

The lower limit π_L is the solution of

$$\sum_{j=r}^{n} \binom{n}{j} \pi_L^j (1 - \pi_L)^{n-j} = 0.025.$$

It can be shown that the left-hand side of this equation is equal to the probability that a variable distributed as F with $2n - 2r + 2$ and $2r$ degrees of freedom exceeds $r(1 - \pi_L)/(n - r + 1)\pi_L$. Therefore

$$\frac{r(1 - \pi_L)}{(n - r + 1)\pi_L} = F_{0.025, 2n - 2r + 2, 2r}.$$

That is,

$$\left. \begin{aligned} \pi_L &= \frac{r}{r + (n - r + 1)F_{0.025, 2n - 2r + 2, 2r}} \\[2em] \pi_U &= \frac{r + 1}{r + 1 + (n - r)F_{0.025, 2r + 2, 2n - 2r}^{-1}} \end{aligned} \right\} \tag{4.10}$$

and similarly,

(Miettinen, 1970).

Example 4.7, continued

With $n = 100$, $p = 0.65$, the exact 95% confidence limits are found to be 0.548 and 0.743.

Method **1** will be found to give 0.548 and 0.741, method **2** gives 0.552 and 0.736, and method **3** gives

$$0.65 \pm 1.96 \sqrt{\left[\frac{(0.65)(0.35)}{100} \right]}$$

$$= 0.65 \pm (1.96)(0.0477)$$

$$= 0.557 \text{ and } 0.743.$$

In this example method **3** is quite adequate.

Example 4.8

As a contrasting example with small numbers, suppose $n = 20$ and $p = 0.25$. The exact 95% confidence limits are 0.087 and 0.491 (see Fig. 4.5).

Method **1** gives 0.096 and 0.494, method **2** gives 0.112 and 0.469, method **3** gives 0.060 and 0.440. Method **3** is clearly less appropriate here than in Example 4.7. In general method **3** should be avoided if either np or $n(1 - p)$ is small (say less than 10). Methods **2** and **3** may also be unreliable when either $n\pi_L$ or $n(1 - \pi_U)$ is less than 5. In this case $n\pi_L$ is about 2 so it is not surprising that the lower confidence limit is not too well approximated by the normal approximation.

Example 4.9

As an example of finding the exact limits using the F distribution consider the data of Fig. 4.5, where $r = 5$ and $n = 20$. Then,

$$\pi_L = 5/(5 + 16F_{0.025, 32, 10})$$

and

$$\pi_U = 6/(6 + 15F_{0.025, 12, 30}^{-1}).$$

The value of $F_{0.025, 32, 10}$ can be obtained by interpolation in Table A4 where interpolation is linear in the reciprocal of the degrees of freedom. Thus,

$$F_{0.025, 32, 10} = 3.37 - (3.37 - 3.08) \times \left(\frac{1}{24} - \frac{1}{32} \right) \Big/ \frac{1}{24}$$

$$= 3.30.$$

Therefore $\pi_L = 0.0865$ and, since $F_{0.025, 12, 30} = 2.41$, $\pi_U = 0.4908$. In this example interpolation was required for one of the F values and then only in the degrees of freedom of the numerator, but in general interpolation would be required for both F values and in both the degrees of freedom of the numerator and denominator. This is tedious and can be avoided by using a method based on the normal approximation except when this method gives values such that either $n\pi_L$ or $n(1 - \pi_U)$ is small (say less than 5).

It was remarked earlier that the discreteness of the distribution of r made inferences from proportions a little different from those based on a variable with a continuous distribution and we now discuss these differences. For a continuous variable an exact significance test would give the result $P < 0.05$ for exactly 5% of random samples drawn from a population in which the null hypothesis were true, and a 95% confidence interval would contain the population value of the estimated parameter for exactly 95% of random samples. Neither of these properties is generally true for a discrete variable. Consider a binomial variable from a distribution with $n = 10$ and $\pi = 0.5$ (Table 2.4, p. 66). Using the exact test, for the hypothesis that $\pi = 0.5$, significance at the 5% level is found only for $r = 0$, 1, 9 or 10 and the probability of one or other of these values is 0.022. Therefore, a result significant at the 5% level would be found in only 2.2% of random samples if the null hypothesis were true. This causes no difficulty if the precise level of P is stated. Thus if $r = 1$ we have that $P = 0.022$, and a result significant at a level of 0.022 or less would occur in exactly 2.2% of random samples. The normal approximation with continuity correction is then the best approximate test, giving, in this case, $P = 0.027$.

A similar situation arises with the confidence interval. The exact confidence limits for the binomial parameter are conservative in the sense that the probability of including the true value is *at least* as great as the nominal confidence coefficient. This fact arises from the debatable decision to include the observed value in the calculation of tail-area probabilities. The limits are termed 'exact' because they are obtained from exact calculations of the binomial distribution, rather than from an approximation, but not because the confidence coefficient is achieved exactly. This problem cannot be resolved, in the same way as for the significance test, by changing the confidence coefficient. First, this is difficult to do but, secondly and more importantly, whilst for a significance test it is desirable to estimate P as precisely as possible, in the confidence interval approach it is perfectly reasonable to specify the confidence coefficient in advance at some conventional value, such as 95%. The approximate limits using the continuity correction also tend to be conservative. The limits obtained by methods **2** and **3**, however, which ignore the continuity correction, will tend to have a probability of inclusion nearer to the nominal value. This suggests that the neglect of the continuity correction is not a serious matter, and may, indeed, be an advantage.

The problems discussed above, due to the discreteness of the distribution, have caused much controversy in the statistical literature, particularly with the analysis of data collected to compare two proportions, to be discussed in §4.9. One approach, suggested by Lancaster (1952, 1961), is to use *mid-P* values, and this approach has been advocated more widely recently (Williams, 1988; Barnard, 1989; Hirji, 1991; Upton, 1992). The mid-P value for a one-sided test is obtained by including in the tail only one-half of the probability of the observed sample.

Thus for a binomial sample with r observed out of n where $r > n\pi_0$, the one-sided mid-P value testing the hypothesis that $\pi = \pi_0$ will be

$$\text{mid-}P_+ = \tfrac{1}{2}P_r + P_{r+1} + \ldots + P_n.$$

It has to be noted that the mid-P value is not the probability of obtaining a significant result by chance when the null hypothesis is true. Again, consider a binomial variable from a distribution with $n = 10$ and $\pi = 0.5$ (Table 2.4, p. 66). For the hypothesis that $\pi = 0.5$, a mid-P value less than 0.05 would be found only for $r = 0, 1, 9$ or 10, since the mid-P value for $r = 2$ is $2[0.0010 + 0.0098 + \tfrac{1}{2}(0.0439)] = 0.0655$, and the probability of one or other of these values is 0.022.

Barnard (1989) has recommended quoting both the P and the mid-P values, on the basis that the former is a measure of the statistical significance when the data under analysis are judged alone, whereas the latter is the appropriate measure of the strength of evidence against the hypothesis under test to be used in combination with evidence from other studies. This arises because the mid-P value has the desirable feature that, when the null hypothesis is true, its average value is 0.5 and this property makes it particularly suitable as a measure to be used when combining results from several studies in making an overall assessment (meta-analysis; Chapter 7). Since it is rare that the results of a single study are used without support from other studies, our recommendation is also to give both the P and mid-P values, but to give more emphasis to the latter.

Corresponding to mid-P values are mid-P confidence limits, calculated as those values which, if taken as the null hypothesis value, give a corresponding mid-P value, that is, the 95% limits correspond to one-sided mid-P values of 0.025.

Where a normal approximation is adequate, P values and mid-P values correspond to test statistics calculated with and without the correction for continuity respectively. Correspondingly, confidence intervals and mid-P confidence intervals can be based on normal approximations, using and ignoring the continuity correction respectively. Thus the mid-P confidence limits for a binomial probability would be obtained using method **2** rather than method **1** (p. 121).

Where normal approximations are inadequate, the mid-P values are calculated by summing the appropriate probabilities. The mid-P limits are more tedious to calculate, as they are not included in standard sets of tables and there is no direct formula corresponding to (4.10). The limits may be obtained fairly readily using a personal computer or programmable calculator by setting up the expression to be evaluated using a general argument, and then by trial and error finding the values that give tails of 0.025.

Example 4.8, continued

The mid-P limits are given by

$$P_0 + P_1 + P_2 + P_3 + P_4 + \tfrac{1}{2}P_5 = 0\cdot975 \text{ or } 0\cdot025$$

where P_i is the binomial probability (as in (2.9)) for i events with $n = 20$ and $\pi = \pi_L$ or π_U. This expression was set up on a personal computer for general π, and starting with the knowledge that the confidence interval would be slightly narrower than the limits of $0\cdot0865$ and $0\cdot4908$ found earlier the exact 95% mid-P confidence limits were found as $0\cdot098$ and $0\cdot470$. Method **2** gives the best approximation to these limits but, as noted earlier, the lower confidence limit is less well approximated by the normal approximation, because $n\pi_L$ is only about 2.

4.8 Comparison of two proportions

As in the comparison of two means, considered in §4.4, we can distinguish between two situations according to whether individual members of the two samples are or are not paired.

Paired case

Suppose there are N observations in each sample, forming therefore N pairs of observations. Denoting the samples by 1 and 2, and describing each individual as A or not A, there are clearly four types of pairs:

	Sample		Number
Type	1	2	of pairs
1	A	A	k
2	A	Not A	r
3	Not A	A	s
4	Not A	Not A	m

If the number of pairs of the four types are as shown above, another way of exhibiting the same results is in the form of a two-way table:

		Sample 2		
		A	Not A	
Sample 1	A	k	r	$k + r$
	Not A	s	m	$s + m$
		$k + s$	$r + m$	N

The proportions of A individuals in the two samples are $(k + r)/N$ in sample 1 and $(k + s)/N$ in sample 2. We are interested in the difference between the two proportions, which is clearly $(r - s)/N$.

Consider first a significance test. The null hypothesis is that the expectation of $(r - s)/N$ is zero, or in other words that the expectations of r and s are equal. This can conveniently be tested by restricting our attention to the $r + s$ pairs in which the two members are of different types. Denote $r + s$ by n. On the null hypothesis, given n disparate or 'untied' pairs, the number of pairs of type 2 (or, indeed, of type 3) would follow a binomial distribution with a parameter equal to $\frac{1}{2}$. The test therefore follows precisely the methods of §4.7. A large-sample test is obtained by regarding

$$z = \frac{r - \frac{1}{2}n}{\frac{1}{2}\sqrt{n}} \tag{4.11}$$

as a standardized normal deviate. A continuity correction may be applied by reducing the absolute value of $r - \frac{1}{2}n$ by $\frac{1}{2}$. This test is sometimes known as McNemar's test. An alternative form of (4.11), with continuity correction included, is

$$z^2 = \frac{(|r - s| - 1)^2}{r + s} \tag{4.12}$$

where z^2 may be regarded as a $\chi^2_{(1)}$ variate. This is one of the few statistical calculations that really can be done in one's head; see also (4.29).

It should be noted that, although the significance test is based entirely on the two frequencies r and s, the estimated difference between the proportions of positives and therefore also its standard error depend also on N. That is, evidence as to the existence of a difference is provided solely by the united pairs; an assessment of the *magnitude* of that difference must allude to the remainder of the data. The distinction between statistical and clinical significance, referred to in §4.2, must be borne in mind.

The calculation of confidence limits for the difference between the two proportions involves accounting for the variation in the number of untied pairs, $r + s$. This may be achieved by deriving the standard error from the properties of the multinomial distribution, which is an extension of the binomial distribution when there are more than two classes. Approximate confidence limits for the difference between the two proportions are then given by taking its standard error to be

$$\frac{1}{N}\sqrt{\left[r + s - \frac{(r - s)^2}{N}\right]} \tag{4.13}$$

(Gardner and Altman, 1989), and using the usual normal theory. When data of this type are obtained in a case–control study emphasis is often directed to estimation of the odds ratio (see (4.15) and (16.17)).

There is a potential discrepancy between the test (4.11) and the confidence limits obtained using (4.13). If the test is just significant at the 5% level, $z = 1{\cdot}96$, the lower confidence limit is higher than zero. This arises because of the second term within the square root of (4.13). The discrepancy will be slight except for large differences between r and s.

Example 4.10

Fifty specimens of sputum are each cultured on two different media, A and B, the object being to compare the ability of the two media to detect tubercle bacilli. The results are shown in Table 4.3. The null hypothesis that the media are equally effective is tested by the standardized normal deviate

$$z = \frac{12 - (\frac{1}{2})(14)}{\frac{1}{2}\sqrt{14}} = \frac{5}{1\cdot871} = 2\cdot67 \quad (P = 0\cdot008).$$

There is very little doubt that A is more effective than B. The continuity correction would reduce the normal deviate to $4\cdot5/1\cdot871 = 2\cdot41$, still a significant result.

The 95% confidence limits for the difference between the proportions of positive sputum on the two media are given by

$$\frac{(12 - 2)}{50} \pm \frac{1\cdot96\sqrt{(14 - 10^2/50)}}{50}$$

$$= 0\cdot20 \pm 0\cdot14$$

$$= 0\cdot06 \text{ and } 0\cdot34.$$

Table 4.3 Distribution of 50 specimens of sputum according to results of culture on two media

Type	Medium A	Medium B	Number of sputa
1	+	+	20
2	+	−	12
3	−	+	2
4	−	−	16
			50

Alternative layout

		Medium B +	Medium B −	Total
Medium A	+	20	12	32
	−	2	16	18
Total		22	28	50

The exact test for the paired case

The approach just considered is based on the normal approximation to a discrete distribution. The situation is similar to that considered in §4.7 except for the complication of the tied pairs, k and m; with the correction for continuity (4.11) corresponds to (4.9) with $\pi_0 = \frac{1}{2}$. The significance test of (4.12) will be satisfactory except for small values of $r + s$ (less than 10), and in such cases an exact test may be carried out on the $r + s$ untied pairs. The confidence limits calculated using (4.13) may not be satisfactory approximations even for values of $r + s$ larger than 10, particularly if r and s differ greatly. There is no completely satisfactory solution. One approach is to base the limits on the 95% confidence limits for the proportion of type 2 pairs out of the $r + s$ untied pairs, which may be obtained exactly or using methods **1** or **2** of §4.7. However this method does not take any account of the variation in $r + s$.

Example 4.10, continued

The exact significance level is given by

$$P = 2 \times (\tfrac{1}{2})^{14}[1 + 14 + (14 \times 13/2)] = 0.013.$$

The mid-P value is obtained by taking only one-half of the last term in the above expression and is 0.007.

The exact 95% confidence limits for the proportion of type 2 pairs (see Table 4.3) out of 14 pairs of type 2 or 3 are 0.5718 and 0.9822. Then the corresponding approximate 95% limits for the difference in proportions out of the total of 50 pairs are

$$(0.5718 - 0.4282) \times \frac{14}{50}$$

and

$$(0.9822 - 0.0178) \times \frac{14}{50}$$

$$= 0.04 \text{ and } 0.27.$$

The exact mid-P 95% confidence limits for the proportion of type 2 pairs are 0.6026 and 0.9753 and these give approximate limits of 0.06 and 0.26 for the difference in proportions.

The exact test may also be obtained using the F distribution as in (16.19).

Unpaired case

Suppose there are two populations in which the probabilities that an individual shows characteristic A are π_1 and π_2. A random sample of size n_1 from the first population has r_1 members showing the characteristic (and a proportion

$p_1 = r_1/n_1$), while the corresponding values for an independent sample from the second population are n_2, r_2, and $p_2 = r_2/n_2$. From (3.11),

$$E(p_1 - p_2) = \pi_1 - \pi_2$$

and

$$\text{var}(p_1 - p_2) = \frac{\pi_1(1 - \pi_1)}{n_1} + \frac{\pi_2(1 - \pi_2)}{n_2}.$$

For confidence limits, π_1 and π_2 are unknown and may be replaced by p_1 and p_2, respectively, to give

$$\text{var}(p_1 - p_2) = \frac{p_1 q_1}{n_1} + \frac{p_2 q_2}{n_2}, \qquad (4.14)$$

where

$$q_1 = 1 - p_1$$

and

$$q_2 = 1 - p_2.$$

Approximate limits then follow by applying the usual normal theory.

Suppose we wish to test the null hypothesis that $\pi_1 = \pi_2$. Call the common value π. Then p_1 and p_2 are both estimates of π, and there is little point in estimating π (as in (4.14)) by two different quantities in two different places in the expression. If the null hypothesis is true, both samples are from effectively the same population, and the best estimate of π will be obtained by pooling the two samples, to give

$$p = \frac{r_1 + r_2}{n_1 + n_2}.$$

This pooled estimate is now substituted for both π_1 and π_2 to give

$$\text{var}(p_1 - p_2) = pq\left(\frac{1}{n_1} + \frac{1}{n_2}\right),$$

writing as usual $q = 1 - p$. The null hypothesis is thus tested approximately by taking

$$z = \frac{p_1 - p_2}{\sqrt{\left[pq\left(\dfrac{1}{n_1} + \dfrac{1}{n_2}\right)\right]}}$$

as a standardized normal deviate.

Example 4.11

In a clinical trial to assess the value of a new method of treatment (A) in comparison with the old method (B), patients were divided at random into two groups. Of 257 patients treated by method A, 41 died; of 244 patients treated by method B, 64 died. Thus, $p_1 = 41/257 = 0.1595$ and $p_2 = 64/244 = 0.2623$.

The difference between the two fatality rates is estimated as $0.1595 - 0.2623 = -0.1028$. For 95% confidence limits we take

$$\text{var}(p_1 - p_2) = \frac{(0.1595)(0.8405)}{257} + \frac{(0.2623)(0.7377)}{244}$$

$$= 0.0005216 + 0.0007930$$

$$= 0.0013146$$

and

$$\text{SE}(p_1 - p_2) = \sqrt{0.0013146} = 0.0363.$$

Thus, 95% confidence limits are

$$-0.1028 \pm (1.96)(0.0363) = -0.0317 \text{ and } -0.1739,$$

the minus sign merely serving to indicate in which direction the difference lies.

For the significance test, we form the pooled proportion

$$p = 105/501 = 0.2096$$

and estimate $\text{SE}(p_1 - p_2)$ as

$$\sqrt{\left[(0.2096)(0.7904)\left(\frac{1}{257} + \frac{1}{244} \right) \right]}$$

$$= 0.0364.$$

Thus, the normal deviate is

$$\frac{-0.1028}{0.0364} = -2.82 \quad (P = 0.005).$$

There is strong evidence of a difference in fatality rates, in favour of A.

Note that, in Example 4.11, the use of p changed the standard error only marginally, from 0.0363 to 0.0364. In fact, there is likely to be an appreciable change only when n_1 and n_2 are very unequal and when p_1 and p_2 differ substantially. In other circumstances, either standard error formula may be regarded as a good approximation to the other, and used accordingly.

In epidemiological studies it is often appropriate to measure the difference in two proportions by their ratio, p_1/p_2, rather than their difference. This measure is referred to as the *risk ratio*, *rate ratio*, or *relative risk* depending on the type of study. In case–control studies the relative risk cannot be evaluated directly but, in many circumstances, the *odds ratio*, defined by

$$OR = \frac{p_1/(1 - p_1)}{p_2/(1 - p_2)} \tag{4.15}$$

is a good approximation to the relative risk (Chapter 16). From the point of view of significance testing it makes no difference which measure is used and the method above or the extensions given in the next section are appropriate.

The confidence limits for the risk ratio and odds ratio both involve the use of logarithms, and the *natural* or Napierian logarithm must be used. In natural logarithms the base is e (= 2·7183); $\log_e x$ is usually written as $\ln x$, and $\ln x = 2·3026 \log_{10} x$. Most pocket calculators have a key for $\ln x$ and for the antilogarithm, the exponential of x, often written as e^x, so that the conversion formula is not normally required.

Writing R for p_1/p_2, we have

$$R = \frac{r_1/n_1}{r_2/n_2} \tag{4.16}$$

$$SE(\ln R) = \sqrt{\left(\frac{1}{r_1} - \frac{1}{n_1} + \frac{1}{r_2} - \frac{1}{n_2}\right)} \tag{4.17}$$

and the 95% confidence interval for R is

$$\exp[\ln R \pm 1·96 SE(\ln R)].$$

For a case–control study (§6.3) we must change the notation since there are no longer samples from the two populations, but instead cases of disease and controls (non-cases) are sampled separately and their exposure to some factor established. Suppose the frequencies are as follows:

		Cases	Controls	
	+	a	c	$a + c$
Factor	–	b	d	$b + d$
		$a + b$	$c + d$	n

Then the observed odds ratio is given by

$$OR = \frac{ad}{bc} \tag{4.18}$$

and

$$SE[\ln(OR)] = \sqrt{\left(\frac{1}{a} + \frac{1}{b} + \frac{1}{c} + \frac{1}{d}\right)}. \tag{4.19}$$

Example 4.12

Liddell *et al.* (1984) reported on a case–control study investigating the association of bronchial carcinoma and asbestos exposure in the Canadian chrysotile mines and mills. The data were as follows:

Asbestos exposure	Lung cancer	Controls
Exposed	148 (*a*)	372 (*c*)
Not exposed	75 (*b*)	343 (*d*)

The calculations are:

$$OR = (148 \times 343)/(75 \times 372) = 1{\cdot}82$$

$$\ln OR = 0{\cdot}599$$

$$SE(\ln OR) = \sqrt{\left(\frac{1}{148} + \frac{1}{75} + \frac{1}{372} + \frac{1}{343}\right)} = \sqrt{0{\cdot}02569} = 0{\cdot}160.$$

95% confidence interval for $\ln OR = 0{\cdot}599 \pm 1{\cdot}96 \times 0{\cdot}160$

$$= 0{\cdot}285 \text{ to } 0{\cdot}913,$$

95% confidence interval for $OR = \exp(0{\cdot}285)$ to $\exp(0{\cdot}913)$

$$= 1{\cdot}33 \text{ to } 2{\cdot}49.$$

These limits are sometimes referred to as *logit limits* (§16.2).

4.9 2 × 2 Tables and χ^2 tests

An alternative way of displaying the data of Example 4.11 is shown in Table 4.4. This is called a *2 × 2*, or sometimes a *fourfold, contingency table*. The total frequency, 501 in this example, is shown in the lower right corner of the table. This total frequency or *grand total* is split into two different dichotomies represented by the two 'horizontal' rows of the table and the two 'vertical' columns. In this example the rows represent the two treatments and the columns represent the two

Table 4.4 2 × 2 Table showing results of a clinical trial

	Outcome		
Treatment	Death	Survival	Total
A	41	216	257
B	64	180	244
Total	105	396	501

outcomes of treatment. There are thus $2 \times 2 = 4$ combinations of row and column categories, and the corresponding frequencies occupy the four *inner cells* in the body of the table. The total frequencies for the two row categories and those for the two columns are shown at the right and at the foot, and are called *marginal totals*.

We have already used a 2×2 table (Table 4.3) to display the results needed for a comparison of proportions in paired samples, but the purpose was a little different from the present approach, which is concerned solely with the *unpaired* case.

We are concerned, in Table 4.4, with possible differences between the fatality rates for the two treatments. Given the marginal totals in Table 4.4 we can easily calculate what numbers would have had to be observed in the body of the table to make the fatality rates for A and B exactly equal. In the top left cell, for example, this *expected* number is

$$\frac{105 \times 257}{501} = 53 \cdot 862,$$

since the overall fatality rate is 105/501 and there are 257 individuals treated with A. Similar expected numbers can be obtained for each of the four inner cells, and are shown in Table 4.5 (where the observed and expected numbers are distinguished by the letters O and E). The expected numbers are not integers and have been rounded off to 3 decimal places. Clearly one could not possibly observe 53·862

Table 4.5 Expected frequencies and contributions to X^2 for data in Table 4.4

| Treatment | | Outcome | | |
		Death	Survival	Total
A	O	41	216	257
	E	53·862	203·138	257
	$O - E$	−12·862	12·862	0
	$(O - E)^2$	165·431	165·431	
	$(O - E)^2/E$	3·071	0·814	
B	O	64	180	244
	E	51·138	192·862	244
	$O - E$	12·862	−12·862	0
	$(O - E)^2$	165·431	165·431	
	$(O - E)^2/E$	3·235	0·858	
Total	O	105	396	501
	E	105	396	
	$O - E$	0	0	

individuals in a particular cell. These expected numbers should be thought of as expectations or mean values over a large number of possible tables with the same marginal totals as those observed, when the null hypothesis is true.

Note that the values of E sum, over both rows and columns, to the observed marginal totals. It follows that the *discrepancies*, measured by the differences $O - E$, add to zero along rows and columns; in other words, the four discrepancies are numerically the same (12·862 in this example), two being positive and two negative.

In a rough sense, the greater the discrepancies, the more evidence we have against the null hypothesis. It would therefore seem reasonable to base a significance test somehow on these discrepancies. It also seems reasonable to take account of the absolute size of the frequencies: a discrepancy of 5 is much more important if $E = 5$ than if $E = 100$.

It turns out to be appropriate to calculate the following index:

$$X^2 = \sum \frac{(O - E)^2}{E},$$
(4.20)

the summation being over the four inner cells of the table. The contributions to X^2 from the four cells are shown in Table 4.5. The total is

$$X^2 = 3·071 + 0·814 + 3·235 + 0·858$$

$$= 7·978.$$

On the null hypothesis, X^2 follows the $\chi^2_{(1)}$ distribution (see §3.4), the approximation improving as the expected numbers get larger. There is one degree of freedom because only one of the values of E is necessary to complete the whole table. Reference to Table A2 shows that the observed value of 7·978 is beyond the 0·01 point of the $\chi^2_{(1)}$ distribution, and the difference between the two fatality rates is therefore significant at the 1% level. The precise significance level may be obtained by taking the square root of 7·978 ($= 2·82$) and referring to Table A1; this gives 0·005.

In §4.8, we derived a standardized normal deviate by calculating the standard error of the difference between the two proportions, obtaining the numerical value of 2·82. This agrees with the value obtained as the square root of X^2. In fact it can be shown algebraically that the X^2 index is always the same as the square of the normal deviate given by the first method. The probability levels given by the two tests are therefore always in agreement.

The X^2 index is often denoted by χ^2, although it seems slightly preferable to reserve the latter for the theoretical distribution, denoting the calculated value by X^2.

There are various alternative formulae for X^2, of which we may note one. Denote the entries in the table as follows:

		Column		
		1	2	
Row	1	a	b	r_1
	2	c	d	r_2
		s_1	s_2	N

Then

$$X^2 = \frac{(ad - bc)^2 N}{r_1 r_2 s_1 s_2}. \tag{4.21}$$

This version is particularly suitable for use with a calculator.

We have, then, two entirely equivalent significance tests. Which the user chooses to use is to some extent a matter of taste and convenience. However, there are two points to be made. First, the standard error method, as we have seen, not only yields a significance test but also leads naturally into the calculation of confidence intervals. This, then, is a strong argument for calculating differences and standard errors, and basing the test on these values rather than on the X^2 index. The main counter-argument is that, as we shall see in Chapter 7, the X^2 method can be generalized to contingency tables with more than two rows and columns.

It is important to remember that the X^2 index can only be calculated from 2×2 tables in which the entries are frequencies. A common error is to use it for a table in which the entries are mean values of a certain variable; this practice is completely erroneous.

A closely related method of deriving a significance test is to work with one of the frequencies in the 2×2 table. With the notation above, the frequency denoted by a could be regarded as a random variable and its significance assessed against its expectation and standard error calculated conditionally on the marginal totals. This method proceeds as follows, using O, E and V to represent the observed value, expected value and variance of a:

$$\left. \begin{aligned} E &= \frac{(a + b)(a + c)}{N} \\ V &= \frac{(a + b)(c + d)(a + c)(b + d)}{N^2(N - 1)} \\ X^2 &= \frac{(O - E)^2}{V}. \end{aligned} \right\} \tag{4.22}$$

Apart from a factor of $(N - 1)/N$, (4.22) is equivalent to (4.21). This form is particularly convenient when combining the results of several studies since the values of O, E and V may be summed over studies before calculating the test statistic. Yusuf *et al.* (1985) proposed an approximate method of estimating the odds ratio and its standard error by

$$
\left.
\begin{aligned}
OR &= \exp\!\left(\frac{O - E}{V}\right) \\[2mm]
SE[\ln(OR)] &= \frac{1}{\sqrt{V}}.
\end{aligned}
\right\}
\tag{4.23}
$$

This method was introduced for the combination of studies where the effect was small, and is known to be biased when the odds ratio is not small (Greenland and Salvan, 1990).

More details of such methods are given in §12.6 and of their application in overviews or meta analyses in §7.2.

Example 4.13

Consider the data of Example 4.12. We have

$$O = 148 \quad E = 123 \cdot 62 \quad V = 42 \cdot 038$$

and (4.23) gives

$$OR = \exp(24 \cdot 38/42 \cdot 038) = 1 \cdot 79$$

$$SE[\ln(OR)] = 0 \cdot 154.$$

These values are close to those found in Example 4.12.

Both the standard-error and the χ^2 tests are based on approximations which are valid particularly when the frequencies are high. In general two methods of improvement are widely used: the application of a continuity correction and the calculation of exact probabilities.

Continuity correction for 2×2 tables

This method was described by F. Yates and is often called *Yates's correction*. The $\chi^2_{(1)}$ distribution has been used as an approximation to the distribution of X^2 on the null hypothesis and subject to fixed marginal totals. Under the latter constraint only a finite number of tables are possible. For the marginal totals of Table 4.4, for example, all the possible tables can be generated by increasing or decreasing one of the entries by one unit at a time, until either that entry or some other reaches zero. (A fuller discussion follows later in this section.) The position therefore is rather like that discussed in §2.7 where a discrete distribution (the binomial) was approximated by a continuous distribution (the normal). In the present case one might base the significance test on the probability of the observed table or one showing a more extreme departure from the null hypothesis. An improvement in the estimation of this probability is achieved by reducing the absolute value of the discrepancy, $O - E$, by $\frac{1}{2}$ before calculating X^2. In Example 4.11, Table 4.5, this would mean taking $|O - E|$ to be 12·362 instead of 12·862, and the corrected value of X^2, denoted by X_c^2, is 7·369, somewhat less than the uncorrected value but still highly significant.

The continuity correction has a relatively greater effect when the expected frequencies are small than when they are large. The use of the continuity correction gives an approximation to the P value in the exact test described below. As in the analogous situations discussed earlier in this chapter (and see also p. 141), we prefer the mid-P value, which corresponds to the *uncorrected* χ^2 test. We therefore recommend that the continuity correction should not routinely be employed.

The continuity-corrected version of (4.21) is

$$X_c^2 = \frac{(|ad - bc| - \frac{1}{2}N)^2 N}{r_1 r_2 s_1 s_2}. \tag{4.24}$$

If the continuity correction is applied in the χ^2 test, it should logically be applied in the standard error test. The procedure there is to calculate $p_1 - p_2$ after the frequencies have been moved half a unit nearer their expected values, the standard error remaining unchanged. Thus, in Example 4.11, we should have $p_{1(c)} = 41 \cdot 5/257 = 0 \cdot 1615$, $p_{2(c)} = 63 \cdot 5/244 = 0 \cdot 2602$, giving $z_{(c)} = -0 \cdot 0987/0 \cdot 0364 = -2 \cdot 71$. Since $(-2 \cdot 71)^2 = 7 \cdot 34$, the result agrees with that for X_c^2 apart from rounding errors.

The exact test for 2 × 2 tables

Even with the continuity correction there will be some doubt about the adequacy of the χ^2 approximation when the frequencies are particularly small. An exact test was suggested almost simultaneously in the mid-1930s by R. A. Fisher, J. O. Irwin and F. Yates. It consists in calculating the exact probabilities of the possible tables described in the previous subsection. The probability of a table with frequencies

a	b	r_1
c	d	r_2
s_1	s_2	N

is given by the formula

$$\frac{r_1! r_2! s_1! s_2!}{N! a! b! c! d!}. \tag{4.25}$$

This is, in fact, the probability of the observed cell frequencies *conditional* on the observed marginal totals, under the null hypothesis of no association between the row and column classifications.

Given any observed table, the probabilities of all tables with the same marginal totals can be calculated, and the *P* value for the significance test calculated by summation. Example 4.14 illustrates the calculations and some of the difficulties of interpretation which may arise.

Example 4.14

The data in Table 4.6, due to M. Hellman, are discussed by Yates (1934).

Table 4.6 Data on malocclusion of teeth in infants (Yates, 1934).

	Infants with:		
	Normal teeth	Malocclusion	Total
Breast-fed	4	16	20
Bottle-fed	1	21	22
Total	5	37	42

There are six possible tables with the same marginal totals as those observed, since neither *a* nor *c* (in the notation given above) can fall below 0 or exceed 5, the smallest marginal total in the table. The cell frequencies in each of these tables are shown in Table 4.7.

Table 4.7 Cell frequencies in tables with the same marginal totals as those in Table 4.6

0	20	20		1	19	20		2	18	20
5	17	22		4	18	22		3	19	22
5	37	42		5	37	42		5	37	42
3	17	20		4	16	20		5	15	20
2	20	22		1	21	22		0	22	22
5	37	42		5	37	42		5	37	42

The probability that $a = 0$ is, from (4.25),

$$P_0 = \frac{20!\,22!\,5!\,37!}{42!\,0!\,20!\,5!\,17!} = 0.03096.$$

Tables of log factorials (Fisher and Yates, 1963, Table XXX) are often useful for this calculation, and many scientific calculators have a factorial key (although it may only function correctly for integers less than 70). Alternatively the expression for P_0 can be calculated without factorials by repeated multiplication and division after cancelling common factors:

$$P_0 = \frac{22 \times 21 \times 20 \times 19 \times 18}{42 \times 41 \times 40 \times 39 \times 38} = 0.03096.$$

The probabilities for $a = 1, 2, \ldots, 5$ can be obtained in succession. Thus,

$$P_1 = \frac{5 \times 20}{1 \times 18} \times P_0$$

$$P_2 = \frac{4 \times 19}{2 \times 19} \times P_1, \text{ etc.}$$

The results are:

a	Probability
0	0.0310
1	0.1720
2	0.3440
3	0.3096
4	0.1253
5	0.0182
	1.0001

This is the complete *conditional distribution* for the observed marginal totals, and the probabilities sum to unity as would be expected. Note the importance of carrying enough significant digits in the first probability to be calculated; the above calculations were carried out with more decimal places than recorded by retaining each probability in the calculator for the next stage.

The observed table has a probability of 0.1253. To assess its significance we could measure the extent to which it falls into the tail of the distribution by calculating the probability of that table or of one more extreme. For a one-sided test the procedure clearly gives

$$P = 0.1253 + 0.0182 = 0.1435.$$

The result is not significant at even the 10% level.

For a two-sided test the other tail of the distribution must be taken into account, and here some ambiguity arises. Many authors advocate that the one-tailed P value should be doubled. In the present example, the one-tailed test gave $P = 0.1435$ and the two-tailed test would give $P = 0.2870$. An alternative approach is to calculate P as the total probability of tables, in either tail, which are at least as extreme as that observed in the sense of having a probability at least as small. In the present example we should have

$$P = 0.1253 + 0.0182 + 0.0310 = 0.1745.$$

The first procedure is probably to be preferred on the grounds that a significant result is interpreted as strong evidence for a difference in the *observed direction*, and there is some merit in controlling the chance probability of such a result to no more than half the two-sided significance level. The tables of Finney *et al.* (1963) enable one-sided tests at various significance levels to be made without computation provided the frequencies are not too great.

To calculate the mid-P value only half the probability of the observed table is included and we have

$$\text{mid-}P = \tfrac{1}{2}(0\cdot1253) + 0\cdot0182 = 0\cdot0808$$

as the one-sided value, and the two-sided value may be obtained by doubling this to give 0.1617.

The results of applying the exact test in this example may be compared with those obtained by the χ^2 test with Yates's correction. We find $X^2 = 2\cdot39$ ($P = 0\cdot12$) without correction and $X_c^2 = 1\cdot14$ ($P = 0\cdot29$) with correction. The probability level of $0\cdot29$ for X_c^2 agrees well with the two-sided value $0\cdot29$ from the exact test, and the probability level of $0\cdot12$ for X^2 is a fair approximation to the exact mid-P value of $0\cdot16$.

Cochran (1954) recommends the use of the exact test, in preference to the χ^2 test with continuity correction, (i) if $N < 20$, or (ii) if $20 < N < 40$ and the smallest expected value is less than 5. With modern scientific calculators and statistical software the exact test is much easier to calculate than previously and should be used for any table with an expected value less than 5.

The exact test and therefore the χ^2 test with Yates's correction for continuity have been criticized over the last 50 years on the grounds that they are conservative in the sense that a result significant at, say, the 5% level will be found in less than 5% of hypothetical repeated random samples from a population in which the null hypothesis is true. This feature was discussed in §4.7 and it was remarked that the problem was a consequence of the discrete nature of the data and causes no difficulty if the precise level of P is stated. Another source of criticism has been that the tests are conditional on the observed margins, which frequently would not all be fixed. For example, in Example 4.14 one could imagine repetitions of sampling in which 20 breast-fed infants were compared with 22 bottle-fed infants but in many of these samples the number of infants with normal teeth would differ from 5. The conditional argument is that, whatever inference can be made about the association between breast-feeding and tooth decay, it has to be made within the context that exactly five children had normal teeth. If this number had been different then the inference would have been made in this different context, but that is irrelevant to inferences that can be made when there are five children with normal teeth. Therefore, we do not accept the various arguments that have been put forward for rejecting the exact test based on consideration of possible samples with different totals in one of the margins. The issues were discussed by Yates (1984) and in the ensuing discussion, and by Barnard (1989) and Upton (1992), and we will not pursue this point further. Nevertheless, the exact test and the corrected χ^2 test have the undesirable feature that the average value of the significance level, when the null hypothesis is true, exceeds 0·5. The mid-P value avoids this problem, and so is more appropriate when combining results from several studies (see §4.7). As for a single proportion, the mid-P value corresponds to an uncorrected χ^2 test, whilst the exact P value corresponds to the corrected χ^2 test.

The confidence limits for the difference, ratio or odds ratio of two proportions based on the standard errors given by (4.14), (4.17) or (4.19) respectively are all approximate and the approximate values will be suspect if one or more of the frequencies in the 2×2 table are small. Various methods have been put forward to give improved limits but all of these involve iterations and are tedious to carry out on a calculator. The odds ratio is the easiest case. Apart from exact limits, which involve an excessive amount of calculation, the most satisfactory limits are those of Cornfield (1956); see Example 16.1 and Breslow and Day (1980, §4.3) or Fleiss (1981, §5.6). For the ratio of two proportions a method was given by Koopman (1984) and Miettinen and Nurminen (1985) which can be programmed fairly readily. The confidence interval produced gives a good approximation to the required confidence coefficient, but the two tail probabilities are unequal due to skewness. Gart and Nam (1988) gave a correction for skewness but this is tedious to calculate. For the difference of two proportions a method was given by Mee (1984) and Miettinen and Nurminen (1985). This involves more calculation than for the ratio limits, and again there could be a problem due to skewness (Gart and Nam, 1990).

4.10 Inferences from counts

Suppose that x is a count, say, of the number of events occurring during a certain period or a number of small objects observed in a biological specimen, which can be assumed to follow the Poisson distribution with mean μ (§2.6). What can be said about μ?

Suppose first that we wish to test a null hypothesis specifying that μ is equal to some value μ_0. On this hypothesis, x would follow a Poisson distribution with expectation μ_0. The departure of x from its expected value, μ_0, is measured by the extent to which x falls into either of the tails of the hypothesized distribution. The situation is similar to that of the binomial (§4.7). Thus if $x > \mu_0$ and the probabilities in the Poisson distribution are $P_0, P_1, \ldots$, the P value for a one-sided test will be

$$P_+ = P_x + P_{x+1} + P_{x+2} + \ldots$$
$$= 1 - P_0 - P_1 - \ldots - P_{x-1}.$$

The possible methods of constructing a two-sided test follow the same principles as for the binomial in §4.7.

Again considerable simplification is achieved by approximating the Poisson distribution by the normal (§2.7). On the null hypothesis, and including a continuity correction,

$$z = \frac{|x - \mu_0| - \frac{1}{2}}{\sqrt{\mu_0}} \tag{4.26}$$

is approximately a standardized normal deviate. Excluding the continuity correction corresponds to the mid-P value obtained by including only $\frac{1}{2}P_x$ in the summation of Poisson probabilities.

Example 4.15

In a study of asbestos workers a large group was followed over several years and 33 died of lung cancer. Making allowance for age, using national death rates, the expected number of deaths due to lung cancer was 20·0. How strong is this evidence that there is an excess risk of death due to lung cancer?

On the null hypothesis that the national death rates applied, the standard error of x is $\sqrt{20\cdot0} = 4\cdot47$. The observed deviation is $33 - 20\cdot0 = 13\cdot0$. With continuity correction, the standardized normal deviate is $(13\cdot0 - 0\cdot5)/4\cdot47 = 2\cdot80$, giving a one-sided normal tail area of 0·0026. The exact one-sided value of P, from the Poisson distribution, is 0·0047, so the normal test exaggerated the significance. Two-sided values may be obtained by doubling these values, and both methods show that the evidence of excess mortality due to lung cancer is strong.

The exact one-sided mid-P value is 0·0037 and the corresponding standardized normal deviate is $13\cdot0/4\cdot47 = 2\cdot91$, giving a one-sided level of 0·0018.

The 95% confidence limits for μ are the two values, μ_L and μ_U, for which x is just significant by a one-sided test at the $2\frac{1}{2}$% level. These values may be obtained from tables of the Poisson distribution (e.g. Pearson and Hartley, 1966, Table 7) and Bailar and Ederer (1964) give a table of confidence factors. Table VIII1 of Fisher and Yates (1963) may also be used.

The normal approximation may be used in similar ways to the binomial case.
1 The tail areas could be estimated from (4.26). Thus approximations to the 95% limits are given by

$$\frac{x - \mu_L - \frac{1}{2}}{\sqrt{\mu_L}} = 1\cdot96$$

and

$$\frac{x - \mu_U + \frac{1}{2}}{\sqrt{\mu_U}} = -1\cdot96.$$

2 If x is large the continuity correction in method **1** may be omitted.
3 Replace $\sqrt{\mu_L}$ and $\sqrt{\mu_U}$ by $\sqrt{x}$. This is only satisfactory for large values (greater than 100).

The exact limits may be obtained by using tables of the χ^2 distribution. This follows from the mathematical link between the Poisson and the χ^2 distributions (see Liddell, 1984). The limits are

$$\mu_L = \tfrac{1}{2}\chi^2_{2x, 0.975}$$

and

$$\mu_U = \tfrac{1}{2}\chi^2_{2x+2, 0.025}.$$

(4.27)

Example 4.15, continued

With $x = 33$ the exact 95% confidence limits are found to be 22·7 and 46·3. Method **1** gives 23·1 and 46·9, method **2** gives 23·5 and 46·3, and method **3** gives 21·7 and 44·3. In this example methods **1** and **2** are adequate. The 95% confidence limits for the relative death rate due to lung cancer, expressed as the ratio of observed to expected, are 22·7/20·0 and 46·3/20·0 = 1·14 and 2·32. The mid-P limits are obtained from method **2** as 23·5/20·0 and 46·3/20·0 = 1·18 and 2·32.

Example 4.16

As an example where exact limits should be calculated, suppose that, in a similar situation to Example 4.15, there were two deaths compared with an expectation of 0·5. Then

$$\mu_L = \tfrac{1}{2}\chi^2_{4, 0.975} = 0.24$$

and

$$\mu_U = \tfrac{1}{2}\chi^2_{6, 0.025} = 7.22.$$

The limits for the ratio of observed to expected deaths are 0·24/0·5 and 7·22/0·5 = 0·5 and 14·4. The mid-P limits of μ may be obtained by trial and error on a programmable calculator or personal computer as those values for which $P(x = 0) + P(x = 1) + \tfrac{1}{2}P(x = 2) = 0.975$ or 0·025. This gives $\mu_L = 0.335$ and $\mu_U = 6.61$ so that the mid-P limits of the ratio of observed to expected deaths are 0·7 and 13·2. The evidence of excess mortality is weak but the data do not exclude the possibility of a large excess.

Suppose that in Example 4.16 there had been no deaths, then there is some ambiguity on the calculation of a 95% confidence interval. The point estimate of μ is zero and, since the lower limit cannot exceed the point estimate and also cannot be negative, its only possible value is zero. There is a probability of zero that the lower limit exceeds the true value of μ instead of the nominal value of $2\tfrac{1}{2}\%$, and a possibility is to calculate the upper limit as $\mu_U = \tfrac{1}{2}\chi^2_{2, 0.05} = 3.00$, rather than as $\tfrac{1}{2}\chi^2_{2, 0.025} = 3.69$, so that the probability that the upper limit is less than the true value is approximately 5%, and the interval has approximately 95% coverage. Whilst this is logical and provides the narrowest 95% confidence interval it seems preferable that the upper limit corresponds to $2\tfrac{1}{2}\%$ in the upper tail to give a uniform interpretation. It turns out that the former value,

$\mu = 3\cdot00$, is the upper mid-P limit. Whilst it is impossible to find a lower limit with this interpretation, this is clear from the fact that the limit equals the point estimate and that both are at the extreme of possible values. This rationale is similar to that in our recommendation that a two-sided significance level should be double the one-sided level.

4.11 Comparison of two counts

Suppose that x_1 is a count which can be assumed to follow a Poisson distribution with mean μ_1. Similarly let x_2 be a count independently following a Poisson distribution with mean μ_2. How might we test the null hypothesis that $\mu_1 = \mu_2$?

One approach would be to use the fact that the variance of $x_1 - x_2$ is $\mu_1 + \mu_2$ (by virtue of (2.16) and (3.9)). The best estimate of $\mu_1 + \mu_2$ on the basis of the available information is $x_1 + x_2$. On the null hypothesis $E(x_1 - x_2) = \mu_1 - \mu_2 = 0$, and $x_1 - x_2$ can be taken to be approximately normally distributed unless μ_1 and μ_2 are very small. Hence,

$$z = \frac{x_1 - x_2}{\sqrt{(x_1 + x_2)}} \tag{4.28}$$

can be taken as approximately a standardized normal deviate.

A second approach has already been indicated in the test for the comparison of proportions in paired samples (§4.8). Of the total frequency $x_1 + x_2$, a portion x_1 is observed in the first sample. Writing $r = x_1$ and $s = x_2$ in (4.11) we have

$$z = \frac{x_1 - \frac{1}{2}(x_1 + x_2)}{\frac{1}{2}\sqrt{(x_1 + x_2)}} = \frac{x_1 - x_2}{\sqrt{(x_1 + x_2)}}$$

as in (4.28). The two approaches thus lead to exactly the same test procedure.

A third approach uses a rather different application of the χ^2 test from that described for the 2×2 table in §4.9. Corresponding to each observed frequency we can consider the expected frequency, on the null hypothesis, to be $\frac{1}{2}(x_1 + x_2)$:

Observed	x_1	x_2
Expected	$\frac{1}{2}(x_1 + x_2)$	$\frac{1}{2}(x_1 + x_2)$

Applying the usual formula (4.20) for a χ^2 statistic, we have

$$X^2 = \frac{[x_1 - \frac{1}{2}(x_1 + x_2)]^2}{\frac{1}{2}(x_1 + x_2)} + \frac{[x_2 - \frac{1}{2}(x_1 + x_2)]^2}{\frac{1}{2}(x_1 + x_2)}$$

$$= \frac{(x_1 - x_2)^2}{x_1 + x_2}. \tag{4.29}$$

As for (4.20) X^2 follows the $\chi^2_{(1)}$ distribution, which we already know to be the distribution of the square of a standardized normal deviate. It is therefore not surprising that X^2 given by (4.29) is precisely the square of z given by (4.28). The third approach is thus equivalent to the other two, and forms a particularly useful method of computation since no square root is involved in (4.29).

Consider now an estimation problem. What can be said about the ratio μ_1/μ_2? The second approach described above can be generalized, when the null hypothesis is not necessarily true, by saying that x_1 follows a binomial distribution with parameters $x_1 + x_2$ (the n of §2.5) and $\mu_1/(\mu_1 + \mu_2)$ (the π of §2.5). The methods of §4.7 thus provide confidence limits for $\pi = \mu_1/(\mu_1 + \mu_2)$, and hence for μ_1/μ_2 which is merely $\pi/(1 - \pi)$. The method is illustrated in Example 4.17.

The difference $\mu_1 - \mu_2$ is estimated by $x_1 - x_2$, and the usual normal theory can be applied as an approximation, with the standard error of $x_1 - x_2$ estimated as in (4.28) by $\sqrt{(x_1 + x_2)}$.

Example 4.17

Equal volumes of two bacterial cultures are spread on nutrient media and after incubation the numbers of colonies growing on the two plates are 13 and 31. We require confidence limits for the ratio of concentrations of the two cultures.

The estimated ratio is $13/31 = 0.4194$. From the Geigy tables a binomial sample with 13 successes out of 44 provides the following 95% confidence limits for π: 0.1676 and 0.4520. Calculating $\pi/(1 - \pi)$ for each of these limits gives the following 95% confidence limits for μ_1/μ_2:

$$0.1676/0.8324 = 0.2013$$

and

$$0.4520/0.5480 = 0.8248.$$

The mid-P limits for π, calculated exactly as described in §4.7, are 0.1752 and 0.4418, leading to mid-P limits for μ_1/μ_2 of 0.2124 and 0.7915.

The normal approximations described in §4.7 can of course be used when the frequencies are not too small.

Example 4.18

Just as the distribution of a proportion, when n is large and π is small, is well approximated by assuming that the number of successes, r, follows a Poisson distribution, so a comparison of two proportions under these conditions can be effected by the methods of this section. Suppose, for example, that, in a group of 1000 men observed during a particular year, 20 incurred a certain disease, whereas, in a second group of 500 men, four cases occurred. Is there a significant difference between these proportions? This question could be answered by the methods of §4.8. As an approximation we could compare the observed proportion of deaths falling into group 2, $p = 4/24$, with the theoretical proportion $\pi = 500/1500 = 0\cdot3333$. The equivalent χ^2 test would run as follows:

	Group 1	Group 2	Total
Observed cases	20	4	24
Expected cases	$\dfrac{1000 \times 24}{1500} = 16$	$\dfrac{500 \times 24}{1500} = 8$	24

With continuity correction

$$X_c^2 = (3\tfrac{1}{2})^2/16 + (3\tfrac{1}{2})^2/8$$
$$= 0\cdot766 + 1\cdot531$$
$$= 2\cdot30 \quad (P = 0\cdot13).$$

The difference is not significant. Without the continuity correction, $X^2 = 3\cdot00$ $(P = 0\cdot083)$.

If the full analysis for the 2×2 table is written out it will become clear that this abbreviated analysis differs from the full version in omitting the contributions to X^2 from the non-affected individuals. Since these are much more numerous than the cases, their contributions to X^2 have large denominators and are therefore negligible in comparison with the terms used above. This makes it clear that the short method described here must be used only when the proportions concerned are very small.

Example 4.19

Consider a slightly different version of Example 4.18. Suppose that the first set of 20 cases occurred during the follow-up of a large group of men for a total of 1000 man-years, whilst the second set of four cases occurred amongst another large group followed for 500 man-years. Different men may have different risks of disease, but, under the assumptions that each man has a constant risk during his period of observation and that the lengths of follow-up are unrelated to the individual risks, the number of cases in each group will approximately follow a Poisson distribution. As a test of the null hypothesis that the mean risks per unit time in the two groups are equal, the χ^2 test shown in Example 4.18 may be applied.

Note, though, that a significant difference may be due to failure of the assumptions. One possibility is that the risk varies with time, and that the observations for one group are concentrated more heavily at the times of high risk than is the case for the other group; an example would be the comparison of infant deaths, where one group might be observed for a shorter period after birth, when the risk is high. Another possibility is that lengths of follow-up are related to individual risk. Suppose, for example, that individuals with high risk were observed for longer periods than those with low risk; the effect would be to increase the expected number of cases in that group.

Further methods for analysing follow-up data are described in Chapter 14.

4.12 Likelihood and Bayesian methods

The statistical methods described earlier in this chapter have all been based on the frequency concept of probability. Reference is made to repeated random samples from the same population, and the probabilities cited in significance tests or confidence limits indicate the relative frequency of certain outcomes ('significant' results, or the inclusion of a parameter value in a confidence interval) in a long series of such repetitions.

We referred in §2.9 to another approach, in which the numerical values allotted to probabilities do not necessarily relate to long-run frequencies, and in which an attempt is made to account for prior knowledge by quantitative measurement. Certainly any sensible use of statistical information must take some account of prior knowledge and of prior assessments about the plausibility of various hypotheses. In a card-guessing experiment to investigate extrasensory perception, for example, a score in excess of chance expectation which was just significant at the 5% level would be regarded by most people with some scepticism: many would prefer to think that the excess had arisen by chance (to say nothing of the possibility of experimental laxity) rather than by the intervention of telepathy or clairvoyance. On the other hand, in a clinical trial to compare an active drug with a placebo, a similarly significant result would be widely accepted as evidence for a drug effect in the observed direction because such findings are commonly made. The question is, though, whether such prior experience can usefully be incorporated in the quantitative assessment of the statistical data, or whether it should be used rather informally in conjunction with the statistical analysis.

It will be useful to discuss this controversy further in terms of a relatively simple example. Denote a normal distribution with mean μ and variance σ^2 by $N(\mu, \sigma^2)$. Suppose we make one observation on a random variable, x, which follows a distribution $N(\mu, 1)$ where μ is unknown. What can be said about μ on the basis of the single observation x? The methods of this chapter would lead us to base a significance test on the standardized normal deviate $x - \mu$, and to obtain confidence limits by taking standardized normal percentiles on either side of x (95% limits being, for instance, $x \pm 1{\cdot}960$).

In discussing Bayes' theorem in §2.8 we noted that the posterior probability of a particular hypothesis was expressed in terms of prior probabilities and likelihoods, the latter being the probabilities of obtaining the observed results on the various alternative hypotheses. Since we are concerned in the present problem with continuous distributions we must consider probability densities rather than probabilities. The likelihoods of the various possible values of μ for a particular observed x are shown in Fig. 4.6. This curve, showing the *likelihood function*, is exactly the same shape as a normal distribution with mean x and variance 1, but it should not be thought of as a probability distribution since the ordinate for each value represents a density from a *different* distribution.

If inferences about parameters are based on Bayes' theorem, the only way in which the observed values of the random variables are used is by their appearance in the likelihood function. Moreover, quite apart from the use of prior probabilities, there are strong logical arguments in favour of basing inferences on the

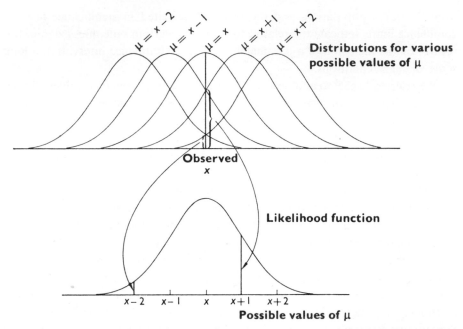

Fig. 4.6. The likelihood function for an observation x from a normal distribution with unit variance. The likelihood for a particular value of μ in the lower diagram is equal to the probability density of x in the distribution with mean μ in the upper diagram.

likelihood function. How might this be done? One reasonable proposal would be to take the value of the parameter with the highest likelihood to be the 'best' estimate of this parameter. This is the method of *maximum likelihood*, advocated and developed by R. A. Fisher, which is the most useful general method of statistical estimation. In our example the value of μ with the highest likelihood is (from Fig. 4.6) x, and we should say that x is the *maximum likelihood estimate* (or *estimator*) of μ.

Secondly, to express a range of likely values of μ around x, we could take all those values whose likelihood is not less than a certain fraction of the maximum likelihood. The width of the interval would depend on the critical ratio. A ratio of 0·146 would, for example, include values of μ within the range $x \pm 1\cdot960$, corresponding exactly to our 95% confidence interval. With this change in interpretation, therefore, we are led to intervals of exactly the same form as the confidence intervals.

This interpretation makes no reference to prior probabilities. We know from Bayes' theorem (2.18) that prior probabilities are converted into posterior probabilities by their interaction with likelihoods. The posterior probability distribution will thus depend on the choice of the prior distribution. In our example it can be shown that if the prior distribution for μ is $N(0, \sigma_0^2)$, the posterior distribution after the observation of the value x is

$$N\left(\frac{x}{1 + 1/\sigma_0^2}, \frac{1}{1 + 1/\sigma_0^2}\right). \tag{4.30}$$

Let us see how this depends on a choice of σ_0^2. If $\sigma_0^2 = 0$, this means that we are initially quite certain that $\mu = 0$; not surprisingly, the mean and variance of the posterior distribution are similarly 0; our initial certainty has in no way been shaken by the observation. At the other extreme the value $\sigma_0^2 = \infty$ would correspond to an initial state of great uncertainty about μ. The posterior distribution is then $N(x, 1)$. This is precisely the lower curve of Fig. 4.6 if we now interpret this curve not as a likelihood function but as a probability distribution. The interval $x \pm 1{\cdot}960$ could now be regarded as the interval which includes the central 95% of the posterior distribution. Here, then, is yet another interpretation of the same numerical result.

The detailed application of Bayesian methods to standard statistical problems is developed in the two volumes by Lindley (1965). It turns out to be widely, but not universally, true that Bayesian methods can be made to correspond (with appropriate changes in interpretation) to the standard frequency methods when a suitable widely dispersed prior distribution is used to indicate a state of initial ignorance. It is interesting that the Bayesian solution to the problem of comparing two means when the variances are unequal (§4.4) yields the Fisher–Behrens rather than the Welch test. One branch of statistics in which there are serious divergencies between the Bayesian and non-Bayesian approaches is that of sequential analysis, discussed in Chapter 15.

In the next section we discuss briefly some further applications of Bayesian methods.

4.13 Some further Bayesian methods

Shrinkage and prediction

In the discussion of (4.30) we noted that the mean of the posterior distribution varied between zero (when the prior variance $\sigma_0^2 = 0$) and x (when $\sigma_0^2 = \infty$). In fact, the posterior mean is always within this range. In other words, the most likely value of μ is *shrunk* from the maximum likelihood estimate x towards the prior mean of zero. The proportionate extent of the shrinkage depends on the ratio of the prior variance to the variance of the likelihood function.

More generally, but still considering a normal prior distribution and likelihood, we could replace x by the mean $\bar{x}$ of a sample of size n, distributed as $N(\mu, \sigma^2/n)$ (where previously we had $\sigma^2/n = 1$), and allow the prior distribution for μ to be $N(\mu_0, \sigma_0^2)$ (where previously we had $\mu_0 = 0$). The posterior distribution for μ is now

$$N\left(\frac{\bar{x} + \mu_0 \sigma^2/n\sigma_0^2}{1 + \sigma^2/n\sigma_0^2}, \frac{\sigma^2/n}{1 + \sigma^2/n\sigma_0^2}\right). \tag{4.31}$$

Two points should be noted. As before, the posterior mean is between the simple estimate $\bar{x}$ and the prior mean μ_0; in other words, the estimate has been shrunk towards the prior mean. Second, the proportionate shrinkage will be very small either if n is very large (when the evidence from the data overwhelms the prior information) or if σ_0^2 is very large (when the prior evidence is very weak). In either of these situations the posterior distribution will be approximately centred around the familiar estimate $\bar{x}$ with the usual variance σ^2/n.

Although these results relate to the specific case of a normal prior distribution and normal likelihood, similar results are found for other distributions, and the normal case often provides a good approximation for other situations. However, shrinkage towards the prior mean generally requires a unimodal prior distribution. If the prior had two or more well-separated modes, as might be the case for some genetic traits, the tendency would be to shrink towards the nearest major mode, and that might be in the opposite direction to the overall prior mean.

As a further example of shrinkage, consider the estimation of a population proportion π from a random sample of size n in which r individuals are affected in some way. The sampling results, involving the binomial distribution, were discussed in §2.5 and §3.3. In the Bayesian approach we need a prior distribution for π. A normal distribution is clearly inappropriate here, since π must lie between 0 and 1. The most convenient and flexible family of distributions for this purpose is that of the *beta distributions*, the density function of which takes the form

$$f(\pi) = \text{constant} \times \pi^{r_0 - 1}(1 - \pi)^{n_0 - r_0 - 1}, \tag{4.32}$$

where the parameters r_0 and $n_0 - r_0$ must both be positive. The mean of the prior distribution is $\pi_0 = r_0/n_0$ and the variance decreases as n_0 increases. Strong prior information is thus represented by high values of n_0.

With (4.32) as the prior distribution, and $p = r/n$ as the observed proportion of affected individuals, the posterior distribution takes the same form as (4.32) with r_0 and n_0 replaced by $r + r_0$ and $n + n_0$, respectively. The posterior mean is thus

$$\tilde{\pi} = \frac{r + r_0}{n + n_0}, \tag{4.33}$$

which lies between p and π_0. The estimate of the population proportion has therefore been shrunk from the sample estimate p towards the prior mean π_0. For very weak prior evidence and a large sample (n_0 small, n large) the posterior estimate will be close to the sample proportion p. For strong prior evidence and a small sample (n_0 large, n small) the estimate will be close to the prior mean π_0.

Consider now the problem of predicting the results of a future random sample from the same population as that from which the current sample was drawn. In the first case considered above, of a normal prior distribution and normal distribution for the data, suppose the future sample is to be of size n_1, and denote the unknown mean of this sample by $\bar{x}_1$. If we knew the value of μ, the distribution of $\bar{x}_1$ would be $N(\mu, \sigma^2/n_1)$. In fact μ is unknown, but its posterior distribution is given by (4.31). The overall distribution of $\bar{x}_1$ is obtained by generating the sampling distribution, with variance σ^2/n_1, for each value of μ in the posterior distribution. The result is a normal distribution with the same mean as in (4.31), but with a variance increased from that in (4.31) by an amount σ^2/n_1. In the simple situation of very weak prior evidence or very large initial sample (either σ_0^2 or n very large), the predictive distribution for $\bar{x}_1$ becomes

$$N\left[\bar{x}, \sigma^2\left(\frac{1}{n} + \frac{1}{n_1}\right)\right].$$

This effectively expresses the facts that, in the absence of prior knowledge, the best guess at $\bar{x}_1$ is $\bar{x}$, that the variation of $\bar{x}_1$ about $\bar{x}$ is essentially that of the difference between the two estimates, and that the variance of this difference is the sum of the separate variances. Bayesian predictive distributions may be useful in situations where investigators are uncertain whether to take further observations, and wish to predict the likely range of error of such observations. An important assumption, of course, is that the future sample, if taken, would be from the same distribution as that already observed, and the validity of this assumption will often be in doubt. For a description of the use of predictive distributions in clinical trials, see for instance Spiegelhalter *et al.* (1986).

The phenomenon of shrinkage, described above, is closely related to that of *regression to the mean*, familiar to epidemiologists and other scientists for many decades. This will be discussed in the context of regression in §5.5.

In contemplating the use of Bayesian methods the crucial question to consider is whether the formal specification of a prior distribution properly reflects the user's uncertainty about the parameters under study. In the estimation of a population proportion, where there might be relevant data from previous surveys, it should not be assumed that the previous sample size and number of affected individuals should automatically be used for n_0 and r_0 in (4.33). The previous survey may have been carried out in different circumstances and on a population differing in important ways from the current population, and its precise relevance may be difficult to determine. In scientific research it may be preferable to present the results of each study as objectively as possible, without prior assumptions, but to take any opportunities that may be available to compare results with previous data and, where appropriate, to combine results from different studies (see §6.5 and §7.2).

There are other situations in which the investigators may wish to introduce their initial views by means of a subjective prior distribution. These may arise particularly when decisions have to be made, for instance about the continuation of a certain line of research. Even though formal decision theory (referred to in

§2.8) may not necessarily be invoked, it will nevertheless be appropriate not only to use the latest study bearing on the question, but to form a judgement using also all other relevant knowledge. Bayesian methods may provide a helpful method of synthesis.

Empirical Bayesian methods

There are many situations where statistics are available for each of a number of groups that share some common feature. The results may differ from group to group, but the common features suggest that the information from the whole data set is to some extent relevant to inferences about any one group, as a supplement to the specific statistics for that group. Some examples are as follows.

1 Biochemical test measurements on patients with a specific diagnosis, where repeated measurements on any one patient may fluctuate and their mean is therefore subject to sampling error, but the results for the whole data set throw some light on the true mean level for that patient.

2 Biological screening tests done on each of a large number of substances to detect possible pharmacological activity. Test results for any one substance are subject to random error, but again the whole data set provides evidence about the distribution of true mean activity levels.

3 Mortality or morbidity rates for a large number of small areas, each of which is subject to random error. Again, some information relevant to a specific area is provided by the distribution of rates for the whole data set, or at least for a subset of adjacent areas.

In studies of this type it seems reasonable to regard the results for the specific group (patient, substance or area, in the above examples) as being drawn from the same prior distribution as all the other groups unless there are distinguishing features that make this assumption unreasonable (such as a special form of disease in **1**, or an important chemical property in **2**). The likelihood to be used in Bayes' theorem will depend on the particular form of data observed for a particular group, and will often follow immediately from standard results for means, proportions, counts, etc. The prior distribution causes more difficulty because it relates to the 'true' values of the parameters for different groups, and these can only be estimated. In **3**, for instance, the 'true' mortality rate for any area can only be estimated from the observed rate. The variability of the observed rates will always be greater than that of the true rates, because of the additional sampling errors that affect the former.

The purpose of empirical Bayes methods is to estimate the prior distribution from the observed data, by adjusting for the sampling errors, and then to use Bayes' theorem to estimate the relevant parameter for any individual group. The general effect is, as in the previous discussion, to shrink the estimates from those obtained from that group alone towards those appropriate for the whole data set.

As before, the proportionate shrinkage depends on the relative magnitudes of the variation between groups and the sampling error of the group in question. In **3**, for instance, a very small area with no observed cases may have an adjusted rate estimate substantially above zero, because of the plausibility that the observed rate of zero was a downwards sampling fluctuation. A large area with a high rate based on a large sample would have a downwards adjustment, but this would be relatively small because the likelihood would play a more dominant part in Bayes' theorem. Some examples of empirical Bayes estimations for area rates are described by Clayton and Kaldor (1987) and Marshall (1991). Breslow (1990) gives a useful survey of empirical Bayes and other Bayesian methods in various medical applications.

5: Regression and Correlation

5.1 Association

In earlier chapters we have been concerned with the statistical analysis of observations on a single variable. In some problems data were divided into two groups, and the dichotomy could, admittedly, have been regarded as defining a second variable. These two-sample problems are, however, rather artificial examples of the relationship between two variables.

In this chapter we examine more generally the association between two quantitative variables. We shall concentrate on situations in which the general trend is linear; that is, as one variable changes the other variable follows *on the average* a trend which can be represented approximately by a straight line. More complex situations will be discussed in Chapters 9 and 10.

The basic graphical technique for the two-variable situation is the *scatter diagram*, and it is good practice to plot the data in this form before attempting any numerical analysis. An example is shown in Fig. 5.1. In general the data refer to a number of *individuals*, each of which provides observations on two variables. In the scatter diagram each variable is allotted one of the two coordinate axes, and each individual thus defines a point, of which the coordinates are the observed values of the two variables. In Fig. 5.1 the individuals are towns and the two variables are the infant mortality rate and a certain index of overcrowding.

The scatter diagram gives a compact illustration of the distribution of each variable and of the relationship between the two variables. Further statistical analysis serves a number of purposes. It provides, first, numerical measures of some of the basic features of the relationship, rather as the mean and standard deviation provide concise measures of the most important features of the distribution of a single variable. Secondly, the investigator may wish to make a prediction of the value of one variable when the value of the other variable is known. It will normally be impossible to predict with complete certainty, but we may hope to say something about the mean value and the variability of the predicted variable. From Fig. 5.1, for instance, it appears roughly that a town with 0·6 persons per room was in 1961 likely to have an infant mortality rate of about 20 per 1000 live births on average, with a likely range of about 14–26. A proper analysis might be expected to give more reliable figures than these rough guesses.

Thirdly, the investigator may wish to assess the significance of the direction of an apparent trend. From the data of Fig. 5.1, for instance, could it safely be

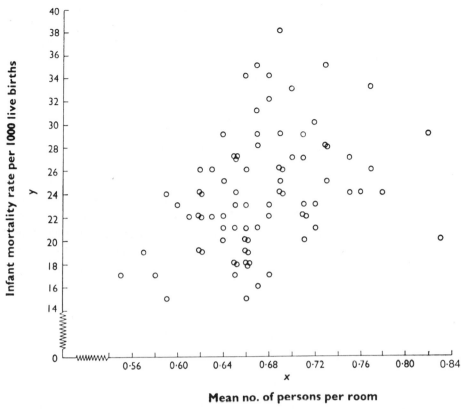

Fig. 5.1 Scatter diagram showing the mean number of person per room and the infant mortality per 1000 live births for the 83 county boroughs in England and Wales in 1961.

asserted that infant mortality increases on the average as the overcrowding index increases, or could the apparent trend in this direction have arisen easily by chance?

Yet another aim may be to correct the measurements of one variable for the effect of another variable. In a study of the forced expiratory volume (FEV) of workers in the cadmium industry who had been exposed for more than a certain number of years to cadmium fumes, a comparison was made with the FEV of other workers who had not been exposed. The mean FEV of the first group was lower than that of the second. However, the men in the first group tended to be older than those in the second, and FEV tends to decrease with age. The question therefore arises whether the difference in mean FEV could be explained purely by the age difference. To answer this question the relationship between FEV and age must be studied in some detail. The method is described in §9.5.

We must be careful to distinguish between *association* and *causation*. Two variables are associated if the distribution of one is affected by a knowledge of the value of the other. This does not mean that one variable *causes* the other. There is a strong association between the number of divorces made absolute in the United Kingdom during the first half of this century and the amount of tobacco imported (the 'individuals' in the scatter diagram here being the individual years). It does not follow either that tobacco is a serious cause of marital discontent, or that those whose marriages have broken down turn to tobacco for solace. Association does not imply causation.

A further distinction is between situations in which both variables can be thought of as random variables, the individuals being selected randomly or at least without reference to the values of either variable, and situations in which the values of one variable are deliberately selected by the investigator. An example of the first situation would be a study of the relationship between the height and the blood pressure of schoolchildren, the individuals being restricted to one sex and one age group. Here the sample may not have been chosen strictly at random, but it can be thought of as roughly representative of a population of children of this age and sex from the same area and type of school. An example of the second situation would arise in a study of the growth of children between certain ages. The nature of the relationship between height and age, as illustrated by a scatter diagram, would depend very much on the age range chosen and the distribution of ages within this range. We return to this point in §5.3.

5.2 Linear regression

Suppose that observations are made on variables x and y for each of a large number of individuals, and that we are interested in the way in which y changes on the average as x assumes different values. If it is appropriate to think of y as a random variable for any given value of x, we can enquire how the expectation of y changes with x. The probability distribution of y when x is known is referred to as a *conditional* distribution, and the conditional expectation is denoted by $E(y|x)$. We make no assumption at this stage as to whether x is a random variable or not. In a study of heights and blood pressures of randomly chosen individuals both variables would be random; if x and y were respectively the age and height of children selected according to age, then only y would be random.

The conditional expectation, $E(y|x)$, depends in general on x. It is called the *regression function* of y on x. If $E(y|x)$ is drawn as a function of x it forms the *regression curve*. Two examples are shown in Fig. 5.2. The regression in Fig. 5.2(b) differs in two ways from that in Fig. 5.2(a). The curve in Fig. 5.2(b) is a straight line—the *regression line* of y on x. Secondly, the variation of y for fixed x is constant in Fig. 5.2(b), whereas in Fig. 5.2(a) the variation changes as x increases. The regression in (b) is called *homoscedastic*, that in (a) being *heteroscedastic*.

The situation represented by Fig. 5.2(b) is important not only because of its simplicity, but also because regressions which are approximately linear and

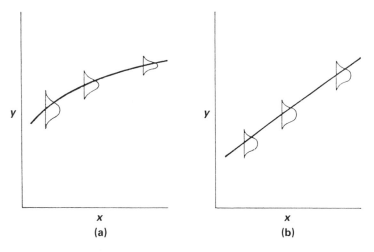

Fig. 5.2 Two regression curves of *y* on *x*: (a) non-linear and heteroscedastic; (b) linear and homoscedastic. The distributions shown are those of values of *y* at certain values of *x*.

homoscedastic occur frequently in scientific work. In the present discussion we shall make one further simplifying assumption—that the distribution of *y* for given *x* is normal.

The model may, then, be described by saying that, for a given *x*, *y* follows a normal distribution with mean

$$E(y|x) = \alpha + \beta x$$

(the general equation of a straight line) and variance σ^2 (a constant). A set of data consists of *n* pairs of observations, denoted by $(x_1, y_2), (x_2, y_2), \ldots, (x_n, y_n)$, each y_i being an independent observation from the distribution $N(\alpha + \beta x_i, \sigma^2)$. How can we estimate the parameters α, β and σ^2, which characterize the model?

Theoretical arguments* lead to the following rule: α and β are estimated by the '*least squares*' estimators, *a* and *b*, namely the quantities which minimize the *residual* sum of squares, $\sum(y_i - Y_i)^2$, where Y_i is given by the estimated regression equation

$$Y_i = a + bx_i. \tag{5.1}$$

This is intuitively an attractive proposal. The regression line is drawn through the *n* points on the scatter diagram so as to minimize the sum of squares of the distances, $y_i - Y_i$, of the points from the line, these distances being measured parallel to the *y*-axis (Fig. 5.3).

---

*The 'least squares' estimators of α and β are also maximum likelihood estimators (see §4.12); furthermore, among all unbiased estimators they have the smallest standard errors.

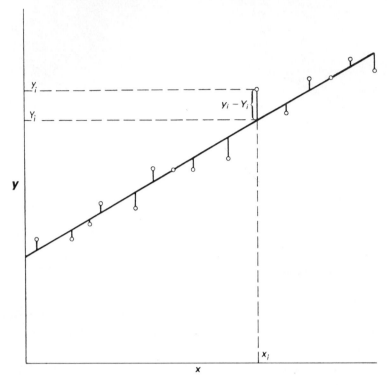

Fig. 5.3 A linear regression line fitted by least squares showing a typical deviation between an observed value y_i and the value Y_i given by the regression line.

It can be shown by elementary calculus that a and b are given by the formulae

$$a = \bar{y} - b\bar{x}, \tag{5.2}$$

$$b = \frac{\sum(x_i - \bar{x})(y_i - \bar{y})}{\sum(x_i - \bar{x})^2}. \tag{5.3}$$

A proof without the use of calculus is as follows. Note first that for any n numbers $p_1, p_2, \ldots, p_n$, the quantity P which minimizes $\sum(p_i - P)^2$ is $P = \bar{p}$. To show this, note that, for any P,

$$\sum(p_i - P)^2 = \sum(p_i - \bar{p})^2 + n(\bar{p} - P)^2 \tag{5.4}$$

(as can be shown by expanding $(p_i - P)^2$ as $[(p_i - \bar{p}) + (\bar{p} - P)]^2$). The right-hand side of (5.4) is a minimum when the second term is zero, i.e. when $P = \bar{p}$.

Now consider $S = \sum(y_i - Y_i)^2 = \sum(y_i - a - bx_i)^2$. For any value of b, the minimum S occurs when

$$a = \sum(y_i - bx_i)/n$$

(from the previous result with $p_i = y_i - bx_i$); that is,

$$a = \bar{y} - b\bar{x}$$

as in (5.2). The regression line can thus be written

$$Y_i = a + bx_i$$
$$= \bar{y} + b(x_i - \bar{x}), \tag{5.5}$$

from which it follows that the line goes through the point $(\bar{x}, \bar{y})$.

We now have to find the value of b minimizing

$$S = \sum [y_i - \bar{y} - b(x_i - \bar{x})]^2$$

$$= \sum (x - \bar{x})^2 \left[b - \frac{\sum (x - \bar{x})(y - \bar{y})}{\sum (x - \bar{x})^2} \right]^2 + \sum (y - \bar{y})^2 - \frac{[\sum (x - \bar{x})(y - \bar{y})]^2}{\sum (x - \bar{x})^2}, \tag{5.6}$$

as may be seen by multiplying out the right-hand side. (The suffix i has been dropped for convenience.) Now the second and third terms of (5.6) do not involve b. The first term is a sum of squares and cannot be negative; it is, however, zero when

$$b = \frac{\sum (x - \bar{x})(y - y)}{\sum (x - \bar{x})^2},$$

which is therefore the required value of b, as in (5.3).

Note that the minimum value of S is given by the last two terms of (5.6), namely

$$\sum (y - \bar{y})^2 - \frac{[\sum (x - \bar{x})(y - \bar{y})]^2}{\sum (x - \bar{x})^2}. \tag{5.7}$$

Finally, it can be shown that an unbiased estimator of σ^2 is

$$s_0^2 = \frac{\sum (y - Y)^2}{n - 2}, \tag{5.8}$$

the residual sum of squares, $\sum (y - Y)^2$ being obtainable from (5.7). The divisor $n - 2$ is often referred to as the residual degrees of freedom, s_0^2 as the *residual mean square*, and s_0 as the *standard deviation about regression*.

The quantities a and b are called the *regression coefficients*; the term is often used particularly for b, the slope of the regression line.

The expression in the numerator of (5.3) is the sum of products of deviations of x and y about their means. A short-cut formula analogous to (1.3) is useful for computational work. By an argument similar to that used to derive (1.3) we find

$$\sum (x_i - \bar{x})(y_i - \bar{y}) = \sum x_i y_i - \frac{(\sum x_i)(\sum y_i)}{n}. \tag{5.9}$$

Note that, whereas a sum of squares about the mean must be positive or zero, a sum of products of deviations about the mean may be negative, in which case, from (5.3), b will also be negative.

The above theory is illustrated in the following example, which will also be used later in the chapter after further points have been considered. All the calculations necessary in a simple linear regression are feasible using a scientific calculator, but nowadays one would usually use either a statistical package on a computer, or a calculator with keys for fitting a regression, and the actual calculations would not be a concern.

Example 5.1

Table 5.1 gives the values for 32 babies of x, the birth weight, and y, the increase in weight between the 70th and 100th day of life expressed as a percentage of the birth weight. A scatter diagram is shown in Fig. 5.4 which suggests an association between the two variables in a negative direction. This seems quite plausible: when the birth weight is low the subsequent rate of growth, *relative to the birth weight*, would be expected to be high, and vice versa. The trend seems reasonably linear.

From Table 5.1 we proceed as follows:

$$n = 32 \qquad \sum x = 3576 \qquad \sum y = 2281$$
$$\bar{x} = 3576/32 \qquad \bar{y} = 2281/32$$
$$= 111 \cdot 75. \qquad\qquad = 71 \cdot 28.$$

$$\sum x^2 = 409\,880 \qquad\qquad \sum xy = 246\,032 \qquad\qquad \sum y^2 = 179\,761$$
$$(\sum x)^2/n = 399\,618 \cdot 00 \qquad (\sum x)(\sum y)/n = 254\,901 \cdot 75 \qquad (\sum y)^2/n = 162\,592 \cdot 53$$
$$\sum(x - \bar{x})^2 = 10\,262 \cdot 00 \quad \sum(x - \bar{x})(y - \bar{y})(y - \bar{y}) = -8869 \cdot 75 \quad \sum(y - \bar{y})^2 = 17\,168 \cdot 47.$$

To predict the weight increase from the birth weight the regression of y on x is needed.

$$b = -\frac{8\,869 \cdot 75}{10\,262 \cdot 00}$$
$$= -0 \cdot 8643.$$

The equation of the regression line is, from (5.5),

$$Y = 71 \cdot 28 - 0 \cdot 8643(x - 111 \cdot 75)$$
$$= 167 \cdot 87 - 0 \cdot 8643x.$$

To draw the line, the coordinates of two points suffice, but it is a safeguard to calculate three. Choosing $x = 80$, 100 and 140 as convenient round numbers falling within the range of x used in Fig. 5.4, we find

Table 5.1 Birth weights of 32 babies and their increases in weight between 70 and 100 days after birth, expressed as percentages of birth weights

x, Birth weight (oz)	y, Increase in weight, 70–100 days, as % of x
72	68
112	63
111	66
107	72
119	52
92	75
126	76
80	118
81	120
84	114
115	29
118	42
128	48
128	50
123	69
116	59
125	27
126	60
122	71
126	88
127	63
86	88
142	53
132	50
87	111
123	59
133	76
106	72
103	90
118	68
114	93
94	91

x	Y
80	98·73
100	81·44
140	46·87

The regression line is now drawn through the three points with these coordinates and is shown in Fig. 5.4.

Note that as x changes from 80 to 120 (i.e. by a factor of $\frac{3}{2}$), y changes on the average from about 100 to 65 (i.e. by a factor of about $\frac{2}{3}$). From the definition of y this implies that *absolute* weight gains are largely independent of x.

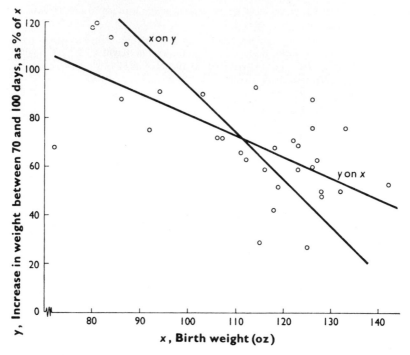

Fig. 5.4 Scatter diagram showing the birth weight, x, and the increase of weight between 70 and 100 days as a percentage of x, for 32 babies, with the two regression lines (Table 5.1).

In situations in which x, as well as y, is a random variable it may be useful to consider the regression of x on y. This shows how the mean value of x, for a given y, changes with the value of y.

The regression line of x on y may be calculated by formulae analogous to those already used, with x and y interchanged. To avoid confusion between the two lines it will be useful to write the equation of the regression of y on x as

$$Y = \bar{y} + b_{y \cdot x}(x - \bar{x}),$$

with $b_{y \cdot x}$ given by (5.3). The regression equation of x on y is then

$$X = \bar{x} + b_{x \cdot y}(y - \bar{y}),$$

with

$$b_{x \cdot y} = \frac{\sum (x - \bar{x})(y - \bar{y})}{\sum (y - \bar{y})^2}.$$

That the two lines are in general different may be seen from Fig. 5.4. Both lines go through the point $(\bar{x}, \bar{y})$ which is therefore their point of intersection. In example 5.1 we should probably be interested primarily in the regression of y on x, since it would be natural to study the way in which changes in weight vary with birth weight and to investigate the distribution of change in weight for a particular value of birth weight, rather than to enquire about the distribution of birth weights for a given weight change. In some circumstances both regressions may be of interest.

5.3 Correlation

When both x and y are random variables it may be useful to have a measure of the extent to which the relationship between the two variables approaches the extreme situation in which every point on the scatter diagram falls exactly on a straight line. Such an index is provided by the *product–moment correlation coefficient* (or simply *correlation coefficient*), defined by

$$r = \frac{\sum (x - \bar{x})(y - \bar{y})}{\sqrt{[\sum (x - \bar{x})^2 \sum (y - \bar{y})^2]}}. \tag{5.10}$$

It can be shown that for any set of data r falls within the range -1 to $+1$. Figure 5.5 shows five sets of data in which the variation in x and that in y remain approximately constant from one set to another. The marked differences between the five scatter diagrams are summarized by the values of r. Figures 5.5(a) and (e) are examples of perfect correlation in which the value of y is exactly determined as a linear function of x. The points lie exactly on a straight line; if both variables increase together, as in (a), $r = +1$, while if one variable decreases as the other increases, as in (e), $r = -1$. In each of these cases the two regression lines coincide. Figure 5.5(c) is a very different situation, in which $r = 0$. The two regression coefficients $b_{y \cdot x}$ and $b_{x \cdot y}$ are also zero and the regression lines are perpendicular. Intermediate situations are shown in (b), where $0 < r < 1$, and (d), where $-1 < r < 0$. Here the two regression lines are set at an angle, but point in the same direction.

From the short-cut formulae for sums of squares and products an alternative formula for the correlation coefficient, more convenient for computation, is

$$r = \frac{\sum xy - (\sum x)(\sum y)/n}{\sqrt{\{[\sum x^2 - (\sum x)^2/n][\sum y^2 - (\sum y)^2/n]\}}}. \tag{5.11}$$

From (5.7) the sum of squares of y about the regression line of y on x is

$$\sum (y - \bar{y})^2 \left\{ 1 - \frac{[\sum (x - \bar{x})(y - \bar{y})]^2}{\sum (x - \bar{x})^2 \sum (y - \bar{y})^2} \right\} = \sum (y - \bar{y})^2 \times (1 - r^2). \tag{5.12}$$

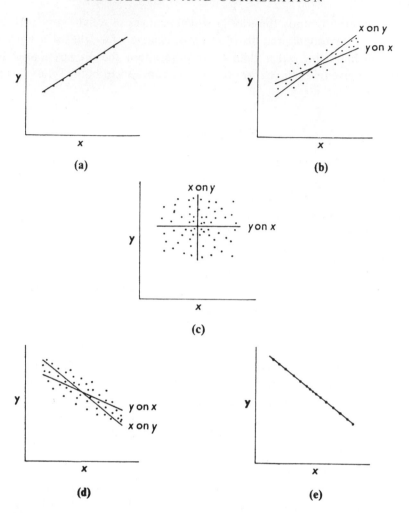

Fig. 5.5 Five scatter diagrams with regression lines illustrating different values of the correlation coefficient. In (a) $r = 1$; (b) $0 < r < 1$; (c) $r = 0$; (d) $-1 < r < 0$; (e) $r = -1$.

This provides a useful interpretation of the numerical value of r. The squared correlation coefficient is the fraction by which the sum of squares of y is reduced to give the sum of squares of deviations from its regression on x. The same result is true if x and y are interchanged in (5.12). In Figs 5.5(a) and (e), $r^2 = 1$, and (5.12) becomes zero. In (c), $r^2 = 0$ and the sum of squares of either variable is unaffected by regression on the other. In (b) and (d) some reductions take place since $0 < r^2 < 1$.

Two other formulae are easily derived from those for the regression and correlation coefficients:

$$b_{y \cdot x} = r \frac{s_y}{s_x} \left. \right\}$$

and   (5.13)

$$b_{x \cdot y} = r \frac{s_x}{s_y},$$

where s_x and s_y are the sample standard deviations of x and y. It follows that

$$b_{y \cdot x} b_{x \cdot y} = r^2.$$

The correlation coefficient has played an important part in the history of statistical methods. It is now of considerably less value than the regression coefficients. If two variables are correlated it is usually much more useful to study the positions of one or both of the regression lines, which permit the prediction of one variable in terms of the other, than to summarize the degree of correlation in a single index.

The restriction of validity of the correlation coefficient to situations in which both variables are observed on a random selection of individuals is particularly important. If, from a large population of individuals, a selection is made by restricting the values of one variable, say x, to a limited range, the correlation coefficient will tend to decrease in absolute value. In the data of Fig. 5.4, for instance, the correlation coefficients calculated on subsets of the data obtained by restricting the range of x values are as follows:

	Range of x		Number of	Correlation
	Lower limit	Upper limit	observations	coefficient
All data	70	150	32	− 0·668
Subsets	85	135	27	− 0·565
	100	120	11	− 0·578
	105	115	6	− 0·325

Conversely, if the study is restricted to individuals with extreme values of x (including both high and low values), then the correlation coefficient will tend to increase in absolute magnitude. For example, restricting attention to individuals whose birth weight was less than 100 oz or greater than 125 oz gives a correlation coefficient of −0·735.

The interpretation of the numerical value of a correlation coefficient calculated from data selected by values of one variable is thus very difficult.

5.4 Sampling errors in regression and correlation

In the regression model of §5.2, suppose that repeated sets of data are generated, each with the same n values of x but with randomly varying values of y. The statistics $\bar{y}$, a and b will vary from one set of data to another. Their sampling variances are obtained as follows:

$$\text{var}(\bar{y}) = \sigma^2/n, \tag{5.14}$$

by an argument similar to that used in §3.2. Note that here σ^2 is the variance of y *for fixed* x, not, as in (3.1), the overall variance of y.

$$\text{var}(b) = \text{var}\left[\frac{\sum y(x - \bar{x})}{\sum (x - \bar{x})^2}\right]$$

(using the fact that $\sum(x - \bar{x})(y - \bar{y}) = \sum(x - \bar{x})y$, the remaining terms vanishing),

$$= \frac{1}{[\sum(x - \bar{x})^2]^2}\sum(x - \bar{x})^2 \text{ var}(y)$$

$$= \frac{\sigma^2}{\sum(x - \bar{x})^2}. \tag{5.15}$$

$$\text{var}(a) = \text{var}(\bar{y} - b\bar{x})$$
$$= \text{var}(\bar{y}) + \bar{x}^2 \text{ var}(b)$$

(since it can be shown that b and $\bar{y}$ have zero covariance)

$$= \sigma^2\left[\frac{1}{n} + \frac{\bar{x}^2}{\sum(x - \bar{x})^2}\right]. \tag{5.16}$$

Formulae (5.14), (5.15) and (5.16) all involve the parameter σ^2. If inferences are to be made from one set of n pairs of observations on x and y, σ^2 will be unknown. It can, however, be estimated by the residual mean square, s_0^2 (5.8). Estimated variances are, therefore,

$$\text{var}(\bar{y}) = s_0^2/n, \tag{5.17}$$

$$\text{var}(b) = s_0^2/\sum(x - \bar{x})^2 \tag{5.18}$$

and

$$\text{var}(a) = s_0^2\left[\frac{1}{n} + \frac{\bar{x}^2}{\sum(x - \bar{x})^2}\right], \tag{5.19}$$

and hypotheses about $\bar{y}$, a or b can be tested using the t distribution on $n - 2$ DF. For example, to test the null hypothesis that $\beta = 0$, i.e. that in the whole population the mean value of y does not change with x, the statistic

$$t = \frac{b}{\text{SE}(b)} \tag{5.20}$$

can be referred to the t distribution on $n - 2\,\mathrm{DF}$, $\mathrm{SE}(b)$ being the square root of (5.18). Similarly, confidence limits for β at, say, the 95% level can be obtained as

$$b \pm t_{n-2,\,0\cdot05}\,\mathrm{SE}(b).$$

An important point about the t statistic (5.20) is seen by writing b as $b_{y \cdot x}$ and using (5.3), (5.7), (5.8) and (5.10). We find

$$t = r\Big/\sqrt{\left(\frac{n-2}{1-r^2}\right)}. \tag{5.21}$$

Since r is symmetric with respect to x and y, it follows that, if, for any set of n paired observations, we calculate the t statistics from $b_{y \cdot x}$ and (by interchanging x and y in the formulae) from $b_{x \cdot y}$, both values of t will be equal to (5.21). In performing the significance test of zero regression and correlation, therefore, it is immaterial whether one tests $b_{y \cdot x}$, $b_{x \cdot y}$ or r. However, we must remember that in some problems only one of the regressions may have a sensible interpretation and it will then be natural to express the test in terms of that regression.

Example 5.1, continued from §5.2

The sum of squares of deviations of y from the regression line is, from (5.7),

$$17\,168\cdot47 - \frac{(-8869\cdot75)^2}{10\,262\cdot00}$$
$$= 17\,168\cdot47 - 7666\cdot39$$
$$= 9502\cdot08.$$

The residual mean square is, from (5.8),

$$s_0^2 = 9502\cdot08/(32-2)$$
$$= 316\cdot74.$$

From (5.18),

$$\mathrm{var}(b) = 316\cdot74/10\,262\cdot00$$
$$= 0\cdot030\,865,$$
$$\mathrm{SE}(b) = \sqrt{0\cdot030\,865}$$
$$= 0\cdot1757.$$

From (5.20),

$$t = -0\cdot8643/0\cdot1757$$
$$= -4\cdot92 \text{ on } 30\,\mathrm{DF}\,(P < 0\cdot001).$$

Alternatively, we could calculate the correlation coefficient

$$r = \frac{-8869 \cdot 75}{\sqrt{[(10\,262 \cdot 00)(17\,168 \cdot 47)]}}$$

$$= -\frac{8869 \cdot 75}{13\,273 \cdot 39}$$

$$= -0 \cdot 668,$$

and, from (5.21),

$$t = -0 \cdot 668 \sqrt{\left(\frac{30}{0 \cdot 554}\right)}$$

$$= -4 \cdot 92,$$

as before.

The sampling error of a correlation coefficient was introduced above in connection with a test of the null hypothesis that its population value is zero. This is the context in which the question usually arises. More rarely we may wish to give confidence limits for the population value in situations in which the individuals providing paired observations can be regarded as randomly drawn from some population. A need arises here to define the nature of the two-dimensional distribution of x and y. A convenient form is the *bivariate normal distribution*, a rough sketch of which is shown in Fig. 5.6. This is a generalization of the

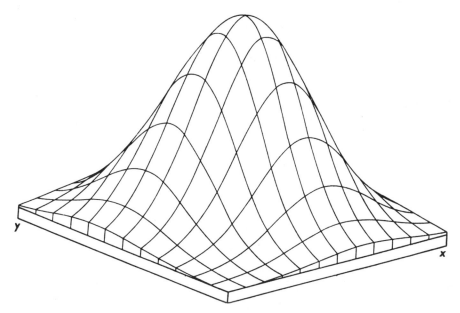

Fig. 5.6 A three-dimensional representation of a bivariate normal distribution, the vertical dimension representing probability density (reprinted from Yule and Kendall, 1950, by permission of the authors and publishers).

familiar univariate normal distribution in which the distribution of y for given x is normal with constant variance, the distribution of x for given y is also normal with constant variance, and both regressions are linear. In large samples from such a distribution the standard error of the correlation coefficient, r, is approximately $(1 - r^2)/\sqrt{n}$, a result which enables approximate confidence limits to be calculated. More refined methods are available for small samples (Geigy Scientific Tables, 1982, Vol. 2, chapter on 'Statistical Methods', §19A).

The utility of these results is limited by the importance of the assumption of bivariate normality, and also by the difficulty, referred to earlier, of interpreting the numerical value of a correlation coefficient.

Errors of prediction

The best estimate of the mean value of y at a given value of x, say x_0, is given by the regression equation

$$Y = a + bx_0 = \bar{y} + b(x_0 - \bar{x}). \tag{5.22}$$

The sampling variance of Y is

$$\text{var}(Y) = \text{var}(\bar{y}) + (x_0 - \bar{x})^2 \, \text{var}(b)$$

$$= \sigma^2 \left[\frac{1}{n} + \frac{(x_0 - \bar{x})^2}{\sum (x - \bar{x})^2} \right],$$

which may be estimated by

$$\text{var}(Y) = s_0^2 \left[\frac{1}{n} + \frac{(x_0 - \bar{x})^2}{\sum (x - \bar{x})^2} \right].$$

Again the t distribution on $n - 2$ DF is required. For instance, 95% confidence limits for the predicted mean are

$$Y \pm t_{n-2,\,0\cdot05}\, s_0 \sqrt{\left[\frac{1}{n} + \frac{(x_0 - \bar{x})^2}{\sum (x - \bar{x})^2} \right]}. \tag{5.23}$$

In (5.23) the width of the confidence interval increases with $(x_0 - \bar{x})^2$, and is therefore a minimum when $x_0 = \bar{x}$. Figure 5.7 shows the limits for various values of x_0 in Example 5.1. The reason for the increase in the width of the interval is that slight sampling errors in b will have a greater effect for values of x_0 distant from $\bar{x}$ than for those near $\bar{x}$. The regression line can be thought of as a rod which is free to move up and down (corresponding to the error in $\bar{y}$) and to pivot about a central point (corresponding to the error in b). Points near the ends of the rod will then be subject to greater oscillations than those near the centre.

A different prediction problem is that of estimating an individual value y_0 of y corresponding to a given x_0. The best single estimate is again the value given by

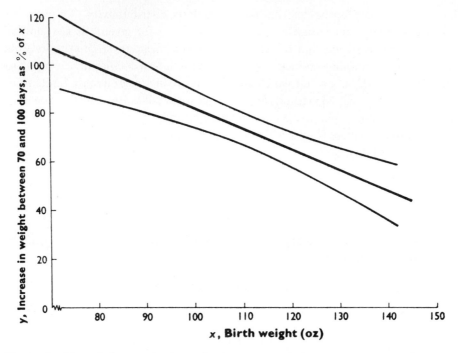

Fig. 5.7 Confidence limits (95%) for the predicted mean value of y for specified values, x_0, of x (data as in Fig. 5.4).

the regression equation, but the limits of error are different from those in the previous case. Two slightly different problems can be distinguished.

1 A single prediction is required. The appropriate limits are not strictly confidence limits because the quantity to be estimated is a value taken by a random variable, not a parameter of a distribution. However, writing

$$y_0 = Y + \varepsilon,$$

where ε is the deviation of y_0 from the predicted value Y, we have

$$\mathrm{var}(y_0) = \mathrm{var}(Y) + \mathrm{var}(\varepsilon)$$

$$= \sigma^2 \left[1 + \frac{1}{n} + \frac{(x_0 - \bar{x})^2}{\sum (x - \bar{x})^2} \right], \tag{5.24}$$

and the limits

$$Y \pm t_{n-2,\,0\cdot05}\, s_0 \sqrt{\left[1 + \frac{1}{n} + \frac{(x_0 - \bar{x})^2}{\sum (x - \bar{x})^2} \right]} \tag{5.25}$$

will include y_0 95% of the time.

2 The object may be to estimate limits within which a certain percentage (say 95%) of the values of y lie when $x = x_0$. Such an interval may be required when a regression has been used to define 'normal' or reference values which are to be used in the assessment of future patients. These limits are

$$\alpha + \beta x_0 \pm 1{\cdot}96\sigma$$

and are estimated by

$$a + bx_0 \pm 1{\cdot}96s_0 = Y \pm 1{\cdot}96s_0. \tag{5.26}$$

These limits are a fixed distance from the regression line and lie wholly within the limits (5.25). When n is very large $t_{n-2,0{\cdot}05}$ is close to $1{\cdot}96$, and the second and third terms inside the square root in (5.25) are very small; (5.25) and (5.26) are then almost the same.

Finally, it should be remembered that prediction from a regression formula may be subject to errors other than those of sampling. The linear model may be an inadequate description of the relationship between the two variables. A visual examination of the scatter diagram will provide a partial check, and analytic methods are described in §9.1. Non-linearity may, of course, exist and remain unsuspected because the data at hand provide no indication of it. The danger of using the wrong model is particularly severe if an attempt is made to extrapolate beyond the range of values observed. In Fig. 5.1, for instance, it would be very dangerous to use the regression of y on x to predict the infant mortality in towns with an overcrowding index of $0{\cdot}4$ or $1{\cdot}0$.

Comparison of variances in two paired samples

We now return to the comparison of two variances, treated in §4.6 in the case of independent samples. Suppose the two samples are of equal size, n, and there is a natural relationship between a particular value x_{1i} of one sample and the corresponding member x_{2i} of the second sample. Define $X_i = x_{1i} + x_{2i}$ and $Y_i = x_{1i} - x_{2i}$, the sum and difference of paired observations. Thus, we have

Pair	Values of x_1	Values of x_2	Sum	Difference
1	x_{11}	x_{21}	X_1	Y_1
2	x_{12}	x_{22}	X_2	Y_2
.	.	.	.	.
.	.	.	.	.
.	.	.	.	.
n	x_{1n}	x_{2n}	X_n	Y_n

Denoting by x'_{ij} the deviation of x_{ij} from its expectation,

$$\text{cov}(X_i, Y_i) = \text{E}[(x'_{1i} + x'_{2i})(x'_{1i} - x'_{2i})]$$

$$= \text{E}[(x'_{1i})^2 - (x'_{2i})^2]$$

$$= \text{var}(x_{1i}) - \text{var}(x_{2i}). \tag{5.27}$$

A test of the equality of $\text{var}(x_{1i})$ and $\text{var}(x_{2i})$ is, therefore, the same as a test of the hypothesis that the covariance of X_i and Y_i is zero, which means that the correlation coefficient also must be zero. The numerator of (5.11) is a multiple of the sample covariance of the two variables. The test of equality of variances may, therefore, be effected by any of the equivalent tests described above for the hypothesis of zero association between X_i and Y_i. This test is due to E. J. G. Pitman. Its adaptation for purposes of estimation is described by Snedecor and Cochran (1989, §10.8).

5.5 Regression to the mean

The term 'regression' was introduced by Sir Francis Galton (1822–1911) to express the fact that for many inherited characteristics, such as height, the measurements on sons are on average closer to the population mean than the corresponding values for their fathers. The regression coefficient of son's height on father's height is less than 1. The regression of father's height on son's height is also less than 1, so that whether one looks forwards or backwards in generations there is a *regression to the mean*.

Similar phenomena are widely observed in various branches of medicine. Suppose, for instance, that a person's systolic blood pressure is determined by the average of five readings to be 162 mmHg. This is somewhat above the likely population mean of, say, 140 mmHg. If a further reading is taken from the same subject, it will *on average* tend to be less than 162 mmHg. Conversely, a subject with a sample mean less than the population mean will tend to show an increase when retested.

The explanation is closely related to the discussion on shrinkage in §4.13, and anticipates a relevant description of *components of variance* in §7.3. Suppose that repeated blood pressure readings on the ith subject follow a distribution with mean μ_i and variance σ^2, and that the values of μ_i vary from one subject to another with a mean μ_0 and variance σ_0^2. (As noted in §7.3, σ^2 and σ_0^2 are 'components of variance' within and between subjects, respectively.) In terms of the discussion of §4.13, the variation between subjects may be thought of as a prior distribution for μ_i, and the distribution of repeated readings on one subject as providing the likelihood. It follows from the discussion in §4.13 that, for a subject with a mean blood pressure of $\bar{x}_i$ based on n observations, the estimate of the true mean μ_i will tend to be shrunk from $\bar{x}_i$ towards the population mean μ_0, as will the mean value of a future set of replicate readings.

Suppose that for each subject two independent samples of size n are taken, with means $\bar{x}_{i1}$ and $\bar{x}_{i2}$ for the ith subject. The correlation coefficient between $\bar{x}_{i1}$ and $\bar{x}_{i2}$ is

$$\rho = \frac{\sigma_0^2}{\sigma_0^2 + \sigma^2/n}. \tag{5.28}$$

If the distributions between and within subjects are normal, the joint distribution of $\bar{x}_1$ and $\bar{x}_2$ will be bivariate normal, as in Fig. 5.6, and (5.28) will also measure the regression coefficient of either of the means on the other one. If there were no within-subject variation ($\sigma^2 = 0$), this regression coefficient would be unity. The regression towards the mean is therefore measured by $1 - \rho$, so the smaller ρ is, the greater is the regression towards the mean. Small values of ρ will occur when σ_0^2 is small in relation to the sampling error of the means, e.g. when there is very little real heterogeneity between subjects. High values of ρ will occur when the prior information is relatively vague and the sampling error relatively small, e.g. for very large samples.

In some studies of medical interventions, subjects are selected by preliminary screening tests as having high values of a relevant test measurement. For example, in studies of cholesterol-lowering agents, subjects may be selected as having serum cholesterol levels above some critical value, either on single or on the mean of repeated determinations. On average, even with no effect of the agent under test, subsequent readings on the same subjects would tend to regress towards the mean. A significant reduction below the pretreatment values thus provides no convincing evidence of a treatment effect. Nevertheless, if precise estimates of the components of variance are available, the extent of regression to the mean can be calculated and allowed for. Gardner and Heady (1973) studied this effect, in relation to cholesterol, blood pressure and daily calorie intake, and gave formulae for the regression effects for various levels of the initial screening cut-off point. As noted above, the effect is reduced by increasing the number of observations made at the initial screen. Johnson and George (1991) extended this work by distinguishing between two sources of within-subject variation: measurement error and physiological fluctuations. The latter type of variation may result in fluctuations that are not independent, showing perhaps cyclical or other trends, a topic discussed in §10.6. In that case, increasing the initial sample size may have a smaller effect on the phenomenon of regression to the mean than would otherwise be so.

Example 5.2

Irwig *et al.* (1991) examined the effects of regression to the mean on the screening of individuals to detect those with high levels of blood cholesterol. They considered three hypothetical populations with the following mean values (all values quoted here and below being in units of mmol/l): A, 5·2; B, 5·8; C, 6·4. These values are based on survey data, as being characteristic of men under 35 years and women under 45 (A); men aged 35–74 and women aged 45–64 (B); and women aged 65 and older (C). The calculations are based on the model described above, but with the assumption (again confirmed by observations) that the log of the cholesterol level, rather than the level itself, is normally distributed between and within subjects, with constant within-subject variance.

Standard guidelines would classify levels less than 5·2 as 'desirable', levels between 5·2 and 6·1 as 'borderline high', and those above 6·1 as 'high'. Irwig *et al.* illustrate the effects of regression to the mean in various ways. For instance, an individual in group B with a single screening measurement of 9·0 would have an estimated true mean of 8·4 with 80% confidence limits of 7·7 and 9·2. If the value of 9·0 was based on three measurements, the estimated true level would be 8·8 (limits 8·3, 9·3)—a less pronounced regression effect than for single measurements.

An important concern is that individuals might be classified on the wrong side of a threshold. For instance, an individual in group A with a screening measurement of 4·9 would have a probability of 0·26 of having a true mean above the threshold of 5·2. For a screening measurement of 5·8 there is a probability of 0·10 that the true level is below 5·2.

Other calculations are concerned with the assessment of an intervention intended to lower blood cholesterol. Suppose that an intervention produces a mean reduction of 13% (this figure being based on the results of a particular study). For an individual in group B with three measurements before and one after the intervention, and a preintervention mean of 7·8, an observed decrease of 25% corresponds to an estimated true decrease of 19%, while an observed decrease of 0% (no apparent change) corresponds to an estimated true decrease of 5%. In each case there is a shift towards the population mean change of 13%.

The authors conclude that the monitoring of changes in cholesterol levels should play only a limited role in patient management, and that interpretation of such changes should take account of regression to the mean. They argue also that the recommended threshold of 5·2 mmol/l is too low since it is likely to be exceeded by the population mean. Many individuals with single measurements below the threshold, who may for that reason receive reassuring advice, may nevertheless have true values above the threshold.

6: The Planning of Statistical Investigations

6.1 General

Statistical investigations—those in which observations are made on groups of individuals—are made necessary by the presence of random variation. If all patients suffering from the common cold experienced well-defined symptoms for precisely 7 days, it might be possible to demonstrate the merits of a purported drug for the alleviation of symptoms by administering it to one patient only. If the symptoms lasted only 5 days, the reduction could safely be attributed to the new treatment. Similarly, if blood pressure were an exact function of age, varying neither from person to person nor between occasions on the same person, the blood pressure at age 55 could be determined by one observation only. Such studies would not be statistical in nature and would not call for statistical analysis. This situation, of course, does not hold. The duration of symptoms from the common cold varies from one attack to another; blood pressures vary both between individuals and between occasions. Comparisons of the effects of different medical treatments must therefore be made on groups of patients; studies of physiological norms require population surveys.

In the planning of a statistical study a number of administrative and technical problems are likely to arise. These will be characteristic of the particular field of research and cannot be discussed fully in the present general context. Two aspects of the planning will almost invariably be present and are of particular concern to the statistician. The investigator will wish the inferences from the study to be sufficiently precise and will also wish the results to be relevant to the questions being asked. Discussions of the statistical design of investigation are concerned especially with the general considerations that bear on these two objectives. Some of the questions that arise are (i) how to select the individuals on which observations are to be made, (ii) how to decide on the numbers of observations falling into different groups, and (iii) how to allocate observations between different possible categories of individuals, such as groups of animals receiving different treatments or groups of people living in different areas.

It is useful to make a conceptual distinction between two different types of statistical investigation, the *experiment* and the *survey*. Experimentation involves a planned interference with the natural course of events so that its effect can be observed. In a survey, on the other hand, the investigator is a more passive observer, interfering as little as possible with the phenomena to be recorded. It is easy to think of extreme examples to illustrate this antithesis, but in practice the distinction is sometimes hard to draw. Consider, for instance, the following series of statistical studies.

1   A survey of the types of motor vehicle passing a checkpoint during a certain period.

2   A public opinion poll.

3   A study of the respiratory function (as measured by various tests) of men working in a certain industry.

4   Observations of the survival times of mice of three different strains after inoculation with the same dose of a toxic substance.

5   A clinical trial to compare the merits of surgery and conservative treatment for patients with a certain condition, the subjects being allotted randomly to the two treatments.

Studies **1** to **3** are clearly surveys, although they involve an increasing amount of interference with nature. Study **5** is equally clearly an experiment. Study **4** occupies an equivocal position. In its statistical aspects it is conceptually a survey, since the object is to observe and compare certain characteristics of three strains of mice. It happens, though, that the characteristic of interest requires the most extreme form of interference—the death of the animal—and the non-statistical techniques involved are more akin to those of a laboratory experiment than to those required in most survey work.

In the next two sections we discuss some of the general principles of the planning of surveys and follow with a discussion of the principles of experimental design.

6.2 The planning of surveys: estimation of population parameters

It is useful to distinguish between *descriptive surveys*, designed to provide esti-mates of some simple characteristics of populations, and *analytical surveys*, designed to investigate associations between certain variables. Examples of the first type are surveys to estimate the prevalence of some illness in a population or the frequency distribution of medical consultations during a certain period. An example of the second type would be a study of the association between the use of a certain drug and the occurrence of a particular adverse effect. The distinction is by no means clear-cut. In a population survey we may be interested also in associations—for example, that between the prevalence of an illness and a per-son's age. Conversely, in an association survey it would be quite reasonable to regard the association in question as a population parameter and to enquire how it varies from one population to another. Nevertheless, in population surveys the main emphasis is on the provision of reliable estimates of the features of a well-defined population; in analytical surveys (to be considered further in §6.3) the definition of the population is less important than the relationship between the variables.

Statistical interest in population surveys arises primarily when these are carried out by sampling methods. Some surveys are, of course, performed by complete enumeration; population censuses are familiar examples. The advantages of sampling lie in the economy of cost, manpower and time. Any of these factors may make complete enumeration out of the question. Furthermore, as noted in §3.1, the smaller scale of a sampling enquiry may permit more reliable observations to be made.

In §3.1 the concept of a sampling frame was introduced and a case was made for some form of random sampling rather than a form of purposive selection such as quota sampling. Simple random sampling, in fact, has formed the model for all the basic results of sampling theory. Some alternative forms of random sampling must now be discussed.

Systematic sampling

When the units or individuals in the population are listed or otherwise ordered in a systematic fashion, it may be convenient to arrange that the units chosen in any one sample occupy related positions in the sampling frame, the first unit being selected at random. For example, in drawing a sample of 1 in 50 of the entries in a card index, the first card may be selected by choosing a number at random from 1 to 50, after which every 50th card would be included. If the initial selection was 39 the selected cards would be those occupying positions 39, 89, 139, 189, . . ., etc. This is called a *systematic sample*. Another example might arise in two-dimensional sampling. Suppose a health survey is to be conducted in geographical units determined by a rectangular grid. If, say, 1 in 25 units are to be selected, the initial 'vertical' and 'horizontal' co-ordinates could be chosen at random, each from the numbers 1 to 5. If the initial random numbers were 5 and 3, the selected units would have the positions shown on p. 178 (the first number being the 'vertical' position and the second the 'horizontal' position).

Systematic sampling is often at least as precise as random sampling. It is particularly dangerous, though, if the ordering of the units in the sampling frame imposes a positive correlation between units whose distance apart is equal to the sampling interval. In the geographical example above, if there were a series of populated valleys running east to west about five sampling units apart, the chosen units might almost all be rather heavily populated or almost all lightly populated. The sampling error of the method would therefore be unusually high. In general it will be difficult to estimate the sampling error from a single systematic sample unless it is assumed that such correlations do not exist and that the sample can therefore be regarded as effectively random. One useful device is to choose

$$\ldots (5,3) \ldots \quad (5,8) \ldots \quad (5,13) \ldots$$

$$\ldots (10,3) \ldots \quad (10,8) \ldots \quad (10,13) \ldots$$

$$\ldots (15,3) \ldots \quad (15,8) \ldots \quad (15,13) \ldots$$

simultaneously several systematic samples by different choices of the starting-point. A mean value or other relevant statistic could then be worked out separately for each systematic sample, and the sampling variance of the overall mean obtained by the usual formula in terms of the variance of the separate means.

Stratified sampling

In this method the population is divided into subgroups, or *strata*, each of which is sampled randomly with a known sample size. Suppose that we wish to estimate the mean value of a certain variable in the population and that strata are defined so that the mean varies considerably from one stratum to another. In simple random sampling the distribution of observations over the strata will vary from sample to sample, and this lack of control will contribute to the variability of the sample mean. In contrast, in repeated sampling with the *same* distribution over the strata this component of variability is irrelevant.

Strata may be defined qualitatively; for example, in a national health survey different regions of the country may be taken as strata. Or they may be defined in terms of one or more quantitative variables, for example as age groups. The fraction of the stratum to be sampled may be constant or it may vary from stratum to stratum. The important points are (i) that the distribution of both the population and the sample over the strata should be known, and (ii) that the between-strata variability should be as high as possible, or equivalently that each stratum should be as homogeneous as possible.

Suppose there are k strata and that in the ith stratum the population size is N_i, and the mean and variance of variable x are μ_i and σ_i^2. A random sample of size n_i is taken from the ith stratum; the sampling fraction n_i/N_i will be denoted by f_i. The sample mean and estimate of variance in the ith stratum are $\bar{x}_i$ and s_i^2. The total population size is

$$N = \sum_{i=1}^{k} N_i,$$

and the total sample size is

$$n = \sum_{i=1}^{k} n_i.$$

The mean value of x in the whole population is clearly

$$\mu = \frac{\sum N_i \mu_i}{N}.$$

The appropriate estimate of μ is

$$\hat{\mu} = \frac{\sum N_i \bar{x}_i}{N}, \tag{6.1}$$

which is easily seen to be unbiased. (Since $E(\bar{x}_i) = \mu_i$, $E(\hat{\mu}) = \sum N_i \mu_i / N = \mu$.) The variance of $\hat{\mu}$ is

$$\text{var}(\hat{\mu}) = \frac{1}{N^2} \sum N_i^2 \, \text{var}(\bar{x}_i)$$

$$= \frac{1}{N^2} \sum \frac{N_i^2 \sigma_i^2}{n_i} (1 - f_i) \tag{6.2}$$

by (3.2), and this may be estimated from the sample as

$$\text{var}(\hat{\mu}) = \frac{1}{N^2} \sum \frac{N_i^2 s_i^2}{n_i} (1 - f_i). \tag{6.3}$$

If all the f_i are small, the terms $1 - f_i$ may be replaced by unity. In general (6.2) will be smaller than the variance of the mean of a random sample because the terms σ_i^2 measure only the variability within strata. Variability between the μ_i is irrelevant.

If n is fixed and the f_i are small, $\text{var}(\hat{\mu})$ becomes a minimum if the n_i are chosen to be as nearly as possible proportional to $N_i \sigma_i$. Thus, if σ_i is constant from one stratum to another, the n_i should be chosen in proportion to N_i, i.e. the sampling fraction should be constant. Strata with relatively large σ_i have correspondingly increased sampling fractions. Usually, little will be known about the σ_i before the survey is carried out and the choice of a constant sampling fraction will be the most reasonable strategy.

If the survey is designed to estimate a proportion, π, the above formulae hold with $\bar{x}_i$ and μ_i replaced by p_i and π_i, the observed and true proportions in the ith stratum, σ_i^2 by $\pi_i(1 - \pi_i)$ and s_i^2 by $n_i p_i(1 - p_i)/(n_i - 1)$ (this being the estimate of variance in a sample of size n_i in which $n_i p_i$ observations are 1 and $n_i(1 - p_i)$ are 0).

Apart from the increased precision in the estimation of the population mean, stratification may be adopted to provide reasonably precise estimates of the means for each of the strata. This may lead to departures from the optimal allocation described above so that none of the sample sizes in the separate strata become too small.

Example 6.1

It is desired to estimate the prevalence of a certain condition (i.e. the proportion of affected individuals) in a population of 5000 people by taking a sample of size 100. Suppose that the prevalence is known to be associated with age and that the population can be divided into three strata defined by age, with the following numbers of individuals:

Stratum, i	Age (years)	N_i
1	0–14	1200
2	15–44	2200
3	45–	1600
		5000

Suppose that the true prevalences, π_i, in the different strata are as follows:

Stratum, i	π_i
1	0·02
2	0·08
3	0·15

It is easily verified that the overall prevalence, π ($= \sum N_i \pi_i / \sum N_i$), is 0·088. A simple random sample of size $n = 100$ would therefore give an estimate p with variance $(0·088)(0·912)/100 = 0·000803$.

For stratified sampling with optimal allocation the sample sizes in the strata should be chosen in proportion to $N_i \sqrt{[\pi_i(1 - \pi_i)]}$. The values of this quantity in the three strata are 168, 597 and 571, which are in the proportions 0·126, 0·447 and 0·427 respectively. The optimal sample sizes are, therefore, $n_1 = 12$, $n_2 = 45$ and $n_3 = 43$, or numbers very close to these (there being a little doubt about the effect of rounding to the nearest integer). Let us call this allocation A. This depends on the unknown π_i, and therefore could hardly be used in practice. If we knew very little about the likely variation in the π_i, we might choose the $n_i \propto N_i$, ignoring the effect of the changing standard deviation. This would give, for allocation B, $n_1 = 24$, $n_2 = 44$ and $n_3 = 32$. Thirdly, we might have some idea that the prevalence (and therefore the standard deviation) increased with age, and therefore adjust the allocation rather arbitrarily to give, say, $n_1 = 20$, $n_2 = 40$ and $n_3 = 40$ (allocation C).

The estimate $\hat{\pi}$ is, in each case, given by the formula equivalent to (6.1).

$$\hat{\pi} = \frac{\sum N_i p_i}{N},$$

where p_i is the estimated prevalence in the ith stratum. The variance of $\hat{\pi}$ is given by the equivalent of (6.2), in which we shall drop the terms f_i as being small:

$$\text{var}(\pi) = \frac{1}{N^2} \sum \frac{N_i^2 \pi_i(1 - \pi_i)}{n_i}.$$

The values of var($\hat{\pi}$) for the three allocations are as follows:

Allocation	var($\hat{\pi}$)
A	0·000714
B	0·000779
C	0·000739

As would be expected, the lowest variance is for A and the highest for B, the latter being only a little lower than the variance for a random sample.

Multistage sampling

In this method the sampling frame is divided into a population of 'first-stage sampling units', of which a 'first-stage' sample is taken. This will usually be a simple random sample, but may be a systematic or stratified sample; it may also, as we shall see, be a random sample in which some first-stage units are allowed to have a higher probability of selection than others. Each first-stage unit thus selected is subdivided into 'second-stage sampling units', which are sampled. The process can continue as long as is appropriate.

There are two main advantages of multistage sampling. First, it enables the resources to be concentrated in a limited number of portions of the whole sampling frame with a consequent reduction in cost. Secondly, it is convenient for situations in which a complete sampling frame is not available before the investigation starts. A list of first-stage units is required, but the second-stage units need be listed only within the first-stage units selected in the sample.

Consider as an example a health survey of men working in a certain industry. There would probably not exist a complete index of all men in the industry, but it might be easy to obtain a list of factories, which could be first-stage units. From each factory selected in the first-stage sample a list of men could be obtained, and a second-stage sample selected from this list. Apart from the advantage of having to make lists of men only within the factories selected at the first stage, this procedure would result in an appreciable saving in cost by enabling the investigation to be concentrated at selected factories instead of necessitating the examination of a sample of men all in different parts of the country.

The economy in cost and resources is unfortunately accompanied by a loss of precision as compared with simple random sampling. Suppose that in the example discussed above we take a sample of 20 factories and second-stage samples of 50 men in each of the 20 factories. If there is systematic variation between the factories, due perhaps to variation in health conditions in different parts of the country or to differing occupational hazards, this variation will be represented by a sample of only 20 first-stage units. A random sample of 1000 men, on the other hand, would represent 1000 random choices of first-stage units (some of which may, of course, be chosen more than once) and would consequently provide a better estimate of the national mean.

A useful device in two-stage sampling is called *self-weighting*. Each first-stage unit is given a probability of selection which is proportional to the number of second-stage units it contains. Second-stage samples are then chosen to have equal size. It follows that each second-stage unit in the whole population has an equal chance of being selected and the formulae needed for estimation are somewhat simplified.

Sometimes, in the final stage of sampling, complete enumeration of the available units is undertaken. In the industrial example, once a survey team has installed itself in a factory it may cost little extra to examine all the men in the factory; it may indeed be useful to avoid the embarrassment that might be caused by inviting some men but not others to participate.

Other considerations

The planning, conduct and analysis of sample surveys give rise to many problems that cannot be discussed here. The books by Moser and Kalton (1971) and Yates (1981) contain excellent discussions of the practical aspects of sampling. Applications to morbidity surveys and public health investigations are described briefly in a report by the World Health Organization (1966). The books by Cochran (1977) and Yates (1981) may be consulted for the main theoretical results.

The statistical theory of sample surveys is concerned largely with the measurement of sampling error. This emphasis may lead the investigator to overlook the importance of non-sampling errors. In a large survey the sampling errors may be so small that systematic non-sampling errors may be much the more important. Indeed, in a complete enumeration, such as a complete population census, sampling errors disappear altogether, but there may be very serious non-sampling errors.

Some non-sampling errors are non-systematic, causing no bias on the average. An example would be random inaccuracy in the reading of a test instrument. These errors merely contribute to the variability of the observation in question and therefore diminish the precision of the survey. Other errors are systematic, causing a bias in a mean value which does not decrease with increasing sample size: for example, in a health survey certain types of illness may be systematically under-reported.

One of the most important types of systematic error is that due to inadequate coverage of the sampling frame, either because of non-cooperation by the individual or because the investigator finds it difficult to make the correct observations. For example, in an interview survey some people may refuse to be interviewed and others may be hard to find or may have moved away from the supposed address or even have died. Individuals who are missed for any of these reasons are likely to be atypical of the population in various relevant respects. Every effort must therefore be made to include the chosen individuals in the enquiry, by persistent attempts to make the relevant observations on all the non-responders or by concentrating on a subsample of them so that the characteristics of the non-responders can at least be estimated.

Reference must finally be made to another important type of study, the *longitudinal survey*. Many investigations are concerned with the changes in certain measurements over a period of time: for example, the growth and development of children over a 10-year period, or the changes in blood pressure during pregnancy. It is desirable where possible to study each individual over the relevant period of time rather than to take different samples of individuals at different points of time. Some of the statistical problems are discussed by Goldstein (1979).

6.3 Surveys to investigate associations

A question commonly asked in epidemiological investigations into the aetiology of disease is whether some manifestation of ill health is associated with certain personal characteristics or habits, with particular aspects of the environment in which a person has lived, or with certain experiences which he has undergone. Examples of such questions are the following.

1 Is the risk of death from lung cancer related to the degree of cigarette smoking, whether current or in previous years?

2 Is the risk that a child dies from acute leukaemia related to whether or not the mother experienced irradiation during pregnancy?

3 Is the risk of incurring a certain illness increased for individuals who were treated with a particular drug during a previous illness?

Sometimes questions like these can be answered by controlled experimentation in which the presumptive personal factor can be administered or withheld at the investigator's discretion; in example **3**, for instance it might be possible for the investigator to give the drug in question to some patients and not to others and to compare the outcomes. In such cases the questions are concerned with causative effects: 'Is this drug a partial *cause* of this illness?' More often, however, the experimental approach is out of the question. The investigator must then be satisfied to observe whether there is an *association* between factor and disease and to take the risk which was emphasized in §5.1 if he or she wishes to infer a causative link.

These questions, then, will usually be studied by surveys rather than by experiments. The precise population to be surveyed is not usually of primary interest here. One reason is that in epidemiological surveys it is usually administratively impossible to study a national or regional population, even on a sample basis. The investigator may, however, have facilities to study a particular occupational group or a population geographically related to a particular medical centre. Secondly, although the mean values or relative frequencies of the different variables may vary somewhat from one population to another, the magnitude and direction of the associations between variables are unlikely to vary greatly between, say, different occupational groups or different geographical populations.

There are two main designs for aetiological surveys—the *case–control* study, sometimes known as a *case–referent* study, and the *cohort* study. In a case–control study a group of individuals affected by the disease in question is compared with a control group of unaffected individuals. Information is obtained, usually in a retrospective way, about the frequency in each group of the various environmental or personal factors which might be associated with the disease. This type of survey is convenient in the study of rare conditions which would appear too seldom in a random population sample. By starting with a group of affected individuals one is effectively taking a much higher sampling fraction of the cases than of the controls. The method is appropriate also when the classification by disease is simple (particularly for a dichotomous classification into the presence or absence of a specific condition), but in which many possible aetiological factors have to be studied. A further advantage of the method is that, by means of the retrospective enquiry, the relevant information can be obtained comparatively quickly.

In a cohort study a population of individuals, selected usually by geographical or occupational criteria rather than on medical grounds, is studied either by complete enumeration or by a representative sample. The population is classified by the factor or factors of interest and followed prospectively in time so that the rates of occurrence of various manifestations of disease can be observed and related to the classifications by aetiological factors. The prospective nature of the cohort study means that it will normally extend longer in time than the case–control study and is likely to be administratively more complex. The corresponding advantages are that many medical conditions can be studied simultaneously and that direct information is obtained about the health of each subject through an interval of time.

Case–control and cohort studies are often called respectively *retrospective* and *prospective* studies. These latter terms are usually appropriate, but the nomenclature may occasionally be misleading since a cohort study may be based entirely on retrospective records. For example, if medical records are available of workers in a certain factory for the past 30 years, a cohort study may relate to workers employed 30 years ago and be based on records of their health in the succeeding 30 years. Such a study is sometimes called a *historical prospective study*.

A central problem in a case–control study is the method by which the controls are chosen. Ideally, they should be on average similar to the cases in all respects except in the medical condition under study and in associated aetiological factors.

Cases will often be selected from one or more hospitals and will then share the characteristics of the population using those hospitals, such as social and environmental conditions or ethnic features. It will usually be desirable to select the control group from the same area or areas, perhaps even from the same hospitals, but suffering from quite different illnesses unlikely to share the same aetiological factors. Further, the frequencies with which various factors are found will usually vary with age and sex. Comparisons between the case and control groups must, therefore, take account of any differences there may be in the age and sex distributions of the two groups. Such adjustments are commonly avoided by arranging that each affected individual is paired with a control individual who is deliberately chosen to be of the same age and sex and to share any other demographic features which may be thought to be similarly relevant.

The remarks made in §6.2 about non-sampling errors, particularly those about non-response, are relevant also in aetiological surveys. Non-responses are always a potential danger and every attempt should be made to reduce them to as low a proportion as possible.

In a cohort study in which the incidence of a specific disease is of particular interest, the case–control approach may be adopted by choosing, for each new case, a control group of randomly selected non-cases. In this approach, termed by Mantel (1973) a *synthetic retrospective study*, care may be needed to avoid the repeated selection of the same individuals as controls for more than one case (Robins *et al.*, 1989).

Example 6.2

Doll and Hill (1950) reported the results of a retrospective study of the aetiology of lung cancer. A group of 709 patients with carcinoma of the lung in 20 hospitals was compared with a control group of 709 patients without carcinoma of the lung and a third group of 637 patients with carcinoma of the stomach, colon or rectum. For each patient with lung cance a control patient was selected from the same hospital, of the same sex and within the same 5-year age group. Each patient in each group was interviewed by a social worker, all interviewers using the same questionnaire.

The only substantial differences between the case and control groups were in their reported smoking habits. Some of the findings are summarized in Table 6.1. The difference in the proportion of non-smokers in the two groups is clearly significant, at any rate for males. (If a significance test for data of this form were required, an appropriate method would be the test for the difference of two paired proportions, described in §4.8.) The group of patients with other forms of cancer had similar smoking histories to those of the control group and differed markedly from the lung cancer group. The comparisons involving this third group are more complicated because the individual patients were not paired with members of the lung cancer or control groups and had a somewhat different age distribution. The possible effect of age had to be allowed for by methods of age standardization (see §12.9).

Table 6.1 Recent tobacco consumption of patients with carcinoma of the lung and control patients without carcinoma of the lung (Doll and Hill, 1950)

| | | Daily consumption of cigarettes | | | | | |
	Non-smoker	1–	5–	15–	25–	50–	Total
Male							
Lung carcinoma	2	33	250	196	136	32	649
Control	27	55	293	190	71	13	649
Female							
Lung carcinoma	19	7	19	9	6	0	60
Control	32	12	10	6	0	0	60

This paper by Doll and Hill is an excellent illustration of the care which should be taken to avoid bias due to unsuspected differences between case and control groups or to different standards of data recording. This study and many others like it strongly suggest an association between smoking and the risk of incurring lung cancer. In such retrospective studies, however, there is room for argument about the propriety of a particular choice of control group; little information is obtained about the time relationships involved, and nothing is known about the association between smoking and diseases other than those selected for study. Doll and Hill (1954, 1956, 1964) carried out a cohort study prospectively by sending questionnaires to all the 59 600 doctors in the United Kingdom in October, 1951. Adequate replies were received from 68·2% of the population (34 440 men and 6197 women). These doctors were followed for 20 years and notifications of deaths from various causes were obtained, only 103 being untraced (Doll and Peto, 1976). Some results for male doctors are shown in Table 6.2. The groups defined by different smoking categories have different age distributions, and the death rates shown in the table have again been standardized for age (§12.9). Cigarette smoking is again shown to be associated with a sharp increase in the death rate from lung cancer, and also shows a less marked association with the death rates from several other causes.

Table 6.2 Standardized annual death rates among male doctors for three causes of death, related to smoking habits (Doll and Peto, 1976)

| | | Standardized death rate per 100 000 men | | | | | |
| | | | | | Current smokers (g per day) | | |
	Number of deaths	Non-smokers	Ex-smokers	Current smokers	1–14	15–24	25–
Lung cancer	441	10	43	104	52	106	224
Chronic bronchitis and emphysema	254	3	44	50	38	50	88
Ischaemic heart disease	3191	413	533	565	501	598	677

This prospective study provides strong evidence that the association between smoking and lung cancer is causative. Many doctors who smoked at the outset of the study stopped smoking during the follow-up period, and by 1971 doctors were smoking less than half as much as people of the same ages in the general population. The death rate from lung cancer for the whole group of male doctors (age-standardized, and expressed as a fraction of the national mortality rate) fell steadily over the 20-year period of follow-up.

The measurement of the degree of association between the risk of disease and the presence of an aetiological factor is discussed in detail in §16.2.

6.4 The design of experiments

We consider now the planning of experiments to compare the effects of various treatments on some type of experimental units. The treatment to be applied to any particular unit is to be decided by the investigator. The following are examples.

1 A comparison of the effects of inoculating animals with different doses of a chemical substance. The units here will be the animals.

2 A prophylactic trial to compare the effectiveness for children of different vaccines against measles. Each child will receive one of the vaccines and may be regarded as the experimental unit.

3 A comparison in one patient suffering recurrent attacks of a chronic disease of different methods of alleviating discomfort. The successive occasions on which attacks occur are now the units for which the choice of treatment is to be made.

4 A study of the relative merits of different programmes of community health education. Each programme would be applied in a different area, and these areas would form the experimental units.

In all such examples a crucial question is how the treatments are to be allotted to the available units. One would clearly wish to avoid any serious disparity between the characteristics of units receiving different treatments. In example **2**, for instance, it would be dangerous to give one vaccine to all the children in one school and another vaccine to all the children in a second school, for the exposure of the two groups of children to measles contacts might be quite different. It would then be difficult to decide whether a difference in the incidence of measles was due to different protective powers of the vaccines or to the different degrees of exposure to infection.

It would be possible to arrange that the groups of experimental units to which different treatments were to be applied were made alike in various relevant respects. For example, in **1**, groups of animals with approximately the same mean weight could be formed; in **2**, children from different schools and of different age groups could be represented equally in each treatment group. But, however careful the investigator is to balance factors which seem important, one can never be sure that the treatment groups do not differ markedly in some factor which is also important but which has been ignored in the allocation.

The accepted solution to this dilemma is that advocated by Fisher in the 1920s and 1930s: the allocation should incorporate an element of *randomization*. In its simplest form this means that the choice of treatment for each unit should be made by an independent act of randomization such as the toss of a coin or the use of random-number tables. This would lead to some uncertainty in the numbers of units finally allotted to each treatment, and if these are fixed in advance the groups may be formed by choosing random samples of the appropriate sizes from the total pool of experimental units. More detailed instructions in the use of random-number tables are given on p. 576.

In clinical trials the total number of patients is often not known in advance since many patients may become available for inclusion in the trial some time after it has started. The simplest method is then to allocate treatment by an independent random choice for each patient. A method by which the numbers allocated to different treatments are kept close together, called *restricted randomization* or *permuted blocks*, is described on p. 576.

Sometimes a form of *systematic allocation*, analogous to systematic sampling, is used as an alternative to random allocation. The units are arranged in a certain order and are then allotted systematically to the treatment groups. In a clinical trial with serial entry, for example, an allocation to two treatment groups might be carried out by strict alternation. This method has much the same advantages and disadvantages as systematic sampling. It is likely to be seriously misleading only if the initial ordering of the units presents some systematic variation of a cyclic type which happens to run in phase with the allocation cycle. In clinical trials this is perhaps unlikely to happen, although if the allocation is systematic and therefore known to the investigator responsible for forming the serial index of patients, he/she may be influenced by this knowledge in deciding the ordering and thereby create a bias (see §6.5). Alternation and other forms of systematic allocation are best avoided in favour of strictly random methods.

A second important principle of experimental design is that of *replication*, the use of more than one experimental unit for each treatment. Various purposes are served by replication. First, an appropriate amount of replication ensures that the comparisons between treatments are sufficiently precise; the sampling error of the difference between two means, for instance, decreases as the amount of replication in each group increases. Secondly, the effect of sampling variation can be estimated only if there is an adequate degree of replication. In the comparison of the means of two groups, for instance, if both sample sizes were as low as two, the degrees of freedom in the t test would only be two (§4.4); the percentage points of t on two degrees of freedom are very high and the test therefore loses a great deal in effectiveness merely because of the inadequacy of the estimate of within-groups variance. Thirdly, replication may be useful in enabling observations to be spread over a wide variety of experimental conditions. In the comparison of two surgical procedures, for instance, it might be useful to organize a cooperative trial in which the methods were compared in each of a number of hospitals, so that the effects of variations in medical and surgical practice and perhaps in the precise type of disease could be studied.

A third basic principle concerns the reduction in random variability between experimental units. The formula for the standard error of a mean, $\sigma/\sqrt{n}$, shows that the effect of random error can be reduced, either by increasing n (more replication) or by decreasing σ. This suggests that experimental units should be as homogeneous as possible in their response to treatment. However, too strenuous an effort to remove heterogeneity will tend to counteract the third reason given above for replication—the desire to cover a wide range of extraneous conditions. In a clinical trial, for example, it may be that a precise comparison could be effected by restricting the age, sex, clinical condition and other features of the patients, but these restrictions may make it too difficult to generalize from the results. A useful solution to this dilemma is to subdivide the units into relatively homogeneous subgroups, called *blocks*. Treatments can then be allocated randomly within blocks so that each block provides a small experiment. The precision of the overall comparisons between treatments is then determined by the random variability *within* blocks rather than that *between* different blocks. This is called a *randomized block* design. More complex designs, allowing simultaneously for more than one source of extraneous variation, are discussed in Chapter 8. Other extensions dealt with in that chapter are designs for the simultaneous comparison of more than one set of treatments; those appropriate for situations similar to that of multistage sampling, in which some units are subdivisions of others; and designs which allow in various ways for the natural restrictions imposed by the experimental material.

Brief references have been made to an important class of controlled experiments—clinical and prophylactic trials. These exemplify most of the general features of experimentation, but also give rise to a number of special problems; they are therefore discussed at greater length in the next section.

6.5 Clinical trials

Clinical trials are controlled experiments to compare the effectiveness, for patients, of different therapeutic measures. The term *clinical trial* is often used in a rather wider sense to include controlled trials of prophylactic measures on individuals who do not yet suffer from the disease under study, and for trials of administrative aspects of medical care, such as the choice of home or hospital care for a particular type of patient. Cochrane (1972), writing particularly about the latter category, uses the term *randomized controlled trial* (RCT). Trials intended as authoritative research studies, with random assignment, are referred to as

Phase III. In drug development, *Phase I* studies are early dose-ranging projects, often with normal volunteers. *Phase II* trials are small screening studies on patients, designed to select agents sufficiently promising to warrant the setting up of larger Phase III trials. *Phase IV* studies are concerned with postmarketing surveillance, and normally take the form of surveys rather than comparative trials.

Clinical and prophylactic trials, strictly controlled by random allocation, date from the mid-1940s. Many of the pioneering collaborative trials organized by the Medical Research Council are reported in Hill (1962). Any proposal for a clinical trial must be carefully scrutinized from an ethical point of view, for no doctor will allow a patient under his or her care to be given a treatment believed to be clearly inferior, unless the condition being treated is extremely mild. There are many situations, though, where the relative merits of rival treatments are by no means clear. Doctors may then agree to random allocation, at least until the issues are resolved. The possibility that the gradual accumulation of data may modify the investigator's ethical stance may lead to the adoption of a *sequential* design (Chapter 15).

The organization of a clinical trial requires careful advance planning. This is particularly so for multicentre trials, which have become increasingly common in the study of chronic diseases, where large numbers of patients are often required, and of other conditions occurring too rarely for one centre to provide enough cases. The aims and methods of the trial should be described in some detail, in a document usually called a *protocol*. This will contain many medical or administrative details specific to the problem under study. It should include clear statements about the types of patient to be admitted, and define precisely the therapeutic measures to be used. The number of patients, the intended duration of the intake and (where appropriate) the length of follow-up should be stated; some relevant methods are described in §6.6. It is not possible to cover here all aspects of the planning and execution of a trial; reference may be made to Hill and Hill (1991, Chapter 23), Schwartz *et al.* (1980), Friedman *et al.* (1985), Shapiro and Louis (1983), Pocock (1983) and Buyse *et al.* (1984). One or two points, though, deserve special attention. The following discussion is directed towards therapeutic trials, although most of the points are equally applicable in the context of trials in preventive medicine or medical care.

Definition of patients

The broad category of disease under study will usually be clear at a very early stage of planning. The fine detail may be less clear. Should the sex and age of the patients be restricted? Should the severity of the disease be narrowly defined? Should patients with certain associated conditions be excluded? These criteria for eligibility must be considered afresh for each trial, but the point made on p. 189, in the discussion on replication, should be borne in mind. It is usually wise to lean in the direction of permissiveness. Not only will this increase the number of patients (provided that the resources needed for their inclusion are available), but it will also permit treatment comparisons to be made separately for different categories of patient. The admission of a broad spectrum of patients in no way prevents their division into more homogeneous subgroups for analysis of the results. However, comparisons based on small subgroups are less likely to detect real differences between treatment effects than tests based on the whole set of data. There is, moreover, the danger that, if too many comparisons are made in different subgroups, one or more of the tests may easily give a significant result purely by chance (see the comments on 'data-dredging' in §7.4). Any subgroups with an a priori claim to attention should therefore be defined in the protocol, and consideration given to them in planning the size of the trial.

Definition of treatments

Again, the therapeutic regimens to be compared are usually known in broad terms from the outset. Should they be defined and standardized down to the last detail? In a multicentre trial different centres may wish to adopt minor variants of the same broad regimen, or to use different concomitant therapy. It will often be better to allow these variations to enter the study, particularly when they are commonly found in medical practice, rather than to introduce a degree of standardization which may not be widely accepted either during the trial or subsequently.

With many therapeutic measures, it is common practice to vary the detailed schedule according to the patient's condition. The dose of a drug, for instance, may depend on therapeutic response or on side-effects. In trials of such treatments there is a strong case for maintaining flexibility; many trials have been criticized after completion, on the grounds that the treatment regimens were unduly rigid.

Assessment of response

The relative merits of the treatments will be compared by measuring one or more responses for each patient at some time(s) after start of treatment. These may be symptoms reported by the patient, signs elicited by the doctor or technical measurements such as biochemical test results. It is often possible that the response measurement could be influenced by a knowledge of which treatment was used, by either the patient, the doctor or any technical assistant involved in the measurement. If no precautions were taken, serious biases might arise. Spurious differences might appear between treatments which were really equally effective, or similar results might be obtained for treatments that really differed in their effect.

In a *single-blind* trial, the identity of the allocated treatment is concealed from the patient. A *double-blind* trial is one in which the doctor, or other technical expert, who assesses response is also unaware of the treatment identities. In drug trials masking is usually done by special formulations of the drugs. Of course, some drugs produce characteristic side-effects which cannot effectively be hidden from the doctor or indeed from a well-informed patient. If the trial is designed to assess the effectiveness of a particular drug in comparison with the absence of the drug, there may be a difference in response which is quite unspecific—due to doing something rather than nothing. An effective control is often provided by a *placebo*—an inert preparation formulated to appear indistinguishable from the supposedly active agent.

Entry and treatment allocation

As already mentioned, the protocol will define the criteria for eligibility of patients for admission to the trial. It may be useful for each centre to keep a log of all patients considered for admission—for example, all patients with the disease in question—to show the extent to which the patients in the trial have been selected from the whole patient population and (if further selection takes place) from the population satisfying the eligibility criteria.

An eligible patient should be admitted formally to the trial, by entry of his or her name into a register and the allocation of a serial number. As soon as possible afterwards, the random treatment allocation should be determined. It is important that the allocation should not be known before admission, since a knowledge or suspicion of the treatment to be used for the next patient may affect the investigator's decision whether or not to admit a particular patient whose entry is under consideration. This clearly precludes systematic allocation systems, and makes it important that future random allocations should in some way be hidden from the investigator. One should also avoid rigid coding systems, such as one in which an active drug is coded as X and the placebo as Y; with such a system if the code is broken for one patient it remains broken for the rest of the trial. It is often satisfactory to use sealed envelopes, bearing the serial number on the outside and containing the treatment allocation inside. In many multicentre trials allocation is made by a telephone call to a data centre where the randomization list is held.

This list should be prepared in advance. As mentioned in §6.4, restricted (permuted-block) randomization may be used, to ensure that the numbers allocated to different treatments keep close together. Such a scheme may be applied separately for each centre, and perhaps also within various subgroups (or *strata*) defined by variables of prognostic importance. Prognostic stratification should be kept to a minimum. It is not necessary to stratify by a large number of factors, since the effect of such variables can be allowed for in the subsequent analysis; in any case, if too many factors are used, many of the strata will be too small to permit adequate balancing of treatments. Indeed, many practitioners of clinical trials prefer not to stratify at all, relying on randomization to provide broad similarity between treatment groups and adjusting later for the effects of prognostic variables.

An alternative to permuted-block randomization, when groups need to be balanced simultaneously for several prognostic variables, is provided by various forms of *minimization*. The aim here is to assign patients in such a way as to minimize (in some sense) the current disparity between the groups, taking account simultaneously of a variety of prognostic variables. Minimization is best implemented with the aid of a computer. For further description see Pocock (1983, pp. 83–86).

Exclusions, withdrawals and protocol departures

After randomization, patients should rarely if ever be excluded from the trial. The chance of exclusion for a particular patient may depend on the treatment received, and to permit the removal of patients from the trial may impair the effectiveness of randomization and lead to biased comparisons.

A few patients may be discovered to contravene the eligibility criteria after randomization: they should be omitted only if it is quite clear that no bias is involved—for example when diagnostic tests have been performed before randomization but the results do not become available until later.

A more serious source of difficulty is the occurrence of departures from the therapeutic procedures laid down in the protocol. Every attempt should be made to encourage participants to follow the protocol meticulously, and types of patients (such as the very old) who could be identified in advance as liable to cause protocol departures should have been excluded by the eligibility criteria. Nevertheless, some departures are almost inevitable, and they may well include withdrawal of the allotted treatment and substitution of an alternative, or defection of the patient from the investigator's care. It would be quite wrong to exclude such cases from the groups to which they were allocated. They are almost certain to be atypical of the whole population, and some forms of protocol departure may well be more likely to arise with one treatment than with another. Moreover, the question being posed in the trial is essentially the comparison of one strategy against another—the strategies of using particular therapeutic regimens where possible, with the realization that departures will necessarily occur in individual patients. The protocol departures are, from this *pragmatic* point of view (Schwartz and Lellouch, 1967), as much a part of the whole treatment policy as are the cases in which the ideal regimen can be maintained.

It is similarly dangerous to omit from the analysis of trials any events or other responses occurring during specified periods after the start of treatment. It may, for example, be thought that a drug cannot take effect before at least a week has elapsed, and that therefore any adverse events occurring during the first week can be discounted. These events should be omitted only if the underlying assumption is universally accepted; otherwise, the possibility of bias again arises. Similarly, adverse events (such as accidental deaths) believed to be unrelated to the disease in question should be omitted only if their irrelevance is beyond dispute (and this is rarely so for accidental deaths!).

The policy of including in the analysis, where possible, all patients in the groups to which they were randomly assigned, is called the *intent(ion)-to-treat* approach. Difficulties will arise if patients have withdrawn from the study before the relevant response can be measured. In trials for which mortality is the major criterion of response, it may be possible to determine each patient's survival status at a specified interval after entry into the trial, from a national death registration system. In other trials, in which the crucial clinical responses are measured at follow-up examinations, there may inevitably be some missing readings. There are no completely satisfactory solutions to this problem. One approach is to carry forward the last available response on each patient. Another is to assign some arbitrarily poor score to the missing response. Brown (1992), for instance, suggests assigning a score equal to the median response observed in a placebo group, and then grouping into one broad response category patients in all groups with that score or worse. Treatment groups may then be compared by the Mann–Whitney test (§13.3). Devices of this type may be useful, even unavoidable, if crucial responses are missing, but they involve the sacrifice of information, and estimation may be biased. The best solution is to avoid withdrawals as far as possible by careful advance planning.

Meta-analysis: overviews

With the recent proliferation of clinical trials it has become increasingly common to find that several trials have been conducted with closely related protocols. The trials are unlikely to be exact replicates: the agents under test may be administered in different ways or at different dosages, or may be different although related substances; the patients will fall into the same broad disease category, but admission criteria such as age or severity of disease may vary. In these situations, treatment comparisons will not be identical from one trial to another, but they may be expected to be similar. The results of any one trial may have too much random error to give a clear indication of the relative efficacy of treatments, whereas the whole data set may present a coherent picture, with a more precise estimate of treatment effect because of the increased sample size.

Studies combining data from related trials are called *meta-analyses* or *over-views*. Some examples are overviews of beta blockade in myocardial infarction

(Yusuf *et al.*, 1985); antiplatelet treatment in vascular disease (Antiplatelet Trialists' Collaboration, 1988); and hormonal, cytotoxic or immune therapy for early breast cancer (Early Breast Cancer Trialists' Collaborative Group, 1992).

Some statistical methods useful for overviews are described in §7.2. One general point is that the data from different trials must not be pooled before treatment comparisons are made. Each trial is a 'block', in the sense of §6.4. Treatment contrasts are made separately for each trial, examined for consistency between trials, and then pooled to provide an overall estimate of a treatment effect.

Care must be taken to ensure that the selection of studies does not introduce bias. It may, for instance, be important to include unpublished as well as published data, since trials showing clear evidence of treatment effects are more likely to be published than those showing no such evidence (a phenomenon known as *publication bias*). For further discussion of the principles underlying overviews, see for instance the papers in Yusuf *et al.* (1987) and also Chalmers *et al.* (1987).

Equivalence testing

In some clinical studies the aim is not to detect possible differences in efficacy, but rather to show that treatments are, within certain narrow limits, equally effective. This situation arises particularly in Phase I studies conducted within the pharmaceutical industry. These *equivalence studies* may concern the serum levels produced by different formulations of the same active agent, or they may involve clinical responses to closely related drugs.

In an equivalence study, a test of the null hypothesis of equal efficacy is irrelevant, for a test with too few observations will be unable to exclude possibly important differences. Suppose the relevant difference in efficacy is measured by a parameter θ, taking the value zero when the treatments are equally effective. It is necessary to define two tolerance limits $\theta_L < 0$ and $\theta_U > 0$, the interval between which is the range of equivalence. The investigator will be in a position to claim equivalence if it can be asserted that $\theta > \theta_L$ and also that $\theta < \theta_U$. These latter assertions would need to be confirmed by standard significance tests against the two tolerance limits, or equivalently by observing that the appropriate confidence interval for θ lies wholly within the range of equivalence (if one-sided tests against the tolerance limits are at, say, the 5% level, the equivalent confidence coefficient has to be 90%).

6.6 The size of a statistical investigation

One of the questions most commonly asked about the planning of a statistical study, and one of the most difficult to answer, is: how many observations should be made? Other things being equal, the greater the sample size or the larger the experiment, the more precise will be the estimates of the parameters and their differences. The difficulty lies in deciding what degree of precision to aim for. An increase in the size of a survey or of an experiment costs more money and takes more time. Sometimes a limit is imposed by financial resources or by the time available, and the investigator will wish to make as many observations as the resources permit, allowing in the budget for the time and cost of the processing and analysis of the data. In other situations there will be no obvious limit, and the investigator will have to balance the benefits of increased precision against the cost of increased data collection or experimentation. In some branches of technology the whole problem can be looked at from a purely economic point of view, but this will rarely be possible in medical research since the benefit of experimental or survey information is so difficult to measure financially.

In any review of these problems at the planning stage it is likely to be important to relate the sample size to a specified degree of precision. We shall consider first the problem of comparing the means of two populations, μ_1 and μ_2, assuming that they have the same known standard deviation, σ, and that two equal random samples of size n are to be taken. If the standard deviations are known to be different the present results may be thought of as an approximation (taking σ^2 to be the mean of the two variances). If the comparison is of two proportions, π_1 and π_2, σ may be taken approximately to be the pooled value

$$\sqrt{\{\tfrac{1}{2}[\pi_1(1 - \pi_1) + \pi_2(1 - \pi_2)]\}}.$$

We now consider three ways in which the precision may be specified.

1   *Given standard error.* Suppose it is required that the standard error of the difference between the observed means, $\bar{x}_1 - \bar{x}_2$, is less than ε; equivalently the width of the 95% confidence intervals might be specified to be not wider than $\pm 2\varepsilon$. This implies

$$\sigma\sqrt{(2/n)} < \varepsilon$$

or

$$n > 2\sigma^2/\varepsilon^2. \qquad (6.4)$$

If the requirement is that the standard error of the mean of one sample shall be less than ε, the corresponding inequality for n is

$$n > \sigma^2/\varepsilon^2. \qquad (6.5)$$

2   *Given difference to be significant.* We might require that if $\bar{x}_1 - \bar{x}_2$ is greater in absolute value than some value d_1, then it shall be significant at some specified level (say at a two-sided 2α level). Denote by $z_{2\alpha}$ the standardized normal deviate exceeded (in either direction) with probability 2α; (for $2\alpha = 0\cdot05$, $z_{2\alpha} = 1\cdot96$). Then

$$d_1 > z_{2\alpha}\sigma\sqrt{(2/n)}$$

or

$$n > 2\left(\frac{z_{2\alpha}\sigma}{d_1}\right)^2. \tag{6.6}$$

3   *Given power against specified difference.* Criterion **2** is defined in terms of a given *observed* difference, d. The true difference, δ, may be either less or greater than d, and it seems preferable to base the requirement on the value of δ. It might be possible to specify a value of δ, say δ_1, which one did not wish to overlook, in the sense that if $\delta > \delta_1$ one would like to get a significant result at, say, the two-sided 2α level. However, a significant difference cannot be guaranteed. Sampling fluctuations may lead to a value of $|d|$ much less than $|\delta|$ and not significantly different from zero. The probability of this is denoted by β and referred to as the *Type II error*, that is the probability of failing to detect a real difference (false negative). The significance level is referred to as the *Type I error*, that is the probability of incorrectly rejecting the null hypothesis (false positive). Whilst the Type I error is controlled at a low value by choice of significance level during analysis, the Type II error can only be controlled at the design stage. One might specify that the Type II error be no greater than some low value, or equivalently that the probability of correctly detecting the difference as significant, $1 - \beta$, should be not less than some high value. This value is called the *power* of study.

   The situation is represented in Fig. 6.1. Positive values of d are significant at the stated level if

$$d > z_{2\alpha}\text{SE}(d), \tag{6.7}$$

that is, d is to the right of the point A. For a power $> 1 - \beta$ the point A must be to the left of a point cutting off a one-sided probability of β on the right-hand distribution. That is,

$$z_{2\alpha}\text{SE}(d) < \delta_1 - z_{2\beta}\text{SE}(d)$$

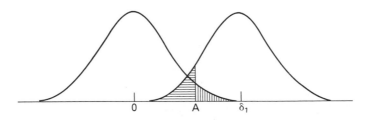

Fig. 6.1 Distributions of d; the left-hand distribution represents the null hypothesis and the right-hand distribution the alternative hypothesis. The vertically shaded area represents the significance level (Type I error) and the horizontally shaded area is the Type II error.

or

$$\delta_1 > (z_{2\alpha} + z_{2\beta})\,\text{SE}(d). \tag{6.8}$$

If d represents the difference, $\bar{x}_1 - \bar{x}_2$, of the means of a continuous variable between two independent groups each of size n then $\text{SE}(d) = \sigma\sqrt{(2/n)}$ and (6.8) becomes

$$n > 2\left[\frac{(z_{2\alpha} + z_{2\beta})\sigma}{\delta_1}\right]^2. \tag{6.9}$$

The distinction between **2** and **3** is important. For instance, if $2\alpha = 0.05$ and $1 - \beta = 0.95$, $z_{2\alpha} = 1.96$ and $z_{2\beta} = 1.64$. If d_1 is put equal to δ_1, the values of n given by (6.9) and (6.6) are thus in the ratio $(1.96 + 1.64)^2 : 1.96^2$ or $3.4 : 1$.

We have assumed, in both **2** and **3**, that the null hypothesis under test specifies a zero value for the true difference, δ. This is usually the case, but there are situations where the null hypothesis specifies a non-zero value, δ_0 for δ. In an equivalence test (§6.5), for instance, one might test against either of the two tolerance limits (θ_L and θ_U in §6.5), requiring high power if the true value of δ is sufficiently far inside the tolerance range (θ_L, θ_U). In general in clinical trials, one might wish to test whether a difference is clearly greater than the minimum 'important' difference (see Fig. 4.1), rather than merely whether it exceeds zero (Meier, 1975; Freedman *et al.*, 1984). The formulae (6.6)–(6.9) still hold, provided that d_1 is interpreted as the difference between $\bar{x}_1 - \bar{x}_2$ and δ_0, and δ_1 is replaced by $\delta_1 - \delta_0$.

Example 6.3

The lung functions of two groups of men are to be compared using the forced expiratory volume (FEV). From previous work the standard deviation of FEV is 0·5 l. A two-sided significance level of 0·05 is to be used and a power of 80% is required against a specified mean difference between the groups of 0·25 l. How many men should there be in each group?

Using (6.9) with $z_{2\alpha} = 1.96$, $z_{2\beta} = 0.842$, $\sigma = 0.5$, and $\delta_1 = 0.25$ gives

$$n > 2\left[\frac{(1.96 + 0.842)(0.5)}{0.25}\right]^2$$

$$= 62.8.$$

Therefore 63 men should be included in each group.

The sample size problem is usually expressed as one of determining *sample size* given the *power* and magnitude of the *specified effect* to be detected. But it could be considered as finding any one of these three items for given values of the other two. This is often a useful approach since the sample size may be limited by other considerations. Then, the relevant questions are: what effect could be detected; or what would the power be? The next example considers the inverse problem of estimating what can be achieved with a given sample size.

Example 6.4

Consider the situation of Example 6.3, but suppose that resources are available to include only 50 men in each group.
(a) What would be the power of the study?
   Substituting in (6.9) with $z_{2\beta}$ as unknown gives

$$50 = 2\left[\frac{(1{\cdot}96 + z_{2\beta})(0{\cdot}5)}{0{\cdot}25}\right]^2,$$

and therefore

$$z_{2\beta} = 0{\cdot}540.$$

From Table A1 this corresponds to a power of

$$1 - 0{\cdot}2946 = 0{\cdot}7054 \text{ or } 71\%.$$

(b) What size of mean difference between the groups could be detected with 80% power?

   Substituting in (6.9) with δ_1 as unknown gives

$$50 = 2\left[\frac{(1{\cdot}96 + 0{\cdot}842)(0{\cdot}5)}{\delta_1}\right]^2,$$

and therefore, $\delta_1 = 0{\cdot}28$. A mean difference of $0{\cdot}28$ l could be detected.
   Note that if the sample size has already been determined for a specified δ_1 the revised value is quickly obtained by noting that the difference that can be detected is proportional to the reciprocal of the square root of the sample size. Thus, since for $\delta_1 = 0{\cdot}25$ the sample size was calculated as $62{\cdot}8$, then for a sample size of 50 we have $\delta_1 = 0{\cdot}25 \times \sqrt{(62{\cdot}8/50)} = 0{\cdot}28$.

   The formulae given above assume a knowledge of the standard deviation, σ. In practice σ will rarely be known in advance, although sometimes the investigator will be able to make use of an estimate of σ from previous data which is felt to be reasonably accurate. The approaches outlined above may be modified in two ways. The first way would be to recognize that the required values of n can be specified only in terms of the ratio of a critical interval $(\varepsilon, d_1 \text{ or } \delta_1)$ to an estimated or true standard deviation $(s \text{ or } \sigma)$. For instance, in **1** we might specify the estimated standard error to be a certain multiple of s; in **2** d_1 might be specified as a certain multiple of s; in **3**, the power might be specified against a given ratio of δ_1 to σ. In **2** and **3**, because the test will use the t distribution rather than the normal, the required values of n will be rather greater than those given by (6.6) or (6.9), but the adjustments will only be important for small samples, that is, those giving 30 or fewer DF for the estimated SD. In this case an adjusted sample size can be given by a second use of (6.9), replacing $z_{2\alpha}$ and $z_{2\beta}$ by the corresponding values from the t distribution, with DF given by the sample size obtained in the initial application of (6.9).

The specification of critical distances as multiples of an unknown standard deviation is not an attractive suggestion. An alternative approach would be to estimate σ by a relatively small pilot investigation and then to use this value in formulae (6.4)–(6.9), to provide an estimate of the total sample size, n. Again, some adjustment is called for because of the uncertainty introduced by estimating σ, but the effect will be small provided that the initial pilot sample is not too small.

The above discussion has been in terms of two independent samples, where the analysis is the two-sample t test (§4.4). If the two groups are paired, the method of analysis would be the paired t test and (6.8) would be used with SE(d) substituted by $\sigma/\sqrt{n}$, where σ is the standard deviation of the differences between paired values and n is the number of pairs. In terms of the methods of analysis of variance, to be introduced in Chapter 7, σ is the 'residual' standard deviation.

The comparison of two independent proportions follows a similar approach. In this case the standard error of the difference depends on the values of the proportions (§4.8). Following approach **3**, specification would be in terms of requiring detection of a difference between true proportions π_1 and π_2, using a test of the null hypothesis that each proportion is equal to the pooled value π. The equation corresponding to (6.9) is

$$ n > \left\{ \frac{z_{2\alpha}\sqrt{[2\pi(1-\pi)]} + z_{2\beta}\sqrt{[\pi_1(1-\pi_1) + \pi_2(1-\pi_2)]}}{\pi_1 - \pi_2} \right\}^2 . \qquad (6.10) $$

This equation is slightly more complicated than (6.9) because the standard error of the difference between two observed proportions is different for the null and alternative hypotheses (§4.8). Use of (6.10) gives sample sizes that are appropriate when statistical significance is to be determined using the uncorrected χ^2 test (4.21). Fleiss *et al.* (1980) show that for the continuity-corrected test (4.24), $2/|\pi_1 - \pi_2|$ should be added to the solution given by (6.10).

Casagrande *et al.* (1978) give tables for determining sample sizes that are based on the exact test for 2×2 tables (§4.9), and Fleiss (1981) gives a detailed set of tables based on a formula that gives a good approximation to the exact values. Table A9 gives the sample size required in each of the two groups, calculated using (6.10) and including the continuity correction for some common situations. Although in general we favour uncorrected tests, Table A9 refers to the corrected version since in those cases where the difference is of practical consequence it would be advisable to aim on the high side.

Example 6.5

A trial of a new treatment is being planned. The success rate of the standard treatment to be used as a control is 0.25. If the new treatment increases the success rate to 0.35, then it is required to detect that there is an improvement with a two-sided 5% significance test and a power of 90%. How many patients should be included in each group?

Using (6.10) with $\pi_1 = 0.25$, $\pi_2 = 0.35$, $\pi = 0.3$, $z_{2\alpha} = 1.96$, and $z_{2\beta} = 1.282$ gives

$$n > \left[\frac{1.96\sqrt{0.42} + 1.282\sqrt{(0.1875 + 0.2275)}}{0.1} \right]^2$$

$$= 439.4.$$

Including Fleiss *et al.*'s correction gives

$$n = 439.4 + 2/0.1$$

$$= 459.4.$$

From Table A9 the sample size is given as 459 (the same value is given in both Casagrande *et al.*'s and Fleiss's tables).

Equivalence testing

In equivalence testing (§6.5) the sample size problem is different. If π_1 and π_2 are the success rates of two treatments, then it would be required with a power of $1 - \beta$ that the confidence interval of the estimate of the difference $\pi_1 - \pi_2$ should be within the range θ_L to θ_U. Often equivalence trials are carried out to determine that a proposed conservative treatment (treatment 2) is at least almost as good as the existing treatment (treatment 1). Then only the upper limit is relevant so a one-sided confidence interval is used. Denoting θ_U by $\delta(> \pi_1 - \pi_2)$ it is required that the upper confidence limit should not exceed δ. With equal numbers of patients in the two groups, the number of patients in each group, n, is given by

$$n = [\pi_1(1 - \pi_1) + \pi_2(1 - \pi_2)] \left[\frac{z_{2\alpha} + z_{2\beta}}{\delta - (\pi_1 - \pi_2)} \right]^2 \qquad (6.11)$$

(Makuch and Simon, 1978). Often it is appropriate to take $\pi_1 = \pi_2 = \pi$ and (6.11) simplifies to

$$n = 2\pi(1 - \pi) \left(\frac{z_{2\alpha} + z_{2\beta}}{\delta} \right)^2. \qquad (6.12)$$

Equation (6.12) also applies in the case where the two treatments are of equal status and it is required that the confidence interval is within $-\delta$ to $+\delta$, but then the value of $z_{2\alpha}$ would be set for a two-sided interval.

Example 6.6

A trial of laparoscopic hernia repair (LHR) in comparison with conventional hernia repair (CHR) is being planned. With conventional repair about 5% of patients will have a recurrence of their hernia due to breakdown of the repair within 5 years. If the breakdown rate is the same after LHR as after CHR then how many patients are required to demonstrate that the recurrence rate with LHR is at most 5% higher than with CHR?

With a power of 80% and using a one-sided 95% confidence interval the number of patients in each group is, from (6.12),

$$2(0{\cdot}95)(0{\cdot}05)\left(\frac{1{\cdot}645 + 0{\cdot}842}{0{\cdot}05}\right)^2 = 235.$$

Thus a total of 470 patients would be required.

Machin and Campbell (1987) give tables for sample size in equivalence testing trials.

Case–control studies

In a case–control study the measure of association is the odds ratio, or approximate relative risk (§4.8 and Chapter 16). For hypothesis testing the data are arranged in a 2×2 table and the significance test is then a comparison of the proportions of individuals in the case and control groups who are exposed to the risk factor. Thus the problem of sample size determination can be converted to that of comparing two independent proportions. The controls represent the general population and we need to specify the proportion of controls exposed to the risk factor, p. The first step is to find the proportion of cases, p', that would be exposed for a specified odds ratio, OR_1.

By definition

$$\frac{p'}{1 - p'} = OR_1 \times \frac{p}{1 - p}.$$

Therefore

$$p' = OR_1 \times \frac{p}{p(OR_1) + 1 - p}. \tag{6.13}$$

To eliminate this step and the need to interpolate in tables such as Table A9, tables have been produced that are indexed by the proportion of exposed in the controls and the specified value of the true odds ratio for which it is required to establish statistical significance. Table A10 is a brief table covering commonly required situations. This table is based on (6.13) and (6.10) with the continuity correction. Schlesselman (1982) gives a more extensive set of tables; these tables give smaller sample sizes than Table A10, since Schlesselman did not include Fleiss's addition for the continuity correction.

Example 6.7

A case–control study is being planned to assess the association between a disease and a risk factor. It is estimated that 20% of the general population are exposed to the risk factor. It is required to detect an association if the relative risk is 2 or greater with 80% power at the 5% significance level. How many cases and controls are required?

Using (6.13) with $p = 0.2$ and $OR_1 = 2.0$ gives $p' = 0.3333$. Then, using (6.10), with $\pi_1 = 0.3333$ and $\pi_2 = 0.2$, and using the continuity correction give $n = 186.5$. So the study should consist of at least 187 cases and the same number of controls. The above calculations can be avoided by direct use of Table A10, which gives $n = 187$.

Inverse formulation

For the inverse problem of determining the power or the size of effect that could be detected with a given sample size, the formulae can be used but the tables are less convenient. Since it is often required to consider what can be achieved with a range of sample sizes, it is convenient to be able to calculate approximate solutions more simply. This can be achieved by noting that, in (6.9), δ_1 is proportional to $1/\sqrt{n}$ and $z_{2\alpha} + z_{2\beta}$ is proportional to $\sqrt{n}$. These relationships apply exactly for a continuous variable but also form a reasonable approximation for comparing proportions.

Example 6.8

In Example 6.5 suppose only 600 patients are available so that $n = 300$.
(a) What size of difference could be detected with 90% power?
Approximately

$$\delta_1 = 0.10 \times \sqrt{(459.4/300)}$$
$$= 0.124.$$

Using (6.10) gives $\delta_1 = 0.126$ so the approximation is good. An increase in success rate to about 37.6% could be detected.
(b) What would be the power to detect a difference of 0.1?
Approximately

$$1.96 + z_{2\beta} = (1.96 + 1.282) \times \sqrt{(300/459.4)}$$
$$= 2.620.$$

Therefore $z_{2\beta} = 0.660$ and the revised power is 74.5%.
Using (6.10) gives $z_{2\beta} = 0.626$ and a revised power of 73.4%.

Unequal-sized groups

It is usually optimal when comparing two groups to have equal numbers in each group. But sometimes the number available in one group may be restricted, e.g.

for a rare disease in a case–control study. In this case the power can be increased to a limited extent by having more in the other group. If one group contains m subjects and the other rm, then the study is approximately equivalent to a study with n in each group where

$$\frac{2}{n} = \frac{1}{m} + \frac{1}{rm}.$$

That is,

$$m = \frac{(r+1)n}{2r}. \tag{6.14}$$

This expression is derived by equating the expressions for the standard error of the difference between two means used in a two-sample t test, and is exact for a continuous variable and approximate for the comparison of two proportions. Fleiss *et al.* (1980) give a formula for the general case of comparing two proportions where the two samples are not of equal size, and their formula is suitable for the inverse problem of estimating power from known sample sizes.

The total number of subjects in the study is

$$\frac{(r+1)^2}{4r} \times 2n,$$

which is a minimum for $r = 1$.

Example 6.9

In Example 6.7 suppose 187 cases are not available. How many cases would be needed if there were two controls per case?

Using (6.14),

$$m = \frac{3(186 \cdot 5)}{4}$$

$$= 139 \cdot 9.$$

That is, 140 cases and 280 controls would be required. Using the more accurate formula given by Fleiss *et al.* (1980), $m = 132 \cdot 8$, so the approximation has overestimated the sample size slightly.

Withdrawals and protocol departures

Some allowance may be made for a proportion of subjects who withdraw or are lost to study during the course of the investigation. If a proportion, θ, are lost so that the outcome variables are not recorded, then the final analysis will be based on $1 - \theta$ times the number of subjects entering the study. To ensure an adequate sample size at the end of the study it would be necessary to start with a sample size, n', given by

$$n' = \frac{n}{1 - \theta},$$

where n is the sample size determined by the methods given earlier in this section.

For a clinical trial comparing an active treatment with a placebo, in which a proportion of patients, ϕ, deviate from the protocol, say by discontinuing their treatment, then, as discussed in §6.5, it is important to continue to observe such patients and to include them in the analysis in the group to which they were randomized. If it is assumed that such patients will respond in the same way as patients on placebo, then the difference between the two treatment groups is reduced by a factor $1 - \phi$, and since the required sample size is proportional to the reciprocal of the square of a specified difference we have

$$n' = \frac{n}{(1 - \phi)^2}$$

(Donner, 1984). As subjects that withdraw or deviate from protocol may be unrepresentative of the total study group, there is the potential of biased comparisons, and this cannot be eliminated by increasing sample size.

Other considerations

The situations considered in this section are relatively simple, those of comparing two groups without any complicating features. The determination of sample size is often facilitated by the use of tables and, in addition to those mentioned earlier, the book by Lemeshow et al. (1990) contains a number of sets of tables. Even in these simple situations it is necessary to have a reasonable idea of the likely form of the data to be collected before sample size can be estimated. For example, when comparing means it is necessary to have an estimate of the standard deviation, or in comparing proportions the approximate size of one of the proportions is required at the planning stage. Such information may be available from earlier studies using the same variables or may be obtained from a pilot study. In more complicated situations more information is required but (6.9) can be used in principle, provided that it is possible to find an expression for σ, the standard deviation relevant to the comparison of interest.

For a comparison of proportions using paired samples, where the significance test is based on the untied pairs (§4.8), it is necessary to have information on the likely effectiveness of the matching, which would determine the proportion of pairs that were tied (Connor, 1987). As such information may be unavailable, the effect of matching is often ignored in the determination of sample size, but this would lead to a larger sample size than necessary if the matching were effective (Parker and Bregman, 1986).

Other more complicated situations include making allowance for confounding variables (Chapter 12), multiple regression (Chapter 10) and survival analysis (Chapter 14). Schlesselman (1982) considers the estimation of sample size in the presence of a confounder (see also Donner, 1984; Woolson *et al.* 1986). Nam (1987) considers the estimation of sample size to detect a trend in proportions where the analysis uses the methods given in §12.2. Freedman (1982) discusses, and gives tables for, the estimation of sample size in clinical trials where the comparison is of the rate at which an event, such as relapse or death, is the outcome measure, a form of survival analysis. Tables for sample size estimation in survival analysis are also given by Lemeshow *et al.* (1990) and Machin and Campbell (1987).

Many investigations are concerned with more than one variable measured on the same individual. In a morbidity survey, for example, a wide range of symptoms, as well as the results of certain diagnostic tests, may be recorded for each person. Sample sizes deemed adequate for one purpose may, therefore, be inadequate for others. In many investigations the sample size chosen would be the largest of the separate requirements for the different variables; it would not matter too much that for some variables the sample size was unnecessarily high. In other investigations, in contrast, this may be undesirable, because either the cost or the trouble incurred by taking the extra observations is not negligible. A useful device in these circumstances is *multiphase sampling*. In the first phase certain variables are observed on all the members of the initial sample. In the second phase a subsample of the original sample is then taken, either by simple random sampling or by one of the other methods described in §6.2, and other variables are observed only on the members of the subsample. The process could clearly be extended to more than two phases.

Some population censuses have been effectively multiphase samples in which the first phase is a 100% sample to which some questions are put. In the second phase, a subsample (say, 1 in 10 of the population) is asked certain additional questions. The justification here would be that complete enumeration is necessary for certain basic demographic data, but that for certain more specialized purposes (perhaps information about fertility or occupation) a 1-in-10 sample would provide estimates of adequate precision. Material savings in cost are achieved by restricting these latter questions to a relatively small subsample.

7: Comparison of Several Groups

7.1 One-way analysis of variance

The body of techniques called the *analysis of variance* forms a powerful method of analysing the way in which the mean value of a variable is affected by classifications of the data of various sorts. This apparent paradox of nomenclature—that the techniques should be concerned with comparisons of means rather than variances—will be clarified when we come to study the method in detail.

We have already, in §4.4, used the *t* distribution for the comparison of the means of two groups of data, distinguishing between the paired and unpaired cases. The *one-way analysis of variance*, the subject of the present section, is a generalization of the unpaired *t* test, appropriate for any number of groups. As we shall see, it is entirely equivalent to the unpaired *t* test when there are just two groups. The analogous extension of the paired *t* test will be described in §8.1.

Some examples of a one-way classification of data into several groups are:
1 the reduction in blood sugar recorded for groups of rabbits given different doses of insulin;
2 the value of a certain lung-function test recorded for men of the same age group in a number of different occupational categories;
3 the volumes of liquid taken up by an experimenter using various pipettes to measure a standard quantity, the repeated measurements on any one pipette being grouped together.

In each of these examples a similar question might be asked: What can be said about the variation in blood-sugar reduction from one dose group to another, in lung-function test from one occupational category to another, or in volume of liquid from one pipette to another? There are, however, important differences in the nature of the classification into groups in these three examples. In **1** the groups are defined by dose of insulin and fall into a natural order; in **2** the groups may not fall in a unique order, but some very reasonable classifications of the groups may be suggested—for instance, according to physical effort, intellectual demand, etc.; in **3** the groups of data will almost certainly fall into no natural order. In the present section we are concerned with situations in which no account is taken of any logical ordering of the groups, either because, as in **3**, there is none, or because a consideration of ordering is deferred until a later stage of the analysis.

Suppose there are k groups of observations on a variable y, and that the ith group contains n_i observations. The numbering of the groups from 1 to k will be quite arbitrary, although if there is a simple ordering of the groups it will be natural to use this in the numbering. Further notation is as follows:

Group	1	2 ... i ... k	All groups combined
Number of observations	n_1	n_2 ... n_i ... n_k	$N = \sum_{i=1}^{k} n_i$
Mean of y	$\bar{y}_1$	$\bar{y}_2$ ... $\bar{y}_i$ ... $\bar{y}_k$	$\bar{y} = T/N$
Sum of y	T_1	T_2 ... T_i ... T_k	$T = \sum_{i=1}^{k} T_i$
Sum of y^2	S_1	S_2 ... S_i ... S_k	$S = \sum_{i=1}^{k} S_i$

Note that the entries N, T and S in the final column are the sums along the corresponding rows, but $\bar{y}$ is not the sum of the $\bar{y}_i$ ($\bar{y}$ will be the *mean* of the $\bar{y}_i$ if all the n_i are equal; otherwise $\bar{y}$ is the *weighted mean* of the $\bar{y}_i$, $\sum n_i \bar{y}_i / \sum n_i$). Let the observations within each group be numbered in some arbitrary way, and denote the jth observation in the ith group by y_{ij}.

When a summation is taken over all the N observations, each contributing once to the summation, we shall use the summation sign

$$\sum_{i,j}$$

or, in the text, $\sum_{i,j}$. When the summation is taken over the k groups, each group contributing once, we shall use the sign

$$\sum_{i}$$

or $\sum_i$, whilst summation over the members of a particular group will be denoted by

$$\sum_{j}$$

or $\sum_j$.

The deviation of any observation from the *grand mean*, $\bar{y}$, may be split into two parts, as follows:

$$y_{ij} - \bar{y} = (y_{ij} - \bar{y}_i) + (\bar{y}_i - \bar{y}). \tag{7.1}$$

The first term on the right of (7.1) is the deviation of y_{ij} from its *group mean*, $\bar{y}_i$, and the second term is the deviation of the group mean from the grand mean. We show below that when each of these terms is squared and summed over all N observations, a similar result holds:

$$\sum_{i,j}(y_{ij} - \bar{y})^2 = \sum_{i,j}(y_{ij} - \bar{y}_i)^2 + \sum_{i,j}(\bar{y}_i - \bar{y})^2. \tag{7.2}$$

This remarkable result means that the 'total' sum of squares about the mean of all N values of y can be partitioned into two parts: (i) the sum of squares of each reading about its own group mean; and (ii) the sum of squares of the deviations of each group mean about the grand mean (these being counted once for every observation). We shall write this result as

$$Total\ SSq = Within\text{-}Groups\ SSq + Between\text{-}Groups\ SSq,$$

'SSq' standing for 'sum of squares'.

Now if there are very large differences between the group means, as compared with the within-group variation, the Between-Groups SSq is likely to be larger than the Within-Groups SSq. If, on the other hand, all the $\bar{y}_i$ are nearly equal and yet there is considerable variation within groups, the reverse is likely to be true. The relative sizes of the Between- and Within-Groups SSq should, therefore, provide an opportunity to assess the variation between group means in comparison with that within groups.

To prove (7.2) we write

$$\sum_{i,j} (y_{ij} - \bar{y})^2 = \sum_{i,j} [(y_{ij} - \bar{y}_i) + (\bar{y}_i - \bar{y})]^2$$

$$= \sum_{i,j} (y_{ij} - \bar{y}_i)^2 + 2\sum_{i,j} (y_{ij} - \bar{y}_i)(\bar{y}_i - \bar{y}) + \sum_{i,j} (\bar{y}_i - \bar{y})^2$$

$$= \sum_{i,j} (y_{ij} - \bar{y}_i)^2 + 2\sum_{i} 0(\bar{y}_i - \bar{y}) + \sum_{i,j} (\bar{y}_i - \bar{y})^2$$

$$= \sum_{i,j} (y_{ij} - \bar{y}_i)^2 + \sum_{i,j} (\bar{y}_i - \bar{y})^2,$$

the transition from the second to the third line following because the middle summation can be done group by group, and for the ith group $\sum_j (y_{ij} - \bar{y}_i) = 0$. The whole summation is therefore zero. Note that the Between-Groups SSq may be written

$$\sum_{i,j} (\bar{y}_i - \bar{y})^2 = \sum_{i} n_i (\bar{y}_i - \bar{y})^2,$$

since the contribution $(\bar{y}_i - \bar{y})^2$ is the same for all the n_i observations in the ith group.

The partitioning of the total sum of squares is most conveniently done by the use of computing formulae analogous to the short-cut formula (1.3) for the sum of squares about the mean of a single sample. These are obtained as follows.

1   *Total SSq.*

$$\sum_{i,j} (y_{ij} - \bar{y})^2 = S - \frac{T^2}{N}, \tag{7.3}$$

by direct application of (1.3).

2 *Within-Groups SSq.*

For the ith group,

$$\sum_j (y_{ij} - \bar{y}_i)^2 = S_i - \frac{T_i^2}{n_i}.$$

Summing over the k groups, therefore,

$$\sum_{i,j} (y_{ij} - \bar{y}_i)^2 = \left(S_1 - \frac{T_1^2}{n_1} \right) + \ldots + \left(S_k - \frac{T_k^2}{n_k} \right)$$

$$= \sum_i S_i - \sum_i (T_i^2/n_i)$$

$$= S - \sum_i (T_i^2/n_i). \tag{7.4}$$

3 *Between-Groups SSq.*

By subtraction, from (7.2),

$$\sum_{i,j} (\bar{y}_i - \bar{y})^2 = \text{Total SSq} - \text{Within-Groups SSq}$$

$$= S - (T^2/N) - \left[S - \sum_i (T_i^2/n_i) \right]$$

$$= \sum_i (T_i^2/n_i) - T^2/N. \tag{7.5}$$

Note that, from (7.5), the Between-Groups SSq is expressible entirely in terms of the group totals, T_i, and the numbers in each group, n_i (and hence in terms of the $\bar{y}_i$ and n_i since $T_i = n_i \bar{y}_i$). This shows clearly that it represents the variation between the group means and not in any way the variation within groups.

Summarizing these results, we have the following formulae for partitioning the total sum of squares:

Between groups	$\sum_i (T_i^2/n_i) - T^2/N$	
Within groups	$S - \sum_i (T_i^2/n_i)$	(7.6)
Total	$S - T^2/N$	

Consider now the problem of testing for evidence of real differences between the groups. Suppose that the n_i observations in the ith group form a random sample from a population with mean μ_i and variance σ^2. As in the two-sample t test, we assume for the moment that σ^2 is the same for all groups. To examine the evidence for differences between the μ_i we shall test the null hypothesis that the μ_i do not vary, being equal to some common unknown value μ. Three ways of estimating σ^2 suggest themselves, as follows.

1 *From the Total SSq.* The whole collection of N observations may be regarded as a random sample of size N, and consequently

$$s_T^2 = \frac{\text{Total SSq}}{N - 1}$$

is an unbiased estimate of σ^2.

2 *From the Within-Groups SSq.* Separate unbiased estimates may be got from each group in turn:

$$\frac{S_1 - T_1^2/n_1}{n_1 - 1}, \frac{S_2 - T_2^2/n_2}{n_2 - 1}, \ldots, \frac{S_k - T_k^2/n_k}{n_k - 1}.$$

A combined estimate based purely on variation within groups may be derived (by an extension of the procedure used in the two-sample t test) by adding the numerators and denominators of these ratios, to give the *Within-Groups mean square* (or *MSq*),

$$s_W^2 = \frac{\text{Within-Groups SSq}}{\sum_i (n_i - 1)} = \frac{\text{Within-Groups SSq}}{N - k}.$$

3 *From the Between-Groups SSq.* Since both s_T^2 and s_W^2 are unbiased,

$$E(s_T^2) = \sigma^2; \text{ hence } E(\text{Total SSq}) = (N - 1)\sigma^2. \tag{7.7}$$

$$E(s_W^2) = \sigma^2; \text{ hence } E(\text{Within-Groups SSq}) = (N - k)\sigma^2. \tag{7.8}$$

Subtracting (7.8) from (7.7),

$$E(\text{Between-Groups SSq}) = (N - 1)\sigma^2 - (N - k)\sigma^2$$
$$= (k - 1)\sigma^2.$$

Hence, a third unbiased estimate is given by the *Between-Groups MSq*,

$$s_B^2 = \frac{\text{Between-Groups SSq}}{k - 1}.$$

The divisor $k - 1$ is reasonable, being one less than the number of groups, just as the divisor for s_T^2 is one less than the number of observations.

These results hold if the null hypothesis is true. Suppose, however, that the μ_i are not all equal. The Within-Groups MSq is still an unbiased estimate of σ^2, since it is based purely on the variation within groups. The Between-Groups MSq, being based on the variation between group means, will tend to increase. In fact, in general, when the μ_i differ

$$E(s_B^2) = \sigma^2 + \frac{\sum_i n_i (\mu_i - \bar{\mu})^2}{k - 1}, \tag{7.9}$$

where $\bar{\mu}$ is the weighted mean of the μ_i, $\sum_i n_i \mu_i / N$. Some indication of whether the μ_i differ can therefore be obtained from a comparison of s_B^2 and s_W^2. On the null hypothesis these two mean squares estimate the same quantity and therefore should not usually be too different; if the null hypothesis is not true s_B^2 is, from (7.9), on average greater than σ^2 and will tend to be greater than s_W^2.

An appropriate test of the null hypothesis, therefore, may be based on the *variance ratio* (VR) s_B^2 / s_W^2, which will be denoted by F. The distribution of F depends on the nature of the distributions of the y_{ij} about their mean $\bar{y}_i$. If the further assumption is made that these distributions are normal, it can be shown that s_B^2 and s_W^2 behave like two *independent* estimates of variance, on $k - 1$ and $N - k$ degrees of freedom, respectively. The relevant distribution, the F distribution, has been discussed in §4.6. Departures from the null hypothesis will tend to give values of F greater than unity. A significance test for the null hypothesis should, therefore, count as significant only those values of F which are sufficiently large; that is, a one-sided test is required. As observed in §4.6, the critical levels of F are tabulated in terms of single-tail probabilities, so the tabulated values (Table A4) apply directly to the present situation (the single-tail form of tabulation in fact arose to serve the needs of the analysis of variance).

If $k = 2$, the situation considered above is precisely that for which the un-paired (or two-sample) t test was introduced in §4.4. The variance ratio, F, will have 1 and $N - 2$ degrees of freedom and t will have $n_1 + n_2 - 2$, i.e. $N - 2$ degrees of freedom. The two solutions are, in fact, equivalent in the sense that (i) the value of F is equal to the square of the value of t; (ii) the distribution of F on 1 and $N - 2$ degrees of freedom is precisely the same as the distribution of the square of a variable following the t distribution on $N - 2$ degrees of freedom. The former statement may be proved algebraically in a few lines. The second has already been noted in §4.6.

If $k = 2$ and $n_1 = n_2 = \frac{1}{2}N$ (i.e. there are two groups of equal size), a useful result is that the Between-Groups SSq (7.5) may be written in the alternative form

$$\frac{(T_1 - T_2)^2}{N}. \tag{7.10}$$

If $k > 2$, we may wish to examine the difference between a particular pair of means, chosen because the contrast between these particular groups is of logical interest. The standard error of the difference between two means, say $\bar{y}_g$ and $\bar{y}_h$, may be estimated by

$$SE(\bar{y}_g - \bar{y}_h) = \sqrt{\left[s_W^2 \left(\frac{1}{n_g} + \frac{1}{n_h} \right) \right]}, \tag{7.11}$$

and the difference $\bar{y}_g - \bar{y}_h$ tested by referring

$$t = \frac{\bar{y}_g - \bar{y}_h}{\text{SE}(\bar{y}_g - \bar{y}_h)}$$

to the t distribution on $N - k$ degrees of freedom (since this is the number of DF associated with the estimate of variance s^2). Confidence limits for the difference in means may be set in the usual way, using tabulated percentiles of t on $N - k$ DF. The only function of the analysis of variance in this particular comparison has been to replace the estimate of variance on $n_g + n_h - 2$ DF (which would be used in the two-sample t test) by the pooled Within-Groups MSq on $N - k$ DF. This may be a considerable advantage if n_g and n_h are small. It has been gained, however, by invoking an assumption that all the groups are subject to the same within-groups variance and if there is doubt about the near-validity of this assumption it will be safer to rely on the data from the two groups alone.

If there are no contrasts between groups which have an a priori claim on our attention, further scrutiny of the differences between means could be made to depend largely on the F test in the analysis of variance. If the variance ratio is not significant, or even suggestively large, there will be little point in examining differences between pairs of means. If F is significant, there is reasonable evidence that real differences exist and are large enough to reveal themselves above the random variation. It then seems natural to see what can safely be said about the direction and magnitude of these differences. This topic will be taken up again in §7.4.

Example 7.1

During each of four experiments on the use of carbon tetrachloride as a worm killer, 10 rats were infested with larvae. Eight days later, five rats were treated with carbon tetrachloride, the other five being kept as controls. After two more days the rats were killed and the number of adult worms counted. It was thought useful to examine the significance of the differences between the means for the four control groups. If significant differences could be established they might be related to definable changes in experimental conditions, thus leading to a reduction of variation in future work. The results and the details of the calculations are shown in Table 7.1. The value of F is 2·27, and comparison with the F table for $v_1 = 3$ and $v_2 = 16$ shows the result to be non-significant at $P = 0·05$. (Actually $P = 0·12$.)

The standard error of the difference between two means is $\sqrt{[2(3997)/5]} = 40·0$. Note that the difference between $\bar{y}_3$ and $\bar{y}_4$ is more than twice its standard error, but since the F value is not significant we should not pay much attention to this particular comparison unless it presents some prior interest (see also §7.4).

Two important assumptions underlying the F test in the one-way analysis of variance are (i) the normality of the distribution of the y_{ij} about their mean μ_i, and (ii) the equality of the variances in the various groups. The F test is not

Table 7.1 One-way analysis of variance: differences between four groups of control rats in counts of adult worms

	Experiment				All groups
	1	2	3	4	
	279	378	172	381	
	338	275	335	346	
	334	412	335	340	
	198	265	282	471	
	303	286	250	318	
T_i	1452	1616	1374	1856	$T = 6298$
n_i	5	5	5	5	$N = 20$
$\bar{y}_i$	290·4	323·2	274·8	371·2	
S_i	434654	540274	396058	703442	$S = 2074428$
T_i^2/n_i	421661	522291	377575	688947	

Between-Groups SSq $= 421\,661 + \ldots + 688\,947 - (6298)^2/20$

$\qquad\qquad\qquad = 2\,010\,474 - 1\,983\,240$

$\qquad\qquad\qquad = 27\,234$

Total SSq $\qquad = 2\,074\,428 - 1\,983\,240$

$\qquad\qquad\qquad = 91\,188$

Within-Groups SSq $= 91\,188 - 27\,234$

$\qquad\qquad\qquad = 63\,954$

Analysis of variance

	SSq	DF	MSq	VR
Between groups	27234	3	9078	2·27
Within groups	63954	16	3997	
Total	91188	19		

unduly sensitive to moderate departures from normality, but it will often be worth considering whether some form of transformation (Chapter 11) will improve matters. The assumption about equality of variances is more serious. It has already been suggested that, for comparisons of two means, where there is doubt about the validity of a pooled within-group estimate of variance, it may be advisable to estimate the variance from the two groups alone. A transformation of the scale of measurement may bring about near-equality of variances. If it fails to do so, an approximate test for differences of means may be obtained by a method described in §7.2.

7.2 The method of weighting

In the one-way analysis of variance we are interested in a series of k means, $\bar{y}_i$, which may have different variances because the group sizes n_i may differ. We ask whether the $\bar{y}_i$ could be regarded as *homogeneous*, in the sense that they could easily differ by sampling variation from some common value, or whether they should be regarded as *heterogeneous*, in the sense that sampling variation is unlikely to explain the differences amongst them.

We now consider a method of wide generality for tackling other problems of this sort. It depends on certain assumptions which may or may not be precisely true in any particular application, but it is nevertheless very useful in providing approximate solutions to many problems. The general situation is that data are available in k groups, each providing an estimate of some parameter. We wish first to test whether there is evidence of heterogeneity between the estimates, and then in the absence of heterogeneity to obtain a single estimate of the parameter from the whole data set.

Suppose we observe k quantities, $Y_1, Y_2, \ldots, Y_k$, and we know that Y_i is $N(\mu_i, V_i)$, where the means μ_i are unknown but the variances V_i are known. To test the hypothesis that all the μ_i are equal to some specified value μ, we could calculate a *weighted* sum of squares

$$G_0 = \sum_i [(Y_i - \mu)^2 / V_i] = \sum_i w_i (Y_i - \mu)^2, \qquad (7.12)$$

where $w_i = 1/V_i$. The quantity G_0 is the sum of squares of k standardized normal deviates and, from (3.6), it follows the $\chi^2_{(k)}$ distribution.

However, to test the hypothesis of homogeneity we do not usually wish to specify the value μ. Let us replace μ by the *weighted* mean

$$\bar{Y} = \frac{\sum_i w_i Y_i}{\sum_i w_i}, \qquad (7.13)$$

and calculate

$$G = \sum_i w_i (Y_i - \bar{Y})^2. \qquad (7.14)$$

The quantity w_i is called a *weight*: note that it is the reciprocal of the variance V_i, so if, for example, Y_1 is more precise than Y_2, then $V_1 < V_2$ and $w_1 > w_2$ and Y_1 will be given the higher weight.

A little algebra gives the alternative formula:

$$G = \sum_i w_i Y_i^2 - \left(\sum_i w_i Y_i \right)^2 \bigg/ \sum_i w_i. \qquad (7.15)$$

Note that if all the $w_i = 1$, (7.14) is the usual sum of squares about the mean, $\bar{Y}$ becomes the usual unweighted mean, and (7.15) becomes the usual short-cut formula (1.3).

It can be shown that, on the null hypothesis of homogeneity, G is distributed as $\chi^2_{(k-1)}$. Replacing μ by $\bar{Y}$ has resulted in the loss of one degree of freedom. High values of G indicate evidence against homogeneity.

If homogeneity is accepted, it will often be reasonable to estimate μ, the common value of the μ_i. The best estimate (in the sense of having the lowest variance) is the weighted mean $\bar{Y}$, defined earlier. Moreover, if the null hypothesis of homogeneity is true, $\text{var}(\bar{Y}) = 1/\sum_i w_i$, and confidence limits for μ may be obtained by using the percentiles of the normal distribution. Thus, 95% limits are

$$\bar{Y} \pm 1{\cdot}96\sqrt{(1/\textstyle\sum_i w_i)}.$$

Let us see how this general theory might be applied to the problem of comparing k independent means, using the notation of §7.1. Write $Y_i = \bar{y}_i$ and $V_i = \sigma^2/n_i$. Then

$$\bar{Y} = \sum_i n_i \bar{y}_i \bigg/ \sum_i n_i = \bar{y},$$

the overall mean; and

$$G = \frac{\sum_i n_i (\bar{y}_i - \bar{y})^2}{\sigma^2} = \frac{\text{Between-Groups SSq}}{\sigma^2}.$$

If σ^2 were known, G could be tested from the $\chi^2_{(k-1)}$ distribution. In practice, we estimate σ^2 by the Within-Groups MSq, s_W^2, and replace G by

$$G' = \frac{\text{Between-Groups SSq}}{s_W^2} = \frac{(k-1)s_B^2}{s_W^2}.$$

This is $k - 1$ times the variance ratio, which we have already seen follows the F distribution on $k - 1$ and $N - k$ DF. For these degrees of freedom the distributions of $(k - 1)F$ and $\chi^2_{(k-1)}$ are exactly equivalent when $N = \infty$ (see §4.6). For reasonably large N the two methods will give closely similar results.

Consider now the possibility mentioned at the end of §7.1, that the groups have different variances σ_i^2. Write $Y_i = \bar{y}_i$ and $V_i = \sigma_i^2/n_i$. Again, the σ_i^2 are unknown, but they may be estimated by

$$s_i^2 = [S_i - (T_i^2/n_i)]/(n_i - 1),$$

and an approximate or *empirical* weight calculated as

$$w_i' = n_i/s_i^2.$$

We calculate the weighted sum of squares (7.15) as

$$G'' = \sum_i w'_i \bar{y}_i^2 - (\sum_i w'_i \bar{y}_i)^2 / \sum_i w'_i.$$

On the null hypothesis of homogeneity of the μ_i, G'' is distributed approximately as $\chi^2_{(k-1)}$, high values indicating excessive disparity between the $\bar{y}_i$. The approximation is increasingly inaccurate for smaller values of the n_i (say, below about 10), and a refinement is given by James (1951) and Welch (1951). For an application of this method in a comparison of sets of pock counts, see Armitage (1957, p. 579).

An important application of the method of weighting occurs in overviews (or meta-analyses) of clinical trials (§6.5). The parameter to be estimated is often the ratio (or odds ratio) of two proportions (e.g. the proportion of patients dying or experiencing a critical event on each of two treatments). A commonly used estimate of the odds ratio (and hence of the ratio of proportions when these are low) is that given by (4.23).

Suppose the log of the odds ratio takes the value μ in each of k trials, and its estimate from the ith trial is

$$Y_i = \frac{O_i - E_i}{V_i}$$

with

$$\text{var}(Y_i) = \frac{1}{V_i},$$

where O_i and E_i are the observed and expected numbers of critical events for one of the treatments, and V_i is calculated, as in (4.22), from the 2×2 table for the trial. Then the weighted mean (7.13) becomes

$$\bar{Y} = \frac{\sum(O_i - E_i)}{\sum V_i}, \tag{7.16}$$

with

$$\text{var}(\bar{Y}) = \frac{1}{\sum V_i}.$$

The heterogeneity statistic (7.15), distributed approximately as $\chi^2_{(k-1)}$, becomes

$$G = \sum \frac{(O_i - E_i)^2}{V_i} - \frac{[\sum(O_i - E_i)]^2}{\sum V_i},$$

the summation being over the k trials.

As noted in §4.9, this method is biased when the treatment effect is large (i.e. when the odds ratio departs greatly from unity). The report by the Early Breast

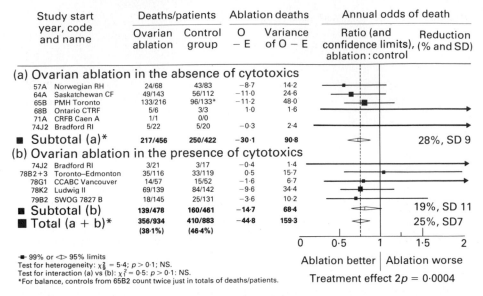

Study start year, code and name	Deaths/patients		Ablation deaths		Annual odds of death	
	Ovarian ablation	Control group	O − E	Variance of O − E	Ratio (and confidence limits), ablation : control	Reduction (% and SD)
(a) Ovarian ablation in the absence of cytotoxics						
57A Norwegian RH	24/68	43/83	−8·7	14·2		
64A Saskatchewan CF	49/143	56/112	−11·0	24·6		
65B PMH Toronto	133/216	96/133*	−11·2	48·0		
68B Ontario CTRF	5/6	3/3	1·0	1·6		
71A CRFB Caen A	1/1	0/0				
74J2 Bradford RI	5/22	5/20	−0·3	2·4		
■ **Subtotal (a)***	**217/456**	**250/422**	**−30·1**	**90·8**		28%, SD 9
(b) Ovarian ablation in the presence of cytotoxics						
74J2 Bradford RI	3/21	3/17	−0·4	1·4		
78B2+3 Toronto–Edmonton	35/116	33/119	0·5	15·7		
78G1 CCABC Vancouver	14/57	15/52	−1·6	6·7		
78K2 Ludwig II	69/139	84/142	−9·6	34·4		
79B2 SWOG 7827 B	18/145	25/131	−3·6	10·2		
■ **Subtotal (b)**	**139/478**	**160/461**	**−14·7**	**68·4**		19%, SD 11
■ **Total (a + b)***	**356/934 (38·1%)**	**410/883 (46·4%)**	**−44·8**	**159·3**		25%, SD7

■ 99% or ◁▷ 95% limits
Test for heterogeneity: $\chi_8^2 = 5\cdot4$; $p > 0\cdot1$; NS.
Test for interaction (a) vs (b): $\chi_1^2 = 0\cdot5$; $p > 0\cdot1$: NS.
*For balance, controls from 65B2 count twice just in totals of deaths/patients.

Ablation better | Ablation worse

Treatment effect $2p = 0\cdot0004$

Fig. 7.1 An overview of mortality results from trials of ovarian ablation in women with early breast cancer below age 50, subdivided by the presence or absence of cytotoxic chemotherapy (Early Breast Cancer Trialists' Collaborative Group, 1992, Fig. 9). In this presentation the area of a black square is proportional to V_i, and thus represents the precision of the estimate from that trial or group of trials. The significance level for a two-sided test is shown as '$2p$'. Reprinted by permission of the authors and publishers.

Cancer Trialists' Collaborative Group (1990) suggests that the bias is not serious if the odds ratio is within twofold in either direction and there are at least several dozen critical events in total. In more doubtful situations it is preferable to apply the method of weighting to the direct estimates of the log odds ratio given by the log of (4.18).

Figure 7.1 shows the results of an overview using these methods. In this example, which is typical of many others, none of the individual trials shows a clear treatment effect, but the results for the various trials are consistent and the pooled values for each of the two subgroups and for the whole data set have narrow confidence ranges, showing clear evidence of an effect.

If the trial results are clearly heterogeneous, the first step should be to see whether this can be explained by known differences between the characteristics of the trials—types of patients, agents under test, etc. If there are just one or two trials inconsistent with the rest, the best course may be to report separately on these and to pool the remainder.

Occasionally, though, there may be general heterogeneity, not explicable by known characteristics and not confined to a small minority of trials. Two alternative approaches may be adopted. The pooled estimate (7.16) may be quoted, with its relatively narrow limits, as appropriate for the particular mix of patients and study characteristics found in these trials, recognizing that a different mix would have given a different result (Yusuf *et al.*, 1985; Early Breast Cancer Trialists' Collaborative Group, 1990). The second approach is to argue that the unexplained variation between trials is a form of random variation, the extent of which can be estimated, and that this needs to be allowed for in quoting the precision of the pooled estimate (DerSimonian and Laird, 1986). This is the so-called 'random-effects' model (see §7.3) and is an example of the empirical Bayes approach described briefly in §4.13. These two approaches are discussed more fully by Berlin *et al.* (1989), Pocock and Hughes (1990) and Whitehead and Whitehead (1991).

7.3 Components of variance

In some studies which lead to a one-way analysis of variance the groups may be of no great interest individually, but may nevertheless represent an interesting source of variation. The result of a pipetting operation, for example, may vary from one pipette to another. A comparison between a particular pair of pipettes would be of little interest; furthermore, a test of the null hypothesis that the different pipettes give identical results on average may be pointless because there may quite clearly be a systematic difference between instruments. A more relevant question here will be: how great is the variation between pipettes as compared with that of repeated readings on the same pipette?

A useful framework is to regard the k groups as being randomly selected from a population of such groups. This will not usually be strictly true, but it serves as an indication that the groups are of interest only as representing a certain type of variation. This framework is often called *Model II*, or the *Random-Effects Model*, as distinct from *Model I*, or the *Fixed-Effects Model*, considered in §7.1.

Suppose, in the first instance, that each group contains the same number, n, of observations. (In the notation of §7.1, all the n_i are equal to n.) Let μ_i be the 'true' mean for the ith group and suppose that in the population of groups μ_i is distributed with mean μ and variance σ_B^2. Readings within the ith group have mean μ_i and variance σ^2. The quantities σ^2 and σ_B^2 are called *components of variance* within and between groups respectively. The situation is illustrated in Fig. 7.2. The data at our disposal consist of a random sample of size n from each of k randomly selected groups.

Consider first the variance of a single group mean, $\bar{y}_i$. We have

$$\bar{y}_i - \mu = (\mu_i - \mu) + (\bar{y}_i - \mu_i),$$

and the two terms in brackets represent independent sources of variation—that of μ_i about μ and that of $\bar{y}_i$ about μ_i. Therefore, using (3.13),

$$\text{var}(\bar{y}_i) = \text{var}(\mu_i) + \text{var}(\bar{y}_i, \text{ given } \mu_i)$$
$$= \sigma_B^2 + (\sigma^2/n). \tag{7.17}$$

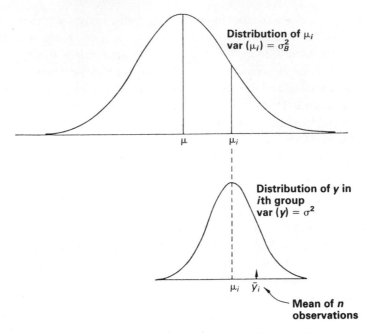

Fig. 7.2 Components of variance between and within groups, with normal distributions for each component of random variation.

Now, the analysis of variance will have the following structure:

	DF	MSq
Between groups	$k - 1$	s_B^2
Within groups	$k(n - 1)$	s_W^2
Total	$nk - 1 \ (= N - 1)$	

The Between-Groups SSq is (with notation for T_i and T as in §7.1)

$$\frac{\sum T_i^2}{n} - \frac{T^2}{N}$$

$$= n\left[\sum \bar{y}_i^2 - \left(\sum \bar{y}_i\right)^2/k\right],$$

summations running from $i = 1$ to k. Thus, the Between-Groups MSq, s_B^2,

$$= n\left[\sum \bar{y}_i^2 - \left(\sum \bar{y}_i\right)^2/k\right]/(k - 1)$$

$= n$ times an unbiased estimate of $\mathrm{var}(\bar{y}_i)$

$= n$ times an unbiased estimate of $\sigma_B^2 + (\sigma^2/n)$, from (7.17),

$=$ an unbiased estimate of $n\sigma_B^2 + \sigma^2$.

That is,

$$E(s_B^2) = \sigma^2 + n\sigma_B^2. \tag{7.18}$$

This important result is similar to (7.9), which is the analogous result for the situation in which the μ_i are fixed.

The Within-Groups MSq is (from §7.1) an unbiased estimate of σ^2. The result (7.18) thus confirms the plausibility of the F test, for the null hypothesis is that $\sigma_B^2 = 0$ and in this case both mean squares are unbiased estimates of σ^2. If $\sigma_B^2 > 0$, s_B^2 will on average be greater than s_W^2, and F will tend to be greater than 1.

To estimate σ_B^2, note that

$$\begin{aligned} E(s_B^2 - s_W^2) &= E(s_B^2) - E(s_W^2) \\ &= (\sigma^2 + n\sigma_B^2) - \sigma^2 \\ &= n\sigma_B^2. \end{aligned}$$

Hence, an unbiased estimate of σ_B^2 is given by

$$\hat{\sigma}_B^2 = \frac{s_B^2 - s_W^2}{n}. \tag{7.19}$$

If $s_B^2 < s_W^2$ (as will often be the case if σ_B^2 is zero or near zero), $\hat{\sigma}_B^2$ is negative. There is a case for replacing $\hat{\sigma}_B^2$ by 0 when this happens, but it should be noted that the unbiased property of (7.19) is then lost.

Example 7.2

Bacharach et al. (1940) carried out an experiment on 'diffusing factor', a substance which, when present in an inoculation into the skin of rabbits, spreads the blister caused by the inoculation. They gave inoculations of the same dose at six sites on the back of each of six animals. Their experimental design permitted a study of the influence of the particular site and the order of administration, but there was no evidence that these factors had any effect and we shall regard the data as forming a one-way classification: between and within animals. The variable analysed is the area of the blister (square centimetres).

An analysis of variance was as follows:

	SSq	DF	MSq	VR
Between animals	12·8333	5	2·5667	4·39
Within animals	17·5266	30	0·5842	
Total	30·3599	35		

We have

$$\begin{aligned} \hat{\sigma}_B^2 &= (2·5667 - 0·5842)/6 \\ &= 0·3304. \end{aligned}$$

The two components of variance are then estimated as follows, where each is expressed as a percentage of the total:

Between animals	$\hat{\sigma}_B^2$	0·3304	36%
Within animals	s_W^2	0·5842	64%
Total	$\hat{\sigma}_B^2 + s_W^2$	0·9146	100%

The sum of the two components is the estimated variance of a single reading from a randomly chosen rabbit, and the analysis shows that of this total variance 36% is estimated to be attributable to systematic differences between rabbits. (For further analysis of these data, see below; also Example 8.5, p. 263.)

Confidence limits for σ^2 are obtained from the Within-Groups SSq by use of the χ^2 distribution, as in §4.5. Confidence limits for σ_B^2 are rather more troublesome. An approximate solution is recommended by Boardman (1974). For $100(1 - \alpha)\%$ confidence limits we need various entries in the F table corresponding to a tabulated one-sided level of $\frac{1}{2}\alpha$. Thus, for 95% confidence limits we need entries corresponding to $P = 0·025$. Denoting the entry for degrees of freedom v_1 and v_2 as F_{v_1, v_2}, and putting $f_1 = k - 1$, $f_2 = k(n - 1)$, we need

$$F_1 = F_{f_1, f_2}$$
$$F_2 = F_{f_1, \infty}$$
$$F_3 = F_{f_2, f_1}$$
$$F_4 = F_{\infty, f_1}$$
$$F = \text{observed value, } s_B^2/s_W^2.$$

Then the upper limit for σ_B^2 is

$$\hat{\sigma}_{BU}^2 = F_4\left(F - \frac{1}{F_3}\right)\left(\frac{s_W^2}{n}\right) \qquad (7.20)$$

and the lower limit is

$$\hat{\sigma}_{BL}^2 = \left(\frac{F - F_1}{F_2}\right)\left(\frac{s_w^2}{n}\right). \qquad (7.21)$$

Note that the lower limit is zero if $F = F_1$, i.e. if F is just significant by the usual test. If $F < F_1$, the lower limit will be negative and in some instances the upper limit may also be negative. For a discussion of this apparent anomaly, see Scheffé (1959, §7.2). The validity of these limits will depend rather heavily on the assumption of normality, particularly for the between-groups variation.

Example 7.2, continued

The 95% confidence limits for σ^2 are (from §4.5)

$$\frac{17\cdot5266}{46\cdot98}$$

and

$$\frac{17\cdot5266}{16\cdot79},$$

i.e.

$$0\cdot373 \text{ and } 1\cdot044,$$

the divisors being the appropriate percentiles of the $\chi^2_{(30)}$ distribution.

For confidence limits for σ^2_B we need the following tabulated values of F, writing $f_1 = 5, f_2 = 30$:

$$F_1 = 3\cdot03, F_2 = 2\cdot57, F_3 = 6\cdot23, F_4 = 6\cdot02,$$

and the observed F is $4\cdot39$. Thus, from (7.20) and (7.21),

$$\hat{\sigma}^2_{BU} = (6\cdot02)\left(4\cdot39 - \frac{1}{6\cdot23}\right)(0\cdot0974) = 2\cdot48$$

and

$$\hat{\sigma}^2_{BL} = \left(\frac{4\cdot39 - 3\cdot03}{2\cdot57}\right)(0\cdot0974) = 0\cdot052.$$

The wide ranges of error associated with these estimates makes it clear that the percentage contributions of 36% and 64% are very imprecise estimates indeed.

If the numbers of observations from the groups are unequal, with n_i from the ith group, (7.19) must be modified as follows:

$$\hat{\sigma}^2_B = \frac{s^2_B - s^2_W}{n_0}, \tag{7.22}$$

where

$$n_0 = \frac{1}{(k-1)}\left[N - \frac{\left(\sum n_i^2\right)}{N}\right].$$

A further difficulty is that (7.22) is not necessarily the best way of estimating σ^2_B. The choice of method depends, however, on the unknown ratio of the variance components which are being estimated, and (7.22) will usually be a sensible method if the n_i are not too different. See Robertson (1962) and Stuart and Ord (1983, §36.26).

7.4 Multiple comparisons

We return now to the fixed-effects model of §7.1. In the analysis of data in this form it will usually be important not to rely solely on the analysis of variance table and its F test, but to examine the differences between groups more closely to see what patterns emerge. It is, in fact, good practice habitually to report the mean values $\bar{y}_i$ and their standard errors, calculated as $s_W/\sqrt{n_i}$, in terms of the Within-Groups MSq s_W^2 unless the assumption of constant variance is clearly inappropriate.

The standard error of the difference between two means is given by (7.11), and the t distribution may be used to provide a significance test or to assign confidence limits as indicated in §7.1. If all the n_i are equal (to n, say), it is sometimes useful to calculate the *least significant difference* (LSD) at a certain significance level. For the 5% level, for instance, this is

$$t_{f_2, 0 \cdot 05} s_W \sqrt{(2/n)},$$

where $f_2 = k(n-1)$, the degrees of freedom within groups. Differences between pairs of means which are significant at this level can then be picked out by eye.

Sometimes interest is focused on comparisons between the group means other than simple differences. These will usually be measurable by a *linear contrast* of the form

$$L = \sum \lambda_i \bar{y}_i, \tag{7.23}$$

where $\sum \lambda_i = 0$. From (3.13),

$$\text{var}(L) = \sum \lambda_i^2 \text{var}(\bar{y}_i),$$

and the standard error of L is thus estimated as

$$\text{SE}(L) = s_W \sqrt{\left(\sum \lambda_i^2 / n\right)}, \tag{7.24}$$

and the usual t test or confidence limits may be applied.

Some examples of linear contrasts are as follows.

1 *A contrast of one group with the mean of several other groups.* One group may have a special identity, perhaps as a control group, and there may be some reason for pooling a set of q other groups (e.g. if related treatments have been applied to these groups). The relevant comparison will then be

$$\bar{y}_c - \left(\sum_{i=1}^{q} \bar{y}_i\right) \Big/ q,$$

which when multiplied by q becomes

$$L_1 = q\bar{y}_c - \sum_{i=1}^{q} \bar{y}_i,$$

a particular case of (7.23) with $\lambda_c = q$, $\lambda_i = -1$ for all i in the set of q groups and $\lambda_i = 0$ otherwise. Note that $\sum \lambda_i = 0$.

2 *A linear regression coefficient.* Suppose that a set of q groups is associated with a variable x_i (for example, the dose of some substance). It might be of interest to ask whether the regression of y on x is significant. Using the result quoted in the derivation of (5.15),

$$L_2 = \sum (x_i - \bar{x}) \bar{y}_i,$$

which again is a particular case of (7.23) with $\lambda_i = x_i - \bar{x}$, and again $\sum \lambda_i = 0$.

3 *A difference between two means.* The difference between $\bar{y}_g$ and $\bar{y}_h$ is another case of (7.23) with $\lambda_g = 1$, $\lambda_h = -1$ and all other $\lambda_i = 0$.

Corresponding to any linear contrast, L, the t statistic, on $k(n-1)$ DF, is from (7.24)

$$t = \frac{L}{\text{SE}(L)} = \frac{L}{s_W \sqrt{(\sum \lambda_i^2 / n)}}.$$

As we have seen, the square of t follows the F distribution on 1 and $k(n-1)$ DF. Thus,

$$F = t^2 = \frac{L^2}{s_W^2 \sum \lambda_i^2 / n} = \frac{s_1^2}{s_W^2},$$

where $s_1^2 = L^2 / (\sum \lambda_i^2 / n)$. In fact, s_1^2 can be regarded as a MSq on 1 DF, derived from a SSq also equal to s_1^2, which can be shown to be part of the SSq between groups of the analysis of variance. The analysis thus takes the following form:

	SSq	DF	MSq	VR
Between groups				
Due to L	$L^2/(\sum \lambda_i^2 / n)$	1	s_1^2	$F_1 = s_1^2/s_W^2$
Other contrasts	$\sum T_i^2/n - T^2/n - L^2/(\sum \lambda_i^2/n)$	$k-2$	s_R^2	$F_2 = s_R^2/s_W^2$
Within groups	$S - \sum T_i^2/n$	$k(n-1)$	s_W^2	
Total	$S - T^2/nk$	$nk - 1$		

Separate significance tests are now provided (i) by F_1 on 1 and $k(n-1)$ DF for the contrast L; as we have seen, this is equivalent to the t test for L; and (ii) by F_2 on $k-2$ and $k(n-1)$ DF for differences between group means other than those measured by L.

Suppose there are two or more linear contrasts of interest:

$$L_1 = \sum \lambda_{1i} \bar{y}_i, \quad L_2 = \sum \lambda_{2i} \bar{y}_i, \text{ etc.}$$

Can the single degrees of freedom for these contrasts all be incorporated in the same analysis of variance? They can, provided the Ls are uncorrelated when the null hypothesis is true, and the condition for this is that for any two contrasts (L_p and L_q, say) the sum of products of the coefficients is zero:

$$\sum_{i=1}^{k} \lambda_{pi} \lambda_{qi} = 0.$$

In this case L_p and L_q are said to be *orthogonal*. If there are k' such orthogonal contrasts, the analysis of variance will run as follows:

	SSq	DF
Between groups		
Due to L_1	$L_1^2 / \left(\sum \lambda_{1i}^2/n \right)$	1
Due to L_2	$L_2^2 / \left(\sum \lambda_{2i}^2/n \right)$	1
$\vdots$	$\vdots$	$\vdots$
Due to $L_{k'}$	$L_{k'}^2 / \left(\sum \lambda_{k'i}^2/n \right)$	1
Other contrasts	$\sum T_i^2/n - T^2/n - \sum_{j=1}^{k'} L_j^2 / \left(\sum \lambda_{ji}^2/n \right)$	$k - k' - 1$
Within groups	$S - \sum T_i^2/n$	$k(n-1)$
Total	$S - T^2/nk$	$nk - 1$

the undesignated summations running from $i = 1$ to k.

The straightforward use of the t or F tests is appropriate for any differences between means or for more general linear contrasts which arise naturally out of the structure of the investigation. However, a difficulty must be recognized. If there are k groups, there are $\frac{1}{2}k(k-1)$ pairs of means which might conceivably be compared and there is no limit to the number of linear contrasts which might be formed. These comparisons are not all independent, but it is fairly clear that, even when the null hypothesis is true, in any set of data *some* of these contrasts are likely to be significant. A sufficiently assiduous search will often reveal some remarkable contrasts which have arisen purely by chance. This may not matter if scrutiny is restricted to those comparisons which the study was designed to throw light on. If, on the other hand, the data are subjected to what is sometimes called a *dredging* procedure—a search for significant contrasts which would not have been thought of initially—there is a real danger that a number of comparisons will be reported as significant, but that they will almost all have arisen by chance.

A number of procedures have been devised to reduce the chance of this happening. They are referred to as methods of making *multiple comparisons* or *simultaneous inference*, and are described in detail by Miller (1981). We mention briefly two methods, one for differences between means and the other for more general linear contrasts.

The first method, based on the distribution of the *studentized range*, is due to Newman (1939) and Keuls (1952). Given a set of p means, each based on n observations, the studentized range, Q, is the range of the $\bar{y}_i$ divided by the estimated standard error. In an obvious notation,

$$Q = \frac{\bar{y}_{max} - \bar{y}_{min}}{s/\sqrt{n}}. \tag{7.25}$$

The distribution of Q, on the null hypothesis that all the μ_i are equal, has been studied and some upper 5% and 1% points are given in Table A5. They depend on the number of groups, p, and the within-groups degrees of freedom, f_2, and are written $Q_{p,0.05}$ and $Q_{p,0.01}$. The procedure is to rank the $\bar{y}_i$ in order of magnitude and to test the studentized range for all pairs of adjacent means (when it actually reduces to the usual t test), for all adjacent triads, all groups of four adjacent means, and so on. Two means are regarded as differing significantly only if all tests for sets of means, including these two, give a significant result. The procedure is most readily performed in the opposite order to that described, starting with all k, following by the two sets of $k - 1$ adjacent means, and so on. The reason for this is that, if at any stage a non-significant Q is found, that set of means need not be used for any further tests. The procedure will, for example, stop after the first stage if Q for all k means is non-significant.

The following example is taken from Miller's book (§6.1). Five means, arranged in order, are 16·1, 17·0, 20·7, 21·1 and 26·5; $n = 5$, $f_2 = 20$, and the standard error $s/\sqrt{5} = 1·2$. The values of $Q_{p,0.05}$ for $p = 2, 3, 4$ and 5 are, respectively, 2·95, 3·58, 3·96 and 4·23. Tests are done successively for $p = 5, 4, 3$ and 2, and the results are as follows, where non-significant groupings are indicated by underlining.

A	B	C	D	E
16·1	17·0	20·7	21·1	26·5

The interpretation is that E differs from {A, B, C, D}, and that within the latter group A differs from C and D, with B occupying an ambiguous position.

In Example 7.1, where we noted that $\bar{y}_3$ and $\bar{y}_4$ differed by more than twice the standard error of the difference, Q calculated for all four groups is

$$(371·2 - 274·8)/\sqrt{(3997/5)} = 96·4/28·3 = 3·41,$$

and from Table A5 $Q_{4,0.05}$ is 4·05, so the test shows no significant difference, as might have been expected in view of the non-significant F test.

The Newman–Keuls procedure has the property that, for a set of groups with equal μ_i, the probability of asserting a significant difference between any of them is at most equal to the chosen level (0·05 in the examples above).

If linear contrasts other than differences are being 'dredged', the infinite number of possible choices suggests that a very conservative procedure should be used, that is, one which indicates significance much less readily than the t test. A method proposed by Scheffé (1959) is as follows. A linear contrast, L, is declared significant at, say, the 5% level if the absolute value of $L/\mathrm{SE}(L)$ exceeds

$$\sqrt{[(k-1)F_{0\cdot05}]}, \tag{7.26}$$

where $F_{0\cdot05}$ is the tabulated 5% point of the F distribution with $k-1$ and $k(n-1)$ DF. When $k = 2$, this rule is equivalent to the use of the t test. For $k > 2$ it is noticeably conservative in comparison with a t test, in that the numerical value of (7.26) may considerably exceed the 5% level of t on $k(n-1)$ degrees of freedom. Scheffé's method has the property that, if the null hypothesis that all μ_i are equal is true, only in 5% of cases will it be possible to find any linear contrast which is significant by this test. Any contrast significant by this test, even if discovered by an exhaustive process of data dredging, may therefore be regarded with a reasonable degree of confidence. In Example 7.1 the contrast between the means for experiments 3 and 4 gives $L/\mathrm{SE}(L) = (371\cdot2 - 274\cdot8)/40\cdot0 = 2\cdot41$; by Scheffé's test the 5% value would be $\sqrt{[3(3\cdot24)]} = 3\cdot12$, and the observed contrast should not be regarded as significant.

It should again be emphasized that the Newman–Keuls and Scheffé procedures, and other multiple-comparison methods, are deliberately conservative in order to reduce the probability of too many significant differences arising by chance in any one study. They are appropriate only when means are being compared in an exploratory way to see what might 'turn up'. When comparisons are made which flow naturally from the plan of the experiment or survey the usual t test is appropriate.

7.5 Comparison of several proportions: the $2 \times k$ contingency table

In §4.8 and §4.9 the comparison of two proportions was considered from two points of view—the sampling error of the difference between the proportions and the χ^2 significance test applied to the 2×2 table. We saw that these two approaches led to equivalent significance tests of the null hypothesis.

Where more than two proportions are to be compared the calculation of standard errors between pairs of proportions raises points similar to those discussed in §7.4: many comparisons are possible and an undue number of significance differences may arise by chance. However, an overall significance test, analogous to the F test in the analysis of variance, is provided by a straightforward extension of the χ^2 test.

Suppose there are k groups of observations and that in the ith group n_i individuals have been observed, of whom r_i show a certain characteristic (say, being 'positive'). The proportion of positives, r_i/n_i, is denoted by p_i. The data may be displayed as follows:

Group	1	2	...	i	...	k	All groups combined
Positive	r_1	r_2	...	r_i	...	r_k	R
Negative	$n_1 - r_1$	$n_2 - r_2$	...	$n_i - r_i$	...	$n_k - r_k$	$N - R$
Total	n_1	n_2	...	n_i	...	n_k	N
Proportion positive	p_1	p_2	...	p_i	...	p_k	$P = R/N$

The frequencies form a $2 \times k$ contingency table (there being two rows and k columns, excluding the marginal totals). The χ^2 test follows the same lines as for the 2×2 table (§4.9). For each of the observed frequencies, O, an expected frequency is calculated by the formula

$$E = \frac{\text{Row total} \times \text{Column total}}{N}.$$
(7.27)

the quantity $(O - E)^2/E$ is calculated, and, finally

$$X^2 = \sum \frac{(O - E)^2}{E}$$
(7.28)

the summation being over the $2k$ cells in the table.

On the null hypothesis that all k samples are drawn randomly from populations with the same proportion of positives, X^2 is distributed approximately as $\chi^2_{(k-1)}$, the approximation improving as the expected frequencies increase in size. An indication of the extent to which the $\chi^2_{(k-1)}$ distribution is valid for small frequencies is given in §7.6. No continuity correction is required, because unless the observed frequencies are very small the number of tables which may be formed with the same marginal totals as those observed is very large, and the distribution of X^2 is consequently more nearly continuous than is the case for 2×2 tables.

An alternative formula for X^2 is of some value. The value of $O - E$ for an entry in the first row of the table (the positives for group i, for instance) is

$$r_i - Pn_i,$$

and this is easily seen to differ only in sign from the entry for the negatives for group i:

$$(n_i - r_i) - (1 - P)n_i = -(r_i - Pn_i).$$

The contribution to X^2 from these two cells is, therefore,

$$(r_i - Pn_i)^2 \left(\frac{1}{Pn_i} + \frac{1}{Qn_i} \right)$$

where $Q = 1 - P$. The expression in the second bracket simplifies to give the following expression for X^2:

$$X^2 = \frac{\sum n_i (p_i - P)^2}{PQ}, \qquad (7.29)$$

the summation now being over the k groups. A little manipulation with the summation in (7.29) gives two equivalent expressions,

$$X^2 = \frac{\sum n_i p_i^2 - NP^2}{PQ}$$

and

$$X^2 = \frac{\sum (r_i^2/n_i) - R^2/N}{PQ}. \qquad (7.30)$$

The last two expressions are more convenient as computing formulae than (7.29).

The expression (7.29) and the results of §7.2 provide an indication of the reason why X^2 follows the $\chi^2_{(k-1)}$ distribution. In the general formulation of §7.2, we can replace Y_i by p_i, V_i by PQ/n_i and w_i by n_i/PQ. The weighted mean $\bar{Y}$ then becomes

$$\frac{\sum (n_i p_i / PQ)}{\sum (n_i / PQ)} = \frac{\sum n_i p_i}{\sum n_i} = \frac{R}{N} = P,$$

and, from (7.14), the test statistic G, distributed as $\chi^2_{(k-1)}$, becomes

$$X^2 = \sum_i \frac{n_i (p_i - P)^2}{PQ}$$

in agreement with (7.29). We have departed from the assumptions underlying (7.14) in two respects: the variation in p_i is binomial, not normal, and the true variance σ_i^2 has been replaced by the estimated variance PQ/n_i. Both these approximations decrease in importance as the expected frequencies increase in size.

Example 7.3

Table 7.2 shows the numbers of individuals in various age groups who were found in a survey to be positive and negative for *Schistosoma mansoni* eggs in the stool.

Table 7.2 Presence or absence of *S. mansoni* eggs in the stool

Age (years)	0–	10–	20–	30–	40–	Total
Positive	14	16	14	7	6	57
Negative	87	33	66	34	11	231
Total	101	49	80	41	17	288

The expected number of positives for the age group 0– is

$$(57)(101)/288 = 19.99.$$

The set of expected numbers for the 10 cells in the table is

					Total
19·99	9·70	15·83	8·11	3·36	57
81·01	39·30	64·17	32·89	13·64	231
Total 101	49	80	41	17	288

The fact that the expected numbers add to the same marginal totals as those observed is a useful check.

The contribution to X^2 from the first cell is

$$(14 - 19.99)^2/19.99 = 1.79,$$

and the set of contributions for the 10 cells is

1·79	4·09	0·21	0·15	2·07
0·44	1·01	0·05	0·04	0·51

giving a total of

$$X^2 = 10.36.$$

The degrees of freedom are $k - 1 = 4$, for which the 5% point is 9·49. The departures from the null hypothesis are thus significant at the 5% level ($P = 0.035$).

In this example the column classification is based on a continuous variable, age, and it would be natural to ask whether the proportions of positives exhibit any smooth trend with age. The estimated proportions, with their standard errors calculated as $\sqrt{(p_i q_i/n_i)}$, are

0·14	0·33	0·18	0·17	0·35,
± 0·03	± 0·07	± 0·04	± 0·06	± 0·12

the last being based on particularly small numbers. No clear trend emerges (a method for testing for a trend is given in §12.2). About half the contribution to X^2 comes from the second age group (10–19 years) and there is some suggestion that the proportion of positives in this group is higher than in the neighbouring age groups.

To illustrate the use of (7.30), call the numbers of positives r_i. Then

$$X^2 = (14^2/101 + \ldots + 6^2/17 - 57^2/288)/(0.1979)(0.8021),$$

where $P = 57/288 = 0.1979$. This gives

$$X^2 = 10.37$$

as before, the discrepancy being due to rounding errors. Note that, if the *negatives* rather than the positives had been denoted by r_i, each of the terms in the numerator of (7.30) would have been different, but the result would have been the same.

7.6 General contingency tables

The form of table considered in the last section can be generalized by allowing more than two rows. Suppose that a total frequency, N, is subdivided by r row categories and c column categories. The null hypothesis, corresponding to that tested in the simpler situations, is that the probabilities of falling into the various columns are independent of the rows; or, equivalently, that the probabilities for the various rows are the same for each column.

The χ^2 test follows closely that applied in the simpler cases. For each cell in the body of the table an expected frequency, E, is calculated by (7.27) and the X^2 index obtained from (7.28) by summation over the rc cells. Various alternative formulae are available, but none is as simple as (7.29) or (7.30) and it is probably most convenient to remember the basic formula (7.28). On the null hypothesis, X^2 follows the $\chi^2_{(f)}$ distribution with $f = (r - 1)(c - 1)$. This number of degrees of freedom may be thought of as the number of arbitrary choices of the frequencies in the body of the table, with the constraint that they should add to the same margins as those observed and thus give the same values of E. (If the entries in $r - 1$ rows and $c - 1$ columns are arbitrarily specified, those in the other row and column are determined by the marginal totals.)

Again, the χ^2 distribution is an approximation, increasingly valid for large expected frequencies. A rough rule (Cochran, 1954) is that the approximation is safe provided that relatively few expected frequencies are less than 5 (say in 1 cell out of 5 or more, or 2 cells out of 10 or more), and that no expected frequency is less than 1. In tables with smaller expected frequencies the result of the significance test should be regarded with caution. If the result is not obviously either significant or non-significant, it may be wise to pool some of the rows and/or columns in which the small expected frequencies occur and recalculate X^2 (with, of course, a reduced number of degrees of freedom). See also the suggestions made by Cochran (1954, p. 420).

Example 7.4

Table 7.3 shows results obtained in a trial to compare the effects of para-amino-salicylic acid (PAS) and streptomycin in the treatment of pulmonary tuberculosis. In each cell of the table are shown the observed frequencies, O, the expected frequencies, E, and the

Table 7.3 Degrees of positivity of sputa from patients with pulmonary tuberculosis treated with PAS, streptomycin or a combination of both drugs (Medical Research Council, 1950)

Treatment		Positive smear	Sputum Negative smear, positive culture	Negative smear, negative culture	Total
PAS	O	56	30	13	99
	E	50·41	23·93	24·66	
	$O - E$	5·59	6·07	−11·66	
Streptomycin		46	18	20	84
		42·77	20·31	20·92	
		3·23	−2·31	−0·92	
Streptomycin and PAS		37	18	35	90
		45·82	21·76	22·42	
		−8·82	−3·76	12·58	
Total		139	66	68	273

discrepancies, $O - E$. For example, for the first cell, $E = (99)(139)/273 = 50·41$. Note that the values of $O - E$ add to zero along each row and down each column, a useful check on the arithmetic.

$$X^2 = (5·59)^2/50·41 + \ldots + (12·58)^2/22·42$$
$$= 17·64.$$

The degrees of freedom for the χ^2 distribution are $(3 - 1)(3 - 1) = 4$, and from Table A2 the 1% point is 13·28. The relationship between treatment and type of sputum is thus significant at the 1% level ($P = 0·0014$). The magnitudes and signs of the discrepancies, $O - E$, show clearly that the main difference is between PAS (tending to give more positive results) and the combined treatment (more negative results).

Fisher's exact test (§4.9) may be extended to a general $r \times c$ table (Mehta and Patel, 1983). The exact probability level is equal to the sum of all probabilities less than or equal to the observed table, where the probabilities are calculated under the null hypothesis that there is no association and all the marginal totals are fixed. This corresponds to a two-tailed test, using the alternative method of calculating the other tail in a 2×2 table (p. 139), but as the test is of general association there are no defined tails. The calculation is available as 'EXACT' in the SAS program PROC FREQ, and is feasible when $n < 5(r - 1)(c - 1)$, and in StatXact (see Chapter 18).

7.7 Comparison of several variances

The one-way analysis of variance (§7.1) is a generalization of the two-sample t test (§4.4). Occasionally one requires a generalization of the F test (used, as in §4.6, for the comparison of two variances) to the situation where more than two estimates of variance are to be compared. In a one-way analysis of variance, for example, the primary purpose is to compare means, but one might wish to test the significance of differences between variances, both for the intrinsic interest of this comparison and also because the analysis of variance involves an assumption that the group variances are equal.

Suppose there are k estimates of variance, s_i^2, having possibly different degrees of freedom, v_i. (If the ith group contains n_i observations, $v_i = n_i - 1$.) On the assumption that the observations are randomly selected from normal distributions, an approximate significance test due to Bartlett (1937) consists in calculating

$$\bar{s}^2 = \sum v_i s_i^2 / \sum v_i$$
$$M = \left(\sum v_i\right) \ln \bar{s}^2 - \sum v_i \ln s_i^2$$

and

$$C = 1 + \frac{1}{3(k-1)}\left[\sum\left(\frac{1}{v_i}\right) - \frac{1}{\sum v_i}\right]$$

and referring M/C to the $\chi^2_{(k-1)}$ distribution. Here 'ln' refers to the *natural* logarithm (see p. 131). The quantity C is likely to be near 1 and need be calculated only in marginal cases. Worked examples are given by Snedecor and Cochran (1989, §13.10).

Bartlett's test is perhaps less useful than might be thought, for two reasons. First, like the F test it is rather sensitive to non-normality. Secondly, with samples of moderate size the true variances σ_i^2 have to differ very considerably before there is a reasonable chance of obtaining a significant test result. To put this point another way, even if M/C is non-significant, the estimated s_i^2 may differ substantially, and so may the true σ_i^2. If possible inequality in the σ_i^2 is important, it may therefore be wise to assume it even if the test result is non-significant. In some situations moderate inequality in the σ_i^2 will not matter very much, so again the significance test is not relevant.

7.8 Comparison of several counts: the Poisson heterogeneity test

Suppose that k counts, denoted by $x_1, x_2, \ldots, x_i, \ldots, x_k$, are available. It may be interesting to test whether they could reasonably have been drawn at random from Poisson distributions with the same (unknown) mean μ. In many microbiological experiments, as we saw in §2.6, successive counts may be expected to follow a Poisson distribution if the experimental technique is perfect. With imperfect technical methods the counts will follow Poisson distributions with *different* means. In bacteriological counting, for example, the suspension may be inadequately mixed, so that clustering of the organisms occurs; the volumes of the suspension inoculated for the different counts may not be equal; the culture media may not invariably be able to sustain growth. In each of these circumstances heterogeneity of the expected counts is present and is likely to manifest itself by excessive variability of the observed counts. It seems reasonable, therefore, to base a test on the sum of squares about the mean of the x_i. An appropriate test statistic is given by

$$X^2 = \frac{\sum (x - \bar{x})^2}{\bar{x}}, \tag{7.31}$$

which, on the null hypothesis of constant μ, is approximately distributed as $\chi^2_{(k-1)}$. The method is variously called the Poisson *heterogeneity* or *dispersion* test.

The formula (7.31) may be justified from two different points of view. First, it is closely related to the test statistic (4.8) used for testing the variance of a normal distribution. On the present null hypothesis the distribution is Poisson, which we know is similar to a normal distribution if μ is not too small; furthermore, $\sigma^2 = \mu$, which can best be estimated from the data by the sample mean $\bar{x}$. Replacing σ_0^2 by $\bar{x}$ in (4.8) gives (7.31). Secondly, we could argue that, given the total count $\sum x$, the frequency 'expected' at the ith count on the null hypothesis is $\sum x/k = \bar{x}$. Applying the usual formula for a χ^2 index, $\sum [(O - E)^2/E]$, immediately gives (7.31). In fact, just as the Poisson distribution can be regarded as a limiting form of the binomial for large n and small p, so the present test can be regarded as a limiting form of the χ^2 test for the $2 \times k$ table (§7.5) when R/N is very small and all the n_i are equal; under these circumstances it is not difficult to see that (7.29) becomes equivalent to (7.31).

Example 7.5

The following data were given by 'Student' (1907), who first emphasized the role of the Poisson distribution in microbiology.

Twenty counts of yeast cells in squares of a haemocytometer were as follows:

2	4	4	8
3	3	5	6
7	7	2	7
4	8	5	4
4	1	5	7

Here

$$k = 20,$$
$$\sum x = 96,$$
$$\bar{x} = 4\cdot8,$$
$$\sum x^2 = 542$$
$$\left(\sum x\right)^2/k = 460\cdot8$$
$$\sum (x - \bar{x})^2 = 81\cdot2.$$
$$X^2 = 81\cdot2/4\cdot8 = 16\cdot92 \text{ on 19 DF} \quad (P = 0\cdot60).$$

There is no suggestion of variability in excess of that expected from the Poisson distribution.

In referring X^2 to the $\chi^2_{(k-1)}$ distribution we should normally do a one-sided test since heterogeneity tends to give high values of X^2. Occasionally, though, departures from the Poisson distribution will lead to reduced variability. In microbiological counting this might be caused by omission of counts differing widely from the average; Lancaster (1950) has shown that unskilled technicians counting blood cells (which under ideal circumstances provide another example of the Poisson theory) tend to omit extreme values or take repeat observations, presumably because they underestimate the extent of random variation. Other causes of reduced variability are an inability to record accurately high counts (for instance, because of overlapping of bacterial colonies), or physical interference between particles which prevents large numbers from settling close together. The latter phenomenon has been noted by Lancaster (1950) in the counting of red blood cells.

The use of the $\chi^2_{(k-1)}$ distribution in the heterogeneity test is an approximation, but is quite safe provided $\bar{x}$ is greater than about 5, and is safe, even for much smaller values of $\bar{x}$ (as low as 2, say) provided k is not too small (>15, say). For very small values of $\bar{x}$, Fisher (1950, 1964) has shown how to obtain an exact test; the method is illustrated by Oldham (1968, §5.15).

Finally, note that, for $k = 2$, (7.31) is equivalent to $(x_1 - x_2)^2/(x_1 + x_2)$, which was used as a $\chi^2_{(1)}$ variate in §4.11.

8: Further Experimental Designs

8.1 Two-way analysis of variance: randomized blocks

In this chapter we consider some further experimental designs and corresponding methods of data analysis. Most of these lead to various forms of analysis of variance. We shall be concerned throughout with studies in which changes in the mean value of some variable are of primary interest, but in which the data have a more complicated structure than the one-way classification into groups considered in §7.1 to §7.4.

The simplest extension is to data classified in two ways: by one set of categories which may be represented, say, as the rows of a table, and by another set forming the columns. This structure arises naturally in the 'randomized block' experimental design, where one classification defines the different treatments and the other consists of the blocks of experimental material. If there are r blocks and c treatments, each block containing c experimental units to which treatments are randomly allocated, there will be a total of $N = rc$ observations on any variable, simultaneously divided into r blocks with c observations in each and c treatment groups with r observations in each.

In other experimental situations both the rows and columns of the two-way table may represent forms of treatment. In a blood-clotting experiment, for instance, clotting times may be measured for each combination of r periods of storage of plasma and c concentrations of adrenalin mixed with the plasma. This is a simple example of a *factorial experiment*, to be discussed more generally in §8.3. The distinction between this situation and the randomized block experiment is that in the latter the 'block' classification is introduced mainly to provide extra precision for treatment comparisons; differences between blocks are usually of no intrinsic interest.

Two-way classifications may arise also in non-experimental work, either by classifying in this way data already collected in a survey, or by arranging the data collection to fit a two-way classification.

We consider first the situation in which there is just one observation at each combination of a row and a column; for the ith row and jth column the observation is y_{ij}. To represent the possible effect of the row and column classifications on the mean value of y_{ij}, let us consider an 'additive model' by which

$$E(y_{ij}) = \mu + \alpha_i + \beta_j, \tag{8.1}$$

where α_i and β_j are constants characterizing the rows and columns. By suitable choice of μ we can arrange that

$$\sum_{i=1}^{r} \alpha_i = 0$$

and

$$\sum_{j=1}^{c} \beta_j = 0.$$

According to (8.1), the effect of being in one row rather than another is to change the mean value by adding or subtracting a constant quantity, irrespective of which column the observation is made in. Changing from one column to another has a similar additive or subtractive effect. Any observed value y_{ij} will in general vary randomly round its expectation given by (8.1). We suppose that

$$y_{ij} = E(y_{ij}) + \varepsilon_{ij}, \tag{8.2}$$

where the ε_{ij} are independently and normally distributed with a constant variance σ^2. The assumptions are, of course, not necessarily true, and we shall consider later some ways of testing their truth and of overcoming difficulties due to departures from the model.

Denote the total and mean for the ith row by R_i and $\bar{y}_{i.}$, those for the jth column by C_j and $\bar{y}_{.j}$, and those for the whole group of $N = rc$ observations by T and $\bar{y}$ (see Table 8.1). As in the one-way analysis of variance, the Total SSq, $\sum (y_{ij} - \bar{y})^2$, will be subdivided into various parts. For any one of these deviations from the mean, $y_{ij} - \bar{y}$, the following is true:

$$y_{ij} - \bar{y} = (\bar{y}_{i.} - \bar{y}) + (\bar{y}_{.j} - \bar{y}) + (y_{ij} - \bar{y}_{i.} - \bar{y}_{.j} + \bar{y}). \tag{8.3}$$

Table 8.1 Notation for two-way analysis of variance data

		Column					Total	Mean, R_i/c
		1	2 ...	j ...	c			
Row	1	y_{11}	$y_{12} \cdots$	$y_{1j} \cdots$	y_{1c}		R_1	$\bar{y}_{1.}$
	2	y_{21}	$y_{22} \cdots$	$y_{2j} \cdots$	y_{2c}		R_2	$\bar{y}_{2.}$
	.	.	.	.	.		.	.
	.	.	.	.	.		.	.
	.	.	.	.	.		.	.
	i	y_{i1}	$y_{i2} \cdots$	$y_{ij} \cdots$	y_{ic}		R_i	$\bar{y}_{i.}$
	.	.	.	.	.		.	.
	.	.	.	.	.		.	.
	.	.	.	.	.		.	.
	r	y_{r1}	$y_{r2} \cdots$	$y_{rj} \cdots$	y_{rc}		R_r	$\bar{y}_{r.}$
Total		C_1	$C_2 \cdots$	$C_j \cdots$	C_c		T	
Mean,	C_j/r	$\bar{y}_{.1}$	$\bar{y}_{.2} \cdots$	$\bar{y}_{.j} \cdots$	$\bar{y}_{.c}$			$(\bar{y} = T/N)$

The three terms on the right-hand side reflect the fact that y_{ij} differs from $\bar{y}$ partly on account of a difference characteristic of the ith row, partly because of a difference characteristic of the jth column and partly by an amount which is not explicable by either row or column differences. If (8.3) is squared and summed over all N observations, we find (the suffixes i, j being implied below each summation sign):

$$\sum (y_{ij} - \bar{y})^2 = \sum (\bar{y}_{i.} - \bar{y})^2 + \sum (\bar{y}_{.j} - \bar{y})^2 + \sum (y_{ij} - \bar{y}_{i.} - \bar{y}_{.j} + \bar{y})^2. \quad (8.4)$$

To show (8.4) we have to prove that all the product terms which arise from squaring the right-hand side of (8.3) are zero. For example, $\sum (\bar{y}_{i.} - \bar{y})(y_{ij} - \bar{y}_{i.} - \bar{y}_{.j} + \bar{y}) = 0$. These results can be proved by fairly simple algebra.

The three terms on the right-hand side of (8.4) are called the Between-Rows SSq, the Between-Columns SSq and the Residual SSq. The first two are of exactly the same form as the Between-Groups SSq in the one-way analysis, and the usual short-cut method of calculation may be used (see (7.5)).

Between rows:
$$\sum (\bar{y}_{i.} - \bar{y})^2 = \sum_{i=1}^{r} R_i^2/c - T^2/N.$$

Between columns:
$$\sum (\bar{y}_{.j} - \bar{y})^2 = \sum_{j=1}^{c} C_j^2/r - T^2/N.$$

The Total SSq is similarly calculated as

$$\sum (y_{ij} - \bar{y})^2 = \sum y_{ij}^2 - T^2/N,$$

and the Residual SSq may be obtained by subtraction:

Residual SSq = Total SSq $-$ Between-Rows SSq $-$ Between-Columns SSq.

$$(8.5)$$

The analysis so far is purely a consequence of algebraic identities. The relationships given above are true irrespective of the validity of the model. We now complete the analysis of variance by some steps which depend for their validity on that of the model. First, the degrees of freedom are allotted as shown in Table 8.2. Those for rows and columns follow from the one-way analysis; if the only classification had been into rows, for example, the first line of Table 8.2 would have been shown as Between groups and the SSq shown in Table 8.2 as Between columns and Residual would have added to form the Within-Groups SSq. With $r - 1$ and $c - 1$ as degrees of freedom for rows and columns, respectively, and $N - 1$ for the Total SSq, the DF for Residual SSq follow by subtraction:

$$(rc - 1) - (r - 1) - (c - 1) = rc - r - c + 1 = (r - 1)(c - 1).$$

Table 8.2 Two-way analysis of variance table

	SSq	DF	MSq	VR
Between rows	$\sum_i R_i^2/c - T^2/N$	$r-1$	s_R^2	$F_R = s_R^2/s^2$
Between columns	$\sum_j C_j^2/r - T^2/N$	$c-1$	s_C^2	$F_C = s_C^2/s^2$
Residual	By subtraction	$(r-1)(c-1)$	s^2	
Total	$\sum_{i,j} y_{ij}^2 - T^2/N$	$rc-1$ $(=N-1)$		

The mean squares for rows, columns and residual are obtain in each case by the formula $MSq = SSq/DF$, and those for rows and columns may each be tested against the Residual MSq, s^2, as shown in Table 8.2. The test for rows, for instance, has the following justification. On the null hypothesis (which we shall call H_R) that all the row constants α_i in (8.1) are equal (and therefore equal to zero, since $\sum \alpha_i = 0$), both s_R^2 and s^2 are unbiased estimates of σ^2. If H_R is not true, so that the α_i differ, s_R^2 has expectation greater than σ^2, whereas s^2 is still an unbiased estimate of σ^2. Hence F_R tends to be greater than 1, and sufficiently high values indicate a significant departure from H_R. This test is valid whatever values the β_j take, since adding a constant on to all the readings in a particular column has no effect on either s_R^2 or s^2.

Similarly, F_C provides a test for the null hypothesis H_C, that all the $\beta_j = 0$, irrespective of the values of the α_i.

If the additive model (8.1) is not true, the Residual SSq will be inflated by discrepancies between $E(y_{ij})$ and the approximations given by the best-fitting additive model, and the Residual MSq will thus be an unbiased estimate of a quantity greater than the random variance. How do we know whether this has happened? There are two main approaches, the first of which is to examine *residuals*. These are the individual expressions $y_{ij} - \bar{y}_{i.} - \bar{y}_{.j} + \bar{y}$. Their sum of squares was obtained, from (8.4), by subtraction, but it could have been obtained by direct evaluation of all the N residuals and by summing their squares. These residuals add to zero along each row and down each column, like the discrepancies between observed and expected frequencies in a contingency table (§7.6), and (as for contingency tables) the number of DF, $(r-1)(c-1)$, is the number of values of residuals which may be independently chosen (the others being then automatically determined). Because of this lack of independence the residuals are not quite the same as the random error terms ε_{ij} of (8.2), but they have much the same distributional properties. In particular, they should not exhibit any striking patterns. Sometimes the residuals in certain parts of the two-way table seem to have predominantly the same sign; provided the ordering of the rows or columns has any meaning this will suggest that the row-effect constants are not the same for all columns. There may be a correlation between the size of the residual and the 'expected' value* $\bar{y}_{i.} + \bar{y}_{.j} - \bar{y}$: this will suggest that a change of scale would provide better agreement with the additive model.

A second approach is to provide replication of observations, and this is discussed in more detail after Example 8.1.

Example 8.1

Table 8.3 shows the results of a randomized block experiment to compare the effects on the clotting time of plasma of four different methods of treatment of the plasma. Samples of plasma from eight subjects (the 'blocks') were assigned in random order to the four treatments.

The correction term, T^2/N, denoted here by CT, is needed for three items in the SSq column, and it is useful to calculate this at the outset. The analysis is straightforward, and

Table 8.3 Clotting times (min) of plasma from eight subjects, treated by four methods

Subject	Treatment				Total	Mean
	1	2	3	4		
1	8·4	9·4	9·8	12·2	39·8	9·95
2	12·8	15·2	12·9	14·4	55·3	13·82
3	9·6	9·1	11·2	9·8	39·7	9·92
4	9·8	8·8	9·9	12·0	40·5	10·12
5	8·4	8·2	8·5	8·5	33·6	8·40
6	8·6	9·9	9·8	10·9	39·2	9·80
7	8·9	9·0	9·2	10·4	37·5	9·38
8	7·9	8·1	8·2	10·0	34·2	8·55
Total	74·4	77·7	79·5	88·2	319·8	
Mean	9·30	9·71	9·94	11·02		(9·99)

Correction term, CT = $(319\cdot8)^2/32$ = 3196·0013

Between-Subjects SSq = $[(39\cdot8)^2 + \ldots + (34\cdot2)^2]/4 - CT$ = 78·9888

Between-Treatments SSq = $[(74\cdot4)^2 + \ldots + (88\cdot2)^2]/8 - CT$ = 13·0163

Total SSq = $(8\cdot4)^2 + \ldots + (10\cdot0)^2 - CT$ = 105·7788

Residual SSq = 105·7788 − 78·9888 − 13·0163 = 13·7737

Analysis of variance

	SSq	DF	MSq	VR	
Subjects	78·9888	7	11·2841	17·20	$(P < 0\cdot001)$
Treatments	13·0163	3	4·3388	6·62	$(P = 0\cdot003)$
Residual	13·7737	21	0·6559	1·00	
Total	105·7788	31			

*This is the value expected on the basis of the average row and column effects, as may be seen from the equivalent expression $\bar{y} + (\bar{y}_{i.} - \bar{y}) + (\bar{y}_{.j} - \bar{y})$.

the F tests show that differences between subjects and treatments are both highly significant. Differences between subjects do not interest us greatly as the main purpose of the experiment was to study differences between treatments. The standard error of the difference between two treatment means is $\sqrt{[2(0.6559)/8]} = 0.405$. Clearly, treatments 1, 2 and 3 do not differ significantly among themselves, but treatment 4 gives a significantly higher mean clotting time than the others.

For purposes of illustration the residuals are shown below:

Subject	1	2	3	4	Total
		Treatment			
1	− 0·86	− 0·27	− 0·10	1·22	− 0·01
2	− 0·33	1·66	− 0·87	− 0·45	0·01
3	0·37	− 0·54	1·33	− 1·15	0·01
4	0·37	− 1·04	− 0·17	0·85	0·01
5	0·69	0·08	0·15	− 0·93	− 0·01
6	− 0·51	0·38	0·05	0·07	− 0·01
7	0·21	− 0·10	− 0·13	− 0·01	− 0·03
8	0·04	− 0·17	− 0·30	0·42	− 0·01
Total	− 0·02	0·00	− 0·04	0·02	− 0·04

The first entry, for example, is calculated from Table 8.3 as

$$8.4 - 9.95 - 9.30 + 9.99 = - 0.86.$$

The sum of squares of the 32 residuals in the body of the table is 13·7744, in agreement with the value found by subtraction in Table 8.3 apart from rounding errors. (These errors account also for the fact that the residuals as shown do not add exactly to zero along the rows and columns.) No particular pattern emerges from the table of residuals, nor does the distribution appear to be grossly non-normal. There are 16 negative values and 16 positive values; the highest three in absolute value are positive (1·66, 1·33 and 1·22), which suggests mildly that the random-error distribution may have slight positive skewness.

If the linear model (8.1) is wrong there is said to be an *interaction* between the row and column effects. In the absence of an interaction the expected differences between observations in different columns are the same for all rows (and the statement is true if we interchange the words 'columns' and 'rows'). If there is an interaction, the expected column differences vary from row to row (and, similarly, expected row differences vary from column to column). With one observation in each row/column cell the effect of an interaction is inextricably mixed with the residual variation. Suppose, however, that we have more than one observation per cell. The variation between observations *within the same cell* provides direct evidence about the random variance σ^2, and may therefore be used as a basis of comparison for the between-cells residual. This is illustrated in the next example.

Example 8.2

In Table 8.4 we show some hypothetical data related to the data of Table 8.3. There are three subjects and three treatments, and for each subject–treatment combination three replicate observations are made. The mean of each group of three replicates will be seen to agree with the value shown in Table 8.3 for the same subject and treatment. Under each

Table 8.4 Clotting time (min) of plasma from three subjects, three methods of treatment and three replications for each subject–treatment combination

Subject	Treatment 2	Treatment 3	Treatment 4	Total	
6	9·8	9·9	11·3		
	10·1	9·5	10·7		
	9·8	10·0	10·7		
	T_{11} 29·7	29·4	32·7	R_1 91·8	
	S_{11} 294·09	288·26	356·67		
7	9·2	9·1	10·3		
	8·6	9·1	10·7		
	9·2	9·4	10·2		
	27·0	27·6	31·2	R_2 85·8	
	243·24	253·98	324·62		
8	8·4	8·6	9·8		
	7·9	8·0	10·1		
	8·0	8·0	10·1		
	24·3	24·6	30·0	R_3 78·9	
	196·97	201·96	300·06		
Total	C_1 81·0	C_2 81·6	C_3 93·9	T 256·5	$\sum y^2$ 2459·85

$$CT = T^2/27 = 2436\cdot75$$

Subjects SSq	$= [(91\cdot8)^2 + \ldots + (78\cdot9)^2]/9 - CT$		$= \ \ 9\cdot2600$
Treatments SSq	$= [(81\cdot0)^2 + \ldots + (93\cdot9)^2]/9 - CT$		$= 11\cdot7800$
Interaction SSq	$= [(29\cdot7)^2 + \ldots + (30\cdot0)^2]/3 - CT - \text{Subj. SSq} - \text{Treat. SSq}$		$= \ \ 0\cdot7400$
Total SSq	$= (9\cdot8)^2 + \ldots + (10\cdot1)^2 - CT = 2459\cdot85 - CT$		$= 23\cdot1000$
Residual SSq	$= \text{Total} - \text{Subjects} - \text{Treatments} - \text{Interaction}$		$= \ \ 1\cdot3200$

Analysis of variance

	SSq	DF	MSq	VR	
Subjects	9·2600	2	4·6300	63·1	
Treatments	11·7800	2	5·8900	80·3	
Interaction	0·7400	4	0·1850	2·52	$(P = 0\cdot077)$
Residual	1·3200	18	0·0733	1·00	
Total	23·1000	26			

group of replicates is shown the total T_{ij}, and the sum of squares, S_{ij} (as indicated for T_{11} and S_{11}).

The Subjects and Treatments SSq are obtained straightforwardly, using the divisor 9 for the sums of squares of row (or column) totals since there are nine observations in each row (or column), and using a divisor 27 in the correction term. The Interaction SSq is obtained in a similar way to the Residual in Table 8.3, but using the totals T_{ij} as the basis of calculation. Thus,

Interaction SSq = SSq for differences between the nine subject/treatment cells

− Subjects SSq − Treatments SSq,

and the degrees of freedom are, correspondingly, $8 - 2 - 2 = 4$. The Total SSq is obtained in the usual way and the Residual SSq follows by subtraction. The Residual SSq could have been obtained directly as the sum over the nine cells of the sum of squares about the mean of each triplet, i.e. as

$$(S_{11} - T_{11}^2/3) + (S_{12} - T_{12}^2/3) + \ldots + (S_{33} - T_{33}^2/3).$$

The F tests show the effects of subjects and treatments to be highly significant. The interaction term is not significant at the 5% level, but the variance ratio is nevertheless rather high. It is due mainly to the mean value for subject 8 and treatment 4 being higher than expected.

The interpretation of significant interactions and the interpretation of the tests for the 'main effects' (subjects and treatments in Examples 8.1 and 8.2) when interactions are present will be discussed in the next section.

In Example 8.2 the number of replications at each row–column combination was constant. This is not a necessary requirement. The number of observations at the ith row and jth column, n_{ij}, may vary, but the method of analysis indicated in Example 8.2 is valid only if the n_{ij} are proportional to the total row and column frequencies; that is, denoting the latter by $n_{i.}$ and $n_{.j}$,

$$n_{ij} = \frac{n_{i.} n_{.j}}{N}. \tag{8.6}$$

In Example 8.2 all the $n_{i.}$ and $n_{.j}$ were equal to 9, N was 27, and $n_{ij} = 81/27 = 3$, for all i and j. If (8.6) is not true, an attempt to follow the standard method of analysis may lead to negative sums of squares for the interaction or residual, which is, of course, an impossible situation. Appropriate methods of analysis are described in §8.8.

If, in a two-way classification without replication, $c = 2$, the situation is the same as that for which the paired t test was used in §4.4. There is a close analogy here with the relationship between the one-way analysis of variance and the two-sample t test noted in §7.1. In the two-way case the F test provided by the analysis of variance is equivalent to the paired t test in that (i) F is numerically equal to t^2; (ii) the F statistic has 1 and $r - 1$ DF while t has $r - 1$ DF, and as noted in §4.6 the distributions of t^2 and F are identical. The Residual MSq in the analysis of variance is half the corresponding s^2 in the t test, since the latter is an estimate of the variance of the difference between two readings.

8.2 The simple crossover design

The crossover design is widely used for clinical trials in which each subject can receive different treatments in successive periods of administration. It is thus most suitable for treatments intended for rapid relief of symptoms in chronic diseases, where the long-term condition of the patient remains fairly stable. In the simplest case, with two treatments, A and B, one randomly chosen group of patients (group I) receives treatments in the order AB, while the other group (group II) receives them in the order BA. There may be different numbers of patients in the two groups.

The design has the following layout:

	Run-in	Period 1	Washout	Period 2
Reading:	z_{ij}	y_{ij1}		y_{ij2}
Group I (n_1)	—	A	—	B
Group II (n_2)	—	B	—	A

Here, the 'readings' are observations of some appropriate measure of the patient's condition (e.g. respiratory test measurement, frequency of attacks of some sort, etc.). The two periods of administration are separated by a 'washout' period to enable the patient's condition to return to a level un-influenced as far as possible by the treatment previously used. (In a drug trial, for instance, it should be long enough to allow for virtual elimination of a drug used in period 1.) The 'run-in' period is optional, but it may provide an opportunity for the patients to settle down and for the investigator to make a 'baseline' observation z_{ij}. The responses y_{ij1} and y_{ij2} will often be made towards the end of the treatment periods, to allow maximal effect of the treatments, but they may be averages or maxima of a series of observations taken throughout the periods.

The notation for the readings is as follows: the subscript i indicates the group ($i = 1$ for group I, $i = 2$ for group II); j identifies the subject within the group; the final subscript indicates the first or second response. The crucial measurements are the active responses y_{ij1} and y_{ij2}, but, as we shall see, the baseline readings z_{ij} may be very useful.

It is possible to analyse such data by an analysis of variance (Hills and Armitage, 1979), although when n_1 and n_2 are unequal the analysis is 'non-orthogonal' (§8.8). It is, in fact, simpler to use t tests, and Example 8.3 illustrates the method on responses from a trial without baseline data.

Example 8.3

In a clinical trial of a new drug for the treatment of enuresis each of 29 patients was given the drug for a period of 14 days and a placebo for a separate period of 14 days, the order of administration being chosen randomly for each patient. Table 8.5 shows the number of dry nights experienced during each treatment period.

A test for the relative effectiveness of drug and placebo could be obtained from the complete series of 29 paired observations. We should need the 29 differences for (drug − placebo). For group I these are the (period 1 − period 2) differences d_{1j} shown in Table 8.5. For group II we should need to change the sign of the differences d_{2j}. Writing $d^*_{1j} = d_{1j}$ and $d^*_{2j} = -d_{2j}$, we can do a t test on the 29 values of d^*_{ij}. This gives

$$\bar{d}^* = 2 \cdot 172,$$

$$s^2 = 11 \cdot 005,$$

$$\text{SE}(\bar{d}^*) = \sqrt{(11 \cdot 005/29)} = 0 \cdot 616,$$

$$t = \bar{d}^*/\text{SE}(\bar{d}^*) = 3 \cdot 53 \text{ on } 28 \text{ DF} \quad (P = 0 \cdot 001).$$

This analysis suggests strongly that the drug increases the number of dry nights as compared with the placebo. However, it is unsatisfactory since it takes no account of the order in which each patient received the two treatments. This might be particularly important if there were a systematic period effect, for example if patients tended to obtain better relief in period 1 than in period 2.

The mean responses in the two periods for the two groups are as follows:

Period	1	2	Diff. (1 − 2)
Group I: Treatment	A $\bar{y}_{11} = 8 \cdot 118$	B $\bar{y}_{12} = 5 \cdot 294$	$\bar{d}_1 = 2 \cdot 824$
Group II: Treatment	B $\bar{y}_{21} = 7 \cdot 667$	A $\bar{y}_{22} = 8 \cdot 917$	$\bar{d}_2 = -1 \cdot 250$

To test for the presence of a treatment effect, we can test the difference between $\bar{d}_1$ and $\bar{d}_2$, since, if there were no treatment effect, the expectations of $\bar{d}_1$ and $\bar{d}_2$ would be equal. This comparison involves a standard two-sample t test, giving

$$t = (\bar{d}_1 - \bar{d}_2)/\text{SE}(\bar{d}_1 - \bar{d}_2) \quad \text{on} \quad n_1 + n_2 - 2 \text{ DF},$$

where

$$\text{SE}(\bar{d}_1 - \bar{d}_2) = \sqrt{\left[s_d^2 \left(\frac{1}{n_1} + \frac{1}{n_2} \right) \right]},$$

and s_d^2 is the pooled within-groups estimate of variance of the d_{ij}. In this example, $\bar{d}_1 - \bar{d}_2 = 4 \cdot 074$, $s_d^2 = 10 \cdot 767$ and $\text{SE}(\bar{d}_1 - \bar{d}_2) = 1 \cdot 237$, giving $t = 4 \cdot 074/1 \cdot 237 = 3 \cdot 29$ on 27 DF ($P = 0 \cdot 003$). The result is close to that given by the earlier, crude, analysis.

To test for a period effect, we test $\bar{d}_1 + \bar{d}_2$, since, if there were no period effect, the expectations of $\bar{d}_1$ and $\bar{d}_2$ would be equal in magnitude but opposite in sign. The same standard error is used as for $\bar{d}_1 - \bar{d}_2$. In the example, this gives $t = 1 \cdot 574/1 \cdot 237 = 1 \cdot 27$ on 27 DF ($P = 0 \cdot 21$), providing no evidence of a period effect.

Table 8.5 Number of dry nights out of 14 nights, experienced by patients with enuresis treated by drug and placebo

Group I

Period:	1	2		
Treatment	A (drug)	B (placebo)	Difference	Sum
Patient			(1 − 2)	(1 + 2)
number, j	y_{1j1}	y_{1j2}	d_{1j}	e_{1j}
1	8	5	3	13
2	14	10	4	24
3	8	0	8	8
4	9	7	2	16
5	11	6	5	17
6	3	5	− 2	8
7	6	0	6	6
8	0	0	0	0
9	13	12	1	25
10	10	2	8	12
11	7	5	2	12
12	13	13	0	26
13	8	10	− 2	18
14	7	7	0	14
15	9	0	9	9
16	10	6	4	16
17	2	2	0	4

Group II

Period:	1	2		
Treatment	B (placebo)	A (drug)	Difference	Sum
Patient			(1 − 2)	(1 + 2)
number, j	y_{2j1}	y_{2j2}	d_{2j}	e_{2j}
1	12	11	1	23
2	6	8	− 2	14
3	13	9	4	22
4	8	8	0	16
5	8	9	− 1	17
6	4	8	− 4	12
7	8	14	− 6	22
8	2	4	− 2	6
9	8	13	− 5	21
10	9	7	2	16
11	7	10	− 3	17
12	7	6	1	13

The magnitude of the treatment effect is estimated as $\frac{1}{2}(\bar{d}_1 - \bar{d}_2) = 2 \cdot 037$ dry nights out of 14, and its standard error as $\frac{1}{2} \text{SE}(\bar{d}_1 - \bar{d}_2) = 0 \cdot 618$. The 95% confidence interval for the treatment effect is thus $2 \cdot 037 \pm (2 \cdot 052)(0 \cdot 618) = 0 \cdot 77$ to $3 \cdot 31$ days. The multiplier here is $t_{27, 0 \cdot 05} = 2 \cdot 052$.

The analysis illustrated in Example 8.3 assumes that the response is affected additively by treatment and period effects. This assumption is not necessarily true. There may be a treatment × period (TP) interaction for any of a number of reasons.

1   If the washout period is too short, the response in period 2 may be affected by the treatment received in period 1 as well as that in period 2.

2   Even if the washout period is sufficiently long for a period 1 drug to be eliminated, its psychological or physiological effect might persist into period 2.

3   If there is a strong period effect, changing the general level of response from period 1 to period 2, the treatment effect might be changed merely because it varies with different portions of the scale of measurement.

A test for the existence of a TP interaction is obtained as follows. If there is no TP interaction, the sum of the two responses for subject j in group i, $e_{ij} = y_{ij1} + y_{ij2}$, should (apart from random error) be the same whether the subject is in group I or group II, since in either case e_{ij} includes contributions for treatments A and B and for periods 1 and 2. If there is an interaction, e_{ij} will tend to be higher in one group than another. For instance, if A is much more effective than B, and there is a strong carry-over effect of A, group I will tend to have the more favourable values of e_{ij}. We can therefore test the difference between the two mean values of e_{ij}, $\bar{e}_1$ and $\bar{e}_2$, again using a two-sample t test. Here, however, the pooled within-group variance estimate s_e^2 is that of the e_{ij}, not (as before) the d_{ij}. Since the e_{ij} vary in part because of variability between subjects, we should expect $s_e^2 > s_d^2$.

Example 8.3, continued

The values of e_{ij} are given in Table 8.5. The two means are $\bar{e}_1 = 13\cdot412$, $\bar{e}_2 = 16\cdot583$. The pooled variance estimate is $s_e^2 = 41\cdot890$ (substantially larger than s_d^2, as expected) and

$$\text{SE}(\bar{e}_1 - \bar{e}_2) = \sqrt{\left[(41\cdot890)\left(\frac{1}{17} + \frac{1}{12}\right)\right]} = 2\cdot440.$$

Thus, $t = (13\cdot412 - 16\cdot583)/2\cdot440 = -1\cdot30$ on 27 DF ($P = 0\cdot20$). There is no clear evidence of a TP interaction, and the earlier analysis therefore seems reasonable.

If there is a TP interaction, there will be little point in testing and estimating the treatment effect from the whole set of data, as in Example 8.3. Period 1 alone provides a perfectly valid test of A versus B, since subjects were randomly allocated to the two treatments. Period 2 is of doubtful value, since the subjects (although originally randomized) have undergone different experiences before entering period 2. The best procedure, therefore, is to do a two-sample test of the y_{ij1} values in period 1, estimating the treatment effect from the difference between the two means, $\bar{y}_{11} - \bar{y}_{21}$. Unfortunately, this comparison is subject to between-subjects variation, and is therefore less precise than the full crossover approach.

A similar drawback applies to the test for interaction. This is based on between-subjects variation, and if the latter is very large the t test will be relatively insensitive. There may then actually be a substantial interaction, large enough to affect markedly the estimate of treatment effect, which nevertheless remains undetected. The analysis outlined above may therefore be somewhat dangerous unless there is strong prior knowledge, obtained perhaps from similar studies in the past, that the interaction is likely to be negligible.

This drawback can be partly overcome by use of the baseline readings z_{ij}. (Armitage and Hills (1982) discuss the use also of second baseline readings made during the washout period.) For each subject, we calculate the difference

$$e'_{ij} = e_{ij} - 2z_{ij},$$

and test the difference in means $\bar{e}'_1 - \bar{e}'_2$ rather than $\bar{e}_1 - \bar{e}_2$. Since the subtraction of $2z_{ij}$ in e'_{ij} removes the general level of response of each subject, the e'_{ij} are not affected by between-subjects variation and can be expected to be less variable than the e_{ij}.

A similar device can be used for the assessment of treatment effect from period 1, when the interaction is present. A corrected response, $y'_{ij1} = y_{ij1} - z_{ij}$, is calculated, and a two-sample t test carried out on the means $\bar{y}'_{11}$ and $\bar{y}'_{21}$. Again, the within-groups variation of the y'_{ij1} values should be less than that of the y_{ij1} values.

Some of the ambiguities of the simple crossover design are removed by larger crossover designs, with more than two periods and perhaps more than two sequence groups (Jones and Kenward, 1989).

8.3 Factorial designs

In §8.1 an example was described of a design for a factorial experiment in which the variable to be analysed was blood-clotting time and the effects of two factors were to be measured: r periods of storage and c concentrations of adrenalin. Observations were made at each combination of storage periods and adrenalin concentrations. There are two factors here, one at r levels and the other at c levels, and the design is called an $r \times c$ *factorial*.

This design contravenes what used to be regarded as a good principle of experimentation, namely that only one factor should be changed at a time. The advantages of factorial experimentation over the one-factor-at-a-time approach were pointed out by Fisher. If we make one observation at each of the rc combinations, we can make comparisons of the mean effects of different periods of storage on the basis of c observations at each period. To get the same precision with a non-factorial design we should have to choose one particular concentration of adrenalin and make c observations for each storage period: rc in all. This would give us no information about the effect of varying the concentration of adrenalin. An experiment to throw light on this factor with the same precision as the factorial design would need a further rc observations, all with the same storage period. Twice as many observations as in the factorial design would therefore be needed. Moreover, the factorial design permits a comparison of the effect of one factor at different levels of the other: it permits the detection of an interaction between the two factors. This cannot be done without the factorial approach.

The two-factor design considered in §8.1 can clearly be generalized to allow the simultaneous study of three or more factors. Strictly, the term 'factorial design' should be reserved for situations in which the factors are all controllable experimental treatments and in which all the combinations of levels are randomly allocated to the experimental units. The analysis is, however, essentially the same in the slightly different situation in which one or more of the factors represents a form of blocking—a source of known or suspected variation which can usefully be eliminated in comparing the real treatments. We shall therefore include this extended form of factorial design in the present discussion.

Notation becomes troublesome if we aim at complete generality, so we shall discuss in detail a three-factor design. The directions of generalization should be clear. Suppose there are three factors: A at I levels, B at J levels and C at K levels. As in §8.1 we consider a linear model whereby the mean response at the ith level of A, the jth level of B and the kth level of C is

$$E(y_{ijk}) = \mu + \alpha_i + \beta_j + \gamma_k + (\alpha\beta)_{ij} + (\alpha\gamma)_{ik} + (\beta\gamma)_{jk} + (\alpha\beta\gamma)_{ijk}, \qquad (8.7)$$

with $\sum_i \alpha_i = \ldots = \sum_i (\alpha\beta)_{ij} = \ldots = \sum_i (\alpha\beta\gamma)_{ijk} = 0$, etc. Here the terms like $(\alpha\beta)_{ij}$ are to be read as single constants, the notation being chosen to indicate the interpretation of each term as an interaction between two or more factors. The constants α_i measure the effects of the different levels of factor A averaged over the various levels of the other factors; these are called the *main effects* of A. The constant $(\alpha\beta)_{ij}$ indicates the extent to which the mean response at level i of A and level j of B, averaged over all levels of C, is not determined purely by α_i and β_j, and it thus measures one aspect of the interaction of A and B. It is called a *first-order interaction term* or *two-factor interaction term*. Similarly, the constant $(\alpha\beta\gamma)_{ijk}$ indicates how the mean response at the triple combination of A, B and C is not determined purely by main effects and first-order interaction terms. It is called a *second-order* or *three-factor interaction term*.

To complete the model, suppose that y_{ijk} is distributed normally about $E(y_{ijk})$ with a constant residual variance σ^2.

Table 8.6 Structure of analysis of variance for three-factor design with replication

		SSq	DF	MSq	VR($= MSq/s^2$)
Main effects					
	A	S_A	$I - 1$	s_A^2	F_A
	B	S_B	$J - 1$	s_B^2	F_B
	C	S_C	$K - 1$	s_C^2	F_C
Two-factor interactions					
	AB	S_{AB}	$(I - 1)(J - 1)$	s_{AB}^2	F_{AB}
	AC	S_{AC}	$(I - 1)(K - 1)$	s_{AC}^2	F_{AC}
	BC	S_{BC}	$(J - 1)(K - 1)$	s_{BC}^2	F_{BC}
Three-factor interaction					
	ABC	S_{ABC}	$(I - 1)(J - 1)(K - 1)$	s_{ABC}^2	F_{ABC}
Residual		S_R	$IJK(n - 1)$	s^2	1
Total		S	$N - 1$		

Suppose now that we make n observations at each combination of A, B and C. The total number of observations is $nIJK = N$, say. The structure of the analysis of variance is shown in Table 8.6. The DF for the main effects and two-factor interactions follow directly from the results for two-way analyses. That for the three-factor interaction is a natural extension. The residual DF are $IJK(n - 1)$ because there are $n - 1$ DF between replicates at each of the IJK factor combinations. The SSq terms are calculated as follows.

1 *Main effects.* As for a one-way analysis, remembering that the divisor for the square of a group total is the total number of observations in that group. Thus, if the total for ith level of A is $T_{i..}$, and the grand total is T, the SSq for A is

$$\sum_i T_{i..}^2/nJK - T^2/N. \tag{8.8}$$

2 *Two-factor interactions.* Form a two-way table of totals, calculate the appropriate corrected sum of squares between these totals and subtract the SSq for the two relevant main effects. For AB, for instance, suppose $T_{ij.}$ is the total for levels i of A and j of B. Then

$$S_{AB} = \left(\sum_{i,j} T_{ij.}^2/nK - T^2/N \right) - S_A - S_B. \tag{8.9}$$

3 *Three-factor interaction.* Form a three-way table of totals, calculate the appropriate corrected sum of squares and subtract the SSq for all relevant two-factor interactions and main effects. If T_{ijk} is the total for the three-factor combination at levels i, j, k of A, B, C respectively,

$$S_{ABC} = \left(\sum_{i,j,k} T_{ijk}^2/n - T^2/N \right) - S_{AB} - S_{AC} - S_{BC} - S_A - S_B - S_C. \tag{8.10}$$

4 *Total.* As usual by

$$\sum_{i,j,k,r} y_{ijkr}^2 - T^2/N,$$

where the suffix r (from 1 to n) denotes one of the n replicate observations at each factor combination.

5 *Residual.* By subtraction. It could also have been obtained by adding, over all three-factor combinations, the sum of squares between replicates:

$$\sum_{i,j,k} \left(\sum_{r=1}^{n} y_{ijkr}^2 - T_{ijk}^2/n \right). \tag{8.11}$$

This alternative formulation unfortunately does not provide an independent check on the arithmetic, as it follows immediately from the other expressions.

The MSq terms are obtained as usual from SSq/DF. Each of these divided by the Residual MSq, s^2, provides an F test for the appropriate null hypothesis about the main effects or interactions. For example, F_A (tested on $I-1$ and $IJK(n-1)$ degrees of freedom) provides a test of the null hypothesis that all the α_i are zero—that is, that the mean responses at different levels of A, averaged over all levels of the other factors, are all equal. Some problems of interpretation of this rather complex set of tests are discussed at the end of this section.

Suppose $n=1$, so that there is no replication. The DF for the residual become zero, since $n-1=0$. So does the SSq, since all the contributions in parentheses in (8.11) are zero, being sums of squares about the mean of a single observation. The 'residual' line therefore does not appear in the analysis. The position is exactly the same as in the two-way analysis with one observation per cell. The usual practice is to take the highest-order interaction (in this case ABC) as the residual term, and to calculate F ratios using this MSq as the denominator. As in the two-way analysis, this will be satisfactory if the highest-order interaction terms in the *model* (in our case $(\alpha\beta\gamma)_{ijk}$) are zero or near zero. If these terms are substantial the makeshift Residual MSq, s_{ABC}^2, will tend to be higher than σ^2 and the tests will be correspondingly insensitive.

Example 8.4

Table 8.7* shows the relative weights of right adrenals (expressed as a fraction of body weight, $\times 10^4$) in mice obtained by crossing parents of four strains. For each of the 16 combinations of parental strains, four mice (two of each sex) were used.

This is a three-factor design. The factors—mother's strain, father's strain and sex—are not, of course, experimental treatments imposed by random allocation. Nevertheless they represent potential sources of variation whose main effects and interactions may be

---

*The data were kindly provided by Drs R. L. Collins and R. J. Meckler. In their paper (Collins and Meckler, 1965) results from both adrenals are analysed.

Table 8.7 Relative weights of right adrenals in mice

Mother's strain	Father's strain 1 ♀	1 ♂	2 ♀	2 ♂	3 ♀	3 ♂	4 ♀	4 ♂	Totals ♀	♂	♀+♂
1	0·93	0·69	1·76	0·67	1·46	0·88	1·45	0·95	12·57	6·57	19·14
	1·70	0·83	1·58	0·73	1·89	0·96	1·80	0·86			
2	1·42	0·50	1·85	0·72	2·14	1·00	1·94	0·63	15·25	6·08	21·33
	1·96	0·74	1·69	0·66	2·17	0·96	2·08	0·87			
3	2·22	0·86	1·96	1·04	1·62	0·82	1·51	0·82	15·32	6·69	22·01
	2·33	0·98	2·09	0·96	1·63	0·57	1·96	0·64			
4	1·25	0·56	1·56	1·08	1·88	1·00	1·85	0·43	13·39	6·32	19·71
	1·76	0·75	1·90	0·80	1·81	1·11	1·38	0·59			
Total	13·57	5·91	14·39	6·66	14·60	7·30	13·97	5·79	56·53	25·66	
	19·48		21·05		21·90		19·76				82·19

CT = 105·5499

Analysis of variance

	DF	SSq	MSq	VR	
Mother's strain, M	3	0·3396	0·1132	2·87	
Father's strain, F	3	0·2401	0·0800	2·03	
Sex of animal, S	1	14·8900	14·8900	376·96	($P < 0.001$)
MF	9	1·2988	0·1443	3·65	($P = 0.003$)
MS	3	0·3945	0·1315	3·33	($P = 0.032$)
FS	3	0·0245	0·0082	0·21	
MFS	9	0·2612	0·0290	0·73	
Residual	32	1·2647	0·0395	1·00	
Total	63	18·7134			

Differences ♀−♂

Mother's strain	Father's strain 1	2	3	4	Total
1	1·11	1·94	1·51	1·44	6·00
2	2·14	2·16	2·35	2·52	9·17
3	2·71	2·05	1·86	2·01	8·63
4	1·70	1·58	1·58	2·21	7·07
Total	7·66	7·73	7·30	8·18	30·87

studied. The DF are shown in the table. The SSq for main effects follow straightforwardly from the subtotals. That for mother's strain, for example, is.

$$[(19·14)^2 + \ldots + (19·71)^2]/16 - CT,$$

where the correction term, CT, is $(82·19)^2/64 = 105·5499$. The two-factor interaction, MF, is obtained as

$$[(4\cdot15)^2 + \ldots + (4\cdot25)^2]/4 - CT - S_M - S_F,$$

where $4\cdot15$ is the sum of the four responses in the first cell $(0\cdot93 + 1\cdot70 + 0\cdot69 + 0\cdot83)$, and S_M and S_F are the SSq for the two main effects. Similarly the three-factor interaction is obtained as

$$[(2\cdot63)^2 + (1\cdot52)^2 + \ldots + (3\cdot23)^2 + (1\cdot02)^2]/2 - CT$$
$$- S_M - S_F - S_S - S_{MF} - S_{MS} - S_{FS}.$$

Here the quantities $2\cdot63$, etc., are subtotals of pairs of responses $(2\cdot63 = 0\cdot93 + 1\cdot70)$. The Residual SSq may be obtained by subtraction, once the Total SSq has been obtained. Alternatively, as a check it may be obtained from the *differences* between replicate observations:

$$[(0\cdot93 - 1\cdot70)^2 + \ldots + (0\cdot43 - 0\cdot59)^2]/2 = 1\cdot2648,$$

the difference from the value obtained by subtraction being due to rounding error.

When, as in this example, one of the factors has only two levels, the calculation of the main effect and the interactions involving this factor may be simplified by considering contrasts between the two levels of the factor. The differences between the totals for the two females and for the two males, at each parental cross, are as shown at the foot of Table 8.7. The SSq for the main effect, S, is, from (7.10), given by $(30\cdot87)^2/64 = 14\cdot8900$ as before. The SSq for MS is

$$[(6\cdot00)^2 + \ldots + (7\cdot07)^2]/16 - 14\cdot8900 = 0\cdot3944,$$

that for FS is

$$[(7\cdot66)^2 + \ldots + (8\cdot18)^2]/16 - 14\cdot8900 = 0\cdot0244,$$

and that for MFS is

$$[(1\cdot11)^2 + \ldots + (2\cdot21)^2]/4 - 14\cdot8900 - S_{MS} - S_{FS} = 0\cdot2614.$$

These SSq agree with those in Table 8.7 apart from rounding errors.

The F tests show the main effects M and F to be non-significant, although each variance ratio is greater than 1. The interaction MF is highly significant. The main effect of sex is highly significant, and also its interaction with M. To elucidate the strain effects it is useful to tabulate the sums of observations for the 16 crosses:

	Father's strain				
Mother's strain	1	2	3	4	Total
1	4·15	4·74	5·19	5·06	19·14
2	4·62	4·92	6·27	5·52	21·33
3	6·39	6·05	4·64	4·93	22·01
4	4·32	5·34	5·80	4·25	19·71
Total	19·48	21·05	21·90	19·76	82·19

Strains 2 and 3 give relatively high readings for both M and F, suggesting a systematic effect which has not achieved significance for either parent separately. The interaction is due partly to the high reading for (M3, F1).

Each of the 16 cell totals is the sum of four readings, and the difference between any two has a standard error $\sqrt{[(2)(4)(0\cdot0395)]} = 0\cdot56$. For M3 the difference between F1 and F3 is significantly positive, whereas for each of the other maternal strains the F1 $-$ F3 difference is negative, significantly so for M2 and M4. A similar reversal is provided by the four entries for M2 and M3, F2 and F3.

The MS interaction may be studied from the previous table of sex contrasts. Each of the row totals has a standard error $\sqrt{[16(0.0395)]} = 0.80$. Maternal strains 2 and 3 show significantly higher sex differences than M1, and M2 is significantly higher also than M4. The point may be seen from the right-hand margin of Table 8.7, where the high responses for M2 and M3 are shown strongly in the female offspring, but not in the males.

This type of experiment, in which parents of each sex from a number of strains are crossed, is called a *diallel cross*. Special methods of analysis are available which allow for the general effect of each strain, exhibited by both males and females, and the specific effects of particular crosses (Bulmer, 1980).

The 2^p factorial design

An interaction term in the analysis of a factorial design will in general have many degrees of freedom, and will represent departures of various types from an additive model. The interpretation of a significant interaction may therefore require careful thought. If, however, all the factors are at two levels, each of the main effects and each of the interactions will have only one degree of freedom, and consequently represent linear contrasts which can be interpreted relatively simply. If there are, say, four factors each at two levels, the design is referred to as a $2 \times 2 \times 2 \times 2$, or 2^4, design, and in general for p factors each at two levels, the design is called 2^p. The analysis of 2^p designs can be simplified by direct calculation of each linear contrast. We shall illustrate the procedure for a 2^3 design.

Suppose there are n observations at each of the 8 ($= 2^3$) factor combinations. Since each factor is at two levels we can, by suitable conventions, regard each factor as being positive or negative—say, by the presence or absence of some feature. Denoting the factors by A, B and C, we can identify each factor combination by writing in lower-case letters those factors which are positive. Thus, (ab) indicates the combination with A and B positive and C negative, while (c) indicates the combination with only C positive; the combination with all factors negative will be written as (1). In formulae these symbols can be taken to mean the totals of the n observations at the different factor combinations.

The main effect of A may be estimated by the difference between the mean response at all combinations with A positive and that for A negative. This is a linear contrast,

$$\frac{(a) + (ab) + (ac) + (abc)}{4n} - \left[\frac{(1) + (b) + (c) + (bc)}{4n}\right] = [A]/4n, \qquad (8.12)$$

where

$$[A] = -(1) + (a) - (b) + (ab) - (c) + (ac) - (bc) + (abc), \qquad (8.13)$$

the terms being rearranged here so that the factors are introduced in order.

The main effects of B and C are defined in a similar way.

The two-factor interaction between A and B represents the difference between the estimated effect of A when B is positive, and that when B is negative. This is

$$\frac{(ab) + (abc) - (b) - (bc)}{2n} - \left[\frac{(a) + (ac) - (1) - (c)}{2n}\right] = [AB]/2n, \quad (8.14)$$

where

$$[AB] = (1) - (a) - (b) + (ab) + (c) - (ac) - (bc) + (abc). \quad (8.15)$$

To avoid the awkwardness of the divisor $2n$ in (8.14) when $4n$ appears in (8.12), it is useful to redefine the interaction as $[AB]/4n$, that is as half the difference referred to above. Note that the terms in (8.15) have a positive sign when A and B are either both positive or both negative, and a negative sign otherwise. Note also that $[AB]/4n$ can be written as

$$\frac{(ab) + (abc) - (a) - (ac)}{4n} - \left[\frac{(b) + (bc) - (1) - (c)}{4n}\right],$$

which is half the difference between the estimated effect of B when A is positive and that when A is negative. This emphasizes the symmetric nature of $[AB]$.

The three-factor interaction $[ABC]$ can similarly be interpreted in a number of equivalent ways. It represents, for instance, the difference between the estimated $[AB]$ interaction when C is positive and when C is negative. Apart from the divisor, this difference is measured by

$$[ABC] = [(c) - (ac) - (bc) + (abc)] - [(1) - (a) - (b) + (ab)]$$
$$= -(1) + (a) + (b) - (ab) + (c) - (ac) - (bc) + (abc), \quad (8.16)$$

and it is again convenient to redefine the interaction as $[ABC]/4n$.

The results are summarized in Table 8.8. Note that the positive and negative signs for the two-factor interactions are easily obtained by multiplying together the coefficients for the corresponding main effects; and those for the three-factor interaction by multiplying the coefficients for $[A]$ and $[BC]$, $[B]$ and $[AC]$, or $[C]$ and $[AB]$.

The final column of Table 8.8 shows the formula for the SSq and (since each has 1 DF) for the MSq for each term in the analysis. Each term like $[A]$, $[AB]$, etc., has a variance $8n\sigma^2$ on the appropriate null hypothesis (since each of the totals (1), (a), etc., has a variance $n\sigma^2$). Hence $[A]^2/8n$ is an estimate of σ^2. In general, for a 2^p factorial, the divisors for the linear contrasts are $2^{p-1}n$, and those for the SSq are $2^p n$.

The significance of the main effects and of interactions may equivalently be tested by t tests. The residual mean square, s^2, has $8(n-1)$ DF, and the variance of each of the contrasts $[A]$, $[AB]$, etc., is estimated as $8ns^2$, to give a t test with $8(n-1)$ DF.

Table 8.8 Calculation of main effects and interactions for 2^3 factorial design

Effect		Multiplier for total								Divisor for contrast	Contribution to SSq
		(1)	(a)	(b)	(ab)	(c)	(ac)	(bc)	(abc)		
Main effects	A	−1	1	−1	1	−1	1	−1	1	$4n$	$[A]^2/8n$
	B	−1	−1	1	1	−1	−1	1	1	$4n$	$[B]^2/8n$
	C	−1	−1	−1	−1	1	1	1	1	$4n$	$[C]^2/8n$
Two-factor interactions	AB	1	−1	−1	1	1	−1	−1	1	$4n$	$[AB]^2/8n$
	AC	1	−1	1	−1	−1	1	−1	1	$4n$	$[AC]^2/8n$
	BC	1	1	−1	−1	−1	−1	1	1	$4n$	$[BC]^2/8n$
Three-factor interaction	ABC	−1	1	1	−1	1	−1	−1	1	$4n$	$[ABC]^2/8n$

Interpretation of factorial experiments with significant interactions

The analysis of a large-scale factorial experiment provides an opportunity to test simultaneously a number of main effects and interactions. The complexity of this situation sometimes gives rise to ambiguities of interpretation. The following points may be helpful.

1 Whether or not two or more factors interact will depend on the scale of measurement of the variable under analysis. Sometimes a simpler interpretation of the data may be obtained by reanalysing the data after a logarithmic or other transformation (see Chapter 11). For instance, if we ignore random error, the responses shown in (a) below present an interaction between A and B. Those shown in (b) present no interaction. The responses in (b) are the square roots of those in (a).

	B		B	
A	Low	High	Low	High
Low	9	16	3	4
High	16	25	4	5
	(a)		(b)	

The search for a scale of measurement on which interactions are small or non-significant is particularly worth trying if the main effects of one factor, as measured at different levels of the other(s), are related closely to the mean responses at these levels. If the estimated main effects of any one factor are in *opposite directions* for different levels of the other(s), transformations are not likely to be useful. This type of effect is called a *qualitative* interaction, and is likely to be more important than a *quantitative* interaction, in which the effect of one variable is changed in magnitude but not direction by the levels of other variables.

2 In a multifactor experiment many interactions are independently subjected to test; it will not be too surprising if one of these is mildly significant purely by chance. Interactions that are not regarded as inherently plausible should therefore be viewed with some caution unless they are highly significant (i.e. significant at a small probability level such as 1%). Another useful device is the 'half-normal plot' (§11.5).

3 If several high-order interactions are non-significant, their SSq are often pooled with the Residual SSq to provide an increased number of DF and hence more sensitive tests of the main effects or low-order interactions.

There remain some further points of interpretation which are most usefully discussed separately according as the factors concerned are thought of as having fixed effects or random effects (§7.3).

Fixed effects

If certain interactions are present they can often best be displayed by quoting the mean values of the variable at each of the factor combinations concerned. For instance, in an experiment with A, B and C at two, three and four levels respectively, if the only significant interaction were BC, the mean values would be quoted at each of the 12 combinations of levels of B and C. These could be accompanied by a statement of the standard error of the difference between two of these means. The reader would then be able to see quickly the essential features of the interaction. Consider the following table of means:

	Level of C			
Level of B	1	2	3	4
1	2·17	2·25	2·19	2·24
2	1·96	2·01	1·89	1·86
3	2·62	2·67	2·83	2·87

(Standard error of difference between two means = 0·05.)

Clearly the effect of C is not detectable at level 1 of B; at level 2 of B the two higher levels of C show a decrease in the mean; at level 3 of B the two higher levels of C show an increase.

In situations like this the main effects of B and C are of no great interest. If the effect of C varies with the level of B, the main effect measures the average effect of C over the levels of B; since it depends on the choice of levels of B it will usually be a rather artificial quantity and therefore hardly worth considering. Similarly, if a three-factor interaction is significant and deemed to exist, the interactions between any two of the factors concerned are rather artificial concepts.

Random effects

If, in the previous example, A and C were fixed-effect factors and B was a random-effect factor, the presence of an interaction between B and C would not preclude an interest in the main effect of C—regarded not as an average over the particular levels of B chosen in the experiment, but as an average over the whole population of potential B levels. Under certain conditions (discussed below) the null hypothesis for the main effect of C is tested by comparing the MSq for C against the MSq for the interaction BC. If C has more than two levels, it may be more informative to concentrate on a particular contrast between the levels of C (say a comparison of level 1 with level 4), and obtain the interaction of this contrast with the factor B.

If one of the factors in a multifactor design is a blocking system, it will usually be natural to regard this as a random-effect factor. Suppose the other factors are controlled treatments (say A, B and C). Then each of the main effects and interactions of A, B and C may be compared with the appropriate interaction with blocks. Frequently the various interactions involving blocks differ by no more than might be expected by random variation, and the SSq may be pooled to provide extra DF.

The situations referred to in the previous paragraphs are examples in which a *mixed model* is appropriate—some of the factors having fixed effects and some having random effects. If there is just one random factor (as with blocks in the example in the last paragraph), any main effect or interaction of the other factors may be tested against the appropriate interaction with the random factor; for example, if D is the random factor, A could be tested against AD, AB against ABD. The justification for this follows by interpreting the interaction terms involving D in the model like (8.7) as independent observations on random variables with zero mean. The concept of a random interaction is reasonable; if, for example, D is a blocking system any linear contrast representing part of a main effect or interaction of the other factors can be regarded as varying randomly from block to block. What is more arguable, though, is the assumption that all the components in (8.7) for a particular interaction, say AD, have the same distribution and are independent of each other. Hence the suggestion, made above, that attention should preferably be focused on particular linear contrasts. Any such contrast, L, could be measured separately in each block and its mean value tested by a t test.

When there are more than two random factors further problems arise because there may be no exact tests for some of the main effects and interactions. For further discussion see Snedecor and Cochran (1989, §16.14).

8.4 Latin squares

Suppose we wish to compare the effects of a treatments in an experiment in which there are two other known sources of variation, each at a levels. A complete factorial design, with only one observation at each factor combination, would require a^3 observations. Consider the following design, in which $a = 4$. The principal treatments are denoted by A, B, C and D, and the two secondary factors are represented by the rows and columns of the table.

	Column			
Row	1	2	3	4
1	D	B	C	A
2	C	D	A	B
3	A	C	B	D
4	B	A	D	C

Only $a^2 (= 16)$ observations are made, since at each combination of a row and a column only one of the four treatments is used. The design is cunningly balanced, however, in the sense that each treatment occurs precisely once in each row and precisely once in each column. If the effect of making an observation in row 1 rather than row 2 is to add a constant amount on to the measurement observed, the differences between the means for the four treatments are unaffected by the size of this constant. In this sense systematic variation between rows, or similarly between columns, does not affect the treatment comparisons and can be said to have been eliminated by the choice of design.

These designs, called *Latin squares*, were first used in agricultural experiments in which the rows and columns represented strips in two perpendicular directions across a field. Some analogous examples arise in medical research when treatments are to be applied to a two-dimensional array of experimental units. For instance, various substances may be inoculated subcutaneously over a two-dimensional grid of points on the skin of a human subject or an animal. In a plate diffusion assay various dilutions of an antibiotic preparation may be inserted in hollows in an agar plate which is seeded with bacteria and incubated, the inhibition zone formed by diffusion of antibiotic round each hollow being related to the dilution used.

In other experiments the rows and columns may represent two identifiable sources of variation which are, however, not geographically meaningful. The Latin square is being used here as a straightforward generalization of a randomized block design, the rows and columns representing two different systems of blocking. Examples are the following.

1   An animal experiment in which rows represent litters and columns represent different days on which the experiment is performed. Individual animals receive different treatments.

2   An extended crossover trial in which rows represent different subjects and columns represent the order of administration of treatments. Here each subject receives the various treatments on different occasions. As in §8.2 the investigator must be satisfied that the response observed on any occasion is influenced only by

the treatment currently given and not by any preceding treatments. It is easy to think of situations in which there is a carry-over, either of the pharmacological effect of a previously administered drug, or (in certain experiments) of the psychological effect of previous treatments. Some Latin squares are balanced for certain residual effects and may be used for their estimation. These are due mainly to E. J. Williams and are described by Cochran and Cox (1957, §4.6a).

Latin squares are sometimes used in situations where either the rows or columns or both represent forms of treatment under the experimenter's control. They are then performing some of the functions of factorial designs, with the important proviso that some of the factor combinations are missing. This has important consequences which we shall note later.

In a randomized block design, treatments are allocated at random within each block. How can randomization be applied in a Latin square, which is clearly a highly systematic arrangement? For any value of a many possible squares can be written down. The safeguards of randomization are introduced by making a random choice from these possible squares. Full details of the procedure are given in Fisher and Yates (1963) and in most books on experimental design. The reader will not go far wrong if he constructs a Latin square of the right size by shifting treatments cyclically by one place in successive rows:

A	B	C	D
D	A	B	C
C	D	A	B
B	C	D	A

and then permutes the rows and the columns randomly.

As an additive model for the analysis of the Latin square, suppose that the response, y_{ijk}, for the ith row, jth column and kth treatment is given by

$$y_{ijk} = \mu + \alpha_i + \beta_j + \gamma_k + \varepsilon_{ijk}, \tag{8.17}$$

where μ represents the general mean, α_i, β_j and γ_k are constants characteristic of the particular row, column and treatment concerned, and ε_{ijk} is a random observation from a normal distribution with zero mean and variance σ^2. The model is, in fact, that of a three-factor experiment without interactions.

The notation for the observations is shown in Table 8.9. The analysis, shown at the foot of Table 8.9, follows familiar lines. The SSq for rows, columns and treatments are obtained by the usual formula in terms of the subtotals, the Total SSq is also obtained as usual, and the residual term is obtained by subtraction:

Residual SSq = Total SSq − (Rows SSq + Columns SSq + Treatments SSq).

The degrees of freedom for the three factors are clearly $a - 1$; the residual DF are found by subtraction to be $a^2 - 3a + 2 = (a - 1)(a - 2)$.

Table 8.9 Notation for Latin square experiment

Row	Column 1	2 ... j ... a	Total	Mean	Treatment	Total	Mean
1			R_1	$\bar{y}_{1..}$	1	T_1	$\bar{y}_{..1}$
2			R_2	$\bar{y}_{2..}$	2	T_2	$\bar{y}_{..2}$
.			.	.	.	.	.
.			.	.	.	.	.
.			.	.	.	.	.
i		y_{ijk}	R_i	$\bar{y}_{i..}$	k	T_k	$\bar{y}_{..k}$
.			.	.	.	.	.
.			.	.	.	.	.
a			R_a	$\bar{y}_{a..}$	a	T_a	$\bar{y}_{..a}$
Total	C_1	$C_2 ... C_j ... C_a$	T			T	
Mean	$\bar{y}_{.1.}$	$\bar{y}_{.2.}$ $\bar{y}_{.j.}$ $\bar{y}_{.a.}$		$\bar{y}$			

Analysis of variance

	SSq	DF	MSq	VR
Rows	$\sum R_i^2/a - T^2/a^2$	$a-1$	s_R^2	$F_R = s_R^2/s^2$
Columns	$\sum C_j^2/a - T^2/a^2$	$a-1$	s_C^2	$F_C = s_C^2/s^2$
Treatments	$\sum T_k^2/a - T^2/a^2$	$a-1$	s_T^2	$F_T = s_T^2/s^2$
Residual	By subtraction	$(a-1)(a-2)$	s^2	
Total	$y_{ijk}^2 - T^2/a^2$	$a^2 - 1$		

The basis of the division of the Total SSq is the following identity:

$$y_{ijk} - \bar{y} = (\bar{y}_{i..} - \bar{y}) + (\bar{y}_{.j.} - \bar{y}) + (\bar{y}_{..k} - \bar{y}) + (y_{ijk} - \bar{y}_{i..} - \bar{y}_{.j.} - \bar{y}_{..k} + 2\bar{y}).$$

(8.18)

When each term is squared and a summation is taken over all of the a^2 observations the four sums of squares are obtained. The product terms such as $\sum (\bar{y}_{.j.} - \bar{y}) \times (\bar{y}_{..k} - \bar{y})$ are all zero as in the two-way analysis of §8.1.

If the additive model (8.17) is correct, the three null hypotheses about equality of the αs, βs and γs can all be tested by the appropriate F tests. Confidence limits for differences between pairs of constants (say, between two rows) or for other linear contrasts can be formed in a straightforward way, the standard errors being estimated in terms of s^2. However, the additive model may be incorrect. If the rows and columns are blocking factors, the effect of non-additivity will be to increase the estimate of residual variance. Tests for differences between rows or between columns are of no great interest in this case, and randomization ensures the validity of the tests and estimates for treatment differences; the extra imprecision is automatically accounted for in the increased value of s^2. If, on the other hand, the rows and the columns are treatments, non-additivity means that some interactions exist. The trouble now is that the interactions cannot be measured independently of the main effects, and serious errors may result. In both sets of circumstances, therefore, additivity of responses is a desirable feature, although its absence is more regrettable in the second case than in the first.

Example 8.5

The experiment of Bacharach *et al.* (1940) discussed in Example 7.2 was designed as a Latin square. The design and the measurements are given in Table 8.10. The object of the experiment was to study the possible effects of order of administration in a series of inoculations on the same animal (the 'treatment' factor, represented here by Roman numerals) and the choice among six positions on the animal's skin (the row factor), and also to assess the variation between animals (the column factor) in comparison with that within animals.

The Total SSq is obtained as usual as

$$1984 \cdot 0000 - 1953 \cdot 6401 = 30 \cdot 3599.$$

The SSq for animal differences is calculated as

$$[(42 \cdot 4)^2 + (51 \cdot 7)^2 + \ldots + (45 \cdot 1)^2]/6 - 1953 \cdot 6401 = 12 \cdot 8333,$$

the other two main effects follow similarly, and the Residual SSq is obtained by subtraction. The VR for order is less than 1 and need not be referred to the F table. That for positions is certainly not significant. The only significant effect is that for animal differences, and further examination of the between-animals component of variance has already been carried out in Example 7.2.

Replication of Latin squares

An important restriction of the Latin square is, of course, the requirement that the numbers of rows, columns and treatments must all be equal. The nature of the experimental material and the purpose of the experiment often demand that the size of the square should be small. On the other hand, treatment comparisons estimated from a single Latin square are likely to be rather imprecise. Some form of replication is therefore often desirable.

Replication in an experiment like that of Example 8.5 may take various forms, for instance: (i) if the six animals in Table 8.10 were from the same litter, the experiment could be repeated with several litters, a new randomization being used for each litter; (ii) if there were no classification by litters, a single design such as that in Table 8.10 could be used with several animals for each column; (iii) if the experiment were repeated with the *same six animals*, on several occasions, again a new randomization should be used for each occasion. In replicated designs of

Table 8.10 Measurements of area of blister (square centimetres) following inoculation of diffusing factor into skin of rabbits in positions a–f on animals' backs, order of administration being denoted by i–vi (Bacharach *et al.*, 1940)

Positions	Animals 1	2	3	4	5	6	Total	Mean
a	iii 7·9	v 8·7	iv 7·4	i 7·4	vi 7·1	ii 8·2	46·7	7·783
b	iv 6·1	ii 8·2	vi 7·7	v 7·1	iii 8·1	i 5·9	43·1	7·183
c	i 7·5	iii 8·1	v 6·0	vi 6·4	ii 6·2	iv 7·5	41·7	6·950
d	vi 6·9	i 8·5	iii 6·8	ii 7·7	iv 8·5	v 8·5	46·9	7·817
e	ii 6·7	iv 9·9	i 7·3	iii 6·4	v 6·4	vi 7·3	44·0	7·333
f	v 7·3	vi 8·3	ii 7·3	iv 5·8	i 6·4	iii 7·7	42·8	7·133
Total	42·4	51·7	42·5	40·8	42·7	45·1	265·2	
Mean	7·067	8·617	7·083	6·800	7·117	7·517		7·367

Order	i	ii	iii	iv	v	vi
Total	43·0	44·3	45·0	45·2	44·0	43·7
Mean	7·167	7·383	7·500	7·533	7·333	7·283

$$\sum y_{ijk}^2 = 1984\cdot0000$$
$$T^2/36 = 1953\cdot6401$$

Analysis of variance

	SSq	DF	MSq	VR	
Rows (Positions)	3·8332	5	0·7667	1·17	
Columns (Animals)	12·8333	5	2·5667	3·91	$(P = 0\cdot012)$
Treatments (Order)	0·5632	5	0·1106	<1	
Residual	13·1302	20	0·6565	1·00	
Total	30·3599	35			

this sort, care needs to be taken to specify the effects to be tested and the correct assignment of degrees of freedom.

8.5 Other incomplete designs

The Latin square may be regarded either as a design which allows simultaneously for two extraneous sources of variation—the rows and columns—or as an incomplete factorial design permitting the estimation of three main effects—rows, columns and treatments—from observations at only a fraction of the possible combinations of factor levels.

Many other types of incomplete design are known. This section contains a very brief survey of some of these designs, with details of construction and analysis omitted. Cox (1958, Chapters 11 and 12) gives a much fuller account of the characteristics and purposes of the various designs, and Cochran and Cox (1957) should be consulted for details of statistical analysis. Most of the designs described in this section have found little use in medical research, examples of their application being drawn usually from industrial and agricultural research. This contrast is perhaps partly due to inadequate appreciation of the less familiar designs by medical research workers, but it is likely also that the organizational problems of experimentation are more severe in medical research than in many other fields, a feature which would tend to favour the use of simple designs.

Graeco-Latin squares

The Latin square generalizes the randomized block design by controlling variation due to two blocking factors. The Graeco-Latin square extends this idea by superimposing on a Latin square a further system of classification which is balanced with respect to the rows, columns and treatments. This is conventionally represented by letters of the Greek alphabet. For example, the following design could be used for an experiment similar to that described in Exampe 8.5:

$A\alpha$	$B\beta$	$C\gamma$	$D\delta$	$E\varepsilon$
$B\delta$	$C\varepsilon$	$D\alpha$	$E\beta$	$A\gamma$
$C\beta$	$D\gamma$	$E\delta$	$A\varepsilon$	$B\alpha$
$D\varepsilon$	$E\alpha$	$A\beta$	$B\gamma$	$C\delta$
$E\gamma$	$A\delta$	$B\varepsilon$	$C\alpha$	$D\beta$

Note that both the 'Latin' (i.e. Roman) letters and the Greek letters form Latin squares with the rows and columns, and also that each Latin letter occurs precisely once with each Greek letter. Suppose that the experimenter wished to compare the effects of five different doses of diffusing factor, allowing simultaneously for the order of administration, differences between animals and differences between positions on the animals' backs. The design shown above could be used, with random allocation of columns to five different animals, rows to five positions, Greek letters to the five places in the order of administration, and Latin letters to the five dilutions.

A general point to remember with Graeco-Latin squares is that the number of DF for the residual mean square is invariably low. Unless, therefore, an estimate of error variance can reliably be obtained from extraneous data, it will often be desirable to introduce sufficient replication to provide an adequately precise estimate of random variation.

Incomplete block designs

In many situations in which a natural blocking system exists, a randomized block design may be ruled out because the number of treatments is greater than the number of experimental units which can conveniently be formed within a block. This limitation may be due to physical restrictions: in an experiment with intradermal inoculations into animals, with an individual animal forming a block, there may be a limit to the number of inoculation sites on an animal. The limitation may be one of convenience; if repeated clinical measurements are made on each of a number of patients, it may be undesirable to subject any one patient to more than a few such observations. There may be a time limit; for example, a block may consist of observations made on a single day. Sometimes when an adequate number of units can be formed within each block this may be undesirable because it leads to an excessively high degree of within-blocks variation.

A possible solution to these difficulties lies in the use of an *incomplete block design*, in which only a selection of the treatments is used in any one block. In general this will lead to designs lacking the attractive symmetry of a randomized block design. However, certain designs, called *balanced incomplete block designs*, retain a considerable degree of symmetry by ensuring that each treatment occurs the same number of times and each pair of treatments occurs together in a block the same number of times.

There are various categories of balanced incomplete block designs, details of which may be found in books on experimental design. The incompleteness of the design introduces some complexity into the analysis. To compare mean effects of different treatments, for example, it is unsatisfactory merely to compare the observed means for all units receiving these treatments, for these means will be affected by differences between blocks. The observed means are therefore adjusted in a certain way to allow for systematic differences between blocks. This is equivalent to obtaining contrasts between treatments solely from within-blocks differences. For details see Cochran and Cox (1957, §9.3).

A further class of designs, *Youden squares* or *incomplete Latin squares*, are similar to balanced incomplete block designs, but have the further feature that a second source of extraneous variation is controlled by the introduction of a column classification. They bear the same relation to balanced incomplete block designs as do Latin squares to randomized block designs.

In a Youden square the row and column classifications enter into the design in different ways. The number of rows (blocks) is equal to the number of treatments, so each column contains all the treatments; the number of columns is less than the number of treatments; so only a selection of treatments is used in each row. Sometimes designs are needed for two-way control of variability, in situations in which both classifications must be treated in an incomplete way. A type of design called a *set of balanced lattice squares* may be useful here. For a brief description see Cox (1958, §11.3(iii)); for details see Cochran and Cox (1957, Chapter 12).

In a balanced incomplete block design all treatments are handled in a symmetric way. All contrasts between pairs of treatments are, for example, estimated with equal precision. Some other incomplete block designs retain some, but not all, of the symmetry of the balanced designs. They may be adopted because of a deliberate wish to estimate some contrasts more precisely than others. Or it may be that physical restrictions on the size of the experiment do not permit any of the balanced designs to be used. *Lattice designs* (not to be confused with lattice squares), in particular, are useful when a large number of treatments are to be compared and where the smallest balanced design is likely to be too large for practical use.

Sometimes it may be necessary to use incomplete block designs which have no degree of symmetry. For some worked examples see Pearce (1965).

Fractional replication and confounding

If the rows and columns of a Latin square represent different treatment factors and the Latin letters represent a third treatment factor, we have an incomplete factorial design. As we have seen in discussing the analysis of the Latin square, one consequence is that the main effects of the factors can be studied only if the interactions are assumed to be absent. There are many other incomplete or *fractional* factorial designs in which only a fraction of all the possible combinations of factor levels are used, with the consequence that not all the main effects or interactions can be separately investigated.

Such designs may be very useful for experiments with a large number of factors in which the number of observations required for a complete factorial experiment is greater than can conveniently be used, or where the main effects can be estimated sufficiently precisely with less than the complete number of observations. If by the use of a fractional factorial design we have to sacrifice the ability to estimate some of the main effects or interactions, it will usually be convenient if we can arrange to lose information about the higher-order interactions rather than the main effects or lower-order interactions, because the former are unlikely to be large without the latter also appearing large, whereas the converse is not true. A further point to remember is that SSq for high-order interactions are often pooled in the analysis of variance to give an estimate of residual variance. The sacrifice of information about some of these will reduce the residual DF, and if this is done too drastically there will be an inadequately precise estimate of error unless an estimate is available from other data.

Fractional factorial designs have been much used in industrial and agricultural work where the simultaneous effects of large numbers of factors have to be studied and where attention very often focuses on the main effects and low-order interactions.

A further way in which a full factorial design can be reduced, in a block experiment, is to arrange that each block contains only a selection of the possible factor combinations. The design is chosen to ensure that some effects, typically main effects and low-order interactions, can be estimated from contrasts *within blocks*, whereas others (of less interest) are estimated from contrasts *between blocks*. The latter are said to be *confounded with blocks*, and are of course estimated with lower precision than the unconfounded effects.

8.6 Split-unit designs

In a factorial design in which confounding with blocks takes place, as outlined at the end of §8.5, two types of random variation are important: the variation between experimental units within a block, and that between blocks. In some simple factorial designs it is convenient to recognize two such forms of experimental unit, one of which is a subdivision of the other, and to arrange that the levels of some factors are spread across the larger units, while levels of other factors are spread across the smaller units within the larger ones.

This principle was first exploited in agricultural experiments, where the designs are called *split-plot designs*. In some field experiments it is convenient to divide the field into 'main plots' and to compare the levels of one factor—say the addition of different soil organisms—by allocating them at random to the main plots. At the same time each main plot is divided into a number of 'subplots', and the levels of some other factor—say different fertilizers—are allocated at random to the subplots within a main plot, exactly as in a randomized block experiment. The comparison of fertilizers would be subject to the random variation between subplots, which would be likely to be less than the variation between main plots, which affects organism comparisons. The organisms are thus compared less precisely than the fertilizers. This inequality of precision is likely to be accepted because of the convenience of being able to spread organisms over relatively large areas of ground.

Similar situations arise in medical and other types of biological experimentation. In general the experimental units are not referred to as 'plots', and the design is therefore more appropriately called a *split-unit design*. Another term is *nested design*. Some examples of the distinction between main units and subunits are as follows:

Main unit	Subunit
Individual human subject or animal	Different occasions with the same subject or animal
Litter	Animals within a litter
Day	Periods during a day

In the first of these instances a split-unit design might be employed to compare the long-term effects of drugs A_1, A_2 and A_3, and simultaneously the short-term effects of drugs B_1, B_2 and B_3. Suppose there are 12 subjects, each of whom must receive one of A_1, A_2 or A_3; and each subject is observed for three periods during which B_1, B_2 and B_3 are to be given in a random order. The design, determined by randomly allocating the As to the different subjects and the Bs to the periods within subjects, might be as follows.

Patient	'A' drug throughout	'B' drug during period		
		1	2	3
1	A_3	B_1	B_3	B_2
2	A_1	B_1	B_2	B_3
3	A_1	B_3	B_1	B_2
4	A_2	B_3	B_2	B_1
5	A_3	B_2	B_3	B_1
6	A_2	B_2	B_1	B_3
7	A_1	B_1	B_2	B_3
8	A_3	B_3	B_1	B_2
9	A_3	B_1	B_3	B_2
10	A_2	B_2	B_1	B_3
11	A_1	B_2	B_1	B_3
12	A_2	B_2	B_1	B_3

The analysis of such designs is illustrated in Example 8.6, using data from a survey rather than an experiment.

Example 8.6

The data in Table 8.11 are taken from a survey on the prevalence of upper respiratory tract infection. The variable to be analysed is the number of swabs positive for *Pneumococcus* during a certain period. Observations were made on 18 families, each consisting of a father, a mother and three children, the youngest of whom was always a preschool child. The children are numbered 1, 2 and 3 in descending order of age. Six families were a random selection of such families living in 'overcrowded' conditions, six were in 'crowded' conditions and six were in 'uncrowded' conditions.

The first point to notice is that two types of random variation are relevant: that between families (the main units in this example) and that between people within families (the subunits). Comparisons between degrees of crowding must be made *between families*; comparisons of family status are made *within families*. With designs of any complexity it is a good idea to start the analysis by subdividing the degrees of freedom. The result is shown in the DF column of Table 8.12. The total DF are 89, since there are 90 observations. These are split (as in a one-way analysis of variance) into 17 ($= 18 - 1$) between families and 72 ($= 18 \times 4$) within families. The between-families DF are split (again as in a one-way analysis) into 2 ($= 3 - 1$) for degrees of crowding and 15 ($= 3 \times 5$) for residual variation within crowding categories. The within-families DF are split into 4 ($= 5 - 1$) for categories of family status, 8 ($= 4 \times 2$) for the interaction between the two main effects, and 60 for

Table 8.11 Numbers of swabs positive for *Pneumococcus* during fixed periods

Crowding category	Family serial number	Family status					
				Child			
		Father	Mother	1	2	3	Total
Overcrowded	1	5	7	6	25	19	62
	2	11	8	11	33	35	98
	3	3	12	19	6	21	61
	4	3	19	12	17	17	68
	5	10	9	15	11	17	62
	6	9	0	6	9	5	29
		41	55	69	101	114	380
Crowded	7	11	7	7	15	13	53
	8	10	5	8	13	17	53
	9	5	4	3	18	10	40
	10	1	9	4	16	8	38
	11	5	5	10	16	20	56
	12	7	3	13	17	18	58
		39	33	45	95	86	298
Uncrowded	13	6	3	5	7	3	24
	14	9	6	6	14	10	45
	15	2	2	6	15	8	33
	16	0	2	10	16	21	49
	17	3	2	0	3	14	22
	18	6	2	4	7	20	39
		26	17	31	62	76	212
Total		106	105	145	258	276	890

Table 8.12 Analysis of variance for data in Table 8.11

	SSq	DF	MSq	VR against:	
				a	b
Between families	1146·09	17			
Crowding		470·49	2	235·24		5·22*
Residual		675·60	15	45·04[b]	1·78	1·00
Within families	3122·80	72			
Status		1533·67	4	383·42	15·17**	
Status × crowding		72·40	8	9·05	0·36	
Residual		1516·73	60	25·28[a]	1·00	
Total	4268·89	89			

$*P = 0.019.$
$**P < 0.001.$

within-families residual variation. The latter number can be obtained by subtraction $(60 = 72 - 4 - 8)$ or by regarding this source of variation as an interaction between the between-families residual variation and the status factor $(60 = 15 \times 4)$. It may be wondered why the interaction between status and crowding is designated as within families when one main effect is between and the other is within families. The reason is that this interaction measures the extent to which the status differences, which are within families, vary from one degree of crowding to another; it is therefore based entirely on within-families contrasts.

The calculation of sums of squares follows familiar lines. Thus,

Correction term CT $= (890)^2/90$	$= 8801 \cdot 11,$
Total SSq $= 5^2 + 7^2 + \ldots + 20^2 - $ CT	$= 4268 \cdot 89,$
Between-Families SSq $= (62^2 + \ldots + 39^2)/5 - $ CT	$= 1146 \cdot 09,$
Within-Families SSq $=$ Total SSq $-$ Between-Families SSq	$= 3122 \cdot 80,$

Subdividing the Between-Families SSq,

Crowding SSq $= (380^2 + 298^2 + 212^2)/30 - $ CT	$= 470 \cdot 49,$
Residual $=$ Between-Families SSq $-$ Crowding SSq	$= 675 \cdot 60.$

Subdividing the Within-Families SSq,

Status SSq $= (106^2 + \ldots + 276^2)/18 - $ CT	$= 1533 \cdot 67,$
S $\times$ C SSq $= (41^2 + \ldots + 76^2)/6 - $ CT $-$ Status SSq $-$ Crowding SSq	$= 72 \cdot 40,$
Residual $=$ Within-Families SSq $-$ Status SSq $-$ S $\times$ C SSq	$= 1516 \cdot 73.$

The variance ratios against the Within-Families Residual MSq show that differences due to status are highly significant; we return to these below. The interaction is not significant; there is therefore no evidence that the relative effects of family status vary from one crowding group to another. The variance ratio of $1 \cdot 78$ between the two residuals is just on the borderline of significance at the 5% level. But we should expect a priori that the between-families residual variance would be greater than that within families, and we must certainly test the main effect for crowding against the between-families residual. The variance ratio, $5 \cdot 22$, is significant.

The means for the different members of the family are:

		Child		
F	M	1	2	3
$5 \cdot 9$	$5 \cdot 8$	$8 \cdot 1$	$14 \cdot 3$	$15 \cdot 3$

The standard error of the difference between two means is $\sqrt{[2(25 \cdot 28)/18]} = 1 \cdot 68$. There are clearly no significant differences between the father, mother and eldest child, but the two youngest children have significantly higher means than the other members of the family.

Split-unit designs more elaborate than the design described above may be useful. For example, the structure imposed on the main units (which in Example 8.6 was a simple one-way classification) could be a randomized block design or something more complex. The subunit section of the analysis would then be correspondingly enlarged by isolation of the appropriate interactions. Similarly,

272   FURTHER EXPERIMENTAL DESIGNS

the subunit structure could be elaborated. Another direction of generalization is in the provision of more than two levels in the hierarchy of nested units. In a study similar to that of Example 8.6, for instance, there might have been several periods of observation for each individual, during which different treatments were administered. There would then be a third section in the analysis, within individuals, with its corresponding residual mean square. In none of these cases should the analysis cause any difficulty once the method illustrated above has been grasped.

The following example illustrates a case in which there are two levels of nested units, but in which the design is very simple. There are no structural factors, the purpose of the analysis being merely to estimate the components of random variation.

Example 8.7

Table 8.13 gives counts of particle emission during periods of 1000 s, for 30 aliquots of equal size of certain radioactive material. Each aliquot is placed twice in the counter. There are three sources of random variation, each with its component of variance, as follows.
1   Variation between aliquots, with a variance component σ_2^2. This may be due to slight variations in size or in radioactivity, or to differences in technique between the 30 occasions on which the different aliquots were examined.
2   Systematic variation between replicate counts causing changes in the expected level of the count, with a variance component σ_1^2. This may be due to systematic biases in counting which affect different counts in different ways, or to inconsistency in the apparatus, due perhaps to variation in the way the material is placed in the counter.
3   Random variation from one time period to another, all other conditions remaining constant; variance component σ_0^2. There is no replication of counts under constant

Table 8.13 Radioactivity counts during periods of 1000 s

Aliquot	Counts		Aliquot	Counts	
1	281	291	16	325	267
2	309	347	17	284	296
3	316	356	18	255	281
4	289	277	19	347	285
5	322	292	20	326	302
6	287	321	21	347	307
7	338	320	22	292	344
8	333	275	23	322	308
9	319	311	24	294	272
10	258	302	25	307	303
11	338	294	26	281	331
12	319	281	27	284	322
13	307	247	28	287	305
14	279	259	29	318	352
15	326	272	30	307	301

conditions, but we know that this form of variation follows the Poisson distribution (§2.6), in which the variance equals the mean. The mean will vary a little over the whole experiment, but to a close approximation we could estimate σ_0^2 by the observed mean for the whole data, 303·6.

The analysis of variance is that for a simple one-way classification and is as follows:

	SSq	DF	MSq	Expected value of MSq
Between aliquots	19 898	29	686·1	$\sigma_0^2 + \sigma_1^2 + 2\sigma_2^2$
Within aliquots	20 196	30	673·2	$\sigma_0^2 + \sigma_1^2$
Total	40 094	59		
Poisson			303·6	σ_0^2

The expected values of the mean squares follow from §7.3, if we note that the within-aliquots variance component is $\sigma_0^2 + \sigma_1^2$ (since differences between replicate counts are affected by variation of both type **2** and type **3**), and that the between-aliquots component is σ_2^2.

The estimates of the variance components are now obtained:

$$\sigma_2^2 = (686·1 - 673·2)/2 = \quad 6·4,$$
$$\sigma_1^2 = 673·2 - 303·6 \quad = 369·6,$$
$$\sigma_0^2 = 303·6.$$

These estimates are, of course, subject to sampling error, but there is clearly no evidence of any large component, σ_2^2, due to aliquot differences. Replicate counts vary, however, by substantially more than can be explained by the Poisson distribution.

8.7 Intraclass correlation

Another situation in which components of variance are used is that in which there are a number of correlated members within classes. This can arise in a number of ways; for example, a class might be a pair of twins, or a class might be a sample or individual with an item measured using a number of different methods. One measure sometimes used in this situation is termed the *intraclass correlation coefficient*.

For a pair of identical twins there is ambiguity in calculating the correlation coefficient using (5.10) since the two values have no particular order that could be used to label them as x and y. This could be done at random but then the result would depend on the randomization used. To avoid this all possibilities are considered and this means that each pair is looked at both ways round, that is as (x, y) and as (y, x). The correlation coefficient is calculated from the $2n$ pairs thus formed and this provides an estimate of the required correlation, although the precision of this estimate would be much closer to that based on a sample of n pairs, not $2n$. The correlation calculated this way achieves its maximum value of

1 only if all the pairs of values fall on a straight line through the origin with slope unity.

Suppose a new method is available for measuring some variable and it is required to assess the agreement between values obtained using the new method and those obtained with an existing method. Data could be collected in which a number of individuals were measured using each method to give a pair of values for each individual. A high correlation about a line not passing through the origin or with a slope different from 1 would not represent useful agreement between the methods as far as the user was concerned, although if this occurred it might be possible to calibrate the new method to give better agreement. Thus, although, unlike the twins, there is no ambiguity on the identification within pairs, we require a measure of correlation that will only equal unity if the two measurements are identical within each individual.

The intraclass correlation coefficient is a measure of the correlation between the values obtained with any two randomly chosen methods within the same individual (class) and has the above property. The correlation calculated from $2n$ pairs as above is approximately equal to the intraclass correlation coefficient except when n is small. The method is closely related to components of variance (§7.3, §8.6), and using this methodology is more convenient and more accurate than forming multiple pairs. In general there may be more than two methods under test, and we suppose that there are m methods each assessed on n subjects. Then the design is equivalent to randomized blocks (§8.1) in which the methods are tested within the subjects, i.e. the blocks. There are three sources of variation, each with its component of variance.

1   Variation between subjects, with a variance component σ_s^2.

2   Systematic variation between methods with a variance component σ_m^2. This variability represents differences between methods.

3   Random variation from one measurement to another with a variance component σ^2, additional to the sources of variation **1** and **2**.

Then the two-way analysis of variance has the form:

	DF	MSq	Expected MSq
Between subjects (classes)	$n - 1$	M_s	$\sigma^2 + m\sigma_s^2$
Between methods	$m - 1$	M_m	$\sigma^2 + n\sigma_m^2$
Residual	$(n - 1)(m - 1)$	M_r	σ^2

The intraclass correlation coefficient is defined as the correlation between any two measurements in the same subject, using randomly chosen methods. All three components of variation contribute to the variance of each measurement and, since the two measurements are for the same subject, the variance component representing variation between subjects is common to the two measurements.

Therefore the intraclass correlation coefficient is

$$\rho_I = \frac{\sigma_s^2}{\sigma_s^2 + \sigma_m^2 + \sigma^2}.$$

Equating the mean squares in the analysis of variance with their expectations gives the following estimate of ρ_I (Bartko, 1966):

$$r_I = \frac{M_s - M_r}{M_s + (m-1)M_r + \dfrac{m}{n}(M_m - M_r)}. \tag{8.19}$$

For $m = 2$ the intraclass correlation coefficient can be obtained as follows. Let x_{i1} and x_{i2} be the values for methods 1 and 2 respectively for subject i. Define $t_i = x_{i1} + x_{i2}$ and $d_i = x_{i1} - x_{i2}$ as the sum and difference of the pair of values. Calculate the mean difference, $\bar{d}$, and the standard deviations of t_i and d_i, s_t and s_d respectively. Then

$$r_I = \frac{s_t^2 - s_d^2}{s_t^2 + s_d^2 + \dfrac{2}{n}(n\bar{d}^2 - s_d^2)}. \tag{8.20}$$

It is easy to see from this form that the systematic difference between the methods reduces the intraclass correlation coefficient, due to the inclusion of $\bar{d}^2$ in the denominator. A closely related index, the concordance correlation coefficient, was given by Lin (1992).

An alternative formulation is appropriate when there is no reason to suppose there are any systematic differences between the values within a class, for example pairs of twins. There is then no entry in the analysis of variance for between methods; M_r is estimated from a one-way analysis of variance (§7.1) with $n(m-1)$ DF and the last term in the denominator of (8.19) is omitted (Snedecor and Cochran, 1989, §13.5).

Another situation where the method may be useful is where a characteristic that cannot be measured objectively is assessed by two or more raters, and the level of agreement between the raters, which may be referred to as the *reliability* of the ratings, is critical to the way the data are used.

Example 8.8

In a study by Bergen *et al.* (1992), tardive dyskinesia was assessed by two assessors on a scale taking integer values from 0 to 28. For one series of assessments there were 168 subjects with the following summary statistics:

$$\bar{t} = 16{\cdot}39, \quad s_t = 7{\cdot}71, \quad \bar{d} = 0{\cdot}28, \quad s_d = 1{\cdot}89.$$

Applying (8.20) gives

$$r_I = \frac{7 \cdot 71^2 - 1 \cdot 89^2}{7 \cdot 71^2 + 1 \cdot 89^2 + \dfrac{2}{168}(168 \times 0 \cdot 28^2 - 1 \cdot 89^2)}$$

$$= 0 \cdot 885.$$

The agreement between the two raters was very good, and the mean difference of 0·28 and variation in the difference (SD 1·89) were small compared with the mean total of 16·4 with standard deviation of 7·7. Therefore it was considered acceptable to combine the assessments of the two raters and use the mean value in the main analysis.

The intraclass correlation coefficient is closely related to the kappa measure of agreement (Chapter 12), used when the ratings are recorded on a categorical scale (Fleiss, 1975).

The intraclass correlation coefficient has the same feature as the product–moment correlation coefficient, namely that its value is influenced by the selection of subjects over which it is defined. If the subjects are highly variable, then the intraclass correlation coefficient will tend to be high, whereas for a more homogeneous group of subjects it will be lower. Another problem is that the intraclass correlation coefficient also combines information from the systematic difference between methods with the random measurement variation. Thus the intraclass correlation coefficient is a measure which combines three features of the data from which it is calculated. This may not matter if the only purpose of calculating the coefficient is to assess agreement between methods within a particular study, but comparisons of intraclass correlation coefficients between studies are difficult to interpret. A fuller evaluation of the agreement between methods is provided by an analysis of the differences, d_i (Altman, 1991, pp. 397–401). A plot of d_i against the mean, $\frac{1}{2}t_i$, allows the determination of whether the systematic difference between the methods or the random variation differ according to the mean value, and if they do not the difference between the methods can be summarized by $\bar{d}$ and s_d. If the random variation increases with the mean value, an analysis of the differences after a logarithmic transformation may be appropriate (§9.3).

8.8 Non-orthogonal two-way tables: some simple cases

Many sets of data follow too unbalanced a design for any of the standard forms of analysis of variance to be appropriate. The trouble here is that the various linear contrasts which together represent the sources of variation in which we are interested may not be orthogonal in the sense of §7.4, and the corresponding sums of squares do not add to the Total SSq. A general discussion of the analysis of non-orthogonal designs must be delayed until §10.4. There are, however, one or two special situations that can conveniently be discussed at this stage. We have referred briefly in §8.5 to the analysis of unbalanced block designs (Pearce, 1965). In this section we discuss some of the simpler problems that arise in two-way tables.

It was stated in §8.1 that two-way data with replication can be analysed by the standard method if the cell frequencies, n_{ij}, are proportionate, i.e. proportional to the row and column marginal frequencies. In many cases this is not so. An attempt to use the standard method of analysis may have misleading or even absurd consequences; for example, an interaction SSq may be calculated as a negative quantity!

There is never any problem in obtaining the Residual SSq, since this is immediately available from the pooled within-cells variation; this depends only on the one-way classification between and within cells, and for this purpose we can have arbitrary cell frequencies. The problem, therefore is to obtain SSq for the main effects of rows and columns and their interaction. The best strategy, in fact, is to test first for interaction. If the interaction is not significant and there is no strong prior supposition that a substantial interaction is present, we may proceed to examine the main effects of rows and columns. If interaction is deemed to be present there is little point in testing the main effects against the Residual SSq. For fixed-effect factors the interaction is best explored by examining cell means and calculating their standard errors from the Residual MSq. For random effects or a mixed model with interaction, it will often be best to study simple contrasts between factor levels.

A useful approximate method is available if the cell frequencies, n_{ij}, are nearly proportionate. They may then be replaced by 'pseudo-frequencies'

$$n'_{ij} = n_{i.}n_{.j}/N,$$

which are exactly proportional to the marginal frequencies. The observed total, T_{ij}, of the values of y in the (i, j)th cell is now replaced by the pseudo-total

$$T'_{ij} = n'_{ij}\bar{y}_{ij},$$

where $\bar{y}_{ij}$ is the observed mean, T_{ij}/n_{ij}. The analysis of variance then proceeds as though the observed frequencies and totals had been n'_{ij} and T'_{ij} (even though the former are likely not to be integers).

Missing readings

We now discuss some devices that can be used if a design is exactly balanced except for a very small number of missing readings. Before discussing any technical matters it is important to stress a general point that arises whenever an intended observation is missing for any reason. The failure to make the observation may be related to its magnitude; for example, a measuring instrument may fail to record particularly high values. Essential information is then lost and no statistical manipulations can remove the bias caused by this failure. We shall assume in this section that the failure is unrelated to the magnitude of the observation that should have been made.

Consider first a two-way table with equal replication (r observations in each cell) except that one cell has a missing reading. The Residual SSq, being an SSq within cells, can be calculated directly from the data. An adequate approximation for the calculation of the SSq for the main effects and interactions is to replace the missing reading by the observed mean value for the affected cell. The design is then balanced and can be analysed in the usual way, except that one degree of freedom is subtracted for the Residual and Total SSq.

In a two-way table without replication (as in a simple randomized block experiment), a similar procedure is followed, but the substituted observation now depends on the row and column effects estimated from the rest of the data. It can be shown that the inserted value should be such as to minimize the Residual SSq in the analysis of variance of the data including that value. This criterion leads to a simple use of differential calculus. An equivalent requirement is that the *residual* for the missing unit, calculated after the substitution, should be zero. In the notation of Table 8.1, suppose the observation y_{ij} is missing. This is replaced by the value

$$y'_{ij} = \frac{rR_i + cC_j - T}{(r-1)(c-1)},\qquad(8.21)$$

where R_i, C_j and T are the totals for the affected row, the affected column and the whole set, *ignoring the missing unit*. The usual analysis is then carried out. The Residual SSq and Total SSq have, respectively, $(r-1)(c-1)-1$ and $rc-2$ DF. The Residual MSq correctly estimates the residual variance. The rows and columns sums of squares are both rather too high. The correction for the test for columns, for example, is to subtract

$$\frac{[R_i - (c-1)y'_{ij}]^2}{c(c-1)^2}\qquad(8.22)$$

from the columns *mean square*. For a comparison between the mean of the affected column and that of another column, the means should be calculated *after* substitution of y'_{ij}. The standard error of the difference between the two means is then

$$\sqrt{\left\{s^2\left[\frac{2}{r} + \frac{c}{r(r-1)(c-1)}\right]\right\}}.\qquad(8.23)$$

Similar methods are available for other designs, such as Latin squares, but are not described here since the availability of general methods for the analysis of non-orthogonal data by the use of computers has made these special methods almost redundant. If there are two or more missing readings in a two-way analysis without replication, the method described above can be used in an iterative way. Again we omit details because it is usually preferable to use the more general methods.

The $2 \times c$ or $r \times 2$ table

We return now to the general case where the n_{ij} are not even approximately proportionate. If there are only two rows or two columns, an exact solution is available without undue complexity.

Suppose there are two rows: a $2 \times c$ table. With the usual notation for cell means we could estimate the row effect in column j by

$$d_j = \bar{y}_{1j} - \bar{y}_{2j}.$$

The variance of d_j is estimated as s^2/w_j, where

$$w_j = \frac{1}{\dfrac{1}{n_{1j}} + \dfrac{1}{n_{2j}}} = \frac{n_{1j}n_{2j}}{n_{1j} + n_{2j}}. \tag{8.24}$$

From §7.2, the best estimate of overall row effect is the weighted mean of the d_j:

$$\bar{d} = \sum_j w_j d_j \Big/ \sum_j w_j, \tag{8.25}$$

and the interaction is represented by the weighted SSq of the d_j about $\bar{d}$,

$$\sum_j w_j(d_j - \bar{d})^2,$$

which can also be written, as in (7.15),

$$\sum_j w_j d_j^2 - \frac{\left(\sum_j w_j d_j\right)^2}{\sum_j w_j}. \tag{8.26}$$

Formula (8.26), then, is the Interaction SSq in the analysis of variance.

If the MSq from (8.26) is not significant, and we are willing to proceed on the assumption of no interaction, the Rows SSq may be obtained. This is given by the second term of (8.26):

$$\left(\sum_j w_j d_j\right)^2 \Big/ \sum w_j. \tag{8.27}$$

An analysis of variance may now be formed from the following SSq terms:

Between cells	By the usual formula, using T_{ij}
Rows (adjusted for columns)	From (8.27)
Columns (unadjusted)	By the usual formula, using C_j
Interaction	From (8.26)
Within cells	By the usual formula.

That the three components of the Between-Cells SSq add up correctly can be verified without too much algebraic difficulty. If the three components are calculated separately, the between-cells term need not be calculated unless it is needed as an arithmetic check. Note that the columns (unadjusted) term is of no great interest in its own right, since if a row effect is present the column means will vary partly because of the variable relative weighting given to the two rows.

For a valid test for columns, the column means can be adjusted for row effects. Alternatively, the adjusted Columns SSq can be calculated by subtraction in an alternative subdivision of the Between-Cells SSq:

(a) *Between cells*	By the usual formula, using T_{ij}
(b) Rows (unadjusted)	By the usual formula, using R_i
(c) Columns (adjusted for rows)	By subtraction, (a) − (b) − (d)
(d) Interaction	From (8.26).

Example 8.9

Table 8.14 shows the number of cerebrovascular accidents experienced during a certain period by 41 men, each of whom had recovered from a previous cerebrovascular accident

Table 8.14 Distributions of numbers of cerebrovascular accidents experienced by males in hypotensive-treated and control groups, subdivided by age

		Age (years)		
	Number of accidents	40– Number of men	50– Number of men	60– Number of men
Control group	0	0	3	4
	1	1	3	8
	2	0	4	1
	3	0	1	0
		1	11	13
Treated group	0	4	7	1
	1	0	4	0
		4	11	1

and was hypertensive. Sixteen of these men received treatment with hypotensive drugs and 25 formed a control group without such treatment. The data are shown in the form of frequency distributions as the variable to be analysed takes only the values 0, 1, 2 and 3. This was not a controlled trial with random allocation, but it was nevertheless useful to enquire whether the difference in the mean numbers of accidents for the two groups was significant, and since the age distributions of the two groups were markedly different it was thought that an allowance for age might be important. The two rows of Table 8.14 represent the two treatment groups and the three columns represent three age groups.

The preliminary steps of the analysis are shown in the body of Table 8.15. The sum T_{ij} and sum of squares S_{ij} for the n_{ij} observations in the ith row and jth column are obtained as usual for a frequency distribution (cf. Tables 1.8 and 1.11). The remaining entries are straightforward.

The next steps are to calculate the Total and Between-Cells SSq. The Total SSq is

$$S - CT = 45 - 20.5122 = 24.4878.$$

The Between-Cells SSq is

$$(1.0000 + 17.8182 + \ldots + 0.0000) - CT = 7.4528.$$

The Within-Cells SSq follows by subtraction.

The Interaction SSq is, from (8.26),

$$5.8949 - 5.8706 = 0.0243,$$

and the Treatments SSq, adjusted for age, is 5.8706. The unadjusted SSq for age follows by subtraction as

$$7.4528 - 5.8706 - 0.0243 = 1.5579,$$

but could also have been obtained directly as

$$\sum_j (C_j^2/n_{.j}) - CT = 22.0702 - 20.5122$$
$$= 1.5580,$$

the discrepancy from 1.5579 being due to rounding error. This analysis, shown on the left at the foot of Table 8.15, provides F tests for treatments and for the interaction T × A. The treatment difference is highly significant; the interaction is very small and far from significant.

To test the age effect adjusted for treatments, calculate the Treatments SSq unadjusted:

$$\sum_i (R_i^2/n_{i.}) - CT = 26.0000 - 20.5122$$
$$= 5.4878,$$

and the adjusted Ages SSq follows by subtraction:

$$7.4528 - 5.4878 - 0.0243 = 1.9407.$$

The F test shows the age effect to be non-significant ($P = 0.15$).

In the original publication (Marshall, 1964) a similar allowance was made for the possible effect of blood pressure, and data from female patients were also included.

Table 8.15 Analysis of data from Table 8.14

Age j		40– 1	50– 2	60– 3	All ages	
Group	*i*				R_i	$n_{i.}$
Control	1	T_{1j} 1	14	10	25	
		n_{1j} 1	11	13		25
		$\bar{y}_{1j}$ 1·0000	1·2727	0·7692		
		S_{1j} 1	28	12		41
		T_{1j}^2/n_{1j} 1·0000	17·8182	7·6923		
Treated	2	T_{2j} 0	4	0	4	
		n_{2j} 4	11	1		16
		$\bar{y}_{2j}$ 0·0000	0·3636	0·0000		
		S_{2j} 0	4	0		4
		T_{2j}^2/n_{2j} 0·0000	1·4545	0·0000		
		C_j 1	18	10	$T = 29$	$S = 45$
		$n_{.j}$ 5	22	14	$N = 41$	
		d_j 1·0000	0·9091	0·7692		
		w_j 0·8000	5·5000	0·9286		
		$w_j d_j$ 0·8000	5·0000	0·7143		
		C_j^2/n_j 0·2000	14·7273	7·1429		

CT, $T^2/N = 20·5122$

Analysis of variance

	SSq	DF	MSq	VR		SSq	DF	MSq	VR
Between cells	7·4528	5							
Treatment (adjusted)	5·8706	1	5·8706	12·06*	Treatment (unadj.)	5·4878	1		
Age (unadj.)	1·5579	2			Age (adjusted)	1·9407	2	0·9704	1·99
T × A	0·0243	2	0·0122	< 1					
Within cells	17·0350	35	0·4867	1·00					
Total	24·4878	40							

*$P < 0.001$.

For an alternative method of analysis, see Example 10.5, p. 349. Both the present analysis and that of Example 10.5 could be criticized for the assumption that the variable being analysed (number of accidents) is normally distributed with constant variance. This is likely to be far from true for a variable taking small integral values, a type of data for which the Poisson distribution is often more appropriate. An alternative approach using a generalized linear model is described in Example 12.11, p. 430.

9: Further Analysis of Straight-Line Data

9.1 Analysis of variance applied to regression

In the last two chapters the analysis of variance has been used to study the effect, on the mean value of a random variable, of various types of classification of the data into qualitative categories. We now return to the linear regression model of Chapter 5, in which the mean value of y is linearly related to a second variable x, and consider the analysis of variance for this situation.

Suppose, as in §5.2, that there are n pairs of values, $(x_1, y_1), \ldots, (x_i, y_i), \ldots, (x_n, y_n)$, and that the fitted regression line of y on x has the equation

$$Y = a + bx, \tag{9.1}$$

with a and b given by (5.2) and (5.3).

The deviation of y_i from the mean $\bar{y}$ can be divided into two parts:

$$y_i - \bar{y} = (y_i - Y_i) + (Y_i - \bar{y}), \tag{9.2}$$

where Y_i is the value of y calculated from the regression line (9.1) with $x = x_i$ (see Fig. 9.1).

It can be shown that when both sides of (9.2) are squared, and the terms summed from $i = 1$ to n, the sum of the products of the terms on the right is zero, and the following relation holds:

$$\sum(y_i - \bar{y})^2 = \sum(y_i - Y_i)^2 + \sum(Y_i - \bar{y})^2. \tag{9.3}$$

The term on the left is the Total SSq; the first term on the right is the SSq of deviations of observed ys about the regression line, and the second is the SSq about the mean of the values Y_i predicted by the regression line. In short,

Total SSq = SSq about regression + SSq due to regression.

In Fig. 9.1(a), most of the Total SSq is explained by the SSq about regression; in Fig. 9.1(b), in contrast, most of the Total SSq is due to regression.

An expression for $\sum(y_i - Y_i)^2$ has already been given in (5.7). From (1.3) and (5.9) the computing formulae shown in Table 9.1 immediately follow (the subscripts i now being dropped).

Suppose, as in §5.2, that the ys are distributed independently and normally, with variance σ^2, about expected values given by

$$E(y) = \alpha + \beta x. \tag{9.4}$$

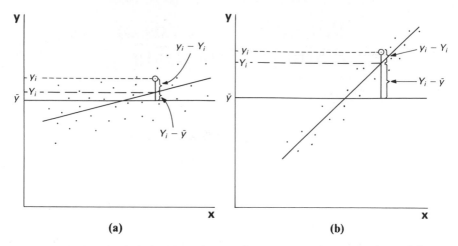

Fig. 9.1 Subdivision of a deviation about the mean into two parts: about regression and due to regression. In (a) the regression of y on x explains a much smaller fraction of the total variation of y than in (b).

Table 9.1 Analysis of variance for linear regression

	SSq	DF	MSq	VR
Due to regression	$\dfrac{\left[\sum xy - (\sum x)(\sum y)/n\right]^2}{\sum x^2 - (\sum x)^2/n}$	1	s_1^2	s_1^2/s_0^2
About regression	By subtraction	$n-2$	s_0^2	
Total	$\sum y^2 - (\sum y)^2/n$	$n-1$		

The null hypothesis that $\beta = 0$ (that is, that the expectation of y is constant, irrespective of the value of x) may be tested by the analysis of variance in Table 9.1. If $\beta = 0$, s_1^2 and s_0^2 are independent unbiased estimates of σ^2. If $\beta \neq 0$, s_0^2 is an unbiased estimate of σ^2 (see (5.8)) but s_1^2 estimates a quantity greater than σ^2. The variance ratio $F = s_1^2/s_0^2$, on 1 and $n-2$ DF, may therefore be used to test whether $\beta = 0$.

The significance of the regression slope has previously been tested by

$$t = \frac{b}{\text{SE}(b)} = \frac{b}{s_0/\sqrt{\sum(x - \bar{x})^2}}$$

on $n-2$ DF (as in (5.18) and (5.20)). Using the formula (5.3) for b, it is easy to see that $F = t^2$, and (as noted, for example, in §4.6 and §7.1) the tests are equivalent.

Example 9.1

The analysis of variance of y, from the data of Example 5.1 (pp. 160 and 167) is as follows:

	SSq	DF	MSq	VR	
Due to regression	7 666·39	1	7666·39	24·2	$(P < 0.001)$
About regression	9 502·08	30	316·74	1·00	
Total	17 168·47	31			

The SSq have already been obtained on pp. 160 and 167. The value of t obtained previously was -4.92; note that $(4.92)^2 = 24.2$, the value of F.

Test of linearity

It is often important to know not only whether the slope of an assumed linear regression is significant, but also whether there is any reason to doubt the basic assumption of the linearity of the regression.

   If the data provide a number of replicate readings of y for certain values of x, a test of linearity is easily obtained. Suppose that, at the value x_i of x, there are n_i observations on y, with a mean $\bar{y}_i$. Each such group of replicates is called an *array*. Figure 9.2 illustrates three different situations. In (a) a linear regression seems to be consistent with the observed data in that the array means $\bar{y}_i$ are reasonably close to the regression line. In (b) and (c), however, the array means deviate from the line by more than can easily be explained by the within-arrays variation. In (b) the deviations seem to be systematic, suggesting that a curved regression line is required. In (c) the deviations seem to be patternless, suggesting perhaps an extra source of variation associated with each array; for example, if each array referred to observations on animals in a single cage, the positioning of the cage in the laboratory might affect the whole array.

   In discussing Fig. 9.2 we have made a rough comparison between the magnitude of deviations of array means from the regression line and the within-arrays variation. The comparison is made formally as follows. For any value y in the array corresponding to x_i, the residual $y - Y_i$ may be divided into two parts:

$$y - Y_i = (y - \bar{y}_i) + (\bar{y}_i - Y_i). \tag{9.5}$$

When both sides are squared and summed over all observations, the sum of products of the two terms on the right vanishes, and we have a partition of the Residual SSq:

$$\sum (y - Y_i)^2 = \sum (y - \bar{y}_i)^2 + \sum (\bar{y}_i - Y_i)^2, \tag{9.6}$$

the summations being taken over all n observations. The first term on the right is the SSq about array means; the second term is the SSq of deviations of array means from the regression line. The first of these is precisely what would be

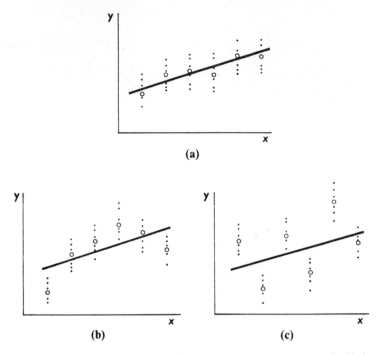

Fig. 9.2 Deviations of array means from linear regression. Those in (a) are explicable by within-arrays variation; those in (b) suggest a systematic departure from linearity; while those in (c) suggest a further source of variation.

Table 9.2 Analysis of variance with test of linearity

	SSq	DF	MSq	VR
Due to regression	(As in Table 9.1)	1	s_1^2	$F_1 = s_1^2/s_3^2$
Deviation of array means from regression	(By subtraction)	$k - 2$	s_2^2	$F_2 = s_2^2/s_3^2$
Within-arrays residual	$\sum y^2 - \sum_i (T_i^2/n_i)$	$n - k$	s_3^2	
Total	$\sum y^2 - (\sum y)^2/n$	$n - 1$		

obtained as the Within-Arrays SSq in a one-way analysis of variance of the ys without reference to the xs.

The computing formulae are given in Table 9.2. Here k is the number of arrays, and T_i is the sum of values of y for the ith array. The variance ratio F_2 tests the deviation of the array means about linear regression, and F_1 tests the departure of β from zero assuming linear regression. If F_2 is not significant and

$n - k$ is rather small, it may be useful to combine the SSq in the second and third lines of the analysis, taking one back to Table 9.1. If F_2 is significant, thought should be given to the question whether the non-linearity is of type (b) or type (c). If it is of type (b), some form of non-linear regression should be fitted (see §10.3). Type (c) may be handled approximately by testing s_1^2 against s_2^2 by a variance ratio $F_1' = s_1^2/s_2^2$ on 1 and $k - 2$ DF.

Example 9.2

In one method of assaying vitamin D, rats are fed on a diet deficient in vitamin D for two weeks so as to develop rickets. The diet is then supplemented by one of a number of different doses of a standard vitamin D preparation or of a test preparation which is to be assayed against the standard. After a further two weeks the degree to which the rickets has been healed is assessed by radiographing the right knee of each animal. The photograph is matched against a standard set of photographs numbered from 0 to 12 (in increasing order of healing).

The results shown in Table 9.3 were obtained with three doses of vitamin D. Each score is the average of four assessments of a single photograph. General experience with this type of assay suggests a linear regression of the score, y, on the log dose, x.

The Total SSq is

$$314 \cdot 2500 - (89 \cdot 00)^2/31 = 58 \cdot 7339,$$

and the Within-Doses Residual SSq is

$$314 \cdot 2500 - (32 \cdot 4000 + 87 \cdot 7813 + 152 \cdot 3269) = 41 \cdot 7418.$$

The calculation of the SSq due to regression makes use of the fact that only three values of x occur. Thus

$$\sum x = 10(0 \cdot 544) + 8(0 \cdot 845) + 13(1 \cdot 146) = 27 \cdot 098,$$

$$\sum (x - \bar{x})^2 = 10(0 \cdot 544)^2 + 8(0 \cdot 845)^2 + 13(1 \cdot 146)^2 - (27 \cdot 098)^2/31 = 2 \cdot 0576$$

and

$$\sum (x - \bar{x})(y - \bar{y}) = (0 \cdot 544)(18 \cdot 00) + (0 \cdot 845)(26 \cdot 50) + (1 \cdot 146)(44 \cdot 50)$$

$$- (27 \cdot 098)(89 \cdot 00)/31 = 5 \cdot 3840,$$

from which

$$\text{SSq due to regression} = (5 \cdot 3840)^2/2 \cdot 0576 = 14 \cdot 0880.$$

The variance ratio for deviations of dose means is not significant, and the conclusion that the regression is effectively linear is reinforced by general experience with this assay method. The regression slope is, of course, highly significant.

If the observations do not fall into arrays at fixed values of x, the testing of linearity is less simple. It is often adequate to form groups along the x-scale, and treat the data as though the arrays corresponded to the midpoints of the groups of x. Alternatively one can use the methods of §10.3 to fit non-linear regression curves.

Table 9.3 Radiographic assessments of bone healing for three doses of vitamin D

Dose (i.u.)	3·5	7	14	
Log dose, x_i	0·544	0·845	1·146	Total
	0	1·50	2·00	
	0	2·50	2·50	
	1·00	5·00	5·00	
	2·75	6·00	4·00	
	2·75	4·25	5·00	
	1·75	2·75	4·00	
	2·75	1·50	2·50	
	2·25	3·00	3·50	
	2·25		3·00	
	2·50		2·00	
			3·00	
			4·00	
			4·00	
T_i	18·00	26·50	44·50	89·00
n_i	10	8	13	31
$\bar{y}_i$	1·8000	3·3125	3·4231	
$\sum y^2$	43·1250	106·3750	164·7500	314·2500
T_i^2/n_i	32·4000	87·7813	152·3269	

Analysis of variance

	SSq	DF	MSq	VR	
Due to regression	14·0880	1	14·0880	9·45	$(P = 0.005)$
Deviations of dose means	2·9041	1	2·9041	1·95	$(P = 0.17)$
Within-doses residual	41·7418	28	1·4908	1·00	
Total	58·7339	30			

9.2 Errors in both variables

In studying the regression of y on x it has not been necessary to consider any form of random variation in the values of x. Clearly, in many sets of data, the values of x do vary randomly—either because the individual units on which the measurements are made are selected by an effectively random process, or because any observation on x is affected by measurement error or some other form of random perturbation. In the standard regression formulation these considerations are irrelevant. There are, however, some questions rather different from those answered by regression analysis, in which random errors in x are relevant. These are, basically, questions involving the values of x which would have been observed had there been no random error.

Suppose that any pair of observed values (x, y) can be regarded as differing by random errors from a pair of 'true values' (X, Y) which are linearly related. Thus

$$Y = \alpha + \beta X, \tag{9.7}$$

where we observe

$$
\left. \begin{array}{r} x = X + \delta \\ y = Y + \varepsilon, \end{array} \right\} \tag{9.8}
$$

and

and δ and ε are distributed independently of each other and also independently of X and Y. Suppose that δ is distributed as $N(0, \sigma_\delta^2)$ and ε as $N(0, \sigma_\varepsilon^2)$ (see Fig. 9.3).

The first point to emphasize is that, if the problem is to predict the behaviour of y or Y in terms of x (the observed value), ordinary regression analysis is appropriate. In many situations this is the case. If y is a measure of clinical change and x is a biochemical measurement, the purpose of an analysis may be to study the extent to which y can be predicted from x. Any value of x used in the analysis will be subject to random variation due to physiological fluctuations and measurement error, but this fact can be disregarded because predictions will be made from values of x which are equally subject to such variation.

Suppose, however, that the purpose is to estimate the value of β, the slope of the line relating Y to X (not to x). This problem is likely to arise in two different circumstances.

1 The 'true' value X may be of much more interest than the 'observed' value, x, because future discussions will be in terms of X rather than x. For instance, in a geographic survey, x may be the mean household size of a certain town as estimated from the survey and y some measure of health in that town. The size of the random error component in x may be peculiar to this particular survey and of

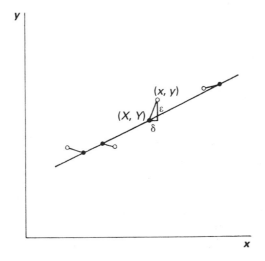

Fig. 9.3 Deviations of observed values from a linear functional relationship with errors in both variables.

no relevance in future work. Any arguments should be based on the effect, on y, of changes in the true mean household size, X.

2 The equation (9.7) may express a *functional relationship* between the true values X and Y, which is of particular scientific importance. For instance, if X and Y are, respectively, the volume and mass of different specimens of a metal, equation (9.7) with $\alpha = 0$ would clearly represent the relationship between X and Y with β measuring the density. The estimation of β would be a reasonable objective, but the complication arises that both X and Y are affected by random measurement errors, so the investigator observes pairs of values (x, y).

The estimation of α and β from pairs of observed values (x, y) is a difficult problem (Kendall, 1951, 1952; Sprent, 1969). One general result is that b, the regression coefficient of y on x, underestimates β on the average. The expected value of b is approximately

$$\beta' = \beta \left[1 - \frac{\sigma_\delta^2}{\text{var}(x)} \right]. \tag{9.9}$$

If σ_δ^2 can be estimated (for example, by a special experimental study involving replicate observations of the same X), the correction term in braces can be estimated, and a correction applied to the estimated slope b.

In many situations no direct estimate of σ_δ^2 will be possible because there is no way of selecting observations with different values of x but the same value of X. Usually the situation here is that a set of pairs (x, y) shows some general linear trend which the investigator wishes to represent by a single straight line without making the distinction between x and y required in a regression analysis. He/She should make quite sure that any subsequent use of the line will not put either variable in the role of a predictor variable, and that a single line will perform a useful function in representing the general trend. If there is insufficient basis for any reasonable assumptions about σ_δ^2 and σ_ε^2, a simple visual approach is probably best: draw a freehand line through the cluster and refrain from any assertions of sampling error.

An interesting special situation is that in which x is a *controlled variable*. Suppose that x is known to differ from X by a random error, as in (9.8), but that the value of x is selected by the experimenter. For example, in drawing liquid into a pipette the experimenter may aim at a specified volume x, and would assume that he/she had carried out the experiment with a value x, although the true value X would differ from x by a random error. If there is no systematic bias, (9.8) will represent the situation, but the important difference between this problem and that considered earlier is that the random error δ is independent of x, whereas previously δ was independent of X. It follows, as Berkson (1950) pointed out, that the regression coefficient of y on x does in this case provide an unbiased estimate of β, and standard methods of regression analysis are appropriate.

9.3 Straight lines through the origin

Sometimes there may be good reason to suppose that a regression line must pass through the origin, in the sense that when $x = 0$ the mean value of y must also be 0. For instance, in a psychological experiment the subject may be asked to guess how far a certain light falls to the left or to the right of a marker. If the guessed distance to the right is y (distances to the left corresponding to $y < 0$) and the true distance is x, a subject whose responses showed no bias to left or right would have $E(y) = 0$ when $x = 0$.

The regression of y on x will then take the form

$$Y = \beta x, \tag{9.10}$$

and the least squares solution is similar to that of the ordinary regression formulae, except that sums of squares and products are not corrected for deviations about mean values. Thus, β is estimated by

$$b = \sum xy / \sum x^2, \tag{9.11}$$

and the SSq about regression is

$$\sum y^2 - (\sum xy)^2 / \sum x^2$$

on $n - 1$(not $n - 2$) DF.

This result assumes, as usual, that the residual variance of y is independent of x. In many problems in which a line through the origin seems appropriate, particularly for variables which take positive values only, this is clearly not so. There is often a tendency for the variability of y to increase as x increases. Two other least squares solutions are useful here.

1   If the residual var(y) increases in proportion to x, the best estimate of β is $b_1 = \sum y / \sum x = \bar{y} / \bar{x}$, the ratio of the two means. An example of this situation would occur in a radioactivity counting experiment where the same material is observed for replicate periods of different lengths. If x_i is a time interval and y_i the corresponding count, Poisson theory shows that $\text{var}(y_i) = E(y_i | x_i) \propto x_i$. The estimate of the mean count per unit time is, as would be expected, $\sum y_i / \sum x_i$, the total count divided by the total time period.

2   If the residual *standard deviation* of y increases in proportion to x, the best estimate of β is $b_2 = \sum (y/x)/n$, the mean of the individual ratios.

Care should be taken to enquire whether a regression line, rather than a functional relationship (§9.2), is really needed in such problems. Suppose that x and y are estimates of a biochemical substance obtained by two different methods. If y is the estimate by the more reliable method, and x is obtained by a rapid but rather less reliable method, it may be reasonable to estimate y from x, and one of the above methods may be appropriate. If the question is rather 'How big are the discrepancies between x and y?' there is no reason to treat the problem as one of the regression of y on x rather than x on y. A useful device here is to rewrite (9.10) as

$$\log Y = \log \beta + \log x,$$

and to take the individual values of $z = \log y - \log x$ as estimates of $\log \beta$ (see also p. 276). If random variation in z is approximately independent of x or y (and this can be checked by simple scatter diagrams), the mean value of z will be the best estimate of $\log \beta$, confidence limits being obtained by the t distribution, as is usual for a mean value. This situation is roughly equivalent to **2** above. If random variation in z depends heavily on x or y, the observations could be grouped and some form of weighted average taken (see §7.2).

9.4 Regression in groups

Frequently data are classified into groups, and within each group a linear regression of y on x may be postulated. For example, the regression of forced expiratory volume on age may be considered separately for men in different occupational groups. Possible differences between the regression lines are then often of interest.

In this section we consider comparisons of the slopes of the regression lines. If the slopes clearly differ from one group to another, then so, of course, must the mean values of y—at least for some values of x. In Fig. 9.4(a), the slopes of the regression lines differ from group to group. The lines for groups (i) and (ii) cross. Those for (i) and (iii) and for (ii) and (iii) would also cross if extended sufficiently far, but here there is some doubt as to whether the linear regressions would remain valid outside the range of values of x observed.

If the slopes do not differ, the lines are parallel, as in Fig. 9.4(b) and (c), and here it becomes interesting to ask whether, as in (b), the lines differ in their height above the x axis (which depends on the coefficient α in the equation $E(y) = \alpha + \beta x$), or whether, as in (c), the lines coincide. In practice the fitted regression lines would rarely have *precisely* the same slope or position, and the question is to what extent differences between the lines can be attributed to random variation. Differences in position between parallel lines are discussed in §9.5. In this section we concentrate on the question of differences between slopes.

Suppose that there are k groups, with n_i pairs of observations in the ith group. Denote the mean values of x and y in the ith group by $\bar{x}_i$ and $\bar{y}_i$, and the regression line calculated as in §5.2 by

$$Y_i = \bar{y}_i + b_i(x - \bar{x}_i). \tag{9.12}$$

If all the n_i are reasonably large, a satisfactory approach is to estimate the variance of each b_i by (5.18) and to ignore the imprecision in these estimates of

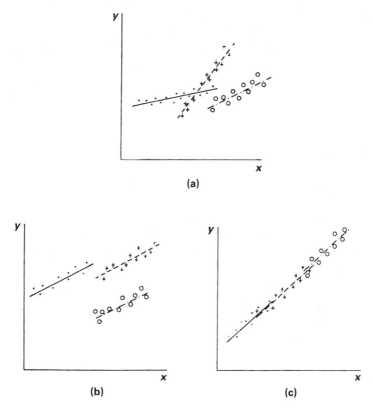

Fig. 9.4 Differences between regression lines fitted to three groups of observations. The lines differ in slope and position in (a), differ only in position in (b), and coincide in (c). (———) (i); (– – –) (ii); (– · –) (iii).

variance. Changing the notation of (5.18) somewhat, we shall denote the residual mean square for the ith group by s_i^2 and the sum of squares of x about $\bar{x}_i$ by $\sum_{(i)} (x - \bar{x}_i)^2$. Note that the parenthesized suffix i attached to the summation sign indicates summation only over the specified group i; that is,

$$\sum_{(i)} (x - \bar{x}_i)^2 = \sum_{j=1}^{n_i} (x_{ij} - \bar{x}_i)^2.$$

Following the method of §7.2, we write

$$w_i = \frac{1}{\text{var}(b_i)} = \frac{\sum_{(i)} (x - \bar{x}_i)^2}{s_i^2}, \tag{9.13}$$

and calculate

$$G = \sum w_i b_i^2 - \left(\sum w_i b_i\right)^2 / \sum w_i. \tag{9.14}$$

On the null hypothesis that the true slopes β_i are all equal, G follows approximately a $\chi^2_{(k-1)}$ distribution. High values of G indicate departures from the null hypothesis, i.e. real differences between the β_i. If G is non-significant, and the null hypothesis is tentatively accepted, the common value β of the β_i is best estimated by the weighted mean

$$\bar{b} = \sum w_i b_i / \sum w_i, \tag{9.15}$$

with an estimated variance

$$\text{var}(\bar{b}) = 1/\sum w_i. \tag{9.16}$$

The sampling variation of $\bar{b}$ is approximately normal.

It is difficult to say how large the n_i must be for this 'large-sample' approach to be used with safety. There would probably be little risk in adopting it if none of the n_i fell below 20.

A more exact treatment is available provided that an extra assumption is made—that the residual variances σ_i^2 are all equal. Suppose the common value is σ^2. We consider first the situation where $k = 2$, as a comparison of two slopes can be effected by use of the t distribution. For $k > 2$ an analysis of variance is required.

Two groups

The residual variance σ^2 can be estimated either as

$$s_1^2 = \frac{\sum_{(1)} (y - Y_1)^2}{n_1 - 2}$$

$$= \frac{\sum_{(1)} (y - \bar{y}_1)^2 - [\sum_{(1)} (x - \bar{x}_1)(y - \bar{y}_1)]^2 / \sum_{(1)} (x - \bar{x}_1)^2}{n_1 - 2}$$

or by the corresponding mean square for the second group, s_2^2. A pooled estimate may be obtained (very much as in the two-sample t test) as

$$s^2 = \frac{\sum_{(1)} (y - Y_1)^2 + \sum_{(2)} (y - Y_2)^2}{n_1 + n_2 - 4}. \tag{9.17}$$

To compare b_1 and b_2 we estimate

$$\text{var}(b_1 - b_2) = s^2 \left[\frac{1}{\sum_{(1)} (x - \bar{x}_1)^2} + \frac{1}{\sum_{(2)} (x - \bar{x}_2)^2} \right]. \tag{9.18}$$

The difference is tested by

$$t = \frac{b_1 - b_2}{\text{SE}(b_1 - b_2)} \text{ on } n_1 + n_2 - 4 \text{ DF}, \qquad (9.19)$$

the DF being the divisor in (9.17).

If a common value is assumed for the regression slope in the two groups, its value β may be estimated by

$$b = \frac{\sum_{(1)}(x - \bar{x}_1)(y - \bar{y}_1) + \sum_{(2)}(x - \bar{x}_2)(y - \bar{y}_2)}{\sum_{(1)}(x - \bar{x}_1)^2 + \sum_{(2)}(x - \bar{x}_2)^2}, \qquad (9.20)$$

with a variance estimated as

$$\text{var}(b) = s^2 / \left[\sum_{(1)}(x - \bar{x}_1)^2 + \sum_{(2)}(x - \bar{x}_2)^2 \right]. \qquad (9.21)$$

Equations (9.20) and (9.21) can easily be seen to be equivalent to (9.15) and (9.16) if, in the calculation of w_i in (9.13), the separate estimates of residual variance s_i^2 are replaced by the common estimate s^2. For tests or the calculation of confidence limits for β using (9.21), the t distribution on $n_1 + n_2 - 4$ DF should be used. Where a common slope is accepted it would be more usual to estimate s^2 as the residual mean square about the parallel lines (9.34), which would have $n_1 + n_2 - 3$ DF.

Example 9.3

Table 9.4 gives age and vital capacity (litres) for each of 84 men working in the cadmium industry. They are divided into three groups: A_1, exposed to cadmium fumes for at least 10 years; A_2, exposed to fumes for less than 10 years; B, not exposed to fumes. The main purpose of the study was to see whether exposure to fumes was associated with a change in respiratory function. However, those in group A_1 must be expected to be older on the average than those in groups A_2 or B, and it is well known that respiratory test performance declines with age. A comparison is therefore needed which corrects for discrepancies between the mean ages of the different groups.

We shall first illustrate the calculations for two groups by amalgamating groups A_1 and A_2 (denoting the pooled group by A) and comparing groups A and B.

The sums of squares and products of deviations about the mean, and the separate slopes b_i are as follows:

Group	i	n_i	$\sum_{(i)}(x - \bar{x}_i)^2$	$\sum_{(i)}(x - \bar{x}_i)(y - \bar{y}_i)$	$\sum_{(i)}(y - \bar{y}_i)^2$	b_i
A	1	40	4397·38	− 236·385	26·5812	− 0·0538
B	2	44	6197·16	− 189·712	20·6067	− 0·0306
Total			10594·54	− 426·097	47·1879	(− 0·0402)

Table 9.4 Ages and vital capacities for three groups of workers in the cadmium industry. x, age last birthday (years); y, vital capacity (litres)

Group A$_1$, exposed > 10 years		Group A$_2$, exposed < 10 years		Group B, not exposed			
x	y	x	y	x	y	x	y
39	4·62	29	5·21	27	5·29	43	4·02
40	5·29	29	5·17	25	3·67	41	4·99
41	5·52	33	4·88	24	5·82	48	3·86
41	3·71	32	4·50	32	4·77	47	4·68
45	4·02	31	4·47	23	5·71	53	4·74
49	5·09	29	5·12	25	4·47	49	3·76
52	2·70	29	4·51	32	4·55	54	3·98
47	4·31	30	4·85	18	4·61	48	5·00
61	2·70	21	5·22	19	5·86	49	3·31
65	3·03	28	4·62	26	5·20	47	3·11
58	2·73	23	5·07	33	4·44	52	4·76
59	3·67	35	3·64	27	5·52	58	3·95
		38	3·64	33	4·97	62	4·60
		38	5·09	25	4·99	65	4·83
		43	4·61	42	4·89	62	3·18
		39	4·73	35	4·09	59	3·03
		38	4·58	35	4·24		
		42	5·12	41	3·88		
		43	3·89	38	4·85		
		43	4·62	41	4·79		
		37	4·30	36	4·36		
		50	2·70	36	4·02		
		50	3·50	41	3·77		
		45	5·06	41	4·22		
		48	4·06	37	4·94		
		51	4·51	42	4·04		
		46	4·66	39	4·51		
		58	2·88	41	4·06		
Sums 597	47·39	1058	125·21			1751	196·33
Number of observations 12		28				44	
$\sum x^2$ 30 613		42 260				75 879	
$\sum xy$ 2 280·01		4 624·93				7 623·33	
$\sum y^2$ 198·8903		572·4599				896·6401	

The SSq about the regressions are

$$\sum{}_{(1)}(y - Y_1)^2 = 26·5812 - (-236·385)^2/4397·38 = 13·8741$$

and

$$\sum{}_{(2)}(y - Y_2)^2 = 20·6067 - (-189·712)^2/6197·16 = 14·7991.$$

Thus,

$$s^2 = (13\cdot8741 + 14\cdot7991)/(40 + 44 - 3) = 0\cdot3584,$$

and, for the difference between b_1 and b_2 using (9·18) and (9·19),

$$t = \frac{-0\cdot0538 - (-0\cdot0306)}{\sqrt{\left[(0\cdot3584)\left(\dfrac{1}{4397\cdot38} + \dfrac{1}{6197\cdot16}\right)\right]}}$$

$$= -0\cdot0232/0\cdot0118$$

$$= -1\cdot97 \text{ on } 80 \text{ DF.}$$

The difference is very nearly significant at the 5% level. This example is continued on p. 300.

The scatter diagram in Fig. 9.5 shows the regression lines with slopes b_A and b_B fitted separately to the two groups, and also the two parallel lines with slope b. The steepness of the slope for group A may be partly or wholly due to a curvature in the regression: there is a suggestion that the mean value of y at high values of x is lower than is predicted by the linear regressions (see p. 300). Alternatively it may be that a linear regression is appropriate for each group, but that for group A the vital capacity declines more rapidly with age than for group B.

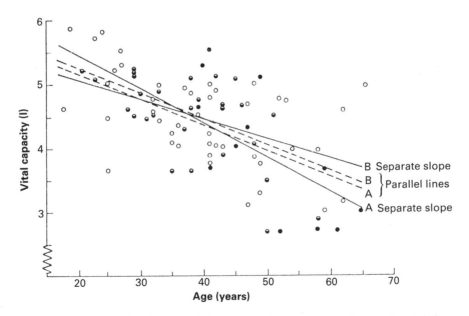

Fig. 9.5 Scatter diagram showing age and vital capacity of 84 men working in the cadmium industry, divided into three groups (Table 9.4). (●) Group A_1; (◐) Group A_2; (○) Group B.

More than two groups

To simplify the notation, denote the sum of squares about the mean of x in the ith group by

$$S_{xxi} \tag{9.22}$$

instead of

$$\sum_{(i)} (x - \bar{x}_i)^2,$$

the sum of products of deviations by S_{xyi}, and so on. Then with any number of groups the pooled slope b is given by the generalization of (9.20):

$$b = \frac{\sum_i S_{xyi}}{\sum_i S_{xxi}}. \tag{9.23}$$

Parallel lines may now be drawn through the mean points $(\bar{x}_i, \bar{y}_i)$, each with the same slope b. That for the ith group will have this equation:

$$Y_{ci} = \bar{y}_i + b(x - \bar{x}_i). \tag{9.24}$$

The subscript c is used to indicate that the predicted value Y_{ci} is obtained using the common slope, b.

The deviation of any observed value y from its group mean $\bar{y}_i$ may be divided as follows:

$$y - \bar{y}_i = (y - Y_i) + (Y_i - Y_{ci}) + (Y_{ci} - \bar{y}_i). \tag{9.25}$$

Again, it can be shown that the sums of squares of these components can be added in the same way. This means that

Within-Groups SSq = Residual SSq about separate lines

+ SSq due to differences between the b_i and b

+ SSq due to fitting common slope b.   (9.26)

The middle term on the right is the one that particularly concerns us now. It can be obtained by noting that the SSq due to the common slope is

$$\left(\sum_i S_{xyi} \right)^2 \bigg/ \sum_i (S_{xxi}); \tag{9.27}$$

this follows directly from (5.7) and (9.23). From previous results,

$$\text{Within-Groups SSq} = \sum_i S_{yyi} \tag{9.28}$$

and Residual SSq about separate lines

$$= \sum_i [S_{yyi} - (S_{xyi})^2/S_{xxi}]. \tag{9.29}$$

From (9.26), (9.27), (9.28) and (9.29),

$$\text{SSq due to differences in slope} = \sum_i \frac{(S_{xyi})^2}{S_{xxi}} - \frac{(\sum_i S_{xyi})^2}{\sum_i S_{xxi}}. \tag{9.30}$$

It should be noted that (9.30) is equivalent to

$$\sum_i W_i b_i^2 - \frac{(\sum_i W_i b_i)^2}{\sum_i W_i}, \tag{9.31}$$

where $W_i = S_{xxi} = \sigma^2/\text{var}(b_i)$, and that the pooled slope b equals $\sum W_i b_i / \sum W_i$, the weighted mean of the b_i. The SSq due to differences in slope is thus essentially a weighted sum of squares of the b_i about their weighted mean b, the weights being (as usual) inversely proportional to the sampling variances (see §7.2).

The analysis is summarized in Table 9.5. There is only one DF for the common slope, since the SSq is proportional to the square of one linear contrast, b. The $k - 1$ DF for the second line follow because the SSq measures differences between k independent slopes, b_i. The residual DF follow because there are $n_i - 2$ DF for the ith group and $\sum_i(n_i - 2) = n - 2k$. The total DF within groups are, correctly, $n - k$. The F test for differences between slopes follows immediately.

Table 9.5 Analysis of variance for differences between regression slopes

	SSq	DF	MSq	VR
Due to common slope	$\dfrac{(\sum_i S_{xyi})^2}{\sum_i S_{xxi}}$	1		
Differences between slopes	$\sum_i \dfrac{(S_{xyi})^2}{S_{xxi}} - \dfrac{(\sum_i S_{xyi})^2}{\sum_i S_{xxi}}$	$k - 1$	s_A^2	$F_A = s_A^2/s^2$
Residual about separate lines	$\sum_i S_{yyi} - \sum_i \dfrac{(S_{xyi})^2}{S_{xxi}}$	$n - 2k$	s^2	
Within groups	$\sum_i S_{yyi}$	$n - k$		

Example 9.3, continued

We now test the significance of differences between the three slopes. The sums of squares and products of deviations about the mean, and the separate slopes, are as follows:

Group	i	n_i	S_{xx}	S_{xy}	S_{yy}	b_i
A_1	1	12	912·25	− 77·643	11·7393	− 0·0851
A_2	2	28	2282·71	− 106·219	12·5476	− 0·0465
B	3	44	6197·16	− 189·712	20·6067	− 0·0306
Total		84	9392·12	− 373·574	44·8936	(− 0·0398)

The SSq due to the common slope is

$$(- 373·574)^2/9392·12 = 14·8590.$$

The Residual SSq about the separate lines using (9.29) are:

$$\sum_{(1)}(y - Y_1)^2 = 5·1310; \sum_{(2)}(y - Y_2)^2 = 7·6050; \sum_{(3)}(y - Y_3)^2 = 14·7991.$$

The total Residual SSq about separate lines is therefore

$$5·1310 + 7·6050 + 14·7991 = 27·5351.$$

The Within-Groups SSq is 44·8936. The SSq for differences between slopes may now be obtained by subtraction, as

$$44·8936 - 14·8590 - 27·5351 = 2·4995.$$

Alternatively, it may be calculated directly as

$$\frac{(- 77·643)^2}{912·25} + \frac{(- 106·219)^2}{2282·71} + \frac{(- 189·712)^2}{6197·16} - \frac{(- 373·574)^2}{9392·12} = 2·4995.$$

The analysis of variance may now be completed.

	SSq	DF	MSq	VR
Common slope	14·8590	1	14·8590	42·09 ($P < 0·001$)
Between slopes	2·4995	2	1·2498	3·54 ($P = 0·034$)
Separate residuals	27·5351	78	0·3530	
Within groups	44·8936	81		

The differences between slopes are more significant than in the two-group analysis. The estimates of the separate slopes, with their standard errors calculated in terms of the Residual MSq on 78 DF, are

$$b_{A1} = - 0·0851 \pm 0·0197, \quad b_{A2} = - 0·0465 \pm 0·0124, \quad b_B = - 0·0306 \pm 0·0075.$$

The most highly exposed group, A_1, provides the steepest slope. Figure 9.6 shows the separate regressions as well as the three parallel lines.

The doubt about linearity suggests further that a curvilinear regression might be more suitable; however, analysis with a quadratic regression line (see §10.3) shows the non-linearity to be quite non-significant.

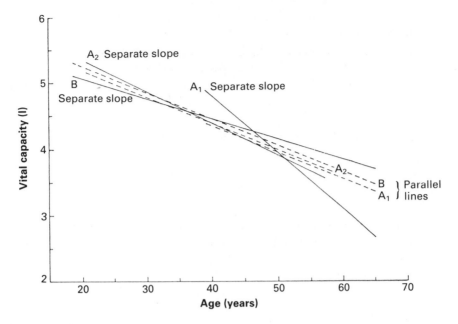

Fig. 9.6 Parallel regression lines and lines with separate slopes, for cadmium workers (Fig. 9.5).

The analysis of variance test can, of course, be applied even for $k = 2$. The results will be entirely equivalent to the t test described at the beginning of this section, the value of F being, as usual, the square of the corresponding value of t.

9.5   The analysis of covariance

If, after an analysis of the type described in the last section, there is no strong reason for postulating differences between the slopes of the regression lines in the various groups, the following questions arise. What can be said about the relative position of parallel regression lines? Is there good reason to believe that the true lines differ in position, as in Fig. 9.4(b), or could they coincide, as in Fig. 9.4(c)? What sampling error is to be attached to an estimate of the difference in positions of lines for two particular groups?

The set of techniques associated with these questions is called the *analysis of covariance*. The relevance of the name will become apparent later in the section.

Before describing technical details it may be useful to note some important differences in the purposes of the analysis of covariance and in the circumstances in which it may be used.

1   *Main purpose.*
    (a) *To correct for bias.* If it is known that changes in x affect the mean value of y, and that the groups under comparison differ in their values of $\bar{x}$, it will

follow that some of the differences between the values of $\bar{y}$ can be ascribed partly to differences between the $\bar{x}$s. We may want to remove this effect as far as possible. For example, if y is FEV and x is age, a comparison of mean FEVs for men in different occupational groups may be affected by differences in their mean ages. A comparison would be desirable of the mean FEVs at the same age. If the regressions are linear and parallel, this means a comparison of the relative position of the regression lines.

(b) *To reduce random variation.* Even if the groups have very similar values of $\bar{x}$, precision in the comparison of values of $\bar{y}$ can be increased by using the residual variation of y about regression on x rather than by analysing the ys alone.

2   *Type of investigation.*

(a) *Uncontrolled study.* In many situations the observations will be made on units which fall naturally into the groups in question—with no element of controlled allocation. Indeed, it will often be this lack of control which leads to the bias discussed in **1**(a).

(b) *Controlled study.* In a planned experiment, in which experimental units are allocated randomly to the different groups, the differences between values of $\bar{x}$ in the various groups will be no greater in the long run than would be expected by sampling theory. Of course, there will occasionally be large fortuitous differences in the $\bar{x}$s; it may then be just as important to correct for their effect as it would be in an uncontrolled study. In any case, even with very similar values of $\bar{x}$, the extra precision referred to in **1**(b) may well be worth acquiring.

Two groups

If the t test based on (9.19) reveals no significant difference in slopes, two parallel lines may be fitted with a common slope b given by (9.23). The equations of the two parallel lines are (as in (9.24)),

$$Y_{c1} = \bar{y}_1 + b(x - \bar{x}_1)$$

and

$$Y_{c2} = \bar{y}_2 + b(x - \bar{x}_2).$$

The difference between the values of Y at a given x is therefore

$$d = Y_{c1} - Y_{c2}$$
$$= \bar{y}_1 - \bar{y}_2 - b(\bar{x}_1 - \bar{x}_2); \tag{9.32}$$

(see Fig. 9.7).

The sampling error of d is due partly to that of $\bar{y}_1 - \bar{y}_2$ and partly to that of b (the term $\bar{x}_1 - \bar{x}_2$ has no sampling error as we are considering x to be

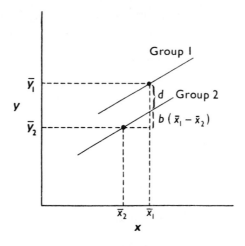

Fig. 9.7 Analysis of covariance for two groups, illustrating formula for vertical difference, d, between parallel lines.

a non-random variable). The three variables, $\bar{y}_1$, $\bar{y}_2$ and b, are independent; consequently

$$\operatorname{var}(d) = \operatorname{var}(\bar{y}_1) + \operatorname{var}(\bar{y}_2) + (\bar{x}_1 - \bar{x}_2)^2 \operatorname{var}(b)$$

$$= \sigma^2 \left[\frac{1}{n_1} + \frac{1}{n_2} + \frac{(\bar{x}_1 - \bar{x}_2)^2}{S_{xx1} + S_{xx2}} \right],$$

which is estimated as

$$s_c^2 \left[\frac{1}{n_1} + \frac{1}{n_2} + \frac{(\bar{x}_1 - \bar{x}_2)^2}{S_{xx1} + S_{xx2}} \right], \tag{9.33}$$

where s_c^2 is the residual mean square about the parallel lines:

$$s_c^2 = \frac{S_{yy1} + S_{yy2} - \dfrac{(S_{xy1} + S_{xy2})^2}{S_{xx1} + S_{xx2}}}{n_1 + n_2 - 3}. \tag{9.34}$$

Note that s_c^2 differs from the s^2 of (9.17). The latter is the residual mean square about separate lines, and is equivalent to the s^2 of Table 9.5. The residual mean square s_c^2 in (9.34) is taken about parallel lines (since parallelism is an initial assumption in the analysis of covariance), and would be obtained from Table 9.5 by pooling the second and third lines of the analysis. The resultant DF would be $(k - 1) + (n - 2k) = n - k - 1$, which gives the $n_1 + n_2 - 3 (= n - 3)$ of (9.34) when $k = 2$.

The standard error of d, the square root of (9.33), may be used in a t test. On the null hypothesis that the regression lines coincide, $E(d) = 0$, and

$$t = d/\text{SE}(d)$$

has $n_1 + n_2 - 3$ DF. Confidence limits for the true difference, $E(d)$, are obtained in the usual way.

Example 9.4

The data of Example 9.3 will now be used in an analysis of covariance. We shall first illustrate the calculations for two groups, the pooled exposed group A and the unexposed group B.

Using the sums of squares and products given earlier we have:

$$S_{xxA} + S_{xxB} = 10\,594 \cdot 54,$$
$$S_{xyA} + S_{xyB} = -426 \cdot 097$$
$$S_{yyA} + S_{yyB} = 47 \cdot 1879.$$

Also

$$n_A = 40, \qquad n_B = 44,$$
$$\bar{x}_A = 41 \cdot 38, \qquad \bar{x}_B = 39 \cdot 80,$$
$$\bar{y}_A = 4 \cdot 315, \qquad \bar{y}_B = 4 \cdot 462.$$

From (9.23),

$$b = -0 \cdot 0402;$$

from (9.32),

$$d = -0 \cdot 0835;$$

from (9.34),

$$s_c^2 = 0 \cdot 3710;$$

from (9.33),

$$\text{var}(d) = 0 \cdot 01779,$$
$$\text{SE}(d) = 0 \cdot 1334,$$

and

$$t = -0 \cdot 0835/0 \cdot 1334 = -0 \cdot 63 \quad \text{on 81 DF.}$$

The difference d is clearly not significant ($P = 0 \cdot 53$).

This analysis is based on the assumption that the regression lines are parallel for groups A and B, but, as noted in Example 9.3, there is at least suggestive evidence that the slopes differ. Suppose we abandon the assumption of parallelism and fit lines with separate slopes, b_A and b_B. The most pronounced difference between predicted values occurs at high ages. The difference at, say, age 60 is

$$d' = \bar{y}_A - \bar{y}_B + b_A(60 - \bar{x}_A) - b_B(60 - \bar{x}_B)$$
$$= -0 \cdot 5306,$$

and

$$\text{var}(d') = \text{var}(\bar{y}_A) + \text{var}(\bar{y}_B) + (60 - \bar{x}_A)^2 \, \text{var}(b_A) + (60 - \bar{x}_B)^2 \, \text{var}(b_B)$$

$$= (0.3584)\left[\frac{1}{40} + \frac{1}{44} + \frac{(18.62)^2}{4397.38} + \frac{(20.20)^2}{6197.16}\right]$$

$$= 0.06896.$$

Thus $t = d'/\text{SE}(d') = -2.02$ on 80 DF ($P = 0.05$).

This test suggests, therefore, that, in spite of the non-significant result in the main analysis of covariance test, there may nevertheless be a difference in mean vital capacity, at least at the higher ages. The statistical significance of this finding is, of course, a reflection of the difference between the slopes, which had a similar level of statistical significance.

More than two groups

Parallel lines may be fitted to several groups, as indicated in §9.4. The pooled slope, b, is given by (9.23) and the line for the ith group is given by (9.24).

The relative positions of the lines are conveniently expressed by the calculation of a *corrected* mean value of y for each group. Suppose the ith group had had a mean value of x equal to some arbitrary constant x_0 rather than $\bar{x}_i$. From (9.24) we should estimate that the mean y would have been

$$\bar{y}'_i = \bar{y}_i + b(x_0 - \bar{x}_i). \tag{9.35}$$

The difference between, say, $\bar{y}'_1$ and $\bar{y}'_2$ can easily be seen to be equal to d, given by (9.32). If all the regression lines coincide, all the $\bar{y}'_i$ will be equal. If the line for group i lies above all the others, at a fixed value of x, $\bar{y}'_i$ will be the highest of the corrected means (see Fig. 9.8).

On the null hypothesis that the true regression lines for the different groups coincide, the corrected means $\bar{y}'_i$ will differ purely by sampling error. The appropriate test is complicated by the fact that the sampling errors of the $\bar{y}'_i$ are not independent since the random variable b enters into each of the expressions (9.35). The procedure is indicated in Table 9.6.

Columns (1) and (3) contain the SSq for straightforward one-way analyses of variance of y and x, respectively. The usual DF are shown in column (4). Column (2) contains a corresponding analysis of the *covariance* of x and y, the feature which provides the name for the whole procedure. This is a technique not previously encountered, but is closely analogous to the corresponding analysis of variance of, say, x, the difference being that any *square* of a quantity involving variable x in the analysis of variance is replaced in the analysis of covariance by the product of the corresponding terms in x and y. Therefore, the sums of squares of y are calculated exactly as in the one-way analysis of variance (§7.1), and the sums of squares of x similarly. The sums of products of x and y are as follows. The notation should be clear.

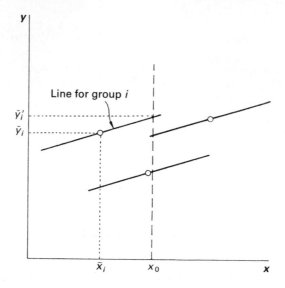

Fig. 9.8 Analysis of covariance with three groups, showing the corrected mean $\bar{y}'$ for the ith group.

Table 9.6 The analysis of covariance for k groups: regression of y on x

Uncorrected sums of squares and products				Corrected			
(1) y^2	(2) xy	(3) x^2	(4) DF	(5) SSq	(6) DF	(7) MSq	(8) VR
Between groups							
$(S_{yy})_B$	$(S_{xy})_B$	$(S_{xx})_B$	$k-1$	(By subtraction)	$k-1$	s_B^2	$F = s_B^2/s_C^2$
Within groups							
$(S_{yy})_W$	$(S_{xy})_W$	$(S_{xx})_W$	$n-k$	$(S_{yy})_W - (S_{xy})_W^2/(S_{xx})_W$	$n-k-1$	s_C^2	
Total							
$(S_{yy})_T$	$(S_{xy})_T$	$(S_{xx})_T$	$n-1$	$(S_{yy})_T - (S_{xy})_T^2/(S_{xx})_T$	$n-2$		

1 Between groups:

$$\frac{(\sum_{(1)}x)(\sum_{(1)}y)}{n_1} + \cdots + \frac{(\sum_{(k)}x)(\sum_{(k)}y)}{n_k} - \frac{(\sum x)_T(\sum y)_T}{n}$$

2 Within groups:

$$(\sum xy)_T - \left[\frac{(\sum_{(1)}x)(\sum_{(1)}y)}{n_1} + \cdots + \frac{(\sum_{(k)}x)(\sum_{(k)}y)}{n_k}\right]$$

3   Total:

$$\left(\sum xy\right)_T - \frac{\left(\sum x\right)_T \left(\sum y\right)_T}{n}$$

The entries in column (5), on the 'Within groups' and 'Total' lines are each obtained by the usual formulae for an SSq about regression, using the entries in columns (1) to (3). These are called *Corrected SSq*. The Corrected Total SSq is, in fact, simply the SSq of residuals about a single regression line fitted to the whole data, and has the usual $n - 2$ DF. The Corrected SSq within groups is the SSq of residuals about parallel regression lines; it is the sum of the SSq in the second and third lines of Table 9.5 and has $n - k - 1$ DF. The Corrected SSq between groups is obtained by subtracting the Corrected SSq within groups from the Corrected Total SSq. The DF can be similarly subtracted, giving $n - 2 - (n - k - 1)$ $= k - 1$. Mean squares follow as usual and lead to an F test.

Why is the Corrected SSq between groups obtained by subtraction and not formed in the same way as the other two corrected terms? We might have expected it to be given by

$$(S_{yy})_B - (S_{xy})_B^2/(S_{xx})_B, \tag{9.36}$$

and to have $k - 2$ DF. In fact (9.36) is a part, but not the whole, of the corrected SSq between groups. Let us write the result of the subtraction carried out in column (5) of Table 9.6. It is

$$[(S_{yy})_T - (S_{xy})_T^2/(S_{xx})_T] - [(S_{yy})_W - (S_{xy})_W^2/(S_{xx})_W]$$

$$= [(S_{yy})_T - (S_{yy})_W] + (S_{xy})_W^2/(S_{xx})_W - (S_{xy})_T^2/(S_{xx})_T$$

$$= [(S_{yy})_B - (S_{xy})_B^2/(S_{xx})_B] + [(S_{xy})_B^2/(S_{xx})_B + (S_{xy})_W^2/(S_{xx})_W - (S_{xy})_T^2/(S_{xx})_T], \tag{9.37}$$

using the fact that $(S_{yy})_T - (S_{yy})_W = (S_{yy})_B$. Now the term in the first set of square brackets in (9.37) is the same as (9.36); it represents deviations of group means about a regression line fitted to the between-groups variation—that is, fitted to the group means. The term in the second set of square brackets in (9.37) is of the same form as (9.30) and represents a difference between the slope of the parallel regression lines fitted *within* groups and that of the *between*-groups regression line fitted to the group means. This latter component has 1 DF because it is a contrast between two random variables, the within-groups slope, $b = (S_{xy})_W/(S_{xx})_W$, and the between-groups slope, $b_B = (S_{xy})_B/(S_{xx})_B$. To summarize this point, then,

Corrected SSq between groups $(k - 1\text{DF})$

= SSq of group means about between-groups regression $(k - 2\text{DF})$

+ SSq for contrast of b and b_B (1DF).   (9.38)

Now, each of the components on the right of (9.38) reflects a type of departure from the null hypothesis of coincident regression lines. This is illustrated in Fig. 9.9. In (a) b and b_B are approximately equal, and the major component of (9.38) is the variation of group means about the between-groups regression. In (b) the means fall on a line but the between-groups and within-groups slopes differ; the major component of (9.38) is now the second term. In (c) both types of variation are important.

The Corrected SSq between groups in Table 9.6 thus provides a general test of departures from the null hypothesis of coincident lines. It could if necessary be subdivided, as in (9.38).

The corrected means (9.35) provide a convenient summary of the relative positions of the parallel lines. The sampling variance of $\bar{y}_i'$ is estimated by

$$\text{var}(\bar{y}_i') = \text{var}(\bar{y}_i) + (x_0 - \bar{x}_i)^2 \text{var}(b)$$

$$= s_c^2 \left[\frac{1}{n_i} + \frac{(x_0 - \bar{x}_i)^2}{(S_{xx})_W} \right],$$ (9.39)

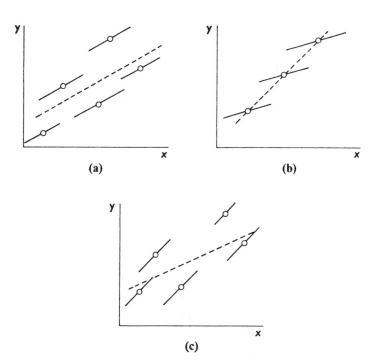

Fig. 9.9 Analysis of covariance: different forms of departure from the null hypothesis of coincident regression lines.

which varies from group to group not only through n_i but also because of the term $(x_0 - \bar{x}_i)^2$, which increases as $\bar{x}_i$ gets further from x_0 in either direction.

The arbitrary choice of x_0 can be avoided by concentrating on differences between the corrected means. For example, the ith and jth groups may be compared by

$$\bar{y}'_i - \bar{y}'_j = (\bar{y}_i - \bar{y}_j) - b(\bar{x}_i - \bar{x}_j), \tag{9.40}$$

as may be seen from (9.35). This does not involve x_0, as is clear from the fact that $\bar{y}'_i - \bar{y}'_j$ is the vertical distance between the parallel regression lines, and is therefore independent of x_0.

$$\text{var}(\bar{y}'_i - \bar{y}'_j) = s_c^2 \left[\frac{1}{n_i} + \frac{1}{n_j} + \frac{(\bar{x}_i - \bar{x}_j)^2}{(S_{xx})_W} \right], \tag{9.41}$$

and a significance test and confidence limits are immediately available, taking the square root of (9.41) as $\text{SE}(\bar{y}'_i - \bar{y}'_j)$, with the t distribution on $n - k - 1$ DF.

Example 9.4, continued

We now use the complete data as an example of an analysis of covariance with three groups. The analysis of covariance is as follows:

	Uncorrected				Corrected			
	y^2	xy	x^2	DF	SSq	DF	MSq	VR
Between groups	2·7473	− 57·390	1254·69	2	0·1616	2	0·0808	0·22 (P = 0·81)
Within groups	44·8936	− 373·574	9392·12	81	30·0347	80	0·3754	
Total	47·6409	− 430·964	10646·81	83	30·1963	82		

$$b = -373 \cdot 574 / 9392 \cdot 12 = -0 \cdot 0398;$$
$$\text{var}(b) = 0 \cdot 3754 / 9392 \cdot 12 = 0 \cdot 00003997;$$
$$\text{SE}(b) = 0 \cdot 00632.$$

Corrected values can be calculated, using (9·35), with $x_0 = 40 \cdot 5$, the overall mean. Thus

$$\bar{y}'_{A1} = 3 \cdot 949 - 0 \cdot 0398(40 \cdot 5 - 49 \cdot 75) = 4 \cdot 32;$$
$$\bar{y}'_{A2} = 4 \cdot 472 - 0 \cdot 0398(40 \cdot 5 - 37 \cdot 79) = 4 \cdot 36;$$
$$\bar{y}'_{B} = 4 \cdot 462 - 0 \cdot 0398(40 \cdot 5 - 39 \cdot 80) = 4 \cdot 43.$$

As in the two-group analysis, it might be more prudent to abandon the assumption of parallelism and compare the positions of the non-parallel lines at, say, age 60. This is left as an exercise for the reader. An alternative, but equivalent, approach to the analysis of these data is given in Example 10.3 (p. 340), using multiple regression.

In considering the possible use of the analysis of covariance with a particular set of data, special care should be given to the identification of the dependent and independent variables. If, in the analysis of covariance of y on x, there are significant differences between groups, it does not follow that the same will be true of the regression of x on y. In many cases this is an academic point because the investigator is clearly interested in differences between groups in the mean value of y, after correction for x, and not in the reverse problem. Occasionally, when x and y have a symmetric type of relation to each other, as in §9.2, both of the analyses of covariance (of y on x, and of x on y) will be misleading. Lines representing the general trend of a functional relationship may well be coincident (as in Fig. 9.10), and yet both sets of regression lines are non-coincident. Here the difficulties of §9.2 apply, and lines drawn by eye may provide the most satisfactory description of the data. For a fuller discussion see Ehrenberg (1968).

The analysis of covariance described in this section is appropriate for data forming a one-way classification into groups. Similar problems arise in the analysis of more complex data. For example, in the analysis of a variable y in a Latin square one may wish to adjust the apparent treatment effects to correct

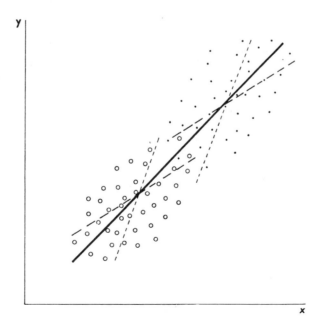

Fig. 9.10 Scatter diagram showing a common trend for two groups of observations but with non-coincident regression lines. (———) Regression of y on x; (– – –) regression of x on y.

for variation in another variable x. In particular, x may be some pretreatment characteristic known to be associated with y; the covariance adjustment would then be expected to increase the precision with which the treatments can be compared. The general procedure is an extension of that considered above and the details will not be given.

The methods presented in this and the previous section were developed before the use of computers became widespread, and were designed to simplify the calculations. Nowadays this is not a problem and the fitting of regressions in groups, using either separate non-parallel lines or parallel lines as in the analysis of covariance, may be accomplished using multiple regression, which is discussed in the next chapter.

10: Multiple Measurements

10.1 Multiple regression

In the earlier discussions of regression in Chapters 5 and 9 we have been concerned with the relationship between the mean value of one variable and the value of another variable, concentrating particularly on the situation in which this relationship can be represented by a straight line.

It is often useful to express the mean value of one variable in terms not of one other variable but of several others. Some examples will illustrate some slightly different purposes of this approach.

1 The primary purpose may be to study the effect on variable y of changes in a particular single variable x_1, but it may be recognized that y may be affected by several other variables x_2, x_3, etc. The effect on y of simultaneous changes in x_1, x_2, x_3, etc., must therefore be studied. In the analysis of data on respiratory function of workers in a particular industry, such as those considered in Examples 9.3 and 9.4, the effect of duration of exposure to a hazard may be of primary interest. However, respiratory function is affected by age, and age is related to duration of exposure. The simultaneous effect on respiratory function of age and exposure must therefore be studied so that the effect of exposure on workers of a fixed age may be estimated.

2 One may wish to derive insight into some causative mechanism by discovering which of a set of variables x_1, x_2, ..., has apparently most influence on a dependent variable y. For example, the stillbirth rate varies considerably in different towns in Britain. By relating the stillbirth rate simultaneously to a large number of variables describing the towns—economic, social, meteorological or demographic variables, for instance—it may be possible to find which factors exert particular influence on the stillbirth rate (see Sutherland, 1946). Another example is in the study of variations in the cost per patient in different hospitals. This presumably depends markedly on the 'patient mix'—the proportions of different types of patient admitted—as well as on other factors. A study of the simultaneous effects of many such variables may explain much of the variation in hospital costs and, by drawing attention to particular hospitals whose high or low costs are out of line with the prediction, may suggest new factors of importance.

3 To predict the value of the dependent variable in future individuals. After treatment of patients with advanced breast cancer by ablative procedures, prognosis is very uncertain. If future progress can be shown to depend on several variables available at the time of the operation, it may be possible to predict which patients have a poor prognosis and to consider alternative methods of treatment for them (Armitage *et al.*, 1969).

The appropriate technique is called *multiple regression*. In general, the approach is to express the mean value of the *dependent* variable in terms of the values of a set of other variables, usually called *independent* variables. The nomenclature is confusing, since some of the latter variables may be either closely related to each other logically (e.g. one might be age and another the square of the age) or highly correlated (e.g. height and arm length). It is preferable to use the terms *predictor* or *explanatory* variables, or *covariates*, and we shall usually follow this practice.

The data to be analysed consist of observations on a set of n individuals, each individual providing a value of the dependent variable, y, and a value of each of the predictor variables, $x_1, x_2, \ldots, x_p$. The number of predictor variables, p, should preferably be considerably less than the number of observations, n, and the same p predictor variables must be available for each individual in any one analysis.

Suppose that, for particular values of $x_1, x_2, \ldots, x_p$, an observed value of y is specified by the linear model:

$$y = \alpha + \beta_1 x_1 + \beta_2 x_2 + \ldots + \beta_p x_p + \varepsilon, \tag{10.1}$$

where ε is an error term. The various values of ε for different individuals are supposed to be independently normally distributed with zero mean and variance σ^2. The constants $\beta_1, \beta_2, \ldots, \beta_p$ are called *partial regression coefficients*; α is sometimes called the *intercept*. The coefficient β_1 is the amount by which y changes on the average when x_1 changes by one unit and all the other x_is remain constant. In general, β_1 will be different from the ordinary regression coefficient of y on x_1 because the latter represents the effect of changes in x_1 on the average values of y with no attempt to keep the other variables constant.

The coefficients $\alpha, \beta_1, \beta_2, \ldots, \beta_p$ are idealized quantities, measurable only from an infinite number of observations. In practice, from n observations, we have to obtain estimates of the coefficients and thus an estimated regression equation:

$$Y = a + b_1 x_1 + b_2 x_2 + \ldots + b_p x_p. \tag{10.2}$$

Statistical theory tells us that a satisfactory method of obtaining the estimated regression equation is to choose the coefficients such that the sum of squares of residuals, $\sum (y - Y)^2$, is minimized. Note that here y is an observed value and Y is the value predicted by (10.2) in terms of the predictor variables. A consequence of this approach is that the regression equation (10.2) is satisfied if all the variables are given their mean values. Thus

$$\bar{y} = a + b_1 \bar{x}_1 + b_2 \bar{x}_2 + \ldots + b_p \bar{x}_p,$$

and consequently a can be replaced in (10.2) by

$$\bar{y} - b_1 \bar{x}_1 - b_2 \bar{x}_2 - \ldots - b_p \bar{x}_p$$

to give the following form to the regression equation:

$$Y = \bar{y} + b_1(x_1 - \bar{x}_1) + b_2(x_2 - \bar{x}_2) + \ldots + b_p(x_p - \bar{x}_p). \qquad (10.3)$$

The equivalent result for simple regression was proved at (5.5).

We are now left with the problem of finding the partial regression coefficients, b_i. An extension of the notation introduced in Chapter 9 will be used; for instance

$$S_{x_j x_j} = \sum x_j^2 - (\sum x_j)^2 / n,$$

$$S_{x_j y} = \sum x_j y - (\sum x_j)(\sum y)/n,$$

and so on.

The method of least squares gives a set of simultaneous linear equations in the b_is as follows:

$$(S_{x_1 x_1})b_1 + (S_{x_1 x_2})b_2 + \ldots + (S_{x_1 x_p})b_p = S_{x_1 y}$$

$$(S_{x_2 x_1})b_1 + (S_{x_2 x_2})b_2 + \ldots + (S_{x_2 x_p})b_p = S_{x_2 y}$$

$$\vdots \qquad\qquad \vdots \qquad\qquad\qquad \vdots$$

$$(S_{x_p x_1})b_1 + (S_{x_p x_2})b_2 + \ldots + (S_{x_p x_p})b_p = S_{x_p y}. \qquad (10.4)$$

These are the so-called *normal equations*; they are the multivariate extension of the equation for b in §5.2. There are p equations for p unknowns, $b_1, b_2, \ldots b_p$, and in general there is a unique solution. The numerical coefficients of the left side of (10.4) form a *matrix* which is symmetric about the diagonal running from top left to bottom right; for example, $S_{x_1 x_2} = S_{x_2 x_1}$. These coefficients involve only the xs. Those on the right involve also the ys.

There are several methods of solving (10.4). Those familiar with matrix algebra will recognize this problem as being soluble in terms of the *inverse matrix* and, since, as we will see later, the inverse matrix is required for purposes of inference, this is the method of choice.

Equation (10.4) may be written in matrix form as

$$\mathbf{S}_{xx}\mathbf{b} = \mathbf{S}_{xy}, \qquad (10.5)$$

where $\mathbf{S}_{xx}$ is a symmetric $p \times p$ matrix with general term $S_{x_i x_j}$, $\mathbf{b}$ is the $p \times 1$ vector of coefficients b_i, and $\mathbf{S}_{xy}$ is the $p \times 1$ vector of terms $S_{x_i y}$. The solution of these equations is

$$\mathbf{b} = \mathbf{S}_{xx}^{-1}\mathbf{S}_{xy} \qquad (10.6)$$

where S_{xx}^{-1} is the inverse matrix of S_{xx}. If the general term of this inverse is c_{ij}, then (10.6) may be written

$$b_1 = c_{11}(S_{x_1y}) + c_{12}(S_{x_2y}) + \ldots + c_{1p}(S_{x_py})$$

$$b_2 = c_{21}(S_{x_1y}) + c_{22}(S_{x_2y}) + \ldots + c_{2p}(S_{x_py})$$

$$\vdots \qquad\qquad \vdots \qquad\qquad \vdots$$

$$b_p = c_{p1}(S_{x_1y}) + c_{p2}(S_{x_2y}) + \ldots + c_{pp}(S_{x_py}). \tag{10.7}$$

The complexity of the calculations increases rapidly with the value of p but, since standard computer programs are available for multiple regression analysis, the complexity of the calculations need not trouble the investigator. For $p = 2$ the calculations may be carried out on a calculator, and the general method is illustrated by considering in detail an example for which $p = 2$.

Example 10.1

The data shown in Table 10.1 are taken from a clinical trial to compare two hypotensive drugs used to lower the blood pressure during operations (Robertson and Armitage, 1959). The dependent variable, y, is the 'recovery time' (in minutes) elapsing between the time at which the drug was discontinued and the time at which the systolic blood pressure had returned to 100 mmHg. The data shown here relate to one of the two drugs used in the trial. The recovery time is very variable, and a question of interest is the extent to which it depends on the quantity of drug used and the level to which blood pressure was lowered during hypotension. The two predictor variables are:

x_1: log (quantity of drug used, mg);

x_2: mean level of systolic blood pressure during hypotension (mmHg).

The 53 patients are divided into three groups according to the type of operation. Initially we shall ignore this classification, the data being analysed as a single group. Possible differences between groups are considered in §10.2.

Table 10.1 shows the values of x_1, x_2 and y for the 53 patients. The columns headed Y and $y - Y$ will be referred to later. Below the data are shown the means and sums of squares and products about the means of the three variables. Equations (10.4) are:

$$\left. \begin{array}{l} 6{\cdot}01758b_1 + 64{\cdot}0958b_2 = 96{\cdot}4392 \\ 64{\cdot}0958b_1 + 3105{\cdot}89b_2 = -704{\cdot}566. \end{array} \right\} \tag{10.8}$$

The inverse matrix can be obtained by applying a standard computer program. Alternatively, for this 2×2 matrix it can be obtained as follows. First calculate the determinant, D, of the matrix,

$$D = (6{\cdot}01758)(3105{\cdot}89) - 64{\cdot}0958^2$$

$$= 18\,689{\cdot}94 - 4108{\cdot}27$$

$$= 14\,581{\cdot}67.$$

316 MULTIPLE MEASUREMENTS

Table 10.1 Data on the use of a hypotensive drug: x_1, log (quantity of drug used, mg); x_2, mean level of systolic blood pressure during hypotension (mmHg); y, recovery time (min)

x_1	x_2	y	Y	$y - Y$	x_1	x_2	y	Y	$y - Y$
Group A: 'Minor' non-thoracic ($n_A = 20$)					Group B (continued)				
2·26	66	7	29·3	− 22·3	2·70	73	39	34·7	4·3
1·81	52	10	28·6	− 18·6	1·90	56	28	27·9	0·1
1·78	72	18	13·6	4·4	2·78	83	12	29·4	− 17·4
1·54	67	4	11·5	− 7·5	2·27	67	60	28·8	31·2
2·06	69	10	22·4	− 12·4	1·74	84	10	4·1	5·9
1·74	71	13	13·4	− 0·4	2·62	68	60	36·3	23·7
2·56	88	21	20·6	0·4	1·80	64	22	19·8	2·2
2·29	68	12	28·5	− 16·5	1·81	60	21	22·9	− 1·9
1·80	59	9	23·4	− 14·4	1·58	62	14	16·1	− 2·1
2·32	73	65	25·7	39·3	2·41	76	4	25·7	− 21·7
2·04	68	20	22·6	− 2·6	1·65	60	27	19·1	7·9
1·88	58	31	26·0	5·0	2·24	60	26	33·1	− 7·1
1·18	61	23	7·3	15·7	1·70	59	28	21·0	7·0
2·08	68	22	25·6	− 1·6					
1·70	69	13	13·9	− 0·9	Group C: Thoracic ($n_C = 13$)				
1·74	55	9	24·8	− 15·8	2·45	84	15	20·9	− 5·9
1·90	67	50	20·0	30·0	1·72	66	8	16·5	− 8·5
1·79	67	12	17·4	− 5·4	2·37	68	46	30·4	15·6
2·11	68	11	24·3	− 13·3	2·23	65	24	29·3	− 5·3
1·72	59	8	21·5	− 13·5	1·92	69	12	19·1	− 7·1
					1·99	72	25	18·6	6·4
Group B: 'Major' non-thoracic ($n_B = 20$)					1·99	63	45	25·0	20·0
1·74	68	26	15·5	10·5	2·35	56	72	38·5	33·5
1·60	63	16	15·8	0·2	1·80	70	25	15·5	9·5
2·15	65	23	27·4	− 4·4	2·36	69	28	29·5	− 1·5
2·26	72	7	25·0	− 18·0	1·59	60	10	17·7	− 7·7
1·65	58	11	20·6	− 9·6	2·10	51	25	36·2	− 11·2
1·63	69	8	12·2	− 4·2	1·80	61	44	22·0	22·0
2·40	70	14	29·7	− 15·7					

Summary statistics for all subjects
$n = 53$
$\sum x_1 = 105·60$ $\sum x_2 = 3516$ $\sum y = 1203$
$\bar{x}_1 = 1·9925$ $\bar{x}_2 = 66·340$ $\bar{y} = 22·698$
$S_{x_1x_1} = 6·01758$ $S_{x_1x_2} = 64·0958$ $S_{x_1y} = 96·4392$
$S_{x_2x_2} = 3105·89$ $S_{x_2y} = -704·566$
$S_{yy} = 13791·2$

Then
$$c_{11} = 3105·89/D$$
$$= 3105·89/14\,581·67$$
$$= 0·213000.$$

$$c_{12} = -(64\cdot0958)/14\,581\cdot67$$
$$= -0\cdot00439564 \ (\text{also} = c_{21}).$$
$$c_{22} = 6\cdot01758/14\,581\cdot67$$
$$= 0\cdot000412681.$$

The inverse matrix is thus

$$\begin{pmatrix} c_{11} & c_{12} \\ c_{21} & c_{22} \end{pmatrix} = \begin{pmatrix} 0\cdot213000 & -0\cdot00439564 \\ -0\cdot00439564 & 0\cdot000412681 \end{pmatrix}.$$

Then, from (10.7),

$$b_1 = (0\cdot213000)(96\cdot4392) + (-0\cdot00439564)(-704\cdot566)$$
$$= 23\cdot6386,$$

and

$$b_2 = (-0\cdot00439564)(96\cdot4392) + (0\cdot000412681)(-704\cdot566)$$
$$= -0\cdot714673.$$

From (10.3), the regression equation is

$$Y = 22\cdot698 + 23\cdot6386(x_1 - 1\cdot9925) - 0\cdot714673(x_2 - 66\cdot340)$$
$$= 23\cdot009 + 23\cdot6386x_1 - 0\cdot714673x_2.$$

The recovery time increases on the average by about 24 min for each increase of 1 in the log dose (i.e. each 10-fold increase in dose), and decreases by 0·71 min for every increase of 1 mmHg in the mean blood pressure during hypotension.

Sampling variation

As in simple regression, the Total SSq of y may be divided into the SSq due to regression and the SSq about regression. For any one observation,

$$y - \bar{y} = (y - Y) + (Y - \bar{y}). \tag{10.9}$$

Squaring and summing,

$$\sum(y - \bar{y})^2 = \sum(y - Y)^2 + 2\sum(y - Y)(Y - \bar{y}) + \sum(Y - \bar{y})^2. \tag{10.10}$$

By substituting for Y using (10.3), and also using (10.4), it can be shown that the middle term on the right of (10.10) is zero so that

$$\sum(y - \bar{y})^2 = \sum(y - Y)^2 + \sum(Y - \bar{y})^2. \tag{10.11}$$

Also, using the same approach, the second term on the right of (10.11) is

$$\sum(Y - \bar{y})^2 = b_1(S_{x_1 y}) + b_2(S_{x_2 y}) + \ldots + b_p(S_{x_p y}). \tag{10.12}$$

The interpretation of (10.11) is the same as that of (9.3) for the case $p = 1$. Figure 9.1 illustrates equation (10.11), although in multiple regression the corresponding figure could not be drawn, since it would be in $(p + 1)$-dimensional space. Thus (10.11) may be written

$$\text{Total SSq} = \text{SSq about regression} + \text{SSq due to regression},$$

the SSq due to regression being most easily calculated from (10.12), and the Residual SSq about regression being obtained by subtraction. This subdivision provides the opportunity for an analysis of variance. The subdivision of DF is as follows:

$$\text{Total} = \text{About regression} + \text{Due to regression}$$
$$n - 1 = (n - p - 1) \qquad + p$$

The variance ratio

$$F = \frac{\text{MSq due to regression}}{\text{MSq about regression}} \tag{10.13}$$

provides a composite test of the null hypothesis that $\beta_1 = \beta_2 = \ldots = \beta_p = 0$, i.e. that all the predictor variables are irrelevant.

The ratio

$$\frac{\text{SSq due to regression}}{\text{Total SSq}} \tag{10.14}$$

is often denoted by R^2 (by analogy with the similar result (5.12) for r^2 in simple regression). The quantity R is called the *multiple correlation coefficient*. R^2 must be between 0 and 1, and so must its positive square root. In general no meaning can be attached to the direction of a multiple correlation with more than one predictor variable, and so R is always given a positive value. The appropriate test for the significance of the multiple correlation coefficient is the F test described above.

R^2 must increase as further variables are introduced into a regression and therefore cannot be used to compare regressions with different numbers of variables. The value of R^2 may be adjusted to take account of the chance contribution of each variable included by subtracting the value that would be expected if none of the variables was associated with y. The adjusted value, R_a^2, is calculated from

$$R_a^2 = R^2 - \frac{p}{n - p - 1}(1 - R^2)$$

$$= \frac{(n - 1)R^2 - p}{n - p - 1}. \tag{10.15}$$

R^2 is not a satisfactory measure of goodness of fit of the fitted regression. Where there are replicate values of y for certain values of the explanatory variables, then the goodness of fit may be assessed by subdividing the SSq about the regression into two components, one representing deviations of the mean of the replicates about the regression, and the other variability within replicates (§9.1 and see Healy, 1984). Without replication, goodness of fit cannot be strictly tested but methods of assessing the adequacy of the model are discussed later in this section.

We have so far discussed the significance of the joint relationship of y with the predictor variables. It is usually interesting to study the sampling variation of each b_j separately. This not only provides information about the precision of the partial regression coefficients, but also enables each of them to be tested for a significant departure from zero. If a particular b_j is not significantly different from zero, it may be thought sensible to call it zero (i.e. to drop it from the regression equation) to make the equation as simple as possible. It is important to realize, though, that if this is done the remaining b_js would be changed; in general new values would be obtained by doing a new analysis on the remaining x_js.

The variance and standard error of b_j are

$$\left.\begin{array}{l} \text{var}(b_j) = s^2 c_{jj}, \\ \text{SE}(b_j) = \sqrt{(s^2 c_{jj})}, \end{array}\right\} \tag{10.16}$$

where s^2 is the Residual MSq about regression. Tests and confidence limits are obtained in the usual way, with the t distribution on $n - p - 1$ DF. We note also, for future reference, that the *covariance* of b_j and b_h is

$$\text{cov}(b_j, b_h) = s^2 c_{jh}. \tag{10.17}$$

Example 10.1, continued

Application of (10.12) gives the value 2783·2. The analysis of variance of y is

	SSq	DF	MSq	VR
Due to regression	2 783·2	2	1392	6·32 $(P = 0.004)$
About regression	11 008·0	50	220·2	
Total	13 791·2	52		

The variance ratio is highly significant and there is thus little doubt that either x_1 or x_2 is, or both are, associated with y. The squared multiple correlation coefficient, R^2, is 2783·2/13 791·2 = 0·2018; $R = \sqrt{0.2018} = 0.45$. Of the total sum of squares of y, about 80% (0·80 = $1 - R^2$) is still present after prediction of y from x_1 and x_2. The predictive value of x_1 and x_2 is thus rather low, even though it is highly significant.

From the analysis of variance, $s^2 = 220.2$. From (10·16),

$$\text{SE}(b_1) = \sqrt{46.89} = 6.85$$

$$\text{SE}(b_2) = \sqrt{0.09086} = 0.301.$$

To test the significance of b_1 and b_2 we have the following values of t on 50 DF:

$$\text{For } b_1: t = 23\cdot64/6\cdot85 = 3\cdot45 \ (P = 0\cdot001)$$
$$\text{For } b_2: t = -0\cdot7147/0\cdot301 = -2\cdot37 \ (P = 0\cdot022).$$

Both partial regression coefficients are thus significant. Each predictor variable contributes separately to the effectiveness of the overall regression.

Analysis of variance test for deletion of variables

The t test for a particular regression coefficient, say b_j, tests whether the corresponding predictor variable, x_j, can be dropped from the regression equation without any significant effect on the variation of y.

Sometimes we may wish to test whether variability is significantly affected by the deletion of a group of predictor variables. For example, in a clinical study there may be three variables concerned with body size: height (x_1), weight (x_2) and chest measurement (x_3). If all other variables represent quite different characteristics, it may be useful to know whether all three of the size variables can be dispensed with. Suppose that q variables are to be deleted, out of a total of p. If two multiple regressions are done, (a) with all p variables, and (b) with the reduced set of $p - q$ variables, the following analysis of variance is obtained:

	DF	
(i) *Due to regression (a)*	p	
(ii) Due to regression (b)		$p - q$
(iii) Due to deletion of q variables		q
(iv) *Residual about regression (a)*	$n - p - 1$	
Total	$n - 1$	

The SSq for (i) and (iv) are obtained from regression (a), that for (ii) from regression (b) and that for (iii) by subtraction: (iii) = (i) − (ii). The variance ratio from (iii) and (iv) provides the required F test.

It is usually very simple to arrange for regressions to be done on several different subsets of predictor variables, using a multiple regression package on a computer. Several tests of the form described above may therefore be done on the same data; the 'TEST' option within the SAS program PROC REG gives the F test for the deletion of the variables.

When only one variable, say, the jth, is to be deleted, the same procedure could in principle be followed instead of the t test. The analysis of variance would be as above with $q = 1$. If this were done, it would be found that the SSq for deletion of x_j was equal to b_j^2/c_{jj}. The variance ratio for deletion of x_j would be

$$F = (b_j^2/c_{jj})/s^2$$
$$= b_j^2/s^2 c_{jj},$$

which is seen from (10.16) to be equal to t^2, thus giving the familiar equivalence between an F test on 1 and $n - p - 1$ DF and a t test on $n - p - 1$ DF.

It will sometimes happen that two or more predictor variables all give non-significant partial regression coefficients, and yet the deletion of the whole group has a significant effect by the F test. This often happens when the variables within the group are highly correlated; any one of them can be dispensed with, without appreciably affecting the prediction of y; the remaining variables in the group act as effective substitutes. If the whole group is omitted, though, there may be no other variables left to do the job. With a large number of interrelated predictor variables it often becomes quite difficult to sort out the meaning of the various partial regression coefficients (see p. 322).

Automatic selection procedures

The difficulty referred to above has led to the development of a number of procedures whereby the computer selects the 'best' subset of predictor variables, the criterion of optimality being somewhat arbitrary; for a fuller discussion see Draper and Smith (1981, Chapter 6). There are four main approaches.

1 *Step-up (forward-entry) procedure.* The computer first tries all the p simple regressions with just one predictor variable, choosing that which provides the highest Regression SSq. Retaining this variable as the first choice, it now tries all the $p - 1$ two-variable regressions obtained by the various possibilities for the second variable, choosing that which adds the largest increment to the Regression SSq. The process continues, all variables chosen at any stage being retained at subsequent stages. The process stops when the increments to the Regression SSq cease to be (in some sense) large in comparison with the Residual SSq.

2 *Step-down (backward-elimination) procedure.* The computer first does the regression on all predictor variables. It then eliminates the least significant and does a regression on the remaining $p - 1$ variables. The process stops when all the retained regression coefficients are (in some sense) significant.

3 *Stepwise procedure.* This is an elaboration of the step-up procedure (**1**), but allowing elimination, as in the step-down procedure (**2**). After each change in the set of variables included in the regression, the contribution of each variable is assessed and, if the least significant makes insufficient contribution, by some criterion, it is eliminated. It is thus possible for a variable included at some stage to be eliminated at a later stage because other variables, introduced since it was included, have made it unnecessary. The criterion for inclusion and elimination of variables could be, for example, that a variable will be included if its partial regression coefficient is significant at the 0·05 level and eliminated if its partial regression coefficient fails to be significant at the 0·1 level.

4 *Best-subset selection procedure.* Methods **1**, **2** and **3** do not necessarily reach the same final choice, even if they end with the same number of retained variables.

None will necessarily choose the best possible regression (i.e. that with the largest Regression SSq) for any given number of predictor variables. Computer algorithms are available for selecting the best subset of variables, where 'best' may be defined as the regression with the largest adjusted R^2 (10.15) or the related Mallows C_p statistic (see Draper and Smith, 1981, §6.2).

All these methods of model selection are available in the SAS program PROC REG under the SELECTION option; method **4** requires much more computer time than the others and may not be feasible for more than a few explanatory variables.

None of these methods provides infallible tactics in the difficult problem of selecting predictor variables. Sometimes certain variables should be retained even though they have non-significant effects, because of their logical importance in the particular problem. Sometimes logical relationships between some of the variables suggest that a particular one should be retained in preference to another. In some cases a set of variables has to be included or eliminated as a group, rather than individually; for example, a set of dummy variables representing a single characteristic (§10.2). In other cases some variables can only logically be included if one or more other variables are also included; for example, an interaction term should only be included in the presence of the corresponding main effects (§10.4). Nevertheless, automatic selection is often a useful exploratory device, even when the selected set of variables has to be modified on common-sense grounds.

Collinearity

We mentioned on p. 321 that difficulties may arise if some of the explanatory variables are highly correlated. This situation is known as *collinearity* or *multi-collinearity*. More generally, collinearity arises if there is an almost linear relationship between some of the explanatory variables in the regression. In this case large changes in one explanatory variable can be effectively compensated for by large changes in other variables, so that very different sets of regression coefficients provide very nearly the same residual sum of squares. This leads to the consequences that the regression coefficients will have large standard errors and, in extreme cases, the computations, even with the precision achieved by computers, may make nonsense of the analysis. The regression coefficients may be numerically quite implausible and perhaps largely useless.

Collinearity is a feature of the explanatory variables independent of the values of the dependent variable. Often collinearity can be recognized from the correlation matrix of the explanatory variables. If two variables are highly correlated, then this implies collinearity between those two variables. On the other hand, it is possible for collinearity to occur between a set of three or more variables without any of the correlations between these variables being particularly large, so it is useful to have a more formal check in the regression calculations. A measure of the collinearity between x_i and the other explanatory variables is provided by the proportion of the variability in x_i that is explained by the other variables, R_i^2, when x_i is the dependent variable in a regression on the other xs. The variance of b_i, in the regression of y on x_1 to x_p, is proportional to the reciprocal of $1 - R_i^2$ (see Wetherill *et al.*, 1986, §4.3), so values of R_i^2 close to 1 will lead to an increased variance for the estimate of b_i. The *variance inflation factor* (VIF) for variable i is defined as

$$\text{VIF} = \frac{1}{1 - R_i^2},$$

and the *tolerance* is the reciprocal of the variance inflation factor, that is,

$$\text{Tolerance} = 1 - R_i^2.$$

Values of the variance inflation factor or tolerance can be printed out as options 'VIF' or 'TOL' in the SAS program PROC REG. A high value of the variance inflation factor, or equivalently a low value of the tolerance, indicates a collinearity problem. Wetherill *et al.* (1986) suggest that, as a rule of thumb, a variance inflation factor higher than 10 is of concern.

The problems of collinearity may be overcome in several ways. In some situations the collinearity has arisen purely as a computational problem and may be solved by alternative definitions of some of the variables. For example, if both x and x^2 are included as explanatory variables and all the values of x are positive, then x and x^2 are likely to be highly correlated. This can be overcome by redefining the quadratic term as $(x - \bar{x})^2$, which will reduce the correlation whilst leading to an equivalent regression. This device is called *centring*. When the collinearity is purely computational, values of the variance inflation factor much greater than 10 can be accepted before there are any problems of computational accuracy, using a modern regression package, such as the SAS program.

In other situations the correlation is an intrinsic feature of the variables; for example, if both diastolic and systolic blood pressure are included, then a high correlation between these two measures may lead to a collinearity problem. The appropriate action is to use only one of the measures or possibly replace them by the mean of the pair. This leads to no real loss because the high correlation effectively means that only one measure is needed to use almost all the information.

In most situations the reasons for collinearity will be readily identified from the variance inflation factors and the nature of the variables, but where this is not the case more complex methods based on the principal components (§10.5) of the explanatory variables may be used (see Kleinbaum *et al.*, 1988).

Another approach, which we shall not pursue, is to use *ridge regression*, a technique that tends to give more stable estimates of regression coefficients, usually closer to zero, than the least-squares estimates. As Draper and Smith (1981, §6.7) point out, this is entirely reasonable from a Bayesian standpoint if one takes the view that numerically large coefficients are intrinsically implausible. In other circumstances the method might be inappropriate.

Adequacy of model

Sometimes, particularly in experimental work, data will be available in groups of replicates, each group corresponding to a particular combination of values of x_1, $x_2, \ldots, x_p$, but providing various values of y. The adequacy of the model can then be tested, as in §9.1, by comparing the variation of the group mean values of y about the predicted values Y, with the variation within groups (obtained from a one-way analysis of variance). The method is a straightforward generalization of that of §9.1. In general, with a total of n observations falling into k groups, the DF are partitioned as follows:

	DF	
(i) *Between groups*	$k - 1$	
(ii) Due to regression		p
(iii) Deviations from regression		$k - p - 1$
(iv) *Within groups*	$n - k$	
Total	$n - 1$	

The SSq for (iii) is obtained by subtraction, (i) − (ii), and the adequacy of the model is tested by the variance ratio from lines (iii) and (iv).

In general, the above approach will not be feasible since the observations will not fall into groups of replicates.

Residual plots

Much information may be gained by graphical study of the residuals, $y - Y$. These values, and the predicted values Y, are often printed in computer output. The values for the data in Example 10.1 are shown in Table 10.1. We now describe some potentially useful scatter diagrams involving the residuals, illustrating these by Fig. 10.1, which relates to Example 10.1.

1 *Plot of $y - Y$ against Y* (Fig. 10.1(a)). The residuals are always uncorrelated with the predicted value, as (10.11) shows. Nevertheless, the scatter diagram may provide some useful pointers. The distribution of the residuals may be markedly non-normal; in Fig. 10.1(a) there is some suggestion of positive skewness. This positive skewness and other departures from normality can also be detected by constructing a histogram of the residuals or a normal plot (§11.5; Example 11.2 is for the data of Example 10.1). The variability of the residuals may not be constant; in Fig. 10.1(a) it seems to increase as Y increases. Both these deficiencies may

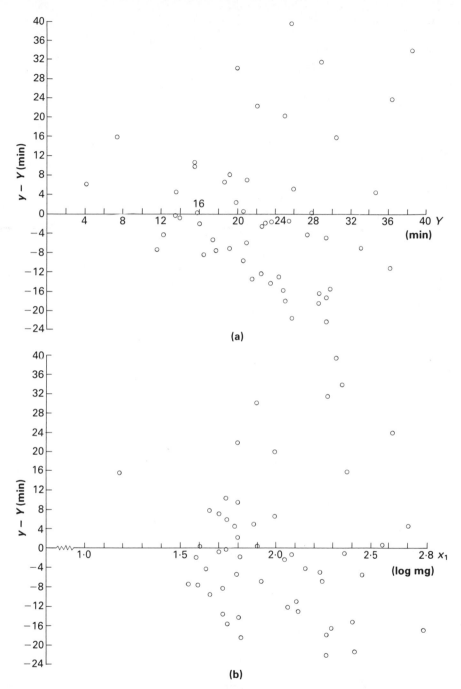

Fig. 10.1 Residuals of recovery time from multiple regression data of Table 10.1 plotted against (a) predicted value; (b) x_1, log quantity of drug; (c) x_2, mean systolic level during hypotension; (d) the product x_1x_2; (e) age.

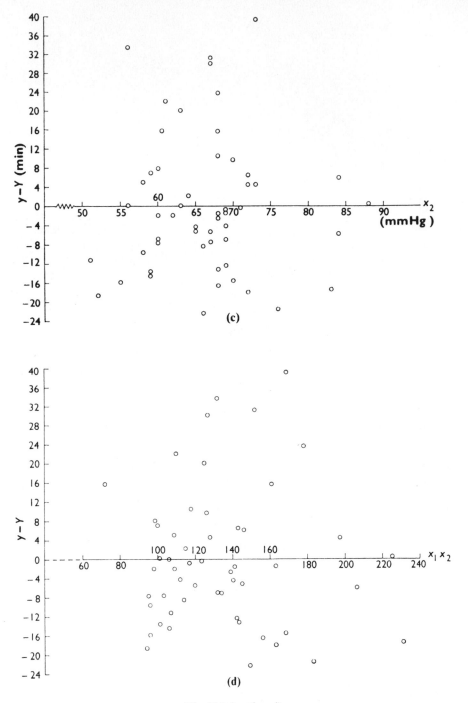

Fig. 10.1 (continued)

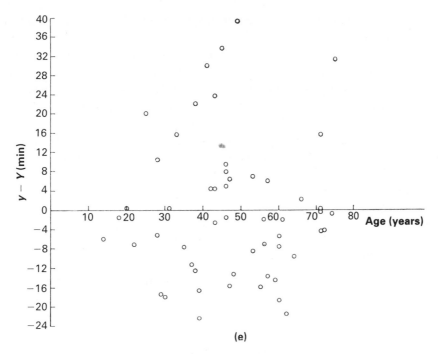

Fig. 10.1 (continued)

sometimes be remedied by transformation of the *y* variable and reanalysis (see Chapter 11). There is some indication in this example that it would be appropriate to repeat the analysis after a logarithmic transformation (§11.3) of *y*. In some cases the trend in variability may call for a weighted analysis (see below). Even though the correlation is zero there may be a marked non-linear trend; if so, it is likely to appear also in the plots of type **2** below.

2 *Plot of y − Y against x_j* (Fig. 10.1(b), (c)). The residuals may be plotted against the values of any or all of the predictor variables. Again, the correlation will always be zero. There may, however, be a non-linear trend, for example with the residuals tending to rise to a maximum somewhere near the mean, $\bar{x}_j$, and falling away on either side, as is perhaps suggested in Fig. 10.1(c); or showing a trend with a minimum value near $\bar{x}_j$. Such trends suggest that the effect of x_j is not adequately expressed by the linear term in the model. The simplest suggestion would be to add a term involving the square of x_j as an extra predictor variable. This so-called *quadratic* regression is described in §10.3.

3 *Plot of y − Y against product $x_j x_h$* (Fig. 10.1(d)). The model (10.1) postulates no interaction between the *x*s, in the sense of §8.3. That is, the effect of changing one predictor variable is independent of the values taken by any other. This would not be so if a term $x_j x_h$ were introduced into the model. If such a term is needed, but has been omitted, the residuals will tend to be correlated with the product $x_j x_h$. Figure 10.1(d) provides no suggestion that interaction is important in our example.

4   *Plot of y − Y against a new variable x'* (Fig. 10.1(e)). If x' is a variable not used in the regression, the presence of correlation in this plot will give a good visual indication that it should be included. In Fig. 10.1(e) we have introduced a variable not previously used in the calculations; i.e. the age of the patient. The diagram gives no suggestion of a correlation. A more sensitive examination is to plot $y − Y$ against the residuals of the regression of x' on the same explanatory variables used in the regression of y; this plot shows the partial association of y and x' for given values of the explanatory variables.

Atkinson (1985) describes methods of checking the adequacy of regression models, particularly by graphical diagnostics.

Statistical checking of residuals

Whilst residual plots can be very informative in identifying possible outliers, more formal methods are also useful. Some *regression diagnostic methods* are directed towards the identification of individual points that are either discrepant from the regression through the remaining points, or have a disproportionate influence on the fitted regression equation, or both. The concepts are illustrated in Fig. 10.2 in terms of a univariate regression, although it is in multivariate regression, where graphical representations are not easy to construct, that these diagnostic methods are most useful. In Fig. 10.2(a) a regression through nine points is shown. Figure 10.2(b) shows an additional point which is distant from the other nine points but nevertheless is near to the regression through these nine points; this point does not influence the slope of the fitted regression. In Fig. 10.2(c), there is an additional point that is distant from the other nine points and lies below the regression line through these nine points; it is not clearly an outlier but inclusion of this point reduces the slope of the fitted line to two-thirds of its value; the additional point is influential in determining the regression. In Fig. 10.2(d) the additional point is again influential in changing the regression but also appears to be an outlier with respect to the regression through the other nine points. Finally, in Fig. 10.2(e) the extra point is within the range of the x values of the other nine points; it is clearly an outlier but does not have a marked effect on the slope of the fitted line. We consider first the identification of outlying points.

For each point the residual is given by $e_i = y_i − Y_i$. The *standardized residual* is defined as $z_i = e_i/s$. At first sight it might seem that e_i is an estimate of ε_i in (10.1). However, this is not strictly the case since the residuals are not independent —this follows because the observed points have been used to fit the regression and the sum of the residuals is zero. Although, if n is much larger than p, the standardized residuals have an average standard deviation of approximately

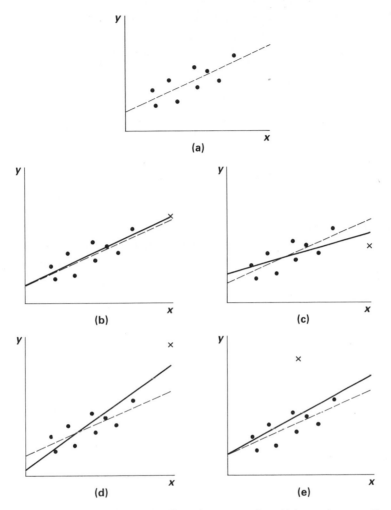

Fig. 10.2 Five regressions illustrating the effect of an extra point which may be an outlier, an influential point, or both. In (a), the regression through nine points is shown. In each of (b)–(e) a tenth point has been added, indicated by ×, and the regression through the set of 10 points (continuous line) is shown together with the regression through the original nine points (broken line).

unity, the standard deviation will vary from point to point. A point that is distant from the other points in terms of the x values is especially important in fixing the regression line, since relatively large changes in the position of the fitted line can be achieved at this point with lesser changes at all the other points; this is illustrated in Fig. 10.2(b), (c) and (d). Such a point is said to have a high *leverage*, where the leverage is a measure of the standardized distance between the point in the multivariate x space and the mean in this space over all the points. The leverage, h_i, lies within the range $1/n$ to 1, and has a mean value of $(p + 1)/n$. The standard error of each residual depends on the leverage, and is estimated as $s\sqrt{(1 - h_i)}$.

This leads to the definition of the *studentized residual*,

$$r_i = \frac{e_i}{s\sqrt{(1 - h_i)}}. \tag{10.18}$$

The studentized residuals are approximately distributed as the t distribution on $n - p - 1$ DF.

A further improvement is possible by noting that if a point, say, the ith point, is an outlier it will have a large residual, which will inflate the estimate of the standard deviation, s. This means that both z_i and r_i will be decreased, so that the fact that the point is an outlier is, paradoxically, making it more difficult to detect that it has a high residual. The way round this is to use an estimate of the standard deviation that is independent of the ith point. Such an estimate can be obtained by fitting the regression to the data excluding the ith point. Denoting this estimate of the standard deviation by $s_{(-i)}$ and defining the residual as

$$t_i = \frac{e_i}{s_{(-i)}\sqrt{(1 - h_i)}} \tag{10.19}$$

gives the *jackknife residual*. From (10.18)

$$t_i = r_i \left(\frac{s}{s_{(-i)}} \right) \tag{10.20}$$

and it can be shown mathematically that

$$t_i = r_i \sqrt{\left(\frac{n - p - 2}{n - p - 1 - r_i^2} \right)} \tag{10.21}$$

so that the jackknife residuals are easily computed for every point without having to fit the n separate regressions, each excluding one point. The jackknife residuals are distributed as the t distribution on $n - p - 2$ DF.

The definition of t_i might seem to be no more than an adjustment using a more appropriate estimate of standard deviation, but it is in fact much more than this. Suppose the residual were redefined as the difference between the observed y_i and the value, $Y_{(-i)}$, that would be predicted for the ith point, using the regression based on all the points except that point. The standard error of this predicted value could be calculated, using the multivariate extension of (5.24). Then define as a standardized residual

$$t_i = \frac{y_i - Y_{(-i)}}{SE(Y_{(-i)})}. \tag{10.22}$$

The residual defined in this way, as an externally studentized residual, is mathematically equivalent to the jackknife residual as defined in (10.21). Therefore each jackknife residual is a standardized residual about the regression, fitted using all the data except the point under consideration. This rather remarkable mathematical property hinges on the leverage. Mathematically inclined readers are referred to the books by Cook and Weisberg (1982) and Belsley *et al.* (1980) for a full mathematical treatment.

These residuals are given in Table 10.2 for the data shown in Fig. 10.2. The column headed D_{10} will be referred to later. Since all the residuals are standardized and independent of the scale on which y and x are measured, these scales have been chosen so that the slope of the line and the standard deviation in Fig. 10.2(a) are both unity. For Fig. 10.2(b) to (e) the residual diagnostic statistics are given for the extra tenth point. When judged against the t distribution with 8 and 7 DF respectively, the studentized and jackknife residuals are clearly not remarkable for either Fig. 10.2(b) or (c). The greater sensitivity of the jackknife residual is shown for Fig. 10.2(d) and (e); the lower values of the studentized residual, r_{10}, in these two cases is a consequence of the increase in standard deviation due to the outlier under test. For Fig. 10.2(d) and (e), the extra point is suggested as a possible outlier by the values of the jackknife residual. We now consider the formulation of a significance test of the residuals.

For Fig. 10.2(d), $t_{10} = 2\cdot84$ and if this is assessed as a t statistic with 7 DF then $P = 0\cdot025$. However, this takes no account of the fact that this residual has been chosen as the largest, in absolute magnitude, and the effect of this is quite considerable and increases with increasing n. The required significance level is then the probability that the largest residual in a set of n residuals will be as large as or larger than the observed value. This probability is the probability that not all 10 residuals are in the central part of the distribution and is given by $P = 1 - (1 - 0\cdot025)^{10} = 0\cdot22$. This is the *Bonferroni correction*. An equivalent means of assessment is to work with a lower critical significance probability, and the largest residual would be significant at the 0·05 level only if the t statistic gave $P < 0\cdot05/n$. For Fig. 10.2(d) we would require $P < 0\cdot005$, so that the largest residual, with a nominal P of 0·025, is not significant. In Fig. 10.2(e) the largest residual has a nominal P of just less than 0·001 and, since this is less than 0·005,

Table 10.2 Residual diagnostic statistics for Fig. 10.2

Fig. 10·2	Fitted slope	s	r_{10}	t_{10}	Leverage h_{10}	Cook's D_{10}
(a)	1·00	1·00				
(b)	1·03	0·94	0·14	0·13	0·54	0·01
(c)	0·64	1·11	− 1·51	− 1·68	0·54	1·37
(d)	1·61	1·37	2·07	2·84	0·54	2·55
(e)	1·21	2·15	2·55	5·49	0·11	0·41

there is significant evidence ($P < 0.05$) that the tenth point is an outlier. Kleinbaum *et al.* (1988) give a table (Table A8) to facilitate the assessment of significance and from this table the significance level is slightly less than 0·01 (critical value 5·41).

Another way of assessing the residuals is to check that they are distributed approximately as the normal distribution. This is discussed in §11.5, and Example 11.3 is an assessment of the normality of the studentized residuals from Example 10.1, using the Kolmogorov–Smirnov and Shapiro–Wilk tests. These tests show that there is significant evidence of non-normality.

The analysis of the residuals has revealed that one of the assumptions of regression analysis does not hold for the data of Example 10.1; that is, there is evidence that the recovery time is not normally distributed with constant variance about the regression line. The distribution of residuals is positively skewed and it was suggested earlier, when discussing Fig. 10.1(a), that it would be appropriate to reanalyse the data after a logarithmic transformation of the *y* variable. This will not be pursued in detail, but this transformation is effective in that there is no evidence of non-normality for the residuals after a regression analysis of log(*y*). The other conclusions from the analysis remain unaltered, so that, in this case, the slight lack of normality did not lead to any unjustified conclusions.

Checking for influential points

A point may be regarded as *influential* if it exerts more than its fair share in determining the values of the regression coefficients. Conceptually the influence of the *i*th point may be envisaged in terms of the changes in the estimates of the regression coefficients when the *i*th point is excluded from the analysis, that is, in terms of the change in the position and slope of the regression in multivariate space. A standardized measure was proposed by Cook (1977) and is known as *Cook's distance*. This measure, D_i, consists of the squares of the changes in each regression coefficient, standardized by the variances and covariances of these regression coefficients. Cook's distance is always positive but has no upper limit. Cook and Weisberg (1982) suggested that values of D_i greater than 1 should be examined. This corresponds to a point whose removal changes the regression coefficients to outside the 50% confidence region of the estimates, using the full data set. The values of the leverage, h_i, are important in determining D_i. It can be shown mathematically that

$$D_i = \frac{r_i^2 h_i}{(p + 1)(1 - h_i)}. \tag{10.23}$$

From Table 10.2 the extra point in both Fig. 10.2(c) and (d) has a Cook's distance greater than 1 and this confirms the impression from the plots that these points are influential in determining the regression coefficients.

The mean value of the leverage is $(p + 1)/n$ and it is sometimes suggested that points with high leverage, say greater than $2(p + 1)/n$, should be scrutinized. Such points are especially distant from the mean position of the points in terms of the x variables. Whilst it is good practice to check data carefully, a point with a high leverage but for which there is no evidence that it is either an outlier or an influential point is not a cause for alarm. Such points are beneficial in reducing the standard errors of the regression coefficients and, if it were possible to supplement a set of data by collecting more data, then a good choice of x values would be those with high leverages.

Example 10.2

Residuals, leverages and Cook's distances are given below for some of the points in Example 10.1. The points with studentized residuals greater than 2 in absolute magnitude have all been included, as well as the points with leverages greater than 0·11 and the two points with the highest Cook's distances.

Patient	x_1	x_2	y	r	t	h	D
A_1	2·26	66	7	−1·53	−1·55	0·035	0·028
A_7	2·56	88	21	0·03	0·03	0·173	0·000
A_{10}	2·32	73	65	2·71	2·90	0·041	0·104
A_{13}	1·18	61	23	1·14	1·14	0·133	0·066
A_{17}	1·90	67	50	2·04	2·11	0·021	0·030
B_{10}	2·78	83	12	−1·27	−1·28	0·150	0·095
B_{11}	2·27	67	60	2·14	2·22	0·034	0·053
B_{12}	1·74	84	10	0·44	0·44	0·200	0·016
C_1	2·45	84	15	−0·42	−0·42	0·121	0·008
C_8	2·35	56	72	2·41	2·53	0·123	0·270
C_{12}	2·10	51	25	−0·81	−0·81	0·133	0·033
C_{13}	1·80	61	44	1·51	1·53	0·029	0·023

The largest studentized residual is 2·71, for the tenth patient in group A. The jackknife residual is 2·90. Is this point an outlier? The jackknife residual is assessed as a t value on 49 DF. This gives $P = 0.0056$ and an adjusted P value of $1 - 0.9944^{53} = 0.26$. Alternatively, referring to Table A8 in Kleinbaum et al. (1988), the critical value for a significance level of 0·1 is 3·28. Since the jackknife residual is less than this, we have $P > 0.1$. The largest residual is not at all exceptional after adjusting for the fact that it is the largest of the 53 residuals.

Examination of Cook's distances for the 53 points shows that there are no points with undue influence on the regression. The largest value of D_i is 0·27 for the eighth subject in group C. This point is the one to the top and left in Fig. 10.1(c).

The mean leverage is $3/53 = 0.057$. There are seven points with a leverage greater than twice this value but only one of these has an exceptional residual. This is the point with the highest Cook's distance identified above, but even for this point the residual is not particularly high, given that there are 53 points. Thus there is no particular concern about points of undue influence or distance from the main set of points.

All the calculations and plots discussed above for the detection of outliers and influential points are conveniently carried out on a computer. For example, values of the residuals, leverage and Cook's distance are all available in the SAS program PROC REG and may be plotted or analysed.

A discussion of the circumstances in which it may be legitimate to exclude outliers is given in §11.6. The same considerations apply to influential points. Certainly data should not be excluded simply because they appear discrepant from the remainder of the data in some way, but such data should be checked especially carefully in case there has been an error at some stage between the data collection and the transfer of data to the computer. When this is not the case it is important to recognize such discrepant data and assess how they influence the interpretations that might be made.

Weighted analysis

Sometimes the various values of y are known to have different residual variances. Suppose the variance of y_i is known, or can be assumed to be σ^2/w_i, where the σ^2 is in general unknown, but the weights w_i are known. In other words, we know the *relative* precisions of the different observations. The correct procedure is to follow the general multiple regression method, replacing all sums like $\sum x_j$ and $\sum y$ by $\sum wx_j$ and $\sum wy$ (the subscript i, identifying the individual observation, has been dropped here to avoid confusion with j, which identifies a particular explanatory variable). Similarly, all sums of squares and products are weighted: $\sum y^2$ is replaced by $\sum wy^2$, $\sum x_j x_k$ by $\sum wx_j x_k$, and in calculating sums of squares and products n is replaced by $\sum w$ (see (7.15)).

The standard t tests, F tests and confidence intervals are then valid. The Residual MSq is an estimate of σ^2, and may, in certain situations, be checked against an independent estimate of σ^2. For example, in the situation discussed on p. 324, where the observations fall into groups with particular combinations of values of predictor variables, y_i may be taken to be the mean of n_i observations at a specified combination of xs. The variance of y_i is then σ^2/n_i, and the analysis may be carried out by weighted regression, with $w_i = n_i$. The Residual MSq will be the same as that derived from line (iii) of the analysis on p. 324, and may be compared (as indicated in the previous discussion) against the Within-Groups MSq in line (iv).

10.2 Multiple regression in groups

When the observations fall into k groups formed by a one-way classification, questions of the types discussed in §§9.4 and 9.5 may arise. Can equations with the same bs (although perhaps different as) be fitted to the different groups, or must each group have its own set of bs? (This is a generalization of the comparison of slopes in §9.4.) If the same bs are appropriate for all groups, can the same a be used (thus leading to one equation for the whole data), or must each group have its own a? (This is a generalization of the analysis of covariance, §9.5.)

The methods of approach are rather straightforward developments of those used previously and will be indicated only briefly. Suppose there are, in all, n observations falling into k groups, with p predictor variables observed throughout. To test whether the same bs are appropriate for all groups, an analysis of variance analogous to Table 9.5 may be derived, with the following subdivision of DF:

	DF
(i) Due to regression with common bs	p
(ii) Differences between bs	$p(k-1)$
(iii) Residual about separate regressions	$n-(p+1)k$
Within groups	$n-k$

The DF agree with those of Table 9.5 when $p = 1$. The SSq within groups is exactly the same as in Table 9.5. The SSq for (iii) is obtained by fitting a separate regression equation to each of the k groups and adding the resulting Residual SSq. The residual for the ith group has $n_i - (p+1)$DF, and these add to $n - (p+1)k$. The SSq for (i) is obtained by a simple multiple regression calculation using the pooled sums of squares and products *within groups* throughout; this is the appropriate generalization of the first line of Table 9.5. The SSq for (ii) is obtained by subtraction. The DF, obtained also by subtraction, are plausible as this SSq represents differences between k values of b_1, between k values of b_2, and so on; there are p predictor variables, each corresponding to $k - 1$ DF.

It may be more useful to have a rather more specific comparison of some regression coefficients than is provided by the composite test described above. For a particular coefficient, b_j, for instance, the k separate multiple regressions will provide k values, each with its standard error. Straightforward comparisons of these, e.g. using (9.14) with weights equal to the reciprocals of the variances of the separate values, will often suffice.

The analysis of covariance assumes common values for the bs and tests for differences between the as. The corrected SSq and their DF are obtained by the following generalization of Table 9.6:

	Corrected SSq	DF
(iv) Between groups	By subtraction	$k-1$
(v) Within groups	Residual about within-groups regression	$n-k-p$
(vi) Total	Residual about total regression	$n-p-1$

The corrected Total SSq (vi) is obtained from a single multiple regression calculation for the whole data; the DF are $n - p - 1$ as usual. That for (v) is obtained as the residual for the regression calculation using *within-groups* sums of squares and products; it is in fact the residual corresponding to the regression term (i) in the previous table, and is the sum of the SSq for (ii) and (iii) in that table. That for (iv) is obtained by subtraction. Corrected means analogous to (9.35) are obtained as

$$\bar{y}_i' = \bar{y}_i + b_1(x_{01} - \bar{x}_{i1}) + b_2(x_{02} - \bar{x}_{i2}) + \ldots + b_p(x_{0p} - \bar{x}_{ip}), \quad (10.24)$$

where $b_1, b_2, \ldots, b_p$ are the coefficients in the within-groups regression and $\bar{x}_{ij}$ is the mean of x_j in the ith group. The corrected difference between two groups—say, groups 1 and 2—is

$$\bar{y}_1' - \bar{y}_2' = (\bar{y}_1 - \bar{y}_2) - \sum_j b_j(\bar{x}_{1j} - \bar{x}_{2j}), \quad (10.25)$$

and its estimated variance is

$$\text{var}(\bar{y}_1' - \bar{y}_2') = s_c^2 \left[\frac{1}{n_1} + \frac{1}{n_2} + \sum_j c_{jj}(\bar{x}_{1j} - \bar{x}_{2j})^2 + 2 \sum_{j \neq h} c_{jh}(\bar{x}_{1j} - \bar{x}_{2j})(\bar{x}_{1h} - \bar{x}_{2h}) \right].$$
$$(10.26)$$

The second summation is taken over all pairs of predictor variables. The general form of (10.26) follows from (3.13) and (3.14), the variances and covariances of the bs being given by (10.16) and (10.17). The cs are the elements of the inverse matrix obtained in the within-groups regression, and s_c^2 the Residual MSq from line (v) on p. 335.

Multiple regression techniques offer an alternative approach to the analysis of covariance, enabling the whole analysis to be done by one application of multiple regression. Consider first the case of two groups. Let us introduce a new variable z, which is given the value 1 for all observations in group 1 and 0 for all observations in group 2. As a model for the data as a whole, suppose that

$$E(y) = \alpha + \delta z + \beta_1 x_1 + \beta_2 x_2 + \ldots + \beta_p x_p. \quad (10.27)$$

Because of the definition of z, (10.27) is equivalent to assuming that

$$E(y) = \begin{cases} \alpha + \delta + \beta_1 x_1 + \beta_2 x_2 + \ldots + \beta_p x_p & \text{for group 1} \\ \alpha + \beta_1 x_1 + \beta_2 x_2 + \ldots + \beta_p x_p & \text{for group 2,} \end{cases} \quad (10.28)$$

which is precisely the model required for the analysis of covariance. According to (10.28) the regression coefficients on the xs are the same for both groups, but there is a difference δ between the intercepts. The usual significance test in the analysis of covariance tests the hypothesis that $\delta = 0$. Since (10.27) and (10.28) are equivalent, it follows from (10.27) that the whole analysis can be performed by a single multiple regression of y on $z, x_1, x_2, \ldots, x_p$. The new variable, z is called a *dummy*, or *indicator*, *variable*. The coefficient δ is the partial regression coefficient of y on z, and is estimated in the usual way by the multiple regression analysis, giving an estimate d, say. The variance of d is estimated as usual from (10.16), and the appropriate tests and confidence limits follow by use of the t distribution. Note that the Residual MSq has $n - p - 2$ DF (since the introduction of z increases the number of predictor variables from p to $p + 1$), and that this agrees with (v) on p. 335 (putting $k = 2$).

When $k > 2$, the procedure described above is generalized by the introduction of $k - 1$ dummy variables. These can be defined in many equivalent ways. One convenient method is as follows. The table shows the values taken by each of the dummy variables for all observations in each group.

	Dummy variables			
Group	z_1	z_2	$\cdots$	z_{k-1}
1	1	0	$\cdots$	0
2	0	1	$\cdots$	0
$\vdots$	$\vdots$	$\vdots$		$\vdots$
$k - 1$	0	0		1
k	0	0		0

The model specifies that

$$E(y) = \alpha + \delta_1 z_1 + \ldots + \delta_{k-1} z_{k-1} + \beta_1 x_1 + \ldots + \beta_p x_p \qquad (10.29)$$

and the fitted multiple regression equation is

$$Y = a + d_1 z_1 + \ldots + d_{k-1} z_{k-1} + b_1 x_1 + \ldots + b_p x_p. \qquad (10.30)$$

The regression coefficients $d_1, d_2, \ldots, d_{k-1}$ represent contrasts between the mean values of y for groups $1, 2, \ldots, k - 1$ and that for group k, after correction for differences in the xs. The overall significance test for the null hypothesis that $\delta_1 = \delta_2 = \ldots = \delta_{k-1} = 0$ was previously done by the F test on $k - 1$ and $n - k - p$ DF ((iv) and (v) on p. 335). The equivalent procedure here is to test the composite significance of $d_1, d_2, \ldots, d_k$ by deleting the dummy variables from the analysis (p. 320). This leads to exactly the same F test.

If the investigator is interested in a contrast between group k and one of the other groups, the appropriate d_i, with its standard error given by the regression analysis, is immediately available; d_i is in fact the same as the difference between corrected means $\bar{y}'_i - \bar{y}'_k$. For a contrast between two groups other than group k, say groups 1 and 2, we use the fact that

$$\bar{y}'_1 - \bar{y}'_2 = d_1 - d_2,$$

and

$$\text{var}(d_1 - d_2) = \text{var}(d_1) + \text{var}(d_2) - 2\text{cov}(d_1, d_2),$$

the variances and covariances being given as usual by (10.16) and (10.17).

Example 10.1, continued

The data of Table 10.1 have so far been analysed as a single group. However, Table 10.1 shows a grouping of the patients according to the type of operation, and we should clearly enquire whether a single multiple regression equation is appropriate for all three groups. Indeed, this question should be raised at an early stage of the analysis, before too much effort is expended on examining the overall regression.

An exploratory analysis can be carried out by examining the residuals, $y - Y$, in Table 10.1. The mean values of the residuals in the three groups are:

$$\text{A: } -2 \cdot 52 \qquad \text{B: } -0 \cdot 46 \qquad \text{C: } 4 \cdot 60.$$

These values suggest the possibility that the mean recovery time, at given values of x_1 and x_2, increases from group A, through group B, to group C. However, the residuals are very variable, and it is not immediately clear whether these differences are significant. A further question is whether the regression coefficients are constant from group to group. If the points in Fig. 10.1(b) and (c) are distinguished by membership of groups A, B or C, there are slight suggestions that the slopes of the relationships vary between groups, but again the situation is far from clear-cut.

As a first step in a more formal analysis, we calculate separate multiple regressions in the three groups. The results are summarized as follows:

	Group A	Group B	Group C
n	20	20	13
$b_1 \pm \text{SE}(b_1)$	$7 \cdot 83 \pm 13 \cdot 78$	$22 \cdot 76 \pm 9 \cdot 19$	$36 \cdot 16 \pm 15 \cdot 86$
$b_2 \pm \text{SE}(b_2)$	$0 \cdot 300 \pm 0 \cdot 553$	$-1 \cdot 043 \pm 0 \cdot 469$	$-1 \cdot 197 \pm 0 \cdot 550$
Res. SSq	3995·8	3190·3	2228·8
Res. MSq (DF)	235·0 (17)	187·7 (17)	222·9 (10)
$\bar{x}_1$	1·9150	2·0315	2·0515
$\bar{x}_2$	66·250	66·850	65·692
$\bar{y}$	18·400	22·800	29·154

The values of $\bar{y}$ show differences in the same direction as was noted from the overall residuals. However, the differences are explained in part by differences in the values of $\bar{x}_1$ and $\bar{x}_2$. Predicted values from the three multiple regressions, for values of x_1 and x_2 equal to the overall means, 1·9925 and 66·340, respectively, are:

$$\text{A: } 19 \cdot 03 \qquad \text{B: } 22 \cdot 44 \qquad \text{C: } 26 \cdot 24,$$

closer together than the unadjusted means shown in the table above.

There are substantial differences between the estimated regression coefficients across the three groups, but the standard errors are large. Using the methods of §9.4, we can test for homogeneity of each coefficient separately, the reciprocals of the variances being used as weights. This gives, as approximate χ^2 statistics on 2 DF, 1·86 for b_1 and 4·62 for b_2, neither of which is significant at the usual levels. We cannot add these $\chi^2_{(2)}$ statistics, since b_1 and b_2 are not independent. For a more complete analysis of the whole data set we need a further analysis, using a model like (10.29). We shall need two dummy variables, z_1 (taking the value 1 in group A and 0 elsewhere) and z_2 (1 in group B and 0 elsewhere). Combining the Residual SSqs from the initial overall regression, the new regression with two dummy variables, and the regressions within separate groups (pooling the three residuals), we have:

	DF	SSq	MSq	VR
Residual from overall regression	50	11 008·0		
Between intercepts	2	421·33	210·7	0·96
Residual from (10.29)	48	10 586·6	220·6	
Between slopes	4	1171·68	292·9	1·37
Residual from separate regressions	44	9414·9	214·0	

In the table above, the SSq between intercepts and between slopes are obtained by subtraction. Neither term is at all significant. Note that the test for differences between slopes is approximately equivalent to $\chi^2_{(4)} = 4 \times 1{\cdot}37 = 5{\cdot}48$, rather less than the sum of the two $\chi^2_{(2)}$ statistics given earlier, confirming the non-independence of the two previous tests. Note also that even if the entire SSq between intercepts were ascribed to a trend across the groups, with 1 DF, the VR would be only $421{\cdot}33/214{\cdot}0 = 1{\cdot}97$, far from significant. The point can be made in another way, by comparing the intercepts, in the model of (10.29), for the two extreme groups, A and C. These groups differ in the values taken by z_1 (1 and 0, respectively). In the analysis of the model (10.29), the estimate d_1, of the regression coefficient on z_1 is $-7{\cdot}39 \pm 5{\cdot}39$, again not significant. Of course, the selection of the two groups with the most extreme contrast biases the analysis in favour of finding a significant difference, but, as we see, even this contrast is not significantly large.

In summary, it appears that the overall multiple regression fitted initially to the data of Table 10.1 can be taken to apply to all three groups of patients.

The between-slopes SSq was obtained as the difference between the residual fitting (10.29) and the sum of the three separate residuals fitting regressions for each group separately. It is often more convenient to do the computations as analyses of the total data set, as follows.

Consider first two groups with a dummy variable for group, z, defined as earlier. Now define new variables w_j, for $j = 1$ to p by $w_j = zx_j$. Since z is zero in group 2 then all the w_j are also zero in group 2; $z = 1$ in group 1 and therefore $w_j = x_j$ in group 1. Consider the following model:

$$E(y) = \alpha + \delta z + \beta_1 x_1 + \ldots + \beta_p x_p + \gamma_1 w_1 + \ldots + \gamma_p w_p. \quad (10.31)$$

Because of the definitions of z and the w_j, (10.31) is equivalent to

$$E(y) = \begin{cases} \alpha + \delta + (\beta_1 + \gamma_1)x_1 + \ldots + (\beta_p + \gamma_p)x_p \text{ for group 1} \\ \alpha + \beta_1 x_1 + \ldots + \beta_p x_p \text{ for group 2,} \end{cases} \quad (10.32)$$

which gives lines of different slopes and intercepts for the two groups. The coefficient γ_j is the difference between the slopes on x_j in the two groups. The overall significance test for the null hypothesis that $\gamma_1 = \gamma_2 = \ldots = \gamma_p = 0$ is tested by deleting the w_j variables from the regression to give the F test on p and $n - 2p - 2$ DF.

When $k > 2$, the above procedure is generalized by deriving $p(k - 1)$ variables, $w_{ij} = z_i x_j$, and an overall test of parallel regressions in all the groups is given by the composite test of the regression coefficients for all the w_{ij}. This is a F test with $p(k - 1)$ and $n - (p + 1)k$ DF.

In the above procedure the order of introducing (or deleting) the variables is crucial. The w_{ij} should only be included in regressions in which the corresponding z_i and x_j variables are also included. Three regressions are fitted in sequence on the following variables:

(i) $x_1, \ldots, x_p$;

(ii) $x_1, \ldots, x_p, \quad z_1, \ldots, z_k$;

(iii) $x_1, \ldots, x_p, \quad z_1, \ldots, z_k, \quad w_{11}, \ldots, w_{kp}$.

These three regressions in turn correspond to Fig. 9.4(c), (b) and (a) respectively.

In this formulation there might be some concern about collinearity since there is likely to be high correlation between terms such as w_{ij} and z_i. For the data of Example 10.1, fitting the full model with eight variables, there were values of the variance inflation factor up to 149. This could have been overcome by centring but the analysis lost no important precision, using the SAS regression PROC REG, so that the collinearity was of no practical concern.

Example 10.3

The three-group analysis of Examples 9.3 and 9.4 may be done by introducing two dummy variables: z_1, taking the value 1 in group A_1 and 0 otherwise; and z_2, taking the value 1 in group A_2 and 0 otherwise. As before, y represents vital capacity and x age. Two new variables are derived: $w_1 = xz_1$ and $w_2 = xz_2$. The multiple regressions of y on x, of y on x, z_1 and z_2, and of y on x, z_1, z_2, w_1 and w_2 give the following analysis of variance table:

	DF	SSq	MSq	VR
(1) Due to regression on x	1	17·4446		
(2) Due to introduction of z_1 and z_2 ($=(4) - (1)$)	2	0·1617	0·0808	0·22
(3) Residual about regression on x, z_1 and z_2	80	30·0347	0·3754	
(4) Due to regression on x, z_1 and z_2	3	17·6063		
(5) Due to introduction of w_1 and w_2 ($=(6) - (4)$)	2	2·4994	1·2497	3·54
(6) Due to regression on x, z_1, z_2, w_1 and w_2	5	20·1057		
(7) Residual about regression on x, z_1, z_2, w_1 and w_2	78	27·5352	0·3530	
Total	83	47·6410		

Apart from rounding errors, lines (5) and (7) agree with the analysis of variance in Example 9.3 on p. 300 and lines (2) and (3) are the same as in Example 9.4 (p. 309).

For the analysis of covariance model, the partial regression coefficients and their standard errors are

$$a = 6.0449$$
$$d_1 = -0.1169 \pm 0.2092$$
$$d_2 = -0.0702 \pm 0.1487$$
$$b_1 = -0.0398 \pm 0.0063 \ (t = -6.29).$$

The coefficients d_1 and d_2 are estimates of the corrected differences between groups A_1 and A_2 respectively, and group B; neither is significant. The coefficient b_1, representing the age effect, is highly significant.

For the model with separate slopes the coefficients are (using c to represent estimates of γ)

$$a = 5.6803$$
$$d_1 = 2.5031 \pm 1.0418$$
$$d_2 = 0.5497 \pm 0.5759$$
$$b_1 = -0.0306 \pm 0.0075$$
$$c_1 = -0.0545 \pm 0.0211$$
$$c_2 = -0.0159 \pm 0.0145.$$

The coefficients c_1 and c_2 represent estimates of the differences in the slope on age between groups A_1 and A_2 respectively, and group B. As noted earlier there are significant differences between the slopes ($F = 3.54$ with 2 and 78 DF, $P = 0.034$). The estimates of the slopes for groups A_1, A_2 and B are $-0.0306 - 0.0545 = -0.0851$, $-0.0306 - 0.0159 = -0.0465$, and -0.0306 respectively, agreeing with the values found earlier by fitting the regressions for each group separately (p. 300).

10.3 Polynomial and other curvilinear regressions

Reference was made in §10.1 to the possibility of creating new predictor variables defined as the squares of existing variables, to cope with non-linear or *curvilinear* relationships. This is an important idea, and is most easily studied in situations in which there is originally only one predictor variable x.

Instead of the linear regression equation

$$\mathrm{E}(y) = \alpha + \beta x \tag{10.33}$$

introduced in §5.2, we consider the *polynomial* model

$$\mathrm{E}(y) = \alpha + \beta_1 x + \beta_2 x^2 + \ldots + \beta_p x^p. \tag{10.34}$$

The highest power of x, denoted here by p, is called the *degree* of the polynomial. Some typical shapes of low-degree polynomial curves are shown in Fig. 10.3. The curve for $p = 2$, when the term in x^2 is added, is called *quadratic*; that for $p = 3$ *cubic*, and that for $p = 4$ *quartic*. Clearly, a wide variety of curves can be

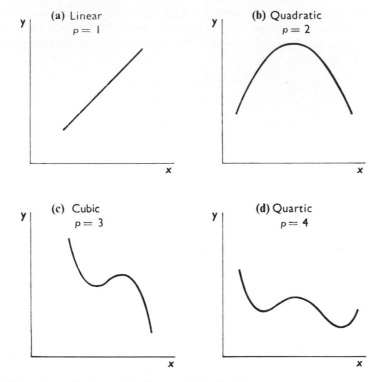

Fig. 10.3 Illustrations of polynomials of up to the fourth degree.

represented by polynomials. The quadratic curve has one peak or trough; the cubic has at most two peaks or troughs; and so on. A particular set of data may be fitted well by a portion of a low-degree polynomial even though no peaks or troughs are present. In particular, data showing a moderate amount of curvature can often be fitted adequately by a quadratic curve.

The general principle of polynomial regression analysis is to regard the successive powers of x as separate predictor variables. Thus, to fit the p-degree polynomial (10.34), we could define $x_1 = x$, $x_2 = x^2$, ..., $x_p = x^p$, and apply the standard methods of §10.1. It will often be uncertain which degree of polynomial is required. Considerations of simplicity suggest that as low an order as possible should be used; for example, we should normally use linear regression unless there is any particular reason to use a higher-degree polynomial. The usual approach is to use a slightly higher degree than one supposes to be necessary. The highest-degree terms can then be dropped successively so long as they contribute, separately or together, increments to the SSq which are non-significant when compared with the Residual SSq. Some problems arising from this approach are illustrated in Example 10.4 below.

Note that, with n observations, all with different values of x, a polynomial of degree $p = n - 1$ would have $n - p - 1 = n - (n - 1) - 1 = 0$ DF. It is always possible to fit a polynomial of degree $n - 1$, so as to pass through n points with different values of x, just as a straight line ($p = 1$) can be drawn through any two points. The Residual SSq is, therefore, also zero, and no significance tests are possible. To provide a test of the adequacy of the model the degree of the polynomial should be considerably lower than the number of observations.

Example 10.4

Table 10.3 gives the population size of England and Wales (in millions) as recorded at decennial censuses between 1801 and 1971; there is a gap in the series at 1941, as no census was taken in that year. It is of some interest to fit a smooth curve to the trend in population size, first, to provide estimates for intermediate years and, secondly, for projection beyond

Table 10.3 Trend in population of England and Wales between 1801 and 1971 fitted by polynomials up to the sixth degree

Year	Population, England and Wales (millions)	Values predicted by polynomial of degree:					
		1	2	3	4	5	6
1801	8·89	6·88	7·42	9·11	9·20	8·61	8·78
11	10·16	9·36	9·71	10·19	10·18	10·63	10·38
21	12·00	11·84	12·02	11·68	11·62	12·20	12·05
31	13·90	14·32	14·36	13·52	13·45	13·73	13·80
41	15·91	16·80	16·72	15·66	15·61	15·50	15·69
51	17·93	19·28	19·10	18·05	18·04	17·64	17·82
61	20·07	21·76	21·51	20·64	20·66	20·18	20·24
71	22·71	24·24	23·94	23·39	23·43	23·06	22·97
81	25·97	26·71	26·40	26·23	26·29	26·16	25·98
91	29·00	29·19	28·88	29·13	29·18	29·34	29·17
1901	32·53	31·67	31·38	32·03	32·06	32·45	32·37
11	36·07	34·15	33·91	34·87	34·88	35·34	35·40
21	37·89	36·63	36·46	37·61	37·58	37·92	38·10
31	39·95	39·11	39·04	40·20	40·14	40·16	40·36
41	—						
51	43·76	44·07	44·26	44·72	44·64	43·95	43·83
61	46·10	46·55	46·91	46·55	46·52	46·00	45·76
71	48·75	49·03	49·58	48·02	48·10	48·73	48·89
(81	49·15)	(51·51	52·28	49·09	49·36	52·82	54·64)
Multiple correlation coefficient		0·9964	0·9966	0·9991	0·9991	0·9997	0·9998
Residual MSq		1·354	1·346	0·365	0·392	0·139	0·109
DF		15	14	13	12	11	10
t for highest-degree term		45·23	1·05	−6·21	0·34	4·78	2·02
P		< 0·001	0·31	<0·001	0·74	<0·001	0·071

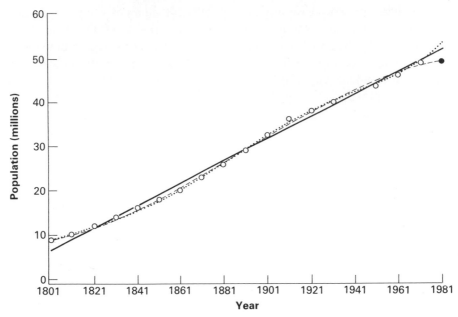

Fig. 10.4 Polynomial regressions fitted to population trend data (Table 10.3). (—) $p = 1$; (– – –) $p = 3$; (……) $p = 5$.

the end of the series, although demographers would in practice use more sophisticated methods of projection. The figure for 1981 is given at the foot of the main series to provide a comparison with estimates obtained by extrapolation from the main series.

The data are plotted in Fig. 10.4. The trend is not too far from linear, but there are obvious systematic deviations which suggest that a polynomial curve might fit quite well.

Table 10.3 shows the predicted values from polynomials up to the sixth degree, and Fig. 10.4 illustrates the fits obtained by linear ($p = 1$), cubic ($p = 3$) and fifth-degree ($p = 5$) curves. The entries at the foot of Table 10.3 show that the Residual MSq is reduced substantially by the introduction of the cubic term, and this curve seems from Fig. 10.4 to provide an excellent fit. However, there are slight systematic fluctuations of groups of adjacent points about the cubic, and Table 10.3 shows that the introduction of the fifth-degree term produces a significant decrease in the Residual MSq (since the t value 8for this coefficient is significant).

The process could be continued beyond this stage, but it is doubtful whether any useful purpose would be achieved. We are left in a slight dilemma. There is no theoretical reason for expecting precisely a polynomial curve plus random error. The cubic is a close approximation to the best-fitting smooth curve, but slight (yet significant) improvement can be made by introducing a higher-degree term. Note that the improvement is evident in the agreement between observed and predicted values within the range 1801–1971. Extrapolation, or prediction outside this range, is a different matter. The cubic curve gives adequate agreement between the predicted and observed value for 1981. The fifth-degree curve is much less satisfactory. This is a rather common finding, and argues strongly for the use of a polynomial with as low a degree as possible for an acceptable fit, even though higher-degree terms provide noticeable reductions in residual variation within the fitted range.

The various powers of x, which form the predictor variables in (10.34), are correlated with each other, often quite highly so. This occasionally causes some computational difficulties due to collinearity (§10.1). Such difficulties can usually be overcome by redefining the powers of x as deviations from their own means or by centring (Healy, 1963).

These intercorrelations of the powers of x mean that the coefficient of a particular power in the fitted regression equation will depend on which other powers are present in the equation, as indeed is usually the case in multiple regression. If the powers were transformed to an equivalent set of predictor variables which were uncorrelated, we should be able to fit successively higher-order polynomials by relatively simple methods, without recalculating the coefficients previously obtained. This is particularly convenient when the xs are equally spaced, as often happens in controlled experiments (where the xs may represent quantities of some substance) or in time series (where the xs may be equally spaced points of time). The method uses what are called *orthogonal polynomials*. Full details and the necessary reference tables are given in Fisher and Yates (1963).

Orthogonal polynomials provide a useful way of incorporating curvilinear regression in the analysis of variance of balanced data. Suppose that a certain factor is represented by a variable x which is observed at k equally spaced values,

$$x_1, x_2 = x_1 + h, \ldots, x_k = x_1 + (k-1)h.$$

Suppose that there are n observations in each group, and that the observed totals of y are

$$T_1, T_2, \ldots, T_k.$$

If $k = 2$, the regression coefficient, b, of y on x, is clearly estimated by

$$\frac{T_2 - T_1}{nh},$$

and the SSq due to regression on 1 DF coincides with the SSq between groups, namely,

$$\frac{(T_2 - T_1)^2}{2n}$$

(as in (7.10)).

If $k = 3$, we could consider a quadratic regression on x which would exactly fit the data, since a quadratic curve can always be found to go through three points.

To obtain the regression equation, define two new variables (the orthogonal polynomials),

$$X_1 = (x - \bar{x})/h$$
$$X_2 = 3X_1^2 - 2, \tag{10.35}$$

so that X_1 takes the values $-1, 0$ and 1, and X_2 takes the values $1, -2$ and 1. The regression equation can be written

$$Y = \bar{y} + b_1 X_1 + b_2 X_2, \tag{10.36}$$

where

$$b_1 = (T_3 - T_1)/2n$$

and

$$b_2 = (T_3 - 2T_2 + T_1)/6n.$$

The equation may be written in terms of x and x^2 by substituting (10.35) in (10.36).

The SSq due to the linear and quadratic terms (which are independent, each on 1 DF, and add to the SSq between groups) are

$$S_1 = \frac{(T_3 - T_1)^2}{2n}$$

and

$$S_2 = \frac{(T_3 - 2T_2 + T_1)^2}{6n}.$$

The method can clearly be generalized for higher values of k (see Table A18 of Snedecor and Cochran, 1989). The most useful features of the generalization are the SSq for the linear and quadratic terms. These take the form $(\sum \lambda_i T_i)^2 / \sum \lambda_i^2$, where for the linear term the λ_is are integers centred about zero (e.g. $-1, 0, 1$ for $k = 3$; $-3, -1, 1, 3$ for $k = 4$). For the quadratic term each λ_i is obtained by squaring the corresponding λ_i for the linear term, subtracting the mean of the values thus obtained and multiplying by a convenient constant if this is necessary to give integer values. These SSq account for 2 DF out of the total $k - 1$ DF between groups. The remaining $k - 3$ DF represent deviations about the quadratic curve and can be tested against the appropriate residual in the analysis. If necessary the cubic and higher terms can be successively isolated until the MSq for deviations reaches a sufficiently low level.

Some forms of curvilinear trend, other than those represented by polynomials, are occasionally encountered. Two examples are illustrated in Fig. 10.5. The first is *asymptotic regression*, in which the regression line approaches an upper or lower limit exponentially. The regression equation is then non-linear in the coefficients and the method of fitting becomes more complicated (see Draper and Smith, 1981, Chapter 10).

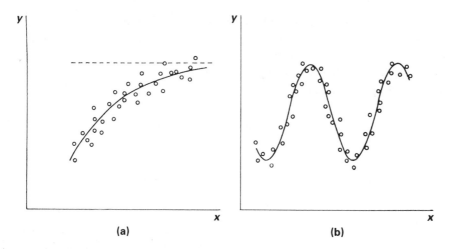

Fig. 10.5 Two forms of non-linear regression: (a) asymptotic; (b) periodic.

The second example shown in Fig. 10.5 is one of *periodic regression*, in which the underlying regression equation has the sinusoidal form

$$Y = \alpha_0 + \alpha_1 \sin(\beta x + \gamma). \qquad (10.37)$$

This represents a cyclical curve with amplitude $\pm \alpha_1$ and wavelength $360/\beta$ (the angles being measured in degrees).

Periodic regression is discussed fully by Bliss (1958). A cyclical trend cannot always be described by a simple sinusoidal curve, and more complex situations are discussed in §10.6 (see particularly Example 10.9). However, the simpler model may sometimes apply, and is useful as a simple alternative to the null hypothesis that no cyclical trend exists.

An example of such a test was presented by Edwards (1961) for testing periodicity in a series of counts made at equally spaced points of time. We describe here a slight variant on Edwards's test, due to Smith (1961). Suppose there are k counts, N_i, with a total count of $N = \sum N_i$. For example, neurological episodes may be classified by the hour of the day ($k = 24$), or congenital abnormalities by the month of birth ($k = 12$).

If the regression equation (10.37) is to have a complete cycle of k time intervals, it can be written in the alternative form

$$\mathrm{E}(N_i) = \alpha_0 + \beta_1 \sin \theta_i + \beta_2 \cos \theta_i,$$

where $\theta_i = (i - \tfrac{1}{2})(360/k)$. Here α_0 represents the mean count, and β_1 and β_2 together determine the amplitude and phase of the sinusoidal curve. With $k = 12$, for example, $\theta_1 = 15°, \theta_2 = 45°$, and so on. Consider now a multiple regression of N_i on $\sin \theta_i$ and $\cos \theta_i$. It can be shown that these two explanatory variables are orthogonal, and the SSq of N_i due to regression is therefore the sum of the two SSqs in simple regressions on the two variables separately. The residual variation of the N_is may be taken to be Poisson, and the residual variance estimated by the mean count, $\bar{N}$. If the regression SSq is divided by $\bar{N}$, the resulting statistic is distributed approximately as $\chi^2_{(2)}$. It is

$$(2/N)\left[\left(\sum N_i \sin \theta_i\right)^2 + \left(\sum N_i \cos \theta_i\right)^2\right].\tag{10.38}$$

St Leger (1976) showed that the approximation of (10.38) to the $\chi^2_{(2)}$ distribution is unsatisfactory for N less than 200 and gave improved values for the significance levels.

Walter and Elwood (1975) extended the method to cope with unequal lengths of time interval and to a variable population at risk. This makes it more appropriate for the second example above, congenital abnormalities by month of birth, since the different number of days in a month and variations between months in the number of births can both be taken into account.

10.4 Multiple regression in the analysis of non-orthogonal data

The analysis of variance was used in Chapter 8 to study the separate effects of various factors, for data classified in designs exhibiting some degree of balance. These so-called *orthogonal designs* enable sums of squares representing different sources of variation to be presented simultaneously in the same analysis. As was observed in §8.8, non-orthogonality in a design often causes considerable complication in the analysis.

Multiple regression, introduced in §10.1, is a powerful method of studying the simultaneous effect on a random variable of various predictor variables, and no special conditions of balance are imposed on their values. The effect of any variable, or any group of variables, can, as we have seen, be exhibited by an analysis of variance. We might, therefore, expect that the methods of multiple regression would be useful for the analysis of data classified in an unbalanced design. In §10.2 the analysis of covariance was considered as a particular instance of multiple regression, the one-way classification into groups being represented by a system of dummy variables. This approach can be adopted for any factor with two or more levels. A significance test for any factor is obtained by performing two multiple regressions: first, including the dummy variables representing the factor and, second, without those variables. For a full analysis of any set of data many multiple regressions may be needed.

Example 10.5

Consider the data in Table 8.14. These were analysed by special methods appropriate to two-way tables, but we could instead have adopted the general approach described above. We define the following dummy variables:

$$x_1 = \begin{cases} 1 & \text{for control group} \\ 0 & \text{for treated group} \end{cases}$$

$$x_2 = \begin{cases} 1 & \text{for age group } 40- \\ 0 & \text{otherwise} \end{cases}$$

$$x_3 = \begin{cases} 1 & \text{for age group } 50- \\ 0 & \text{otherwise.} \end{cases}$$

These represent the main effects of the two factors, treatment and age, and to allow for possible interaction we need two other variables,

$$x_4 = x_1 x_2$$

and

$$x_5 = x_1 x_3.$$

The dependent variable, y, is the number of accidents; the frequency distributions of y are shown in Table 8.14. The total number of observations is 41. As an example of the specification of the variables, the single subject in the control 40− group has the following values:

x_1	x_2	x_3	x_4	x_5	y
1	1	0	1	0	1

To obtain the necessary SSq for the analysis of variance shown in Table 8.15, we need the multiple regressions shown in Table 10.4. For many computer programs these can all be requested as part of the same job.

The Residual SSq (a) is 17·0350, the same as the Within-Cells Residual of Table 8.15, since the five dummy variables, x_1 to x_5, exactly account for the differences between the six cells. The difference between (b) and (a) is 0·0243 on 2 DF, the same as the SSq for the interaction $T \times A$ in Table 8.15. Having seen, by the F test given in Table 8.15, that the interaction is non-significant, we test treatments by the difference (c) − (b), which is 5·8706 on 1 DF, essentially the same as the adjusted Treatments SSq in Table 8.15. As a test for age, (d) − (b) = 1·9407 on 2 DF, again agreeing with the adjusted Age SSq in Table 8.15.

Table 10.4 Multiple regressions required for analysis of data in Table 8.14

Regression	Residual SSq	DF
y on x_1, x_2, x_3, x_4, x_5	17·0350 (a)	35
y on x_1, x_2, x_3	17·0593 (b)	37
y on x_2, x_3	22·9299 (c)	38
y on x_1	19·0000 (d)	39

Many statistical packages have programs for performing this sort of analysis. The name *general linear model* is often used, and should be distinguished from the more complex *generalized linear model* to be described in §12.8. In interpreting the output of such an analysis, care must be taken to ensure that the test for the effect of a particular factor is not distorted by the presence or absence of correlated factors. In particular, for data with a factorial structure, the warning given on p. 258, against the testing of main effects in the presence of interactions involving the relevant factors, should be heeded.

Freund *et al.* (1986) describe four different ways in which sums of squares can be calculated in general linear models. Briefly, Type I is appropriate when factors are introduced in a predetermined order; Type II shows the contribution of each factor in the presence of all others except interactions involving that factor; in Types III and IV, any interactions defined in the model are retained even for the testing of main effects. The authors' advocacy of Type III runs counter to the advice given above, although no difficulty would arise if the model were explicitly defined without interactions. Type II corresponds to a more commendable strategy of testing interactions in the presence of main effects, and either testing main effects without interactions (if the latter can safely be ignored) or not testing main effects at all (if interactions are regarded as being present).

10.5 Multivariate methods

In multiple regression each individual provides observations simultaneously on several variables; thus the data are *multivariate*. Yet only one of these, the dependent variable, is regarded as a *random* variable and the purpose of the analysis is to explain as much as possible of the variation in this dependent variable in terms of the multiple predictor variables. Multiple regression is, therefore, an extension of the other methods considered so far in this book and essentially involves no new concepts beyond those introduced in Chapter 5 for a simple linear regression with just one independent variable. The function of the predictor variables in multiple regression is to classify the individual in a way which is rather similar to the qualitative classifications in an experimental design.

Multivariate analysis is a collection of techniques appropriate for the situation in which the random variation in several variables has to be studied simultaneously. The subject is extensive and is treated in several textbooks; there are useful introductory texts by Kendall (1980), Chatfield and Collins (1980) and Krzanowski (1988), and a more advanced text by Mardia *et al.* (1979). The subject cannot be explored in detail in the present book but this section contains a brief survey of some methods which have been found useful in medical research.

A general point to note is that tests of significance play a much less important role in multivariate analysis than in univariate analysis. As noted in comment 3 on p. 97, a univariate significance test is often useful as giving an immediate indication of the likely direction of any departure from the null hypothesis. With multivariate data, no such simple interpretation is possible. If, for instance, a significance test shows that two multivariate samples are unlikely to come from the same population, it may not be at all obvious in what respect they differ—whether, for instance, there are clear differences for each of the component variates, or for only some of them. The main emphasis in the methods to be described below is therefore on estimation—that is, on the attempt to describe the nature of the data structure. Nevertheless, significance tests sometimes play a modest role, particularly in preliminary analyses of data before more searching methods are applied, and we shall describe a few of the more useful techniques.

Principal components

Often observations are made on a medium or large number of separate variables on each individual even though the number of different characteristics it is required to determine of the individuals is much less. For example, on p. 10 part of a questionnaire is given in which six different questions are asked about stress or worry. The purpose of these separate questions may be to obtain information on an individual's overall stress or worry, with no particular interest in what has contributed to the stress. The separate questions are asked only because no single question would be adequate. In some cases sufficient may be known of the field of application to allow a combined variable or score to be calculated; for example, the answers to the six stress questions considered above could be combined by averaging to give a single variable, 'stress'. In other cases some analysis is required to determine which variables might be sensibly combined.

Suppose we have observations on p variables, $x_1, x_2, \ldots, x_p$, made on each of n individuals. We could ask whether it is possible to combine these variables into a small number of other variables which could provide almost all the information about the way in which one individual differed from another. One way of expressing this is to define new variables,

$$y_1 = a_{11}x_1 + a_{12}x_2 + \ldots + a_{1p}x_p,$$
$$y_2 = a_{21}x_1 + a_{22}x_2 + \ldots + a_{2p}x_p. \tag{10.39}$$

etc., so that y_1 has the highest possible variance and so represents better than any other linear combination of the xs the general differences between individuals. (If no restrictions are placed on the a_{ij}s, this is a pointless requirement, since larger values of the coefficients will lead to a larger variance of y_1; we therefore standardize their general magnitude by requiring that $\sum_{j=1}^{p} a_{ij}^2 = 1$). Then we could choose y_2 such that it is uncorrelated with y_1 and has the next largest variance; and so on. If $p = 3$, the individual observations can be visualized as a three-dimensional scatter diagram with n points, perhaps clustered in the shape of an airship. The first *principal component*, y_1, will represent distances along the length of the airship. The second component, y_2, represents distances along the widest direction perpendicular to the length (say side to side); the third and last component, y_3, will then represent distances from top to bottom of the airship. There are in general p principal components, but the variation of all but a few may be quite small. If, in the previous example, the airship were very flat, almost like a disc, y_3 would show very little variation, and an individual's position in the whole diagram would be determined almost exactly by y_1 and y_2.

The method of analysis involves the calculation of latent roots of the covariance or correlation matrix. Most computers have standard programs that can be used. An important point to note is that if the scale of measurement for any variable is changed, even by a multiplying factor, the whole results are changed. This fact has led some workers to standardize each variable initially by dividing by its standard deviation; this is equivalent to working with the correlation matrix.

The interpretation of any of the components, the jth, say, defined by (10.39) involves consideration of the relative values of the coefficients a_{ij} for that component. If all the coefficients were about equal, then the component could be interpreted as an average of all the variables. If some of the coefficients were small, then the corresponding variables could be ignored and the component interpreted in terms of a subset of the original variables. The application of the method will only have produced a useful reduction in the dimensionality of the data if the components have an interpretation that appears to represent some meaningful characteristics. Thus, interpretation is to some extent subjective and involves knowledge of the field of application.

Since interpretation of each component is in terms of the original variables, it may be more informative to assess each component in terms of its correlations with the original variables rather than in terms of the coefficients a_{ij}. For principal components calculated from the correlation matrix these correlations are obtained by multiplying each component by the square root of the corresponding latent root. These correlations are termed the *component correlations* or *loadings*, although the latter term is sometimes used for the coefficients of (10.39).

Another aspect of the analysis is the choice of the number of components to include. Whilst various methods have been suggested, there is no universally accepted method and the decision is usually made with the interpretation of the components in mind. It is seldom worth including an extra component if that component cannot be given a meaningful interpretation.

Once a decision has been made on the number of components to include, the data have effectively been reduced to that number of dimensions; for example, if two components are accepted, then the observations are regarded as lying in two-dimensional space and the remaining $p - 2$ dimensions of the original variables are ignored. A point in two-dimensional space is represented by two coordinates with respect to two axes; using the representation (10.39) the point would be (y_1, y_2). There are, however, many ways of constructing the axes. Restricting attention to orthogonal axes, that is, axes at right angles to one another, the pair of axes could be rotated together about the origin and would remain an orthogonal pair of axes. The coordinates of a point would change, to (y_1', y_2'), say, but the geometrical configuration of the points would be unaltered. Corresponding to (10.39) we should have

$$y_1' = a_{11}' x_1 + a_{12}' x_2 + \ldots + a_{1p}' x_p,$$
$$y_2' = a_{21}' x_1 + a_{22}' x_2 + \ldots + a_{2p}' x_p,$$

(10.40)

etc. If a rotation could be found so that the components defined in (10.40) were more readily interpretable than those of (10.39), then the analysis would be improved. Several criteria for choosing a rotation have been suggested but the most widely used is the *varimax* method. In this method the aim is that for each component the coefficients should divide into two groups, with those in one group as large as possible and those in the other as near zero as possible. That is, each component is expressed in terms of a subset of the original variables with the minimum contamination from variables not in the subset. The rotated components are no longer principal and the relationship between the coefficients of (10.40) and the component correlations is more complicated than for principal components. Provided that the components are scaled to have unit variance before the rotation procedure is applied, then the rotated components are uncorrelated with one another.

Equations (10.39) or (10.40) can be used to assign values to each component for each individual. These values are termed the *component scores* and can be used in further steps of the analysis instead of the full set of x variables. Sometimes, for example, the component scores are used as a reduced set of independent variables in a regression analysis of some other variables not considered in the principal component analysis.

Example 10.6

Cockcroft *et al.* (1982) recorded answers to 20 questions designed to characterize patients with chronic respiratory disability in a clinical trial according to the influence of their illness on everyday living. The answers were recorded by marking a line joining two opposite statements (this is called a *visual analogue scale*) and analysed after a transformation of the proportional distance of the mark from one end of the line. The correlation matrix of the variables is given in Table 10.5; an abbreviated version of the statement at the favourable end of each line is also shown.

The first principal component accounts for 29.9% of the total variation in the 20 variables, the second for 17.1%, the third for 10.0%, the fourth for 6.8%, the fifth for 6.5%, the sixth for 5.7%, whilst the remaining 14 components account for 24% of the total variation.

Table 10.5 Correlation matrix of 20 variables

Variable	1	2	3	4	5	6	7	8	9
1 Physical health good									
2 Optimistic about future	0·17								
3 Never breathless	0·44	0·05							
4 Breathlessness does not distress me	0·35	0·14	0·40						
5 Rarely cough	0·45	0·02	0·37	0·36					
6 Coughing does not trouble me	0·35	0·07	0·37	0·42	0·92				
7 Never wheezy	0·44	0·07	0·55	0·42	0·61	0·64			
8 Hardly ever feel ill	0·64	0·23	0·37	0·67	0·55	0·59	0·57		
9 Condition has improved	0·42	−0·13	0·34	0·35	0·70	0·67	0·56	0·45	
10 Never worry about future	−0·06	0·46	0·11	0·42	0·04	0·11	−0·14	0·10	−0·12
11 Confident could cope	0·16	0·33	0·21	0·49	0·27	0·30	0·03	0·29	0·00
12 Health depends on me	0·23	0·31	0·18	0·15	−0·08	0·08	0·27	0·23	−0·17
13 Worth trying anything	0·06	0·23	−0·04	0·13	0·06	0·10	−0·04	0·01	0·11
14 Wife happy with my condition	0·41	−0·06	0·29	0·38	0·44	0·46	0·62	0·37	0·68
15 Feel like going out	−0·09	0·03	−0·38	−0·01	−0·18	−0·10	−0·44	−0·18	−0·17
16 Relaxing with other people	0·10	0·15	0·22	0·09	−0·12	−0·05	−0·06	−0·07	−0·08
17 Support the family	0·38	0·16	0·24	0·28	0·52	0·46	0·38	0·46	0·52
18 Making a useful contribution	0·39	0·33	0·26	0·31	0·13	0·13	0·12	0·48	0·01
19 Accept my condition	0·37	0·36	0·45	0·56	0·08	0·10	0·34	0·46	0·07
20 Feel happy	−0·02	0·61	−0·29	0·02	−0·27	−0·26	−0·22	0·05	−0·32

Variable	10	11	12	13	14	15	16	17	18	19
1 Physical health good										
2 Optimistic about future										
3 Never breathless										
4 Breathlessness does not distress me										
5 Rarely cough										
6 Coughing does not trouble me										
7 Never wheezy										
8 Hardly ever feel ill										
9 Condition has improved										
10 Never worry about future										
11 Confident could cope	0·71									
12 Health depends on me	0·26	0·46								
13 Worth trying anything	0·32	0·21	−0·02							
14 Wife happy with my condition	0·01	0·11	0·20	−0·11						
15 Feel like going out	0·12	−0·02	−0·20	0·31	−0·29					
16 Relaxing with other people	0·24	0·15	−0·01	0·59	−0·07	0·50				
17 Support the family	0·03	0·04	−0·03	0·03	0·43	−0·13	−0·09			
18 Making a useful contribution	0·21	0·63	0·50	0·09	0·05	−0·18	0·05	0·09		
19 Accept my condition	0·52	0·27	0·17	0·08	0·30	−0·26	0·22	0·25	0·23	
20 Feel happy	0·28	0·18	0·04	−0·03	−0·23	0·20	0·07	−0·11	0·18	0·27

Table 10.6 Component correlations (loadings) of the first three principal components

Variable		Component			Rotated component		
		1	2	3	1	2	3
1	Physical health good	**0·67**	0·02	−0·01	**0·59**	0·32	−0·07
3	Never breathless	**0·63**	−0·02	−0·08	**0·55**	0·28	−0·14
4	Breathlessness does not distress me	**0·69**	0·28	0·10	**0·53**	**0·51**	0·13
5	Rarely cough	**0·76**	−0·31	0·24	**0·86**	0·00	0·04
6	Coughing does not trouble me	**0·77**	−0·23	0·26	**0·84**	0·07	0·08
7	Never wheezy	**0·77**	−0·29	−0·12	**0·77**	0·13	−0·29
8	Hardly ever feel ill	**0·81**	0·08	−0·08	**0·67**	0·45	−0·12
9	Condition has improved	**0·68**	−0·47	0·30	**0·86**	−0·19	0·04
14	Wife happy with my condition	**0·66**	−0·29	−0·04	**0·69**	0·06	−0·21
17	Support the family	**0·59**	−0·19	0·13	**0·63**	0·06	0·00
2	Optimistic about future	0·22	**0·66**	−0·08	−0·07	**0·68**	0·15
10	Never worry about future	0·23	**0·74**	0·14	−0·04	**0·69**	0·38
11	Confident could cope	0·43	**0·64**	−0·04	0·13	**0·75**	0·16
12	Health depends on me	0·29	0·41	−0·47	−0·01	**0·61**	−0·31
18	Making a useful contribution	0·43	0·49	−0·32	0·12	**0·70**	−0·15
19	Accept my condition	**0·52**	0·44	−0·13	0·27	**0·64**	0·10
20	Feel happy	−0·14	**0·61**	−0·15	−0·40	**0·50**	0·00
13	Worth trying anything	0·09	0·37	**0·68**	0·10	0·15	**0·76**
15	Feel like going out	−0·33	0·27	**0·68**	−0·23	−0·12	**0·76**
16	Relaxing with other people	0·01	0·43	**0·64**	0·00	0·18	**0·75**

In Table 10.6 the first three components are given. The variables have been reordered, and component correlations exceeding 0·5 are given in bold type, to show the main features of each component. The first component is correlated more with variables 1, 3, 4, 5, 6, 7, 8, 9, 14 and 17 and may be interpreted as 'physical health'. The second component is correlated with variables 2, 10, 11, 12, 18, 19 and 20 and may be interpreted as 'optimism'. The third component is correlated with variables 13, 15 and 16 and may be interpreted as 'socializing'. The identification of the components in terms of the original variables is clearer for the rotated components. These three components accounted for 57% of the total variation and, since no clear interpretation was made of the next component, attention was restricted to these three.

In the above example the dimensionality of the data was reduced from 20 to 3 by the use of principal component analysis. It would appear that the method was highly effective. However, the original questions were chosen to represent a few characteristics and, before the data were collected, groupings of the questions were perceived that were similar to those of the components extracted. Although it may be argued that the weights, a_{ij}, of the different variables in the components (10.39) are optimum, this may only be so for the particular data set. Quantitatively, the components are not necessarily generalizable outside the data set, even though qualitatively they may be. For the sake of wider generalizability and standardization amongst research workers it may be preferable to choose equal weights in each component after verifying that the subsets of variables defining each component are reasonable.

Factor analysis

This method has been used considerably by psychologists. It is closely related to principal component analysis, but differs in that it assumes a definite model for the way in which the observed variables, x_i, are influenced by certain hypothetical underlying factors. Suppose the xs are educational tests applied to children and that each test reflects to a differing extent certain factors; for example, general intelligence, verbal facility, arithmetical ability, speed of working, etc. Imagine that each individual has a certain value for each of these common factors, $f_1, f_2, f_3, \ldots$, which are uncorrelated, but that these cannot be measured directly. The factor-analysis model is

$$x_1 = b_{11} f_1 + b_{12} f_2 + b_{13} f_3 + \ldots + \mu_1 + \varepsilon_1,$$
$$x_2 = b_{21} f_1 + b_{22} f_2 + b_{23} f_3 + \ldots + \mu_2 + \varepsilon_2, \tag{10.41}$$

etc. Here μ_i is the mean of x_i and ε_i is the residual specific to the ith test after taking account of the contributions of the factors. The values of the factors $f_1, f_2, f_3, \ldots$ vary from one subject to another, but have zero mean and unit variance, and are assumed to be uncorrelated with one another and with the residuals. The quantities b_{ij} are constants, like regression coefficients, indicating how much each test is affected by each factor. The b_{ij} are referred to as the *factor loadings*; where the x_i are standardized to zero mean and unit variance, then the factor loading b_{ij} is the correlation between the ith test and the jth factor. The variance in x_i that is explained by the factor model (10.41) is called the *communality*; for standardized x_i the communality is the proportion of variance explained.

The factor loadings, the communalities and the number of factors required have to be estimated from the data, usually from the sample correlation matrix. Of course, multiple regression methods cannot be used because the values of the

fs are unknown. A good general account is that of Lawley and Maxwell (1971). If the basic model can be justified on psychological grounds, a factor analysis may be expected to throw some light on the number of factors apparently affecting the test scores and to show which tests are closely related to particular factors. The place of factor analysis in other scientific fields is very doubtful. It is often used in situations for which simpler multivariate methods, with fewer assumptions, would be more appropriate. For example, the interpretation placed on the factor loadings is usually very similar to that placed on the coefficients of the first few principal components.

Discriminant analysis

Suppose there are k groups of individuals, with n_i individuals in the ith group, and that on each individual we measure p variables, $x_1, x_2, \ldots, x_p$. A rule is required for discriminating between the groups, so that, for any new individual known to come from one of the groups (the particular group being unknown), the rule could be applied and the individual assigned to the most appropriate group. This situation might arise in taxonomic studies, the xs being physical measurements and the groups being species. The rule would then allocate a new individual to one or other of the species on the basis of its physical characteristics. Another example might arise in differential diagnosis. Observations would be made on patients known to fall into particular diagnostic groups. The object would be to obtain a rule for allotting a new patient to one of these groups by measuring the same variables. In each of these examples, and in all applications of discriminant functions, the original classification into groups must be made independently of the x variables. In the diagnostic situation, for example, the patients' diagnoses may be determined by authoritative but arduous procedures, and one may wish to see how reliably the same diagnoses can be reached by using variables (the xs) which are cheaper or less harrowing for the patient. Alternatively, the correct diagnoses may have become available only after the lapse of time, and one may wish to determine these as far as possible by variables measurable at a much earlier stage of the disease.

Consider first the situation with $k = 2$, denoting the two groups by A and B. We shall approach this problem from three different points of view, all of which we shall find leading to the same solution.

(a) Fisher's linear discriminant function

Suppose we look for a linear function

$$z = b_1 x_1 + b_2 x_2 + \ldots + b_p x_p. \tag{10.42}$$

If this is going to discriminate well between the groups we should expect the mean values of z in the two groups to be reasonably far apart in comparison with the variation of z within groups. We could therefore try to find values of the bs such that the ratio

$$D^2 = \frac{(\bar{z}_A - \bar{z}_B)^2}{\text{variance of } z \text{ within groups}} \qquad (10.43)$$

is as large as possible. The estimated variance of z will, in general, be different in the two groups, but a pooled estimate could be calculated as in the two-sample t test.

The solution of this problem is as follows:

1 Calculate the pooled sums of squares and products of the xs within groups, divide by $n_A + n_B - 2$ to obtain the matrix of within-group variances and covariances, and obtain the inverse matrix with general term c_{ij}. Here n_A and n_B are the numbers of individuals in groups A and B respectively.

2 Calculate the bs as follows:

$$\left. \begin{aligned}
b_1 &= c_{11}(\bar{x}_{A1} - \bar{x}_{B1}) + c_{12}(\bar{x}_{A2} - \bar{x}_{B2}) + \ldots + c_{1p}(\bar{x}_{Ap} - \bar{x}_{Bp}) \\
b_2 &= c_{21}(\bar{x}_{A1} - \bar{x}_{B1}) + c_{22}(\bar{x}_{A2} - \bar{x}_{B2}) + \ldots + c_{2p}(\bar{x}_{Ap} - \bar{x}_{Bp}) \\
&\;\vdots \\
b_p &= c_{p1}(\bar{x}_{A1} - \bar{x}_{B1}) + c_{p2}(\bar{x}_{A2} - \bar{x}_{B2}) + \ldots + c_{pp}(\bar{x}_{Ap} - \bar{x}_{Bp}).
\end{aligned} \right\} \qquad (10.44)$$

Here, $\bar{x}_{Ai}$ is the mean of x_i in group A and so on.

To use (10.42) for allocating future individuals to one of the two groups we need an end-point, or cut-point, to discriminate between A and B. A completely symmetrical rule would be to use the mean, z_0, of $\bar{z}_A$ and $\bar{z}_B$. From (10.42),

and
$$\left. \begin{aligned}
\bar{z}_A &= b_1 \bar{x}_{A1} + b_2 \bar{x}_{A2} + \ldots + b_p \bar{x}_{Ap} \\
\bar{z}_B &= b_1 \bar{x}_{B1} + b_2 \bar{x}_{B2} + \ldots + b_p \bar{x}_{Bp},
\end{aligned} \right\} \qquad (10.45)$$

whence

$$z_0 = b_1 \left(\frac{\bar{x}_{A1} + \bar{x}_{B1}}{2} \right) + b_2 \left(\frac{\bar{x}_{A2} + \bar{x}_{B2}}{2} \right) + \ldots + b_p \left(\frac{\bar{x}_{Ap} + \bar{x}_{Bp}}{2} \right). \qquad (10.46)$$

If $\bar{z}_A > \bar{z}_B$ the allocation rule is: allocate an individual to A if $z > z_0$ and to B if $z < z_0$. Many computer programs calculate the value of z for each individual in the two original samples. It is thus possible to count how many individuals in the two groups would have been wrongly classified by the allocation rule. This unfortunately gives an over-optimistic picture, because the allocation rule has been determined to be the best (in a certain sense) for these two particular samples, and it is likely to perform rather less well on the average with subsequent observations from the two groups (see Hills, 1966).

The allocation rule based on z_0 is intended to get close to minimizing the sum of two probabilities of misclassification—that of allocating an A individual to group B, and that of allocating a B individual to group A. Two situations lead to some modifications. In the first, suppose that the individuals come from a population in which it is known, from past experience, that the proportion in category A, p_A, is different from that in category B, p_B ($= 1 - p_A$). Then it would be reasonable to take account of this by moving the cut-point to increase the probability of allocation to the group with the higher prior probability. This is a situation where Bayes' theorem (§2.8) may be applied to adjust the prior probabilities, using the observations on an individual to obtain posterior probabilities. If this approach is taken, then the cut-point would be increased by $\ln(p_B/p_A)$, again assuming $\bar{z}_A > \bar{z}_B$ (otherwise the cut-point would be decreased). Secondly, the consequences of misclassification might not be symmetric. In diagnostic screening (see §16.4), for example, the consequences of missing a case of disease (false negative) might be more serious than wrongly classifying a disease-free individual to the disease category (false positive). In the former case, treatment may be delayed by several months and the prognosis be much poorer, whilst in the latter the individual may only experience the inconvenience of attending for more tests before being classified as disease-free. If the consequences of the two types of misclassification can be given a score, then the aim of the discrimination would be to minimize the expected value of this score for each individual. Often the scores are called costs but this terminology does not imply that the scores need to be expressible in monetary terms. If c_A is the penalty for failing to classify an A individual into group A, and c_B is similarly defined, then the cut-point should be increased by $\ln(c_B/c_A)$. Thus only the ratio of the two penalties is required.

Another way of assessing the effectiveness of the discrimination is to calculate the ratio D^2 from (10.43). Its square root, D, is called the *generalized distance*, or *Mahalanobis distance*, between the two groups. If D is greater than about 4 the situation is like that in two univariate distributions whose means differ by more than 4 standard deviations: the overlap is quite small, and the probabilities of misclassification are correspondingly small. An alternative formula for D^2, equivalent to (10.43), is:

$$D^2 = \sum b_i(\bar{x}_{Ai} - \bar{x}_{Bi}). \qquad (10.47)$$

(b) Likelihood rule

If there were only one variable, x, following a continuous distribution in each group, it would be natural to allocate an individual to the group which gave the higher probability density for the observed value of x; another way of expressing this is to say that the allocation is to the group with the higher likelihood. If there are several xs we cannot easily depict the probability density, but given the mathematical form of the distribution of the xs this density, or likelihood, can be calculated. One particular form of distribution is called the *multivariate normal distribution*; it implies, among other things, that each x separately follows a normal distribution and that all regressions of one variable on any set of other variables are linear. If the xs followed multivariate normal distributions with the same variances and correlations for group A as for group B, but with different means, the ratio of the likelihoods of A and B would be found to depend on a linear function

$$z = \beta_1 x_1 + \beta_2 x_2 + \ldots + \beta_p x_p,$$

and the βs would be estimated from the two initial samples precisely by the bs as calculated in (a). The rule described above, in which the allocation is to A or B according as $z > z_0$ or $z < z_0$, is equivalent to asking which of the two groups is estimated to have the higher likelihood.

In practice, of course, multivariate distributions are not normal, and are perhaps less likely to be nearly normal than are univariate distributions. Nevertheless, the discriminant function (10.42) is likely to be a good indication of the relative likelihoods of the two groups.

(c) Regression with a dummy dependent variable

Suppose we define a variable y which takes the value 1 in group A and 0 in group B. Putting all the observations into one group, we could do the multiple regression of y on $x_1, x_2, \ldots, x_p$. This would give a linear function of the xs which would predict the observed values of y as well as possible. If the multiple correlation coefficient is reasonably high, the predicted values of y for groups A and B should therefore be rather well separated (clustering near the observed values of 1 and 0). The estimated regression function can be shown to be (apart from a constant factor) the same as the linear discriminant function obtained by method (a). This is a useful identity since method (c) can be carried out on a computer with a multiple regression program, whereas method (a) requires a special program.

A further advantage of the regression approach is that the usual variance ratio test for the significance of the multiple regression can be interpreted also as a valid test for the discriminant function. The null hypothesis is that in the two groups from which the samples are drawn the xs have exactly the same joint distribution; in that case, of course, no discrimination is possible. Furthermore, the usual t tests for the partial regression coefficients give a useful indication of the importance of particular variables in the discrimination.

Although multiple regression provides a useful way of calculating the discriminant function, it is important to realize that the usual model for multiple regression is no longer valid. Usually, in multiple regression, y is a random variable and the xs are arbitrary variables. In the present problem the xs are random variables and y is an arbitrary score characterizing the two groups. A related point is that the average value of y for a particular set of xs should not be interpreted as the probability that an individual with these xs falls in group A rather than in group B; if the regression equation were interpreted in this way it might lead to some predicted probabilities greater than 1 or less than 0.

The usual analysis of variance of y corresponding to the multiple regression analysis provides a useful method of estimating the generalized distance, D:

$$D^2 = \frac{(n_A + n_B)(n_A + n_B - 2)}{n_A n_B} \times \frac{\text{SSq due to regression}}{\text{SSq about regression}}. \qquad (10.48)$$

Computer programs for the whole calculation are widely available and, as for all multivariate methods, the availability of appropriate software is generally essential. However, to illustrate the method, an example with two variables will be worked through.

Example 10.7

The data shown in Table 10.7 relate to 79 infants affected by haemolytic disease of the newborn, of whom 63 survived and 16 died. For each infant there is recorded the cord haemoglobin concentration, x (measured in g/100 ml) and the bilirubin concentration, y (mg/100 ml). It is required to predict by means of these two measurements whether any particular infant is more likely to die or to survive.

We follow method (a). The within-groups covariance matrix and its inverse are

$$\begin{pmatrix} 8\cdot3641 & -1\cdot6851 \\ -1\cdot6851 & 1\cdot6061 \end{pmatrix}$$

and

$$\begin{pmatrix} 0\cdot151602 & 0\cdot159057 \\ 0\cdot159057 & 0\cdot789510 \end{pmatrix}.$$

The means, and their differences and means, are

	$\bar{x}$	$\bar{y}$
Survivals	13·897	3·090
Deaths	7·756	4·831
Difference, $S - D$	6·141	-1·741
Mean, $\frac{1}{2}(S + D)$	10·827	3·961

From (10.44),

$$b_1 = (0\cdot151602)(6\cdot141) + (0\cdot159057)(-1\cdot741) = 0\cdot6541$$
$$b_2 = (0\cdot159057)(6\cdot141) + (0\cdot789510)(-1\cdot741) = -0\cdot3978.$$

Table 10.7 Concentrations of haemoglobin and bilirubin for infants with haemolytic disease of the newborn (x haemoglobin (g/100 ml); y bilirubin (mg/100 ml))

Survivals ($n = 63$)

x	y	x	y	x	y	x	y
18·7	2·2	15·8	3·7	14·3	3·3	11·8	4·5
17·8	2·7	15·8	3·0	14·1	3·7	11·6	3·7
17·8	2·5	15·8	1·7	14·0	5·8	10·9	3·5
17·6	4·1	15·6	1·4	13·9	2·9	10·9	4·1
17·6	3·2	15·6	2·0	13·8	3·7	10·9	1·5
17·6	1·0	15·6	1·6	13·6	2·3	10·8	3·3
17·5	1·6	15·4	4·1	13·5	2·1	10·6	3·4
17·4	1·8	15·4	2·2	13·4	2·3	10·5	6·3
17·4	2·4	15·3	2·0	13·3	1·8	10·2	3·3
17·0	0·4	15·1	3·2	12·5	4·5	9·9	4·0
17·0	1·6	14·8	1·8	12·3	5·0	9·8	4·2
16·6	3·6	14·7	3·7	12·2	3·5	9·7	4·9
16·3	4·1	14·7	3·0	12·2	2·4	8·7	5·5
16·1	2·0	14·6	5·0	12·0	2·8	7·4	3·0
16·0	2·6	14·3	3·8	12·0	3·5	5·7	4·6
16·0	0·8	14·3	4·2	11·8	2·3		
						875·5	194·7

Deaths ($n = 16$)

x	y	x	y
15·8	1·8	7·1	5·6
12·3	5·6	6·7	5·9
9·5	3·6	5·7	6·2
9·4	3·8	5·5	4·8
9·2	5·6	5·3	4·8
8·8	5·6	5·3	2·8
7·6	4·7	5·1	5·8
7·4	6·8	3·4	3·9
		124·1	77·3

Sums of squares and products within groups

	S_{xx}	S_{xy}	S_{yy}
Survivals	500·6593	−108·4219	96·6943
Deaths	143·3794	−21·3281	26·9744
Pooled	644·0387	−129·7500	123·6687
Var./cov.	8·3641	−1·6851	1·6061

The discriminant function is

$$z = 0.6541x - 0.3978y. \tag{10.49}$$

From (10.46),

$$z_0 = (0.6541)(10.827) + (-0.3978)(3.961) = 5.506.$$

The symmetric allocation rule would predict survival if $z > 5.506$ and death if $z < 5.506$.

The position is shown in Fig. 10.6, where the diagonal line represents critical points for which $z = z_0$. It is clear from Fig. 10.6 that discrimination by z is much better than by y alone, but hardly better than by x alone. This is confirmed by a count of the numbers of individuals misclassified by x alone (using a critical value of 10.83), by y alone (critical value 3.96) and by z:

	Group to which individual is allocated						
Actual	By x		By y		By z		
group	S	D	S	D	S	D	Total
S	53	10	47	16	54	9	63
D	2	14	5	11	2	14	16

It seems, therefore, that discrimination between deaths and survivals is improved little, if at all, by the use of bilirubin concentrations in addition to those of haemoglobin.

To calculate D, we find using (10.47)

$$D = (0.6541)(6.141) + (-0.3978)(-1.741)$$

$$= 4.709,$$

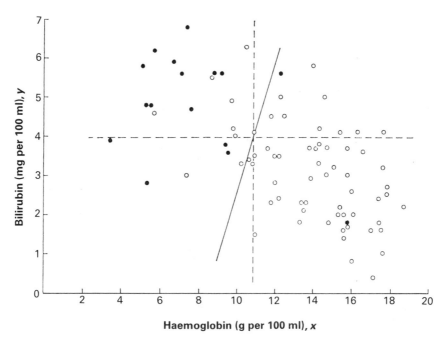

Fig. 10.6. Scatter diagram of haemoglobin and bilirubin values for infants with haemolytic disease (Table 10.7) showing a line of discrimination between deaths (●) and survivals (○).

and

$$D = \sqrt{4 \cdot 709} = 2 \cdot 17.$$

For two normal distributions with equal variance, separated by 2·17 standard deviations, the proportion of observations misclassified by the midpoint between the means would be the single tail area beyond a normal deviate of 1·085, which is 0·139. As it happens the proportion of misclassification by z is given above as $11/79 = 0 \cdot 139$, but the closeness of the agreement is fortuitous!

The reader with access to a multiple regression program is invited to analyse these data by method (c), using (10.48) as an alternative formula for D^2.

If the proportions of survivors and deaths in the sample were considered typical of the individuals to whom the discrimination rule would be applied in the future then the cut-point would be increased by $\ln(16/63)$, i.e. by $-1 \cdot 371$, to 4·135. This would reduce the number of individuals misclassified in the sample to eight, but four of these would be deaths misclassified as survivors. If it were more important to classify probable deaths correctly, perhaps to give them more intensive care, then the cut-point would be increased and the number of deaths misclassified as survivors would be reduced at the expense of a larger increase in the number of survivors misclassified as deaths.

In the discussion so far it has been assumed that it was known which variables should be included in the discriminant function (10.42). Usually a set of possible discriminatory variables is available and it is required to find the minimum number of such variables which contribute to the discrimination. Many computer programs include a stepwise procedure, similar to that in multiple regression (see p. 321), to achieve this.

The likelihood rule was derived assuming that the xs had a multivariate normal distribution. Although the method may prove adequate in some cases when this assumption breaks down, an alternative approach may be preferable. In particular, if the xs contain categorical variables, then the use of logistic regression (see §12.8) would be appropriate. The data of Example 10.7 are analysed using this approach on p. 430.

In most examples of discriminant analysis, there will be little point in testing the null hypothesis that the two samples are drawn from identical populations. The important question is *how* the populations differ. There are, though, some studies, particularly those in which two treatments are compared by multivariate data, in which a preliminary significance test is useful in indicating whether there is much point in further exploration of the data. Usually we are interested in possible differences in the mean values of the variates, and the appropriate test is based on Hotelling's two-sample T^2 statistic. This assumes that the data follow a multivariate normal distribution, but is reasonably robust against departures from normality.

Using the same notation as before, calculate

$$T^2 = \left(\frac{n_A n_B}{n_A + n_B}\right) D^2. \tag{10.50}$$

This is the square of the highest possible value of t that could be obtained in a two-sample t test for any linear combination of the p variables. If the null hypothesis is true,

$$\frac{(n_A + n_B - p - 1)}{(n_A + n_B - 2)p} T^2 \tag{10.51}$$

follows the F distribution on p and $n_A + n_B - p - 1$ DF. If $p = 1$, (10.51) reduces to the square of the usual t statistic.

In Example 10.7, there is no real point in carrying out a significance test, since Fig. 10.6 shows clearly that the two bivariate distributions differ significantly. However, as an illustration of the calculations, we have

$$T^2 = \left(\frac{63 \times 16}{79}\right) \times 4.709 = 60.08$$

and, since $p = 2$, $76T^2/(77 \times 2) = 29.65$ is referred to the F distribution on 2 and 76 DF, giving $P < 0.001$. The difference is highly significant, as expected. In most applications of Hotelling's T^2 test, it is useful to explore further any significant result by calculating the discriminant function to show the best way in which the variates combine to reveal the difference between the groups.

Paired data: Hotelling's one-sample T^2 statistic

In most problems of discrimination, particularly where the object is to obtain allocation rules, the individuals from the two populations will not be paired or matched in any way. However, in the related situations discussed earlier, where treatments are compared on multivariate data, the individual observations might well be paired. For example, two treatments might be administered on different occasions and several clinical responses observed for each treatment application; or, with a single treatment, observations might be made before and after the administration.

In studies of this type it is natural to work with the differences, either between two treatments or between the readings before and after treatment. Each subject will provide a multivariate set of differences, $d_1, d_2, \ldots, d_p$, and the natural questions to ask are (i) is there any evidence that the expected values of the differences are other than zero? and (ii) if so, what is the nature of these effects?

The procedure is a simple variant on the two-sample methods described above. Suppose there are n subjects, each providing a multivariate set of p differences, d_i. The corrected sums of squares and products of the ds are calculated in the usual way, and the estimated variances and covariances are obtained by dividing by $n - 1$. The inverse matrix is obtained, with general term c_{ij}. The coefficients b_i in the discriminant function are calculated as in (10.44), but with the terms $\bar{x}_{Ai} - \bar{x}_{Bi}$ in (10.44) replaced by the mean differences $\bar{d}_i$. The test statistic is then obtained as

$$T^2 = n \sum b_i \bar{d}_i. \tag{10.52}$$

Finally, if the null hypothesis is true,

$$\frac{(n-p)T^2}{p(n-1)} \tag{10.53}$$

follows the F distribution on p and $n - p$ DF. If the result is significant, the coefficients in the discriminant function will indicate the way in which the variates combine to yield the most significant effect.

Example 10.8

Table 10.8 shows selected data from a small pilot trial to compare the efficacy and safety of various treatments to prevent anaemia in premature infants during the first few months of life. The table refers to 10 infants receiving one particular treatment, and presents measurements on four variables made when the infants were aged about 25 and 50 days. Haemoglobin is a measure of the efficacy of treatment, while the three other variables are recorded for monitoring the safety of the treatment.

Measurements at younger ages show clear trends in some of these and other physiological measurements, but between 25 and 50 days the position seems more stable. The purpose of the present analysis is to ask whether there is clear evidence of change during this later period, and if so to identify its nature.

The lower part of Table 10.8 shows the changes, d_i, in the variables from 25 to 50 days. The log transformation for leucocytes was carried out because this variable (particularly in other data sets) shows positive skewness (see §11.3). The multiplying factors for d_2 and d_3 were introduced to avoid too great a disparity in the ranges of magnitude of the four measures of change.

As a preliminary step we note the means and standard errors of the four differences, together with the results of t tests for the hypotheses that the population mean of each difference is zero:

	Mean ± SE (mean)	t	P
d_1	-0.53 ± 0.46	-1.15	0.28
d_2	-0.03 ± 0.39	-0.08	0.94
d_3	-0.59 ± 0.49	-1.20	0.26
d_4	3.10 ± 1.95	1.59	0.15

Table 10.8 Efficacy and safety measurements for 10 premature infants receiving treatment for the prevention of anaemia

Age (days):	Haemoglobin (g/dl)		Platelets ($\times 10^9$/l)		Leucocytes ($\times 10^9$/l)		Systolic blood pressure (mmHg)	
	25	50	25	50	25	50	25	50
Patient number								
1	10·5	10·5	700	596	8·0	9·8	71	65
2	10·4	11·4	363	370	16·0	7·6	54	68
3	10·4	10·2	456	645	10·9	16·1	67	69
4	15·6	13·3	260	301	8·6	8·0	77	82
5	16·3	13·9	387	385	8·4	11·1	60	60
6	11·2	10·2	375	431	13·1	12·6	65	75
7	11·8	10·3	472	337	15·0	10·4	71	69
8	12·8	12·8	469	244	16·2	9·9	61	63
9	10·3	9·1	381	505	16·3	13·0	72	70
10	8·9	11·2	526	539	11·8	8·7	57	65

Changes from day 25 to day 50

	Haemoglobin d_1	Platelets $\times 10^{-2}$ d_2	log Leucocytes $\times 10$, d_3	Systolic BP d_4
1	0·0	− 1·0	0·9	− 6
2	1·0	0·1	− 3·2	14
3	− 0·2	1·9	1·7	2
4	− 2·3	0·4	− 0·3	5
5	− 2·4	0·0	1·2	0
6	− 1·0	0·6	− 0·2	10
7	− 1·5	− 1·4	− 1·6	− 2
8	0·0	− 2·2	− 2·1	2
9	− 1·2	1·2	− 1·0	− 2
10	2·3	0·1	− 1·3	8

None of the mean differences is individually significant, but three exceed their standard errors, and in view of possible correlations between the four differences it seems worth pursuing a multivariate test.

The matrix of covariances between the d_i is

$$\begin{pmatrix} 2·1401 & − 0·1188 & − 0·8941 & 3·5922 \\ − 0·1188 & 1·4868 & 0·7914 & 1·8811 \\ − 0·8941 & 0·7914 & 2·4099 & − 4·6011 \\ 3·5922 & 1·8811 & − 4·6011 & 37·8778 \end{pmatrix}$$

and its inverse is

$$
\begin{pmatrix}
0{\cdot}59389 & 0{\cdot}03210 & 0{\cdot}12918 & -0{\cdot}04223 \\
0{\cdot}03210 & 1{\cdot}20462 & -0{\cdot}65584 & -0{\cdot}14254 \\
0{\cdot}12918 & -0{\cdot}65584 & 0{\cdot}93359 & 0{\cdot}13373 \\
-0{\cdot}04223 & -0{\cdot}14254 & 0{\cdot}13373 & 0{\cdot}05373
\end{pmatrix}.
$$

Both matrices are obtained by standard computer programs.

The coefficients b_i in the discriminant function are obtained by cross-multiplying the rows of the inverse matrix by the column of means, giving $(-0{\cdot}5228, -0{\cdot}1081, -0{\cdot}1851, 0{\cdot}1143)$. From (10.52), with $n = 10$,

$$T^2 = 7{\cdot}439,$$

and, with $p = 4$ in (10.53), the test statistic is

$$6 \times 7{\cdot}439/36 = 1{\cdot}24.$$

For $F = 1{\cdot}24$ on 4 and 6 DF, $P = 0{\cdot}39$. There is thus no strong evidence of departures from zero in the set of four mean differences.

Note that the main contributions to the test statistic come from the variables d_1 and d_4, which are positively correlated but have means with opposite signs. If the analysis is performed with these two variables alone, the test statistic (as F on 2 and 8 DF) becomes $2{\cdot}80$, with $P = 0{\cdot}12$. However, the enhanced significance is misleading, since these variables were selected only after the first analysis had been performed, as being likely to be the most sensitive pair.

Discrimination with more than two groups: MANOVA

The linear discriminant function can be generalized to the situation where there are $k(>2)$ groups in two different ways. The first approach leads to what are known as *canonical variates*. We saw from (10.43) that when $k = 2$ the linear discriminant function maximizes the ratio of the difference in means *between* the groups to the standard deviation *within* groups. A natural generalization of this criterion is to maximize the ratio of the SSq between groups to the SSq within groups. This requirement is found to lead to a standard technique of matrix algebra—the calculation of *eigenvalues* or *latent roots* of a matrix. The appropriate equation, in fact, has several solutions. One solution, corresponding to the highest latent root, gives the coefficients in the linear function which maximizes the ratio of SSqs. This is called the first *canonical variate*, W_1. If one wanted as good discrimination as possible from one linear function, this would be the one to choose. The second canonical variate, W_2, is the function with the highest ratio of SSqs, subject to the condition that it is uncorrelated with W_1 both between and within groups. Similarly, W_3 gives the highest ratio subject to being uncorrelated with W_1 and W_2. The number of canonical variates is the smaller of p or $k - 1$. Thus the linear discriminant function (10.42) is for $k = 2$ the first and only canonical variate.

If most of the variation between groups is explained by W_1 and W_2, the ratios of SSqs corresponding to the later canonical variates will be relatively small. It is then convenient to plot the data as a scatter diagram with W_1 and W_2 as the two axes. This will give a clear picture of any tendency of the groups to form clusters. It may also be interesting to see which of the original variables are strongly represented in each canonical variate. The magnitudes of the coefficients depend on the scales of measurement, so their relative sizes are of no great interest, although it should be noted that the method is scale-invariant. Some computer programs print the correlations between each canonical variate and each x_i, a feature which helps to give some insight into the structure of the canonical variates. Discrimination takes place in the two-dimensional space defined by W_1 and W_2 and an individual is allocated to the group for which the distance between the individual's data point and the group mean is least.

As in the two-group situation, the identification of canonical variates is usually more important than a significance test of the null hypothesis that the populations are identical. Nevertheless, such a test may be useful, particularly as an initial screening step. The appropriate method for testing changes in means of multivariate normal data is the *multivariate analysis of variance* (*MANOVA*). We shall not describe this in detail here; books such as Krzanowski (1988) give full descriptions. In contrast to the two-sample Hotelling's T^2, there are in the general case ($k > 2$) several alternative test statistics, which fortunately usually lead to similar conclusions. MANOVA can, like the univariate analysis of variance, be used for more complex data structures, such as factorial designs, and can be extended to allow for covariates, as a generalization of the analysis of covariance. Computer programs usually give details of the significance tests for the various factors, and also identify the relevant canonical variates. For an example of the use of MANOVA in the analysis of data from dental clinical trials, see Geary *et al.* (1992).

Returning to the problem of discrimination, a second generalization of the linear discriminant function is to use approach (b) of p. 360 and allocate an individual to the group with highest likelihood. This is equivalent to forming the likelihood ratio of every pair of groups. There are $\frac{1}{2}k(k - 1)$ pairs of groups, but only $k - 1$ likelihood ratios are needed. For example, if L_j is the log likelihood for the jth group, we could take

$$
\begin{aligned}
Z_1 &= L_1 - L_2 \\
Z_2 &= L_2 - L_3 \\
&\vdots \\
Z_{k-1} &= L_{k-1} - L_k,
\end{aligned}
$$

and any difference between pairs of L_js (which is, of course, the log of the corresponding likelihood ratio) can be expressed in terms of the Zs. This could be done by calculating linear discriminant functions by the methods given earlier, for each of the $k - 1$ pairs of groups. The only modification is to calculate pooled within-groups variances and covariances from all k groups, and to use the inverse of this pooled matrix in the calculation of each discriminant function. The procedure can be simplified by calculating a discriminant score for each group. This score is the log likelihood, omitting any terms common to all groups. Allocation is then to the group with the highest score. The method is also equivalent to allocating an individual to the group with nearest mean, in the sense of generalized distance. Computer programs exist for the whole procedure.

This likelihood ratio approach is more appropriate than that of canonical variates if the main purpose is to form an allocation rule. If the purpose is to gain insight into the way in which groups differ, using as few dimensions as possible, then canonical variates are the more appropriate method.

Although the two methods do not usually give identical results, there is a close relationship between them. Using the first canonical variate gives the same discrimination as the likelihood method if the group means are collinear in p-dimensional space. Thus, as noted earlier, the two methods are identical for $k = 2$ because the two group means may be regarded as collinear. If, for example, $k = 3$ and $p > 1$, there will be $k - 1 = 2$ canonical variates, W_1 and W_2, and 2 independent likelihood ratio discriminators, say $Z_1 = L_1 - L_2$ and $Z_2 = L_2 - L_3$. (Note that $L_3 - L_1 = -(Z_1 + Z_2)$.) If the observations are plotted (i) with W_1 and W_2 as axes, and (ii) with Z_1 and Z_2 as axes, it will be found that the scatter diagrams are essentially similar, differing only in the orientation and scaling of the axes. Thus, the use of both canonical variates is equivalent to the likelihood approach. In general, using $k - 1$ canonical variates gives the same discrimination as the likelihood approach. However, the idea behind using canonical variates is to reduce the dimensionality and the only advantage of this approach is if it is possible to use just a few variates without any material loss in discriminating ability. For further discussion of this point see Marriott (1974).

Scoring systems, using canonical variates

Suppose that a variable is measured on a p-point scale from 1 to p. For example, a patient's response to treatment may be graded in categories ranging from 'much worse' (scored 1) to 'much better' (scored p). This sequence of equidistant integers may not be the best scale on which to analyse the data. The best method of scoring will depend on the criterion we wish to optimize. Suppose, for example, that patients were classified into k treatment groups. It would be reasonable to choose a system of scoring which maximized differences between treatments as compared with those within treatments. For this purpose consider a set of p dummy variables, $x_1, x_2, \ldots, x_p$, such that if a patient is graded into category j, his/her value of x_j is 1 and that of all the other x_is is 0. Now choose the first canonical variate of the xs, say

$$g = l_1 x_1 + l_2 x_2 + \ldots + l_p x_p.$$

Then g will take the value l_j in category j, and will define the system which maximizes the ratio of the Between-Groups SSq to the Within-Groups SSq. There is, however, no guarantee that the scores follow in magnitude the natural order of the categories. Bradley *et al.* (1962) have shown how the ratio of SSq can be maximized subject to there being no reversals of the natural order.

The investigator might want a scoring system which was as closely correlated as possible with some other variable. For instance, in dose–response experiments in serology, a reaction may be classified as $- -, -, 0, +$ or $+ +$, and it may be useful to replace these categories by a score which forms a good linear regression on the log dose of some reagent. The approach is similar to that in the previous problem, the ratio of SSq to be maximized being that of the SSq due to regression to the Total SSq (for an example see Ipsen, 1955).

Cluster analysis

Component analysis and factor analysis are 'internal' methods of analysis, in that the individuals are not classified by any criteria other than the variables used in the analysis. In some problems no initial grouping is imposed on the data, but the object of the analysis is to see whether the individuals can be formed into any natural system of groups. The number of groups may not be specified in advance. The individuals could, of course, be grouped in an entirely arbitrary way, but the investigator seeks a system such that the individuals within a group resemble each other (in the values taken by the variables) more than do individuals in different groups. This specification is rather vague, and there are several ways of defining groups to make it more explicit. In addition to chapters in Chatfield and Collins (1980), Kendall (1980) and Krzanowski (1988), an introductory text is Everitt (1980), whilst a more mathematical treatment is in Mardia *et al.* (1979, Chapter 13).

Two broad approaches may be distinguished. The first is to do a principal component analysis of all the data. If most of the variation is explained by the first two or three components, the essential features of the multidimensional scatter can be seen by a two-dimensional scatter diagram, or perhaps a two-dimensional representation of a three-dimensional model. Any clustering of the individuals into groups would then become apparent—at least in its main features—although the precise definitions of the groups might be open to question. If the scatter is not largely represented by the first two or three components, the method will be very much less useful.

A closely related approach is that of *correspondence analysis* (extensively developed in France under the title '*analyse des correspondances*'). Here the variables are categorical, and can be represented by dummy, or indicator, variables, as on p. 336. Linear functions of the indicator variables are chosen in such a way that the multidimensional scatter is most closely approximated by a diagram in a small number of dimensions (normally two). The individuals in a particular response category can be represented by a point in this diagram, and it may then be possible to identify interesting clusters of individuals. A very full account is given by Greenacre (1984), who lists (pp. 317, 318) some references to medical applications.

The second approach, that of *numerical taxonomy*, is discussed in detail by Sneath and Sokal (1973). The idea here is to calculate an index of similarity or dissimilarity for each pair of individuals. The precise definition of this index will depend on the nature of the variables. If all the variables are recorded on a continuous scale, a suitable index of dissimilarity might be the distance in multidimensional space between the two points whose coordinates are the values of the variables of two individuals; this index is the Euclidean distance. If, as in some clinical applications, the variables are dichotomies (expressing the presence or absence of some feature), a suitable similarity index might be the proportion of variables for which the two individuals show the same response. Alternative measures are discussed fully by Sneath and Sokal. When the similarity indices have been calculated, some form of sorting is carried out so that pairs of individuals with high values of the index are sorted into the same group. These procedures can be effected by a computer once a method of forming clusters has been chosen.

A medical application which suggests itself is the definition of a system of related diseases. Hayhoe *et al.* (1964), for instance, have studied the classification of the acute leukaemias from this point of view. Whether the methods are really useful will depend largely on whether the classifications subsequently perform any useful function. For example, in the definition of disease categories, one would hope that any system suggested might lead to suggestions about aetiology, recommendations about future treatment, or at the very least a useful system for tabulating vital statistics. One of the problems in medical applications is how to define generally any groups that may have been formed by a clustering procedure. Lists of particular individuals placed in the groups in any one study are, of course, of insufficient general interest, and some more general definitions are required.

Cluster analysis may also be used to cluster variables rather than individuals, that is, to arrange the variables into groups such that the variables in each group measure a similar or closely related feature of the individuals whilst the separate groups represent different features. This objective is similar to that of principal component analysis and, where the variables are measured on a continuous scale, principal component analysis is probably to be preferred. For example, if cluster analysis is applied to the data of Example 10.6, the arrangements of variables into clusters is very similar to the groups extracted using principal components.

The different methods of defining clusters will generally give different results when applied to the same data. The most appropriate method in a particular case depends on the structure in the data, which is often unknown. In effect each method imposes implicit assumptions on the type of clustering expected and if these assumptions are invalid the results may be meaningless. For this reason we suggest that cluster analysis should only be used in circumstances where other multivariate methods are inappropriate, and the results must be interpreted with a great deal of caution.

Finally, the method of cluster analysis should not be confused with the problem of determining whether cases of disease occur in clusters in time, space or families. This problem gives rise to different methods discussed in §16.5.

Multidimensional scaling

Suppose data are available on a set of individuals and it is possible to derive an index of similarity, or dissimilarity, between every pair of individuals. This index would be of the same type as those considered in the discussion of cluster analysis. Then multidimensional scaling is a method of arranging the individuals in a space of a few dimensions so that the distances between the points in this space are nearly the same as the measures of dissimilarity. In particular, if two dimensions provide an adequate representation then it is possible to plot the individuals on a two-dimensional graph, and examination of how the individuals are arranged on this graph might lead to some useful interpretation. For example, the individuals might occur in clusters.

The method is, like many multivariate methods, an attempt to reduce dimensionality. If the dissimilarities are measured using a set of continuous variables, then the method of principal components has a similar aim.

For more details on this method see Chatfield and Collins (1980).

Concluding remarks

All the multivariate methods rely on a large amount of computation and have only been widely applicable in the last two decades. Computer programs have made generally accessible several methods of analysis which previously entailed heroic feats of arithmetic. There is a risk that multivariate methods may be applied blindly in circumstances different from those for which they were designed, and that incorrect conclusions may be drawn from them.

The majority of data sets are multivariate and therefore multivariate analysis of some sort is often required. In choosing an approach it is essential to keep uppermost in mind the objective of the research and only to use a method of analysis if it is appropriate for that objective. In many cases the objective is to examine the relationship between an outcome variable and a number of possible explanatory variables. In this case the method of multiple regression (§10.1) is appropriate. If the outcome variable is binary, then the conceptually similar method of multiple logistic regression (§12.8) would be required. Discriminant analysis is often used in the latter case but would only be the most appropriate method if there were some reason to classify future individuals.

Of the methods discussed in this section the most widely used in medical research are principal components, factor analysis and discriminant analysis. Some of the other methods we have mentioned briefly not because we think they have wide applicability in medical research, but to provide readers with some indication of their characteristics since their use is sometimes reported in the literature. There is overlap in the aims of several of the methods and the temptation of trying several methods in the hope that something 'of interest' may emerge should be resisted.

10.6 Time series

Some statistical investigations involve long series of observations on one or more variables, made at successive points of time. Three medical examples are: (i) a series of mortality rates from a certain cause of death, recorded in a particular community over a period of, say, 100 years; (ii) haemodynamic measurements on a pregnant woman, made at intervals of 1 minute during a period of 1 hour; and (iii) a continuous trace from an electroencephalogram (EEG) over 5 minutes. The widespread use of automatic analysers and other devices for the automatic recording of clinical measurements has led to an enormous increase in the output of data of this sort—often much more data than can conveniently be analysed and interpreted.

The first purpose of a statistical analysis of time series data is to describe the series by a model which provides an appropriate description of the systematic and random variation. This may be useful merely as a summary description of a large and complex set of data, for example by identifying any points of time at which changes in the characteristics of the series occurred, or by noting any periodic effects. Or it may be necessary to describe the structure of the series before any valid inferences can be made about the effects of possible explanatory variables. Again, some features revealed by a statistical analysis, such as a periodic effect, or a relation between movements in several time series, may provide insight into biological mechanisms.

Time series analysis may, however, have a more operational role to play. In the monitoring of clinical measurements, one may wish to predict future observations by taking into account recent changes in the series, perhaps taking remedial action to forestall dangerously large changes. Prediction and control is important also in vital statistics, for example in the monitoring of congenital malformations.

The problem in time series analysis can be regarded as one of regression—the measurement in question being a dependent variable, with time as an explanatory variable—but the methods outlined in Chapters 5 and 9, and in earlier sections of this chapter, are unlikely to be very useful. In the first place the trends exhibited by long-term series are unlikely to be representable by the simple mathematical functions considered hitherto. Secondly, although individual observations are likely to show apparently random fluctuations about any long-term trend, these deviations are unlikely to be independently distributed. If one observation on a physiological variable is somewhat above a general trend, it is likely that neighbouring observations will also be somewhat higher than expected. This form of correlation between the random components of neighbouring observations is called *serial correlation*. Sometimes the effect may be in the opposite direction. In a series of notifications of an infectious disease in successive years, a high value in one year may be associated with a low value in adjacent years, because a high proportion of the population acquires immunity during years of high incidence. Sometimes, also, the apparent effect of serial correlation may extend to observations separated by several time units, although it is usually found that the longer the 'lag' between paired observations, the lower in absolute magnitude is the serial correlation.

To overcome these problems a number of methods of statistical analysis have been developed. They are based on rather more complicated models than those underlying the simpler regression methods, and their details are too complex to be described at all fully here. We shall give a brief outline of one or two general approaches. For further details, see Chatfield (1989) or Diggle (1990).

It is convenient to distinguish between analyses in the *time domain* and those in the *frequency domain*. The two approaches are, in fact, mathematically equivalent, in that one form of analysis can be derived from the other. However, they emphasize different features of a time series and can usefully be considered separately. The time domain is concerned with relationships between observations at different times, in particular with serial correlations at different lags. In the frequency domain, the observations are regarded as being composed of contributions from periodic terms at different frequencies, and the analysis is concerned with the relative amplitudes at different frequencies, as in the spectral decomposition of light.

Before considering these two approaches further it is worth making one or two elementary points.

1 In the analysis of any time series it is good practice to plot the data before doing any computations. A visual inspection may reveal features of the data, such as heterogeneity of different sections or a grossly non-normal distribution, which

should affect the choice of method of analysis (in the latter case perhaps by suggesting an initial transformation of the data).

2 Look for extreme outliers, and enquire whether there are special reasons for any aberrant readings which may justifiably lead to their exclusion.

3 Many series exhibit an obvious long-term trend. It is often useful to remove this at the outset, either by fitting a linear or other simple curve or by taking differences between successive observations. Time series analysis may then be applied to the residuals from the fitted curve or the successive differences.

The time domain

An important class of models is that of *autoregressive series*. Here the expected value of the dependent variable at any time depends to some extent on the values at previous points of time. In the simplest model of this sort, the *first-order autoregressive* (or *Markov*) scheme, the dependence is only on the immediately preceding observation. If Y_t denotes the deviation from the long-run mean at time t, the first-order process may be expressed by the equation

$$Y_t = \rho Y_{t-1} + \varepsilon_t,$$

where the ε_t are random errors, independently distributed around a mean of zero. If the series is to be stationary, i.e. to retain the same statistical properties throughout time, the coefficient ρ must lie between -1 and $+1$. If the variance of Y_t is σ^2, the variance of ε_t will be $\sigma^2(1 - \rho^2)$. The correlation between adjacent values of Y_t is ρ, and that between values separated by a lag of k time units is ρ^k. Thus, values of ρ near $+1$ lead to series in which observations at neighbouring points of time tend to be close together, while longer stretches of the series exhibit wandering characteristics. This type of behaviour illustrates the danger of applying standard statistical methods to different portions of a time series. With a high value of ρ, it would be quite easy to find two sets, each of, say, five adjacent observations, such that there was relatively little variation within each set, but quite a large difference between the two means. A two-sample t test might show a 'significant' difference, but the probability level would have no useful meaning because the assumption of independence which underlies the t test is invalid. This point is particularly important when the two sets differ in some specific feature, such as the occurrence of an intervention of some sort between the two time periods. A 'significant' difference cannot be ascribed to the effect of the intervention, since it may be merely a reflection of the structure of a time series which, in the long run, is stationary. By contrast, values of ρ near -1 show marked oscillation between neighbouring values, as was indicated as a possibility on p. 376.

The first-order process has been suggested by Wilson *et al.* (1981) as a representation of repeated blood pressure measurements taken at 5-minute intervals.

However, their analysis dealt only with short series, and it is not clear that the model would be appropriate for longer series. More general autoregressive series, with dependence on more than one preceding reading, were used by Marks (1982) in a study of the relations between different hormone levels in rats receiving hormone injections following oophorectomy. This paper illustrates the way in which autoregressive models, in which preceding values act as explanatory variables, can also incorporate other explanatory variables such as the current or earlier values in other time series.

Another broad class of models is that of *moving-average* schemes. If x_1, x_2, x_3, etc. are independent random variables, the quantities

$$y_2 = \tfrac{1}{3}(x_1 + x_2 + x_3), \; y_3 = \tfrac{1}{3}(x_2 + x_3 + x_4), \text{ etc.}$$

are examples of simple moving averages. Note that y_2 and y_3 are correlated, because of the common terms x_2 and x_3, but y_2 and y_5 are not correlated, because they have no terms in common. The y_t series is a simple example of a moving-average scheme, more general schemes being obtainable by altering the number of xs in each y and also their weights. Although time series are not usually formed explicitly by taking simple moving averages, observed series may nevertheless be found to behave in a similar way, showing positive correlations between a short range of neighbouring observations. A wide variety of different models for time series may be obtained by combining auto-regressive and moving-average features. For a discussion of some ways of distinguishing between different models, see Box and Jenkins (1976).

Reference was made earlier to the problem of monitoring time series of clinical and other measurements with a view to the detection of changes in the statistical pattern. Most medical applications have adapted methods derived from industrial quality control, in which observations are usually assumed to vary independently. Thus, Weatherall and Haskey (1976) describe methods for monitoring the incidence of congenital malformations, using quality control charts designed to detect outlying readings, and cumulative sum (cusum) methods designed to detect changes in the mean incidence rate. In this application the random variation may be assumed to follow the Poisson distribution. Rowlands *et al.* (1983) describe the application of similar methods to control data used in routine radioimmunoassays of progesterone. In many situations the assumption of serial independence will not be valid. Smith *et al.* (1983) and Trimble *et al.* (1983) describe a Bayesian approach to the monitoring of plasma creatinine values in individual patients following a kidney transplant. By formulating a specific model for their data they provide posterior probabilities that, at any stage, the process is in a state of steady evolution, that there has been a change in the level of response, or in the slope, or that the current observation is an outlier.

The frequency domain

In this approach the time series is decomposed into a number of periodic components of a sinusoidal form, as in the periodic regression model of §10.3. Inferences are then made about the amplitudes of waves of different frequencies. The first approach to be discussed here, harmonic analysis, is concerned with periodic fluctuations with predetermined frequencies. The second approach, spectral analysis, allows the whole frequency band to be studied simultaneously.

Harmonic analysis

If k observations are available at equally spaced points of time, the whole set of data can be reproduced exactly in terms of k parameters, namely one parameter for the general mean and $k - 1$ parameters representing the amplitude and phase of a series of sinusoidal curves. If k is odd there will be $\frac{1}{2}(k - 1)$ of these components; if k is even there will be $\frac{1}{2}k$ components, one of which has a predetermined phase. The periods of these components are (in terms of the time interval between observations) k, $k/2$, $k/3$, $k/4$, and so on. If the observations are supposed to follow a trend with less than the full set of parameters, and if the random variance is known or can be estimated, the amplitudes of different components can be tested for significance so that simple models with fewer parameters can be regarded as providing an adequate description of the data.

Example 10.9

Pocock (1974) describes a harmonic analysis of a 5-year series of weekly records of sickness absence in an industrial concern. There were $k = 261$ weekly observations. Periods of $261/j$ will be fractions of a year if j is a multiple of 5 ($j = 5$ being a complete year). Collectively, therefore, these frequencies represent a 'seasonal' trend, repeated in each of the 5 years. Other frequencies with significant amplitudes represent significant departures from the overall seasonal pattern in particular years. Significance tests can be carried out on the plausible assumption that random variation follows a Poisson distribution, the variance of which can be estimated by the overall mean. In Fig. 10.7, the irregular line shows the seasonal trend, composed of 26 frequencies. The smooth curve is a single sinusoidal curve with a period of 1 year. A comparison of the two curves shows that the seasonal trend is nearly sinusoidal, but that there are clear departures from the simple curve, particularly at annual holiday periods.

Spectral analysis

Here the time series is effectively decomposed into an infinite number of periodic components, each of infinitesimal amplitude, so the purpose of the analysis is to

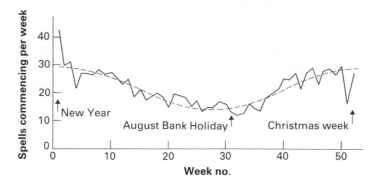

Fig. 10.7. The estimated seasonal trend in weekly spells of sickness absence (1960–64) (from Pocock, 1974).

estimate the contributions of components in certain ranges of frequency. A spectral analysis may show that contributions to the fluctuations in the time series come from a continuous range of frequencies, and the pattern of spectral densities may suggest a particular time-domain representation. Or the spectral analysis may suggest one or two dominant frequencies, leading to a subsequent harmonic analysis. A further possibility is that the spectrum may be a mixture of discrete and continuous components, as, for example, in a time series in which a harmonic term is combined with an autoregressive error term.

Various features of a spectral decomposition may provide useful summary statistics for a time series. Gevins (1980), for instance, reviews a considerable body of work in which spectral analyses of series of human brain electrical potentials have been used to discriminate between different clinical states or as a basis for various forms of pattern recognition and cluster analysis.

10.7 Repeated measurements and growth curves

Many investigations are characterized by repeated measurements of the same type, made on each of a number of subjects at successive points of time. Three examples of such data are as follows.

1 Measurements of respiratory function at three successive hours after application of a bronchoconstricting agent. The subjects may have been randomly assigned to receive different doses of a bronchodilator.

2 Blood pressure measurements on the same patients on five successive days.

3 Physical measurements on schoolchildren at four successive annual examinations.

Small series of observations of this sort, on any one subject, may show a smooth trend, which may or may not be consistent over different subjects, and they will almost certainly show some degree of random variation. However many of the methods of analysis described in earlier chapters are not strictly applicable because the random fluctuations on successive occasions on the same subject are unlikely to be independent. Each series is, in fact, a time series, but the methods outlined in §10.6 are not likely to be very useful because the series are typically too short for appropriate models to be identified.

We discuss briefly here some approaches which may be followed in different situations. For other useful general discussions, see Oldham (1968) and Healy (1981).

Treatments varying with time

In many investigations the different occasions on which measurements are made provide the opportunity to apply different treatments, and the main purpose of the analysis is to compare the effects of these treatments. If the treatments are administered in a random order for each subject, it is always possible to regard the experiment as having a randomized block design, with subjects as 'blocks' and occasions as 'plots'; the methods of analysis described in §8.1 may then be applied.

However, if there are systematic differences in response on different occasions, it may be advantageous to take this source of variation into account in the analysis. With two treatments and two occasions the design is the simple cross-over discussed in §8.2. When there are more than two treatments and periods Latin square designs are often appropriate, with subjects as 'rows', occasions as 'columns' and treatments playing their usual role. As was emphasized in §8.4, the element of randomization in the choice of a particular Latin square ensures that the inferences about treatment effects are valid, whether or not the response follows an additive model.

Treatments not changing with time

In many other investigations each subject receives the same treatment throughout the whole time period, during which responses are measured on different occasions. Different subjects may receive different treatments, or may be categorized in other ways. An example would be an experiment involving the glucose-tolerance test, in which blood-sugar measurements are made at hourly intervals after a glucose meal. The subjects may be categorized by their clinical diagnosis and also by the possible administration of oral hypo-glycaemic agents.

In studies of this sort the emphasis may be on (i) a precise description of the trend in response with time, or (ii) the contrasts between different groups of subjects, or both. We discuss cases (i) and (ii) separately.

Time trends and growth curves

Two examples of this type of study were mentioned briefly in the reference to longitudinal surveys in §6.2: the growth and development of children over a 10-year period, and the changes in blood pressure during pregnancy. Where there is a clear and systematic trend in the response with time, this trend is often referred to as the *growth curve*. The trend may be approximately linear, but frequently there will be clear evidence of curvature and a natural suggestion is that a low-order polynomial should be fitted. However, the methods described in §10.3 are not immediately applicable, because of the possible serial correlation. Simple methods, such as the fitting of polynomials to the mean responses at different time-points, are likely to provide a reasonable estimate of the average trend, but will not give a correct estimate of its precision. Two general approaches are as follows.

1 Separate polynomials may be fitted to the responses for each subject, e.g. by using orthogonal polynomials (§10.3). The linear, quadratic and, if necessary, higher-order terms may be averaged over subjects, and the overall growth curve built up from these average terms. The precision of this average curve can be worked out by standard methods, but it must be remembered that any two components, such as the mean response and the linear term, will in general be correlated; their correlation will be the same as the observed correlation between these components in different subjects.

Darby and Fearn (1979) adopted a similar approach in a longitudinal study of blood pressure in children. They used Bayesian methods, and were able to show that their analysis provided much better predictions of future readings for individual children than were obtained from simple regression lines for each child separately. This is because of the large random error associated with extrapolations from regression lines fitted to small series of observations.

2 The set of observations for any one subject on different occasions may be regarded as a single multivariate observation. The variances and covariances of the responses on different occasions can be estimated directly from the data. If a polynomial is fitted to each subject's data, the coefficients of the various terms (linear, quadratic, etc.) are linear functions of the original observations, and their variances and covariances can also be obtained. The coefficients for the average curve may be obtained by averaging the corresponding values for individual subjects, and the standard error of the estimated mean response at any time-point may be calculated. Details are given by Grizzle and Allen (1969) and Morrison (1976).

A simple variant on this procedure was suggested by Hills (1968). If the overall trend is linear, the first differences (i.e. differences between successive observations) should be about equal, apart from random fluctuations, and the second differences (i.e. differences between first differences) should be near zero on the average. Similarly, if the trend is quadratic, the third differences should be near zero on the average. The appropriateness of adding additional terms to a polynomial can therefore be tested by assessing the average departure from zero of differences of increasing order. This can be achieved by a standard multivariate test (Hotelling's T^2 test), provided that the random errors are not grossly non-normal.

Assessing the effects of between-subjects factors

Suppose there are m groups, each containing r subjects, and that each subject provides responses on k successive occasions. The main purpose of the investigation will probably lie in the comparison of the m groups, but the nature of the time trend may also be of interest. Superficially, this looks like a split-unit experiment, with subjects as 'units', and one may be tempted to allocate degrees of freedom (DF) in an analysis of variance as follows:

Between subjects	$mr - 1$
Groups	$m - 1$
Residual	$m(r - 1)$
Within subjects	$mr(k - 1)$
Occasions	$k - 1$
Groups × Occasions	$(m - 1)(k - 1)$
Residual	$m(r - 1)(k - 1)$.

However, the variance-ratio tests usually employed in a split-unit analysis (§8.6) are inappropriate here. The usual F test for groups, based on the 'Between subjects' part of the table, is valid, because the responses for different subjects are independent. However, the usual F tests from the 'Within subjects' part are invalid, because they do not allow for the possible serial correlation between the successive observations on the same subject. An approximate adjustment may be made by reducing the within-subjects DF (Box, 1954; Greenhouse and Geisser, 1959). More precise multivariate methods are described by Greenhouse and Geisser (1959) and Morrison (1976).

A common method of analysis is to carry out a separate analysis at each time at which measurements are made. This approach is not usually appropriate since it leads to a multiplicity of comparisons, takes no account of the fact that the same individuals have been measured at each time, and ignores correlations between successive observations in the same subject (Matthews *et al.*, 1990). In many situations a more revealing approach is to carry out univariate analyses on each of a number of indices summarizing important features of the time trend. For example, in an experiment in which pain threshold is measured immediately before administration of an analgesic, and at every hour for the following 3 hours, one might be particularly interested in (i) the final response, (ii) the linear trend in the last three responses, and (iii) the maximum increase above the pre-treatment response. For each of these summary indices a standard univariate analysis is appropriate. The outcomes of these analyses will not be independent, since the indices will, in general, be correlated. In the example mentioned above, all three indices are likely to be positively correlated. If all three analyses showed a significant difference between groups, therefore, they could not be regarded as providing three independent pieces of evidence. If necessary an overall assessment could be made using Hotelling's T^2 to compare two groups or MANOVA if there are more than two groups (§10.5). Another example of a summary measure is where the concentration of a drug is measured at intervals over a period of time. The total uptake of the drug may be of interest and can be measured by the area under the response curve for each subject (Matthews *et al.*, 1990).

In a univariate analysis of any one summary index, the DF would be allocated as follows:

$$
\begin{array}{ll}
\text{Groups} & m - 1 \\
\text{Residual} & m(r - 1).
\end{array}
$$

If, as in the example above, the first reading on a subject is pretreatment, the groups would not be expected to differ significantly on this first occasion, although subsequent readings might be affected differentially by treatments. In that case, any index calculated from the second and subsequent readings could be analysed by an analysis of covariance, using the pretreatment reading as a covariate.

A useful discussion of analyses of this type is given by Yates (1982). The experiment discussed by Yates had no division of subjects into groups, but it had the additional feature that each of r subjects provided a set of k repeated measurements at each of s levels of a certain factor (in that case, ambient temperature). The DF for any summary index are:

$$
\begin{array}{ll}
\text{Subjects} & r - 1 \\
\text{Temperatures} & s - 1 \\
\text{Residual} & (r - 1)(s - 1).
\end{array}
$$

A standard randomized block analysis would be valid provided that the temperatures were allocated in random order. Alternatively, as discussed at the beginning of this section, the temperatures could be applied in a systematic order, following a crossover or Latin square design.

Recent developments are given in papers presented at the 1986 Workshop on Methods for Longitudinal Data Analysis in Epidemiological and Clinical Studies, published in *Statistics in Medicine* (1988; **7 (1/2)**) and at the 1991 Symposium on Longitudinal Data Analysis, published in *Statistics in Medicine* (1992; **11 (14/15)**).

One way of incorporating correlation between successive measures is that of autoregressive modelling. Each value of the dependent variable, except the first, is regressed on variables of interest, with the value of the dependent variable on the previous occasion included as a covariate. The inclusion of this covariate means that the correlation of successive values within individuals is taken into account. Except at the end of each individual's series, each value of the dependent variable is in two regressions, first as the dependent variable and secondly as a covariate. Rosner and Muñoz (1988) showed that this method can be adapted to take account of missing and unequally spaced visits. Bergen *et al.* (1992) applied this method to data from up to five annual examinations of patients on neuroleptic medication, to relate the AIMS score, a measure used in studies of tardive dyskinesia, with a number of patient characteristics and the medication in each year interval. In this study 235 patients contributed 678 pairs of examinations; 646 of these pairs were 1 year apart and 32 were 2 years apart because of a missed visit. The regression coefficient on the value at the previous visit 1 year earlier, which is an estimate of the correlation between successive visits, was 0·6, and after allowing for this the effects of other variables were assessed.

Another approach is based on a *generalized estimating equation.* Zeger *et al.* (1988) illustrated this method on data consisting of four annual examinations of 527 children, where the objective of the analysis was to determine whether the probability that a child had respiratory infection was associated with the mother's smoking habits. Various patterns of correlation between successive visits were used and the estimates and test statistics were similar for the different patterns; however, an assumption of no correlation between successive visits leads to concluding incorrectly that there is strong evidence of an effect due to the mother's smoking.

11: Data Editing

11.1 Preliminary remarks

The phrase 'data editing' may conjure up a picture of the statistician as a skilful manipulator of evidence, able, by careful selection of data, to provide unassailable support for any stated hypothesis. Our purpose here is much less sinister. All statistical methods are founded on certain assumptions, for example about the forms of distributions or of relationships between variables. These assumptions are very rarely likely to be exactly true. It is not unreasonable to suppose, however, that in any particular instance they are sufficiently nearly true to make the relevant methods of analysis valid and useful. Frequently the data, as originally observed, will present some feature which is clearly incompatible with the theoretical model. One course of action might be to try to develop a special theory for this situation; this is often the way in which new developments in statistical methodology come about. More usually it will be found possible to look at the data in a rather different way, for instance by using a different scale of measurement for one or more variables, and then to use standard methods of analysis.

The next three sections are concerned with various methods of transforming variables to different scales. Section 11.5 describes simple methods for checking whether data are approximately normally distributed. In §11.6 we discuss the more contentious question of the detection of *outliers*—observations differing so widely from what the rest of the data would lead one to expect that a gross error may be suspected.

Most of the procedures described in this chapter are appropriate at a very early stage of examination of the data, before detailed analyses are carried out. It is useful to emphasize the great value, in this preliminary data screening, of simple descriptive tools—frequency distributions, mean values, scatter diagrams, etc. In particular, the value of graphical methods such as scatter diagrams can hardly be overstated. A number of graphical devices are described in detail below.

11.2 Transformations in general

By a transformation we mean a change to a different scale of measurement for some variable. *Linear* transformations, which involve at most a change in origin and a scaling factor (such as the change from °F to °C in measuring temperature), may be useful in simplifying arithmetic (e.g. working units, §1.5); or they may

386

satisfy the investigator because the new scale is more readily understood than the old. However, they rarely affect the essential features of a statistical analysis. More important are non-linear transformations, in which equal increments on the original scale do not correspond to equal increments on the new scale. Examples are the logarithm and the square root.

There are five main purposes of transformations, the first three of which are the most important:

1   to stabilize variances;
2   to linearize relationships;
3   to make distributions more normal;
4   to simplify the handling of data with other awkward features;
5   to enable results to be presented in an acceptable scale of measurement.

Variance-stabilizing transformations

Many statistical methods require that the residual variance for different subgroups of data should be constant. If this is not so, an approximate solution may be available in which the subgroups are differentially weighted, as explained in §7.2. A simpler solution would be to transform to a scale in which residual variances were approximately constant. Suppose the original variable is x and the transformed variable is y, this being some definite function of x. Then (3.17) shows that, for var(y) to be constant, the following relationship should be approximately true:

$$\frac{dy}{dx} = \frac{\text{constant}}{\sqrt{[\text{var}(x)]}}. \tag{11.1}$$

If var(x) is known as a function of x (or, more strictly, of E(x)), (11.1) enables y to be found as a function of x, i.e. it defines the appropriate transformation. Some examples are discussed in the next section.

Linearizing transformations

If a regression line, say of v on u, is clearly non-linear, a satisfactory solution may be to fit a curvilinear function as in §10.3. Again, however, it may be simpler to transform one or both variables so as to give a nearly linear relationship. The problem is particularly acute when the dependent variable is a proportion, which necessarily lies between 0 and 1; regression curves similar to that shown in Fig. 11.2(a) (p. 393) are often encountered. Transformations for proportions are discussed separately in §11.4.

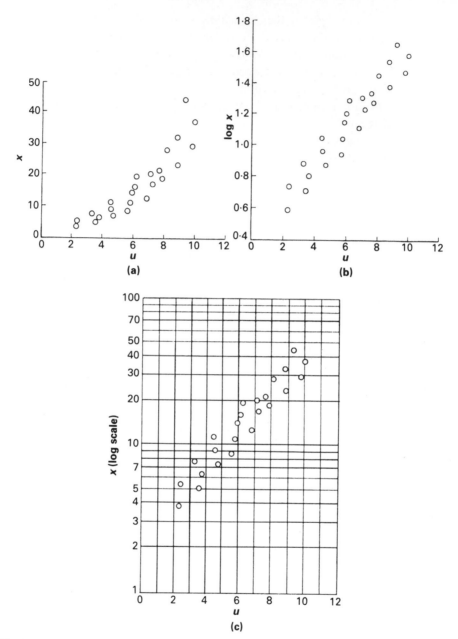

Fig. 11.1 Scatter diagram of hypothetical data plotted (a) with arithmetic scale for the ordinate, x; (b) with arithmetic scale for log x; (c) with logarithmic scale for x (using semilogarithmic paper).

Normalizing transformations

A similar point arises here. Non-normal variation can be incorporated into a theoretical model, but the resulting methods of analysis are often very complex. Fortunately, many of the standard methods of analysis are *robust* (i.e. insensitive to non-normality), and this particular reason for transformation is less cogent than the other two. If the three principal criteria discussed here conflicted in the transformations required to satisfy them, the need for normality would present the weakest case. Fortunately, it often happens that the same transformation simultaneously stabilizes variance, produces linear relationships and provides more nearly normal distributions (see Fig. 11.1).

Methods of checking departures from normality are described in §11.5.

11.3 Logarithmic and power transformations

In the logarithmic transformation we change from one variable, x, to another variable, y, by the equation

$$y = \log x. \tag{11.2}$$

In many branches of medical science, e.g. microbiology and haematology, it is customary to use *common* logarithms, to base 10. If necessary this usage can be indicated by writing $\log_{10} x$. In purely mathematical work, and in many formulae arising in statistics, the *natural* logarithm is more convenient (§4.8).

The logarithmic transformation (whether with common or natural logarithms) can only be made for positive values of x, because $\log 0 = -\infty$ and logs of negative numbers do not exist. As x increases, larger and larger changes in x are needed to give equal changes in y, as shown by the following example (where y is the common logarithm):

x	2	20	200	2000
y	0·3	1·3	2·3	3·3

We should expect, therefore, that the logarithmic transformation would tend to stabilize variances when, in the original data, $\text{var}(x)$ tended to increase markedly with x. In fact, (11.1) shows that $\text{var}(y)$ will be approximately constant when $\text{var}(x) \propto [\text{E}(x)]^2$. Equivalent statements are that the standard deviation of x is proportional to the mean, or that the coefficient of variation of x is constant.

Secondly, if x is related to a variable u by a trend with a consistently increasing slope, (11.2) will often result in a more nearly linear relationship between y and u, by 'compressing' the upper part of the scale of x.

Thirdly, if the distribution of a variable x, taking positive values, is positively skew, (11.2) will reduce this skewness and may result in a more nearly normal distribution for y.

Figures 11.1(a) and (b) illustrate a situation in which the logarithmic transformation from x to y simultaneously helps to stabilize variance, linearize the relationship with u and provide more normal distributions. This sort of situation is often found when a variable x is restricted to positive values and can vary over a wide range; examples are survival times and quantities or concentrations of some substance. Figure 11.1(c) illustrates the use of a *logarithmic scale* for x. The quantities marked on the vertical axis are values of x, but the distances between them are proportional to the distances between the corresponding values of y. The effect is precisely the same as in (b), where the logarithms, y, were looked up in tables and then plotted on an ordinary arithmetic scale. Graph paper with scales marked as in (c) can be bought; it is called *semilogarithmic* paper. Another variety, sometimes called *double-logarithmic* paper, has logarithmic scales along both axes. Graphs are often drawn using a computer, in which case the transformed variables are computed and plotted.

The relation between the logarithmic transformation and the geometric mean has been described in §1.5, where particular reference was made to the use of the transformation in microbiological and serological work. If confidence limits are required for a geometric mean, they should be obtained in the usual way on the log scale, and then converted back to the original scale.

With logarithms it is usually adequate to work to two decimal places at most.

Power transformations are defined by the equation

$$y = x^c. \tag{11.3}$$

Again, these are used mainly for a variable x taking positive values only. Equation (11.3) represents a family of transformations, distinguished by the value of c. Values of c less than 1 produce transformations with properties rather similar to those of the logarithmic transformation. Indeed, the statistical properties of the latter are equivalent to those of the power transformation (11.3) as c gets very close to zero. This can best be seen from a standardized version of (11.3), used, for instance, by Box and Cox (1964):

$$y = \frac{x^c - 1}{c}. \tag{11.4}$$

As c approaches zero, y approaches $\ln x$.

Two particular values of $c < 1$ require comment.

1 $c = \frac{1}{2}$: *the square-root transformation.* This is, from (11.1), the appropriate variance-stabilizing transformation when $\text{var}(x) \propto \text{E}(x)$. We know from (2.16) that this is true of counts following the Poisson distribution, and the square-root transformation is therefore often used for such data; for example, for the analysis of microbiological counts or counts of random events like accidents. From (3.17), if x follows a Poisson distribution (with $\text{var}(x) = E(x)$), and $y = \sqrt{x}$, then $\text{var}(y) \simeq \frac{1}{4}$. This provides a useful check on whether residual variation between counts, after eliminating the effect of various known factors, is down to the level expected from Poisson theory. In an analysis of variance of y, for example, the Residual MSq could be compared with a theoretical value of $\frac{1}{4}$ (on effectively infinite DF).

2 $c = -1$: *the reciprocal transformation.* This stabilizes variance if $\text{var}(x)$ is proportional to $\{E(x)\}^4$—a rather spectacular form of increase in variance. A feature of the reciprocal transformation is that high values of x correspond to values of y close to zero, and beyond a certain value of x further increases in x cause only trivial decreases in y. This is particularly useful in the analysis of survival time data in animal experiments in which most observations result in a reasonably short survival time but occasional animals survive for long periods. Little is lost if the observation period is 'truncated' at a moderately high value at which y can be given the value zero (Smith and Westgarth, 1957). Suppose, for example, that most animals died between 5 and 15 days after a certain treatment. The following reciprocal values could be used in an analysis.

Survival time x (days)	Reciprocal y
5	0·20
10	0·10
15	0·07
20	0·05
30	0·03
> 30	0

If a series of measurements is transformed to reciprocals, the arithmetic mean may be calculated on the transformed scale and converted back to the original scale by taking the reciprocal again. The resulting quantity is known as the *harmonic mean*. It bears the same relation to the reciprocal transformation as the geometric mean (§1.5) bears to the logarithmic transformation.

Power transformations with $c > 1$ are useful when the sorts of rectification required are the opposite of those for which the logarithmic transformation and the power transformations with $c < 1$ are appropriate. The *square transformation*, $y = x^2$, may, for example, be useful if $\text{var}(x)$ tends to decrease with increasing x, if a curvilinear relationship bends downwards rather than upwards (as in Fig. 10.5(a)) and if the distribution of x is negatively skew.

In considering linearity requirements the possibility of transforming other variables should not be forgotten. For instance, if a scatter diagram of x on

u shows the type of curvature referred to above (the trend in x curving downwards as u increases), it may be better to use a logarithmic or square-root transformation of u rather than a square transformation of x.

11.4 Transformations for proportions

In some sets of data the context seems to require one of the standard methods of analysis—t test, analysis of variance, regression, etc.—but the problem is complicated because the basic obserations are proportions for which the basic form of random variation might be expected to be binomial. In a study of insecticides applied under different controlled conditions, a known number of flies might be exposed under each set of conditions and a count made of the number killed. Such data give rise to many of the difficulties described in §11.2. The variance of an observed proportion depends on the expected proportion, as well as on the denominator of the fraction (see (2.13)). Regression curves are unlikely to be linear, because the scale of the proportion is limited by the values 0 and 1 and changes in any relevant explanatory variable (such as dose of an insecticide) at the extreme ends of its scale are unlikely to produce much change in the proportion. A *sigmoid* regression curve as in Fig. 11.2(a) is, in fact, likely to be found. Finally, the binomial distribution of random error is likely to be skew in opposite directions as the proportion approaches 0 or 1.

Two transformations are commonly used for proportions. They have very similar effects, and instances in which one is clearly superior to the other are rare.

Probit transformation

For any proportion p, suppose y' is the *normal equivalent deviate* (NED) such that a proportion p of the standard normal distribution falls to the left of y'. That is, if Φ is the cumulative distribution function of a standardized normal variable (§2.3 and §2.7), so that $\Phi(y') = p$, then

$$y' = \Phi^{-1}(p). \tag{11.5}$$

The *probit* of p is defined as

$$y = 5 + y'. \tag{11.6}$$

The addition of 5 was included in the original definition to avoid negative probits in hand calculations, but now (11.5) is also often referred to as the probit transformation. Probits may be obtained from Table A1, using (11.5). Any table of the normal distribution giving y' in terms of p may of course be used. Table IX of Fisher and Yates (1963) uses probits directly rather than NEDs.

The range of the probit scale is infinite, and there is an obvious problem if the data contain some observations with $p = 0$ or $p = 1$, since the corresponding

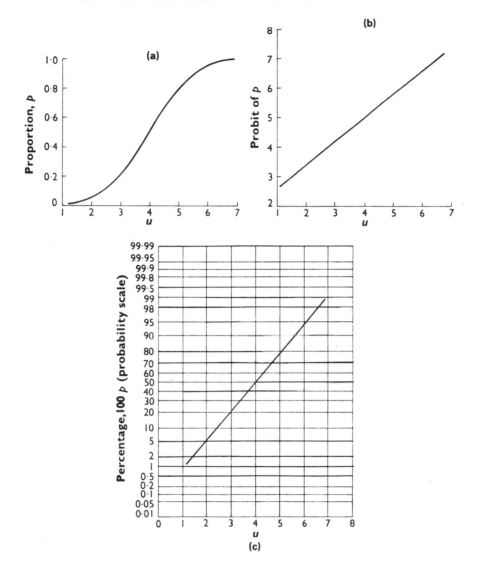

Fig. 11.2. Hypothetical response curve plotted (a) with arithmetic scale for the ordinate, p; (b) with an arithmetic scale for the probit of p; (c) with 'probability' scale for p (using probability paper).

values of y, $-\infty$ and ∞, cannot conveniently be used in standard methods of analysis. In approximate solutions and graphical studies a useful device is to calculate y from an adjusted value of p derived by assuming that $\frac{1}{2}$ (rather than 0) positive or negative response occurred. That is, if $p = r/n$, calculate $p' = 1/(2n)$ when $r = 0$ and $p' = (2n - 1)/2n$ when $r = n$, and obtain y from p'.

A further point is that the probit transformation does not stabilize variances, even for observations with constant n. Some form of weighting is therefore desirable in any analysis. A rigorous approach is provided by the method called *probit analysis* (see §17.4; also Finney, 1971).

The effect of the probit transformation in linearizing a relationship is shown in Fig. 11.2. Figure 11.2(c) illustrates the use of *probability paper*, in which the distances between points on the vertical scale are proportional to the corresponding distances on the probit or NED scale. The use of probability paper is analogous to that of logarithmic paper. The shape of the curve (in this case, exactly a straight line) is the same as that in Fig. 11.2(b), in which the probit values are plotted on an arithmetic scale. Another variety, *log probability paper*, combines the same vertical scale as in Fig. 11.2(c) with a logarithmic scale for u.

Logit transformation

The *logit* of p is defined as

$$y = \ln \frac{p}{1 - p}. \tag{11.7}$$

Occasionally (Fisher and Yates, 1963; Finney, 1978) the definition incorporates a factor $\frac{1}{2}$, so that $y = \frac{1}{2}\ln[p/(1 - p)]$; this has the effect of making the values rather similar to those of the NED (i.e. probit $-$ 5). The effect of the logit (or *logistic*) transformation is very similar indeed to that of the probit transformation. Methods of analysis using logits are discussed more fully in the context of generalized linear models in §12.8.

11.5 Goodness of fit of frequency distributions

It is often useful to regard a random variable as following a standard distributional form; common examples are the normal, binomial and Poisson distributions. The observed frequencies at different values, or in different grouping intervals, of the variables will not be precisely those expected by theory, and the question arises whether the discrepancy between observed and expected frequencies can easily be explained by sampling fluctuation.

In the examples mentioned above, a theoretical probability distribution can be fitted by using certain simple statistics calculated from the data. For a normal distribution, for instance, we need to estimate the mean μ and variance σ^2 by the sample mean $\bar{x}$ and estimate of variance s^2 (after application of Sheppard's correction if necessary). For the binomial the parameter π is estimated by the sample frequency r divided by n (using the notation of §2.5). For the Poisson the parameter μ is estimated by $\bar{x}$ (see §2.6). Expected values of the frequencies can now be calculated, from exact formulae in the case of the binomial and Poisson distributions and from tables in the case of the normal distribution.

Suppose the frequency for any value or grouping interval is denoted by O_i, and the expected value by E_i. Then, if E_i is a small fraction of the total frequency, the random variation of O_i about E_i is approximately represented by a Poisson distribution. Unless E_i is quite small, $(O_i - E_i)/\sqrt{E_i}$ can be taken as approximately a standardized normal deviate, and $(O_i - E_i)^2/E_i$ as a $\chi^2_{(1)}$ variate. If there were k such frequencies, and if all the deviations $O_i - E_i$ were independent, we should expect from the general theory of §3.4 that the familiar statistic

$$X^2 = \sum \frac{(O_i - E_i)^2}{E_i} \tag{11.8}$$

would follow the $\chi^2_{(k)}$ distribution. In fact, the deviations are not independent, if only because the values of E_i will have been chosen to add to the same total, n, as the values of O_i. Furthermore, the expected frequencies E_i have been calculated in terms of parameter estimates which closely fit the data. It turns out that, with efficient methods of estimating parameters, the degrees of freedom for (11.8) are $k - k_0$, where k_0 is

(1 + the number of parameters independently estimated from the data).

The term 1 accounts for the equality of observed and expected totals. Like most methods this is an approximation, and it is wise not to use more than a small proportion of values of E_i less than about 5; values smaller than about 2 are best avoided. This can be done by pooling adjacent cells with small values of E_i.

Example 11.1

Table 2.3 on p. 65 shows certain observed frequencies of bacterial counts, with expected frequencies calculated from the Poisson distribution with the same mean as that observed. No cells have very small frequencies, although if the original table had shown frequencies for $x = 7$ and > 7 separately they would probably have had to be pooled for the χ^2 test. The value of X^2 is 6·02, and the degrees of freedom are 6, since there are eight groups, and one parameter and the total frequency have been estimated from the data. The discrepancies are not significant (from Table A2 $0·25 < P < 0·5$, or $P = 0·42$). As mentioned on p. 65, this suggests that the anticlumping treatment has been effective.

The χ^2 test using (11.8) is a 'portmanteau' test, sensitive to a variety of types of departure from the assumed distributional form. If interest centres round a particular form of divergence from the postulated model, the χ^2 test of goodness of fit is likely to be too insensitive. In studying the departures of microbiological counts from a Poisson distribution, for example, it will often be important to test for increased variability, and this can best be done by the Poisson heterogeneity test (7.31) of §7.8.

Testing normality

Although one should not expect real data to follow exactly a normal distribution, it is usually convenient if continuous variables do not depart too drastically from normality. Transformations to improve the approximation to normality have been discussed earlier. It is useful to have a quick visual device for checking the approximate normality of an observed distribution, either in an initial study of the raw data or after transformation. This may be done by plotting the cumulative distribution on probability paper (see §11.4). If the observations are grouped, the boundary points between the groups may be plotted horizontally and the cumulative frequencies below each boundary point are plotted on the transformed probability scale. Any systematic departure from a normal distribution will produce a systematic deviation from a straight line in this graph. If the observations are not grouped, one can either (i) introduce a convenient system of group intervals; (ii) arrange the individual observations in order of magnitude and plot on probability paper, the ordinate for the ith observation out of n being the proportion $p' = (2i - 1)/2n$; or (iii) plot the individual observations *on ordinary graph paper* against the so-called *normal scores* (see §13.3).

Normal plots are particularly useful for checking the adequacy of fit of a model, such as a multiple regression, in which the error terms are normally distributed. If the model is fitted by standard methods, the residuals should behave rather like a sample from a normal distribution, and this can be checked from a normal plot. Most computer packages will provide listings of residuals and many will provide normal plots.

Example 11.2

Residuals after fitting a multiple regression are given in Table 10.1 (p. 316). Are these normally distributed? It is preferable to work with the studentized residuals, r, which have mean 0 and standard deviation 1. The normal probability plot is shown in Fig. 11.3,

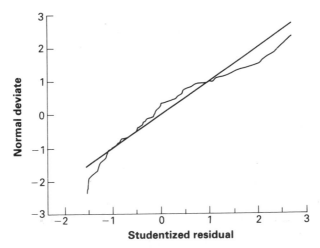

Fig. 11.3. Normal plot of studentized residuals. The cumulative probability is plotted on the ordinate in terms of the normal deviate against the residual on the abscissa.

plotted following method (ii) and showing the normal deviate, rather than p' on the ordinate. This figure shows some deviations from normality, with a deficit of low values and an excess of high values, that is, an indication of positive skewness.

A further application of normal plots arises in 2^p factorial experiments, where it is often useful to test the joint significance of a large number of main effects and interactions (see p. 257). On the null hypothesis that none of the relevant effects are present, the observed contrasts should follow approximately a normal distribution. The signs of the contrasts are, however, arbitrary, and it is useful to have a visual test which ignores these signs. In the *half-normal plot* (Daniel, 1959) the observed contrasts are put into order of absolute magnitude (ignoring sign) and plotted on the upper half of a sheet of probability paper. The value $\frac{1}{2}(1 + p')$, which lies between $\frac{1}{2}$ and 1, is used for the ordinate. The half-normal plot should indicate which, if any, of the contrasts suggest the presence of real effects.

The χ^2 test of goodness of fit when used for a continuous variable involves forming groups in such a way that the assumptions necessary for the test statistic to be approximately distributed as a χ^2 are satisfied, and there is no unique way of doing this. An alternative test which avoids this is the Kolmogorov–Smirnov test. The basis of this test is a comparison of the observed and hypothesized distribution functions. The observations, x, are first put into ascending order and then the observed distribution function, $S(x)$, is calculated at each point. The hypothesized distribution function, $F(x)$, is calculated. Then the Kolmogorov–Smirnov test statistic is

$$T = \max_{(x)} |F(x) - S(x)| \qquad (11.9)$$

where $\max_{(x)}$ indicates the maximum value over the whole range of x, and the vertical lines indicate that the sign of the difference is ignored. This test statistic is referred to tables, for example, Table A14 in Conover (1980).

The Kolmogorov–Smirnov test in its original form applies when $F(x)$ is completely specified independently of the data. Usually this is not the case. When testing if a series of observations fits a normal distribution, the particular normal distribution would be the one with mean and standard deviation estimated from the data, and a modified version of the Kolmogorov–Smirnov test, due to H. W. Lilliefors, is used. The test statistic is calculated exactly as in (11.9) but the critical values are different. Table A15 of Conover (1980) gives critical values for n up to 30, and for larger values of n the critical values for a two-sided test at levels of 0·10, 0·05 and 0·01 are $0·805/\sqrt{n}$, $0·886/\sqrt{n}$ and $1·031/\sqrt{n}$ respectively.

Example 11.3

Consider the studentized residuals used in Example 11.2. The concept of the test can be expressed in graphical form (Fig. 11.4) by plotting $F(r)$ and $S(r)$ against r, where $S(r)$ is plotted as a series of steps. Again the positive skewness is revealed by the plot.

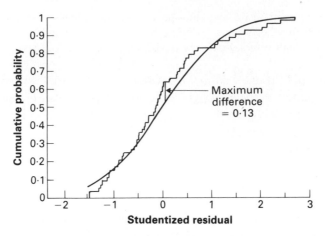

Fig. 11.4. Plot of observed and expected distribution functions plotted against studentized residual.

The value of the test statistic is the maximum vertical difference between the two distribution functions, and this equals 0.131. This exceeds the critical value for a significance level of 5%, $0.886/\sqrt{53} = 0.122$, but not that for a level of 1%, 0.142. Therefore there is evidence ($P < 0.05$) that the assumption that the observed values are normally distributed with constant variance about the predicted values does not hold.

Another test for normality that is commonly used is the Shapiro–Wilk test. The basis for this test is to compare two measures of the variability of the data, which would be equal for a normal distribution but not otherwise. The first such measure is the sum of squares about the mean, whilst the second is the square of a weighted sum of differences between pairs of values, where each pair consists of corresponding values from each side of the median. The data values are denoted by $x_1, x_2, \ldots, x_n$, and after sorting into ascending order by $x_{(1)}, x_{(2)}, \ldots, x_{(n)}$. Then the test statistic is

$$W = \frac{\left[\sum_{i=1}^{k} a_i(x_{(n-i+1)} - x_{(i)}) \right]^2}{\sum_{i=1}^{n} (x_i - \bar{x})^2} \tag{11.10}$$

where k is the integral part of $\frac{1}{2}n$. The coefficients a_i depend on n and are tabulated by Conover (1980, Table A17). The test statistic has to be in the range $0 < W \leq 1$, and would be 1 for a normal distribution. Low values of W indicate non-normality and critical values are given by Conover (1980, Table A18).

Example 11.4

The gains in weight of seven rats on a low-protein diet are 70, 85, 94, 101, 107, 118 and 132 g (Table 4.2). The sum of squares about the mean, 101·0, is 2552·0. The difference between the two extreme values, $132 - 70 = 62$ is a measure of variability, as are the differences between the next two extreme values, $118 - 85 = 33$, and the next $107 - 94 = 13$. These differences are combined, using coefficients from Table A17 of Conover, to give

$$(0·6233)(62) + (0·3031)(33) + (0·1401)(13) = 50·47,$$

and

$$W = (50·47)^2/2552·0 = 0·9981.$$

Referring to Table A18 in Conover (1980) we find that these seven values are exceptionally close to a normal distribution, $P > 0·99$.

Both the Shapiro–Wilk and Lilliefors modification of the Kolmogorov–Smirnov test are extremely tedious to calculate by hand and would normally be obtained using statistical software; for example, SAS allows the calculation of one or other of these test statistics in its UNIVARIATE procedure.

Example 11.3, continued

The value of W is 0·9320, $P = 0·006$. This test also shows significant evidence of non-normality.

Although tests of normality have a place in checking the assumptions of an analysis their importance should not be overestimated since many of the methods are valid because the sample size is sufficient to take care of non-normality through operation of the cental limit theorem. For example, a two-sample t test (§4.4) is exactly correct if the two samples are from normal distributions with equal variances, and otherwise is approximately valid where the approximation improves with increasing n_1 and n_2, and the closer the distributions are to normality. The larger n_1 and n_2 then the more non-normality can be tolerated, but it is precisely in this situation that non-normality is easiest to detect. It is likely that the value of the Shapiro–Wilk statistic, W, is more relevant than its statistical significance.

11.6 Outlying observations

Occasionally a single observation is affected by a gross error, either of measurement or recording, or due to a sudden lapse from the general standards of investigation applying to the rest of the data. It is important to detect such errors if possible, partly because they are likely to invalidate the assumptions underlying standard methods of analysis and partly because gross errors may seriously distort estimates, such as mean values.

Recording errors can often be reduced by careful checking of all the steps at which results are copied on to paper, and by minimizing the number of transcription steps between the original record and the final data. Frequently the original measurement will come under suspicion. The measurement may be repeatable (for example, the height of an individual if a short time has elapsed since the first measurement), or one may be able to check it by referring to an authoritative document (such as a birth certificate, if age is in doubt). A much more difficult situation arises when an observation is strongly suspected of being erroneous but no independent check is available. Possible courses of action are discussed below, at (b) and (c). First we discuss some methods of detecting gross errors.

(a) *Logical checks*

Certain values may be seen to be either impossible or extremely implausible by virtue of the meaning of the variable. Frequently the range of variation is known sufficiently well to enable upper and/or lower limits to be set; for example, an adult man's height below, say, 140 cm or above 205 cm would cause suspicion. Other results would be impossible because of relationships between variables; for example, a child aged 10 years cannot be married. Checks of this sort can be carried out routinely, once the rules of acceptability have been defined. They can readily be performed by computer, possibly when the data are being entered (§1.3); indeed, editing procedures of this sort should form a regular part of the analysis of large-scale bodies of data by computer.

(b) *Statistical checks*

Certain observations may be found to be unusual, not necessarily on a priori grounds, but at least by comparison with the rest of the data. Whether or not they are to be rejected or amended is a controversial matter to be discussed below; at any rate, the investigator will probably wish to have his/her attention drawn to them.

A good deal of statistical checking can be done quite informally by graphical exploration and the formation of frequency distributions. If most of the observations follow an approximately normal distribution, with one or two aberrant values falling well away from the main distribution, the *normal plot* described in §11.5 is a useful device. Sometimes observations are unusual only when considered in relation to other variables; for example, in an anthropometric survey of schoolchildren, a weight measurement may be seen to be unusually low or high in relation to the child's height; checking-rules for weights in terms of heights will be much more effective than rules based on weights alone (Healy, 1952). The detection of outliers that are apparent only when other variables are considered forms part of the diagnostic methods used in multiple regression (§10.1).

Should a statistically unusual reading be rejected or amended? If there is some external reason for suspicion, for example that an inexperienced technician made the observation in question, or that the air-conditioning plant failed at a certain point during an experiment, common sense would suggest the omission of the observation and (where appropriate) the use of missing-reading techniques (§8.8). When there is no external reason for suspicion there are strong arguments for retaining the original observations. Clearly there are some observations which no reasonable person would retain—for example, an adult height recorded as 30 cm. However, the decision will usually have to be made as a subjective judgement on ill-defined criteria which depend on one's knowledge of the data under study, the purpose of the analysis and so on. A full treatment of this topic, including descriptions of more formal methods of dealing with outliers, is given by Barnett and Lewis (1984).

(c) Robust estimation

In some analyses the question of rejection or correction of data may not arise, yet it may be suspected or known that occasional outliers occur, and some safeguard against their effect may be sought. For the estimation of a location parameter, for example, one might seek an estimator which is less influenced than the mean by occasional outliers. In §1.5 we commended the sample median on these grounds. This approach is called *robust estimation*, and a wide range of such estimators has been suggested. One of the most widely used is the *trimmed mean*, obtained by omitting some of the most extreme observations (for example, a fixed proportion in each tail) and taking the mean of the rest. These estimators are remarkably efficient for samples from normal distributions, and better than the sample mean for distributions 'contaminated' with a moderate proportion of outliers. The choice of method (e.g. the proportion to be trimmed from the tails) is not entirely straightforward, and the precision of the resulting estimator may be difficult to determine.

Similar methods are available for more complex problems, although the choice of method is, as in the simpler case of the mean, often arbitrary, and the details of the analysis may be complicated. In multiple regression, for example, it may be suspected that occasional large deviations occur more frequently than they should if errors were normally distributed. Methods of robust regression are available which give less weight to extreme residuals than does the method of least squares. See Draper and Smith (1981, §6.14) for a brief discussion.

12: Further Analysis of Categorical Data

12.1 Introduction

Categorical data show the frequencies with which observations fall into various categories or combinations of categories. Some of the basic methods of handling this type of data have been discussed in earlier sections of the book, particularly §§2.5, 3.3, 4.7, 4.8, 7.5 and 7.6. In the present chapter we gather together a number of more advanced techniques for dealing with categorical data. It is useful at this stage to make a distinction between three different types of classification into categories, according to the types of variable described in §1.4.

1 *Nominal* variables, in which no ordering is implied.

2 *Ordinal* variables, in which the categories assume a natural ordering although they are not necessarily associated with a quantitative measurement.

3 *Quantitative* variables, in which the categories are ordered by their association with a quantitative measurement.

It is often useful to consider both ordinal and quantitative variables as *ordered*, and to distinguish particularly between nominal and ordered data. But data can sometimes be considered from more than one point of view. For instance, quantitative data might be regarded as merely ordinal if it seemed important to take account of the ordering but not to rely too closely on the specific underlying variable. Ordered data might be regarded as purely nominal if there seemed to be differences between the effects of different categories which were not related to their natural order. We need, therefore, methods which can be adapted to a wide range of situations.

Many of the χ^2 tests introduced earlier have involved test statistics distributed as χ^2 on several degrees of freedom. In each instance the test was sensitive to departures from a null hypothesis, which could occur in various ways. In a $2 \times k$ contingency table, for instance, the null hypothesis postulates equality between the expected proportions of individuals in each column which fall into the first row. There are k of these proportions, and the null hypothesis can be falsified if any one of them differs from the others. These tests may be thought of as 'portmanteau' techniques, able to serve many different purposes. If, however, we were particularly interested in a certain form of departure from the null hypothesis, it might be possible to formulate a test which was particularly sensitive to this situation, although perhaps less effective than the portmanteau χ^2 test in detecting other forms of departure. Sometimes these specially directed tests can be

402

achieved by subdividing the total χ^2 statistic into portions which follow χ^2 distributions on reduced numbers of degrees of freedom.

The situation is very similar to that encountered in the analysis of variance, where an SSq can sometimes be subdivided into portions, on reduced numbers of DF, which represent specific contrasts between groups (§7.4).

In §§12.2 and 12.3 we describe methods for detecting trends in the probabilities with which observations fall into a series of ordered categories. In §12.4 a similar method is described for a single series of counts. In §12.5 two other situations are described, in which the χ^2 statistic calculated for a contingency table is subdivided to shed light on specific ways in which categorical variables may be associated. In §§12.6 and 12.7 some of the methods described earlier are generalized for situations in which the data are stratified (i.e. divided into subgroups), so that trends can be examined within strata and finally pooled.

Many of the techniques described in these sections make use of the χ^2 distributions, which have been used extensively in earlier chapters. These χ^2 methods are, however, almost exclusively designed for significance testing. In many problems involving categorical data the estimation of relevant parameters which describe the nature of possible associations between variables is much more important than the performance of significance tests of null hypotheses. Section 12.8 is devoted to a general approach to modelling the relationships between variables, of which some particular cases are relevant to categorical data. In §12.9 we describe methods of standardization, particularly in relation to vital statistical data.

More comprehensive treatments of the analysis of categorical data are contained in the monographs by Agresti (1990), Cox and Snell (1989), Fienberg (1980) and Fleiss (1981).

12.2 Trends in proportions

Suppose that, in a $2 \times k$ contingency table of the type discussed in §7.5, the k groups fall into a natural order. They may correspond to different values, or groups of values, of a quantitative variable like age; or they may correspond to qualitative categories, such as severity of a disease, which can be ordered but not readily assigned a numerical value. The usual $\chi^2_{(k-1)}$ test is designed to detect differences between the k proportions of observations falling into the first row. More specifically one might ask whether there is a significant trend in these proportions from group 1 to group k.

For convenience of exposition we shall assign the groups to the rows of the table, which now becomes $k \times 2$ rather than $2 \times k$.

Let us assign a quantitative variable, x, to the k groups. If the definition of groups uses such a variable, this can be chosen to be x. If the definition is qualitative, x can take integer values from 1 to k. The notation is as follows:

Group	Variable x	Frequency			Proportion positive
		Positive	Negative	Total	
1	x_1	r_1	$n_1 - r_1$	n_1	p_1
2	x_2	r_2	$n_2 - r_2$	n_2	p_2
$\vdots$					
i	x_i	r_i	$n_i - r_i$	n_i	p_i
$\vdots$					
k	x_k	r_k	$n_k - r_k$	n_k	p_k
All groups combined		R	$N - R$	N	$P(=R/N)$

The numerator of the χ^2 statistic, X^2, is, from (7.29),

$$\sum n_i(p_i - P)^2,$$

a weighted sum of squares of the p_i about the (weighted) mean P (see discussion below (7.30)). It also turns out to be a straightforward sum of squares, between groups, of a variable y taking the value 1 for each positive individual and 0 for each negative. This SSq can be divided (as in §9.1) into an SSq due to regression of y on x and an SSq due to departures from linear regression. If there is a trend of p_i with x_i, we might find the first of these two portions to be greater than would be expected by chance. Dividing this portion by PQ, the denominator of (7.29), gives us a $\chi^2_{(1)}$ statistic, X_1^2, which forms part of X^2 and is particularly sensitive to trend.

A little algebraic manipulation (Armitage, 1955) provides the following formula for X_1^2:

$$X_1^2 = \frac{N(N\sum r_i x_i - R\sum n_i x_i)^2}{R(N-R)[N\sum n_i x_i^2 - (\sum n_i x_i)^2]}. \tag{12.1}$$

The difference between the two statistics,

$$X_2^2 = X^2 - X_1^2, \tag{12.2}$$

may be regarded as a $\chi^2_{(k-2)}$ statistic testing departures from linear regression of p_i on x_i. As usual, both of these tests are approximate, but the approximation (12.2) is likely to be adequate if only a small proportion of the expected frequencies are less than about 5. The trend test (12.1) is adequate in these conditions but also more widely, since it is based on a linear function of the frequencies, and is likely to be satisfactory provided that only a small proportion of expected frequencies are less than about 2 and that these do not occur in adjacent rows. An exact test can be constructed following the same rationale as that used in Fisher's exact test for a 2×2 table (§4.9). Conditional on the marginal totals, the test involves evaluation of the probability that $\sum r_i x_i$ is as at least as large as the observed value (Agresti, 1990, §4.8.2). The exact method involves a large amount of calculation and is only feasible with appropriate statistical software (see Chapter 18).

Example 12.1

In the analysis of the data summarized in Table 12.1 it would be reasonable to ask whether the proportion of patients accepting their general practitioner's invitation to attend screening mammography tends to decrease as the time since their last consultation increases. The first step is to decide on scores representing the four time-period categories. It would be possible to use the midpoints of the time intervals, 3 months, 9 months, etc., but the last interval, being open, would be awkward. Instead, we shall use equally spaced integer scores, as shown in the table.

From (12.1),

$$X_1^2 = \frac{(278)[(278)(49) - (86)(236)]^2}{(86)(192)[(278)(530) - (236)^2]}$$

$$= (1 \cdot 2383 \times 10^{10})/(0 \cdot 15132 \times 10^{10})$$

$$= 8 \cdot 18,$$

which, as a $\chi_{(1)}^2$ variate, is highly significant ($P = 0 \cdot 004$).

The overall $\chi_{(3)}^2$ statistic, from (7.28) or (7.30), is calculated as

$$X^2 = 8 \cdot 92.$$

The test for departures from a linear trend thus gives

$$X_2^2 = X^2 - X_1^2$$

$$= 8 \cdot 92 - 8 \cdot 18$$

$$= 0 \cdot 74$$

as a $\chi_{(2)}^2$ variate, which is clearly non-significant. There is thus a definite trend which may well result in approximately equal decreases in the proportion of attenders as we change successively to the categories representing longer times since the last consultation.

Table 12.1 Numbers of patients attending or not attending screening mammography, classified by time since last visit to the general practitioner (Irwig et al., 1990)

Time since last visit	Score x	Attendance		Total	Proportion attending
		Yes	No		
< 6 months	0	59	97	156	0.378
6–12 months	1	10	31	41	0·244
1–2 years	2	12	36	48	0·250
> 2 years	3	5	28	33	0·152
		86	192	278	

A number of other formulae are equivalent or nearly equivalent to (12.1). The regression coefficient of y on x, measuring the rate at which the proportion p_i changes with the score x_i, is estimated by the expression

$$b = \frac{NT}{N\sum n_i x_i^2 - (\sum n_i x_i)^2},$$
(12.3)

where

$$T = \sum r_i x_i - \frac{R\sum n_i x_i}{N} = \sum x_i(r_i - e_i),$$
(12.4)

the cross-product of the scores x_i and the discrepancies $r_i - e_i$ in the contingency table between the frequencies in the first column (i.e. of positives) and their expected values from the margins of the table. Here r_i and e_i correspond to the O and E of (7.28), e_i being calculated as Rn_i/N. On the null hypothesis of no association between rows and columns, for fixed values of the marginal totals, the exact variance of T is

$$\operatorname{var}(T) = \frac{R(N-R)[N\sum n_i x_i^2 - (\sum n_i x_i)^2]}{N^2(N-1)}.$$
(12.5)

A $\chi^2_{(1)}$ test for the trend in proportions is therefore provided by the statistic

$$X^2_{1a} = \frac{T^2}{\operatorname{var}(T)} = \frac{(N-1)[\sum x_i(r_i - e_i)]^2}{(N-R)[\sum e_i x_i^2 - (\sum e_i x_i)^2/R]}.$$
(12.6)

In fact, $X^2_{1a} = (N-1)X^2_1/N$, so the two tests are very nearly equivalent. The distinction is unimportant in most analyses, when N is fairly large, but (12.6) should be used when N is rather small. In particular, it is preferable in situations to be considered in §12.7, where data are subdivided into strata, some of which may be small.

If the null hypothesis is untrue, (12.5) overestimates $\operatorname{var}(T)$, since it makes use of the total variation of y rather than the variation about regression on x. For the regression of a binary variable y on x, an analysis of variance could be calculated, as in Table 9.1. In this analysis the sum of squares about regression turns out to be $R(N-R)(N-X_1^2)/N^2$, and, using (5.18), $\operatorname{var}(b)$ may be calculated as

$$\operatorname{var}(b) = \frac{R(N-R)(N-X_1^2)}{N(N-2)[N\sum n_i x_i^2 - (\sum n_i x_i)^2]}.$$

For the calculation of confidence limits for the slope, therefore, the formula below (5.20) may be used, with the percentile of the t distribution on $N - 2$ DF (which in most applications will be close to the standardized normal value), and with $SE(b) = \sqrt{var(b)}$. The results of these calculations for the data used in Example 12.1 are:

$b = -0.0728$, $SE(b) = 0.0252$, with 95% confidence limits $(-0.122, -0.023)$.

Note that $b^2/var(b) = 8.37$, a little higher than X_1^2, as would be expected.

By analogy with the situation for simple regression (see the paragraph below (5.21)), the test for association based on the regression of y on x, as in (12.1) and (12.6), should give the same significance level as that based on the regression of x on y. Since y is a binary variable the latter regression is essentially determined by the difference between the mean values of x at the two levels of y. In many problems, particularly where y is clearly the dependent variable, this difference is of no interest. In other situations, for example when the columns of the table represent different treatments and the rows are ordered categories of a response to treatment, this is a natural way of approaching the data. The standard method for comparing two means is, of course, the two-sample t test. The method now under discussion provides an alternative to the t test, which may be preferable for categorical responses since the data are usually far from normal.

The difference between the mean scores for the first and second columns of the table (i.e. for positive and negative responses) is

$$d = \frac{NT}{R(N - R)},\tag{12.7}$$

where T is given by (12.4). Since $d^2/var(d) = X_{1a}^2$, as given by (12.6), it can easily be checked that

$$var(d) = \sigma_x^2\left(\frac{1}{R} + \frac{1}{N - R}\right),\tag{12.8}$$

where σ_x^2 is the variance of x, given by

$$\sigma_x^2 = \frac{\sum n_i x_i^2 - \frac{(\sum n_i x_i)^2}{N}}{N - 1}.\tag{12.9}$$

Note that (12.9) is the variance of x for the complete data, not the variance within the separate columns. If the null hypothesis is not true, (12.8) will overestimate the variance of d, and confidence limits for the difference in means calculated from (12.8) will tend to be somewhat too wide.

The test for the difference in means described above is closely related to the Wilcoxon and Mann–Whitney distribution-free tests described later (see §13.3).

12.3 Trends in larger contingency tables

Tests for trend can also be applied to contingency tables larger than the $k \times 2$ table considered in §12.2. The extension to more than two columns of frequencies gives rise to two possibilities: the columns may be nominal (i.e. unordered) or ordered. In the first case we might wish to test for differences in the mean row scores between the different columns; this would be an alternative to the one-way analysis of variance, just as the χ^2 test based on (12.7) and (12.8) is an alternative to the two-sample t test. In the second case, of ordered column categories, the problem might be to test the regression of one set of scores on the other, or equivalently the correlation between the row and column scores. Both situations are illustrated by an example, the methods of analysis following closely those described by Yates (1948).

Example 12.2

Sixty-six mothers who had suffered the death of a newborn baby were studied to assess the relationship between their state of grief and degree of support (Tudehope *et al.*, 1986). Grief was recorded on a qualitative ordered scale with four categories and degree of support on an ordered scale with three categories (Table 12.2). The overall test statistic (7·28) is 9·96 (6 DF), which is clearly not significant. Nevertheless, examination of the contingency table suggests that those with good support experienced less grief than those with poor support, whilst those with adequate support were intermediate, and that this effect is being missed by the overall test. The aim of the trend test is to produce a more sensitive test on this specific aspect.

We first ignore the ordering of the columns, regarding them as three different categories of a nominal variable. The calculations proceed as follows.

1   Assign scores to rows (x) and columns (y): integer values starting from 1 have been used. Denote the row totals by R_i, $i = 1$ to r, the column totals by C_j, $j = 1$ to c, and the total number of subjects by N.

Table 12.2 Numbers of mothers by state of grief and degree of support (data of Tudehope *et al.*, 1986)

Grief state	Row score x_i	Support			Total R_i	Sum of column scores Y_i
		Good	Adequate	Poor		
I	1	17	9	8	34	59
II	2	6	5	1	12	19
III	3	3	5	4	12	25
IV	4	1	2	5	8	20
Total, C_j		27	21	18	66	123
Col. score, y_j		1	2	3		
Sum of row scores, X_j		42	42	42	126	
Mean score, $\bar{x}_j$		1·56	2·00	2·33		

2   For each column calculate the sum of the row scores, X_j, and the mean score $\bar{x}_j$. For the first column,

$$X_1 = (17 \times 1) + (6 \times 2) + (3 \times 3) + (1 \times 4) = 42,$$

$$\bar{x}_1 = 42/27 = 1{\cdot}56.$$

This calculation is also carried out for the column of row totals to give 126, which serves as a check on the values of X_j, which sum over columns to this value. This total is the sum of the row scores for all the mothers, i.e. $\sum x = 126$.

3   Calculate the sum of squares of row scores for all the mothers,

$$\sum x^2 = (34 \times 1) + (12 \times 4) + (12 \times 9) + (8 \times 16)$$

$$= 318.$$

Correct this sum of squares for the mean,

$$S_{xx} = 318 - 126^2/66 = 77{\cdot}455.$$

4   A test of the equality of the mean scores $\bar{x}_j$ may now be carried out. The test statistic is

$$X^2 = (N-1)\left[\sum(X_j^2/C_j) - \left(\sum x\right)^2/N\right]/S_{xx} \qquad (12.10)$$

$$= \frac{65}{77{\cdot}455}\left(\frac{42^2}{27} + \frac{42^2}{21} + \frac{42^2}{18} - \frac{126^2}{66}\right)$$

$$= 5{\cdot}70.$$

This may be regarded as a $\chi^2_{(c-1)}$, i.e. a $\chi^2_{(2)}$ statistic. This is not quite significant at the 5% level ($P = 0{\cdot}058$), but is sufficiently close to allow the possibility that a test for the apparent trend in the column means, $\bar{x}_j$, may be significant. We now, therefore, make use of the column scores, y_j.

5   Repeat steps **2** and **3**, working across rows instead of down columns; it is not necessary to calculate the mean scores.

$$\sum y = 123,$$

$$\sum y^2 = 273,$$

$$S_{yy} = 273 - 123^2/66$$

$$= 43{\cdot}773.$$

6   Calculate the sum of products of the sum of row scores, X_j, and the corresponding column scores, y_j.

$$\sum X_j y_j = (42 \times 1) + (42 \times 2) + (42 \times 3) = 252.$$

This total is $\sum xy$ over all mothers and should be corrected for the means,

$$S_{xy} = 252 - (123 \times 126)/66$$

$$= 17{\cdot}182.$$

7   The test statistic for the trend in the mean scores, $\bar{x}_j$, is

$$X^2 = (N-1)S_{xy}^2/(S_{xx}S_{yy}) \qquad (12.11)$$

$$= 65 \times 17{\cdot}182^2/(77{\cdot}455 \times 43{\cdot}773)$$

$$= 5{\cdot}66.$$

This is approximately a $\chi_{(1)}^2$ statistic and is significant ($P = 0{\cdot}017$). In this example most of the difference between column means lies in the trend. This is clear from examination of the column means, and the corresponding result for the test statistics is that the overall test statistic of $5{\cdot}70$ (2 DF) for equality of column means may be subdivided into $5{\cdot}66$ (1 DF) for linear trend and, by subtraction, $0{\cdot}04$ (1 DF) for departures from the trend.

Note that the test statistic (12.11) is $N-1$ times the square of the correlation coefficient between the row and column scores, and this may be a convenient way of calculating it on a computer. When $r = 2$, (12.10) tests the equality of c proportions, and is identical with (7.30) except for a multiplying factor of $(N-1)/N$; (12.11) tests the trend in the proportions and is identical with (12.6).

Both (12.10) and (12.11) are included in the SAS program PROC FREQ, the former as the 'ANOVA statistic' and the latter as the 'Mantel–Haenszel chi-square'.

12.4 Trends in counts

In many problems of the type considered in §12.2, the proportions under consideration are very small. If, for instance, the frequencies in the 'positive' column of the table on p. 404 are much smaller than those in the 'negative' column, almost all the contribution to the test statistic comes from the first column. In the limit, as the p_i become very small and the n_i become very large, both (12.1) and (12.6) take the form

$$X_{1P}^2 = \frac{[\sum x_i(r_i - e_i)]^2}{\sum e_i x_i^2 - (\sum e_i x_i)^2/R} . \qquad (12.12)$$

The subscript P is used for this test statistic because in this limiting situation the observed frequencies r_i can be regarded as Poisson variates with means (under the null hypothesis) e_i, the expected values. In some applications the expected values are proportional to subject-years of exposure for individuals in each category (see §14.9).

Example 12.3

In the data shown in Table 12.3, the expected frequencies of maternal deaths are calculated in proportion to the numbers of mothers in the different time periods, so as to add to the

Table 12.3   Maternal mortality in New South Wales, for primiparae aged 40 and over (Wilcocks and Lancaster, 1951)

Years	Score, x_i (midpoint − 1900)	Number of mothers	Maternal deaths Observed, r_i	Expected, e_i
1894–1900	− 2·5	346	10	6·603
1901–07	4·5	454	9	8·664
1908–10	9·5	272	3	5·191
1911–20	16·0	1133	23	21·621
1921–30	26·0	1546	32	29·503
1931–37	34·5	909	17	17·347
1938–42	40·5	699	13	13·339
1943–48	46·0	1296	20	24·732
Total		6655	127	127·000

observed total of 127. The total $\chi^2_{(7)}$ statistic, calculated as $\sum (r_i - e_i)^2/e_i$, is 3·91, clearly non-significant. Even if the whole of this quantity were ascribed to linear regression, it would barely reach the 5% significance level on 1 DF. However, there is a suggestion of an excess of deaths in the early years and a deficit later. In fact, application of (12.12) gives $X^2_{1P} = 1·27\,(P = 0·26)$. There is clearly no strong evidence for a gradual decline in the rate of maternal mortality in this particular population.

12.5   Other components of χ^2

Most of the χ^2 statistics described earlier in this chapter can be regarded as components of the total χ^2 statistic for a contingency table. Two further examples of the subdivision of χ^2 statistics are given below.

Hierarchical classification

In §12.2, the numerator of the $\chi^2_{(k-1)}$ statistic (7.29) was regarded as the SSq between groups of a dummy variable y, taking the values 0 and 1. We proceeded to subdivide this in a standard way. Other types of subdivision encountered in Chapters 7 and 8 may equally be used if they are relevant to the data under study. For example, if the k groups form a factorial arrangement, and if the n_i are equal or are proportional to marginal totals for the separate factors, the usual techniques could be used to separate SSq and hence components of the $\chi^2_{(k-1)}$ statistic, representing main effects and interactions.

Another situation, in which no conditions need be imposed on the n_i, is that in which the groups form a hierarchical arrangement.

Example 12.4

Table 12.4 Proportions of houseflies killed in experiments with two insecticides

Insecticide:	A					B					
Batch:	A1		A2			B1		B2			
					Total					Total	Total
Test:	1	2	1	2	A	1	2	1	2	B	A + B
Flies:											
Killed	49	43	43	48	183	41	44	39	39	163	346
Surviving	2	5	4	1	12	5	8	11	9	33	45
Total	51	48	47	49	195	46	52	50	48	196	391
Proportion killed					0·9385					0·8316	0·8849

Table 12.4 shows proportions of houseflies killed by two different insecticides. There are two batches of each insecticide, and each of the four batches is subjected to two tests. The overall $\chi^2_{(7)}$ test gives

$$X^2_{(7)} = (2^2/51 + \ldots + 9^2/48 - 45^2/391)/(0·8849)(0·1151)$$

$$= 1·6628/0·1019 = 16·32 \text{ on } 7 \text{ DF},$$

which is significant ($P = 0·022$). This can be subdivided as follows:

Between tests (4 DF):

$$X^2_{(4)} = \frac{(2^2/51 + 5^2/48 - 7^2/99) + \ldots + (11^2/50 + 9^2/48 - 20^2/98)}{0·1019}$$

$$= 2·75 \ (P = 0·60);$$

Between batches (2 DF):

$$X^2_{(2)} = \frac{(7^2/99 + 5^2/96 - 12^2/195) + (13^2/98 + 20^2/98 - 33^2/196)}{0·1019}$$

$$= 2·62 \ (P = 0·27);$$

Between insecticides (1 DF):

$$X^2_{(1)} = \frac{(12^2/195 + 33^2/196 - 45^2/391)}{0·1019}$$

$$= 10·95 \ (P < 0·001).$$

As a check, $X^2_{(1)} + X^2_{(2)} + X^2_{(4)} = 16·32$, agreeing with $X^2_{(7)}$. There is thus clear evidence of a difference in toxicity of the two insecticides, but no evidence of differences between batches or between tests.

A few remarks about this analysis.

1 Since a difference between A and B has been established it would be logical, in calculating $X^2_{(2)}$ and $X^2_{(4)}$, to use separate denominators for the contributions from the two insecticides. Thus, in calculating $X_{(2)}^2$ the first term in the numerator would have a denominator $(0.9385)(0.0615) = 0.0577$, and the second term would have a denominator $(0.8316)(0.1684) = 0.1400$. The effect of this correction is usually small. If it is made, the various χ^2 indices no longer add exactly to the total.

2   In entomological experiments it is common to find significant differences between replicate tests, perhaps because the response is sensitive to small changes in the environment and all the flies used in one test share the same environment (for example, being often kept in the same box). In such cases comparisons between treatments must take account of the random variation between tests. It is useful, therefore, to have adequate replication. The analysis can often be done satisfactorily by measuring the proportion of deaths at each test and analysing these proportions with or without one of the standard transformations.

3   An experiment of the size of that shown in Table 12.4 is not really big enough to detect variation between batches and tests. Although the numbers of flies are quite large, more replication both of tests and of batches is desirable.

Larger contingency tables

The hierarchical principle can be applied to larger contingency tables (§7.6). In an $r \times c$ table, the total χ^2 statistic, X^2, can be calculated from (7.28). It has $(r-1)(c-1)$ DF, and represents departures of the cell frequencies from those expected by proportionality to row and column totals. It may be relevant to ask whether proportionality holds in some segment of the whole table; then in a second segment chosen after collapsing either rows or columns in the first segment; then in a third segment; and so on. If, in performing these successive χ^2 calculations, one uses expected frequencies derived from the whole table, the various χ^2 statistics can be added in a natural way. If, however, the expected frequencies are derived separately for each subtable, the various components of χ^2 will not add exactly to the total. The discrepancy is unlikely to be important in practice.

Example 12.5

Table 12.5, taken from Example 11.10.2 of Snedecor and Cochran (1989), shows data from a study of the relationship between blood groups and disease. The small number of AB patients have been omitted from the analysis. The overall $\chi_{(4)}^2$ test for the whole table gives $X^2 = 40.54$, a value which is highly significant. A study of the proportions in the three blood groups, for each group of subjects, suggests that there is little difference between the controls and the patients with gastric cancer, or between the relative proportions in groups A and B, but that patients with peptic ulcer show an excess of group O. These comparisons can be examined by a subdivision of the 3×3 table into a hierarchical series of 2×2 tables as shown in Fig. 12.1(a)–(d). The sequence is deliberately chosen so as to reveal the possible association between group O and peptic ulcer in the subtable (d). The arrows indicate a move to an enlarged table by amalgamation of the rows or columns of the previous table.

Table 12.5 Frequencies (and percentages) of ABO blood groups in patients with peptic ulcer, patients with gastric cancer and controls (Snedecor and Cochran, 1989, Ex. 11.10.2)

Blood group	Peptic ulcer	(%)	Gastric cancer	(%)	Controls	(%)	Total
O	983	(55)	383	(43)	2892	(48)	4258
A	679	(38)	416	(47)	2625	(43)	3720
B	134	(7)	84	(10)	570	(9)	788
Total	1796	(100)	883	(100)	6087	(100)	8766

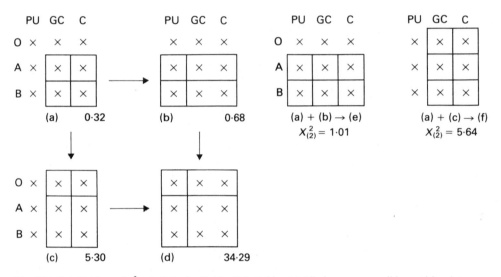

Fig. 12.1 Subdivision of $\chi^2_{(4)}$ statistic for Table 12.5. Tables (a)–(d) show one possible partition into separate $\chi^2_{(1)}$ statistics. Tables (e) and (f) show two ways of combining contrasts.

The corresponding values of $X^2_{(1)}$ are shown in the diagram, and are reproduced here:

Row comparison	Column comparison	$X^2_{(1)}$
(a) A vs. B	GC vs. C	0·32
(b) A vs. B	PU vs. (GC, C)	0·68
(c) O vs. (A, B)	GC vs. C	5·30
(d) O vs. (A, B)	PU vs. (GC, C)	34·29
		40·59

As noted earlier, the total of the X^2_1 statistics is a little different from the X^2_4 value of 40·54 for the whole table, but the discrepancy is slight. The value of X^2_1 for (c) gives $P = 0·021$, giving rise to some doubt about the lack of association of blood groups and gastric cancer. The outstanding contrast is that between the proportions of group O in the peptic ulcer patients and in the other subjects.

The process of collapsing rows and columns could have been speeded up by combining some of the 1 DF contrasts into 2 DF contrasts. For example, (a) and (b) could have been combined in a 2 × 3 table, (e). This gives an $X^2_{(2)}$ of 1·01, scarcely different from the sum of 0·32 and 0·68, representing the overall association of blood groups A and B with the two disease groups and controls. Or, to provide an overall picture of the association of blood groups with gastric cancer, (a) and (c) could have been combined in a 3 × 2 table, (f). This gives an $X^2_{(2)}$ of 5·64 (very close to 0·32 + 5·30), which is, of course, less significant than the $X^2_{(1)}$ of 5·30 from (c).

There are many ways of subdividing a contingency table. In Example 12.5, the elementary table (a) could have been chosen as any one of the 2 × 2 tables forming part of the whole table. The choice, as in that example, will often be data-dependent, that is, made after an initial inspection of the data. There is, therefore, the risk of data-dredging, and this should be recognized in any interpretation of the analysis. In Example 12.5, of course, the association between group O and peptic ulcer is too strong to be explained away by data-dredging.

12.6 Combination of 2 × 2 tables

Sometimes a number of 2 × 2 tables, all bearing on the same question, are available, and it seems natural to combine the evidence for an association between the row and column factors. For example, there may be a number of retrospective studies, each providing evidence about a possible association between a certain disease and a certain environmental factor. Or, in a multicentre clinical trial, each centre may provide evidence about a possible difference between the proportions of patients whose condition is improved with treatment A and treatment B. These are examples of *stratification*. In the clinical trial, for example, the data are *stratified* by centre, and the aim is to study the effect of treatment on the patients' improvement *within the strata*.

How should such data be combined? The first point to make is that it may be quite misleading to pool the frequencies in the various tables, and examine the association suggested by the table of pooled frequencies. An extreme illustration is provided by the following hypothetical data.

Example 12.6

The frequencies in the lower left-hand corner of Table 12.6 are supposed to have been obtained in a retrospective survey in which 1000 patients with a certain disease are compared with 1000 control subjects. The proportion with a certain characteristic A is very slightly higher in the control group than in the disease group. If anything, therefore, the data suggest a negative association between the disease and factor A, although of course the difference would be far from significant. However, suppose the two groups had not been matched for sex, and that the data for the two sexes separately were as shown in the

Table 12.6 Retrospective survey to study the association between a disease and an aetiological factor; data subdivided by sex

		Observed frequencies			Expected frequencies	
		Disease	Control	Total	Disease	Control
Male	A	160	80	240	144	96
	Not A	440	320	760	456	304
		600	400	1000	600	400
Female	A	240	330	570	228	342
	Not A	160	270	430	172	258
		400	600	1000	400	600
Male	A	400	410	810	(372)	(438)
+ female	Not A	600	590	1190	(628)	(562)
		1000	1000	2000		

upper left part of the table. For each sex there is a positive association between the disease and factor A, as may be seen by comparing the observed frequencies on the left with the expected frequencies on the right. The latter are calculated in the usual way, separately for each sex; for example $144 = (240)(600)/1000$. What has happened here is that the control group contains a higher proportion of females than the disease group, and females have a higher prevalence of factor A then do males. The association suggested by the pooled frequencies is in the opposite direction from that suggested in each of the component tables. A variable like sex in this example, related both to the presence of disease and to a factor of interest, is called a *confounding variable*.

How should the evidence from separate tables be pooled? There is no unique answer. The procedure to be adopted will depend on whether the object is primarily to test the significance of a tendency for rows and columns to be associated in one direction throughout the data, or whether the association is to be measured, and if so in what way.

In some situations it is natural or convenient to study the association in each table by looking at the difference between two proportions. Suppose that, in the ith table, we are interested in a comparison between the proportion of individuals classified as 'positive', in each of two categories A and B, and that the frequencies in this table are as follows:

	A	B	Total A + B
Positive	r_{Ai}	r_{Bi}	$r_{.i}$
Negative	$n_{Ai} - r_{Ai}$	$n_{Bi} - r_{Bi}$	$n_{.i} - r_{.i}$
Total	n_{Ai}	n_{Bi}	$n_{.i}$
Proportion +ve	$p_{Ai} = r_{Ai}/n_{Ai}$	$p_{Bi} = r_{Bi}/n_{Bi}$	$p_{0i} = r_{.i}/n_{.i}$
			$q_{0_i} = 1 - p_{0i}$

The differences which interest us are

$$d_i = p_{Ai} - p_{Bi}. \tag{12.13}$$

These differences could be pooled in the form of a weighted mean

$$\bar{d} = \sum_i w_i d_i \bigg/ \sum_i w_i. \tag{12.14}$$

Cochran (1954) suggested the use of the weights defined as follows:

$$w_i = \frac{n_{Ai} n_{Bi}}{n_{Ai} + n_{Bi}}. \tag{12.15}$$

These have the property that in general more weight is given to tables with larger numbers provided they are reasonably balanced between categories A and B. It can be shown that this system of weights is the best for detecting small systematic differences between p_{Ai} and p_{Bi} of such a magnitude that the difference between their logits (11.7) is constant. This is a plausible requirement because a differential effect between A and B is likely to produce a larger d_i when the ps are near $\frac{1}{2}$ than when they are near 0 or 1.

Using the usual formula appropriate to the null hypothesis:

$$\mathrm{var}(d_i) = p_{0i} q_{0i} (n_{Ai} + n_{Bi})/n_{Ai} n_{Bi}, \tag{12.16}$$

we find

$$\mathrm{var}(\bar{d}) = \sum_i w_i p_{0i} q_{0i} \bigg/ \left(\sum w_i \right)^2,$$

$$\mathrm{SE}(\bar{d}) = \sqrt{\mathrm{var}(\bar{d})},$$

and, on the null hypothesis, $\bar{d}/\mathrm{SE}(\bar{d})$ can be taken as approximately a standardized normal deviate; or its square, $\bar{d}^2/\mathrm{var}(\bar{d})$, as a $\chi^2_{(1)}$ variate. An equivalent formula for the normal deviate is

$$\sum w_i d_i \bigg/ \sqrt{\left(\sum w_i p_{0i} q_{0i} \right)}.$$

Example 12.7

Table 12.7 shows some results taken from a trial to compare the mortality from tetanus in patients receiving antitoxin and in those not receiving antitoxin. The treatments were allocated at random, but by chance a higher proportion of patients in the 'No antitoxin' group had a more severe category of disease (as defined in terms of incubation period and period of onset of spasms). The third category (unknown severity) is clearly numerically unimportant, but may as well be included in the calculations. The overall results favour the use of antitoxin, but this may be due partly to the more favourable distribution of cases.

Table 12.7 Mortality from tetanus in a clinical trial to compare the effects of using and not using antitoxin, with classification of patients by severity of disease (from Brown *et al.*, 1960)

	No antitoxin		Antitoxin	
Severity group	Deaths/ total	Proportion deaths	Deaths/ total	Proportion deaths
I (most severe)	22/26	0·8462	15/21	0·7143
II (least severe)	6/11	0·5455	4/18	0·2222
III (unknown)	1/1	1·0000	1/2	0·5000

Cochran's test proceeds as follows.

Group	p_{0i}	d_i	$p_{0i}q_{0i}$	w_i
I	37/47 = 0·7872	0·1319	0·1675	11·62
II	10/29 = 0·3448	0·3233	0·2259	6·83
III	2/3 = 0·6667	0·5000	0·2222	0·67
				19·12

$$\bar{d} = 4·0758/19·12 = 0·2132,$$
$$SE(\bar{d}) = (\sqrt{3·6381})/19·12 = 0·0997,$$
$$\bar{d}/SE(\bar{d}) = 2·14,$$

beyond the 5% level of significance ($P = 0·032$).

Another approach to the problem of combining 2×2 tables is known as the Mantel–Haenszel method (Mantel and Haenszel, 1959). The number of positive individuals in group A, r_{Ai}, may be compared with its expected frequency

$$e_{Ai} = r_{.i}n_{Ai}/n_{.i}.$$

The variance of the discrepancy between observed and expected frequencies is

$$\text{var}(r_{Ai} - e_{Ai}) = \frac{n_{Ai}n_{Bi}r_{.i}(n_{.i} - r_{.i})}{n_{.i}^2(n_{.i} - 1)}. \tag{12.17}$$

A test for the association in the ith table is given by the $\chi^2_{(1)}$ statistic

$$X^2_{MH} = \frac{(r_{Ai} - e_{Ai})^2}{\text{var}(r_{Ai} - e_{Ai})}, \tag{12.18}$$

which is, in fact, equal to (4.22) and to the usual χ^2 statistic (4.21) multiplied by the factor $(n_{.i} - 1)/n_{.i}$, which is near unity for large sample sizes. If desired, a continuity correction analogous to (4.24) can be obtained by subtracting $\frac{1}{2}$ from the absolute value of the discrepancy before squaring in the numerator of (12.18).

To test the association in the set of tables combined we merely add the discrepancies and their variances, to obtain the combined statistic

$$X^2_{MH} = \frac{[\sum(r_{Ai} - e_{Ai})]^2}{\sum \text{var}(r_{Ai} - e_{Ai})}, \tag{12.19}$$

which is distributed approximately as a χ^2 with 1 DF. Were it not for the multiplying factors $(n_{.i} - 1)/n_{.i}$ this formula would agree exactly with the expression $\bar{d}^2/\text{var}(\bar{d})$ in Cochran's method (Radhakrishna, 1965). For this reason the present approach is often called the Cochran–Mantel–Haenszel method.

Example 12.7, continued

For the data in Table 12.7 the calculations for the Mantel–Haenszel test proceed as follows:

Group	r_{Ai}	e_{Ai}	$r_{Ai} - e_{Ai}$	$\text{var}(r_{Ai} - e_{Ai})$
I	22	20·468	1·532	1·988
II	6	3·793	2·207	1·598
III	1	0·667	0·333	0·222
	29	24·928	4·072	3·808

$$X^2_{MH} = (4·072)^2/3·808 = 4·35,$$

$$X_{MH} = 2·09,$$

a little less significant than the standardized deviate of 2.14 given earlier by the Cochran method, the change being due to the multiplying factors used in the variance calculations. With the continuity correction,

$$X^2_{MHc} = 3·35, \; X_{MHc} = 1·83 \; (P = 0·067).$$

The Mantel–Haenszel test is valid even when some or all of the strata have small total frequencies. A particular case is when each stratum consists of a matched pair. Then (12.19) is equivalent to McNemar's test, (4.12). The test is likely to be valid provided that $\sum e_{Ai}$ and the corresponding totals in the other three cells all exceed 5. When this is not the case an exact treatment is possible. This is an extension of the exact test in a single 2×2 table (§4.9). The one-tailed significance level is the probability that $\sum r_{Ai}$ is equal to or greater than its observed value where for any value of $\sum r_{Ai}$ the probability is calculated by considering all the possible combinations of tables over the strata that produce this total (Mehta et al., 1985; Hirji et al., 1988; Agresti, 1990, §7.4.4). The calculations are only feasible with appropriate software (see Chapter 18).

12.7 Combination of larger tables

The sort of problem considered in §12.6 can arise with larger tables. The investigator may be interested in the association between two categorical factors, with r and c categories respectively, and data may be available for k subgroups or strata, thus forming k separate tables. We can distinguish between (i) row and column factors both nominal; (ii) one factor (say, columns) nominal, and the other ordinal; and (iii) rows and columns both ordinal. In each case the Mantel–Haenszel method provides a useful approach. The general idea is to obtain discrepancies between observed frequencies and those expected if there were no association between rows and columns within strata. For a fuller account, see Kuritz *et al.* (1988).

When both factors are nominal, the question is whether there is an association between rows and columns, forming a reasonably consistent pattern across the different strata. A natural approach is to obtain expected frequencies from the margins of each table by (7.27), to add these over the k strata, and to compare the observed and expected total frequencies in the rc row–column combinations. One is tempted to do an ordinary χ^2 test on these pooled frequencies, using (7.28). However, this is not quite correct, since the expected frequencies have not been obtained directly from the pooled marginal frequencies. The simple statistic, X^2 from (7.28), does not follow the χ^2 distribution with $(r-1)(c-1)$ DF: the correct DF should be somewhat lower, making high values of X^2 more significant than would at first be thought. The effect is likely to be small, and it will often be adequate to use this as a convenient, although conservative, approximation, realizing that effects are somewhat more significant than they appear.

A correct χ^2 test involves matrix algebra, and is described, for instance by Kuritz *et al.* (1988), and for tables with $r = 2$ rows by Breslow and Day (1980, §4.5). The test is implemented by various computer programs, e.g. as the 'general association statistic' in the SAS program PROC FREQ. With only one stratum the test statistic is $(N-1)/N$ times the usual statistic (7.28). For $r = c = 2$, so that a series of 2×2 tables are being combined, the test statistic is identical with the Mantel–Haenszel statistic (12.19).

For the second case, of ordinal rows and nominal columns, we need a generalization of the $\chi^2_{(c-1)}$ test for equality of mean scores $\bar{x}_j$ given by (12.10). One solution is the 'ANOVA statistic' in the SAS program PROC FREQ. The case with $c = 2$ is of particular interest, being the stratified version of the test for trends in proportions dealt with in §12.2 (Mantel, 1963). Using the index h to denote a particular stratum, the quantities T_h and $\text{var}(T_h)$ are calculated from (12.4) and (12.5), and the overall trend is tested by the statistic

$$X^2 = \frac{(\sum_h T_h)^2}{\sum_h \text{var}(T_h)}, \tag{12.20}$$

approximately distributed as $\chi^2_{(1)}$.

Example 12.8

Table 12.8 Combination of trends in proportions of operating theatre staff with antibodies to humidifier fever antigens

Length of exposure (years)	Score x	Age (years)							
		−34 ($h = 1$)		35–44 ($h = 2$)		45– ($h = 3$)		Total	
		Antibodies							
		+	−	+	−	+	−	+	−
< 1	1	0	9	2	5	0	3	2	17
1–5	2	3	7	2	2	6	1	11	10
> 5	3	3	0	4	2	5	6	12	8
		6	16	8	9	11	10	25	35
$\sum x_{ih} r_{ih}$		15		18		27		60	
$\sum x_{ih} e_{ih}$		10·36		15·53		26·19		52·08	
T_h		4·64		2·47		0·81		7·92	
var (T_h)		2·15		3·43		2·87		8·45	

Table 12.8 gives some data from a study by Cockcroft *et al.* (1981). Staff who worked in an operating theatre were tested for antibodies to humidifier antigens. The objective was to establish if there was a relationship between the prevalence of antibodies and the length of time worked in the theatre. Age was related to length of exposure and to antibodies and it was required to test the association of interest after taking account of age. The calculations are shown in Table 12.8. The test statistic is

$$X^2 = (7·92)^2/8·45$$

$$= 7·42 \text{ (1 DF)}.$$

Thus there was evidence of an association after allowing for age ($P = 0·006$); if age had been ignored the association would have appeared stronger ($X^2_{1a} = 9·53$ using (12.6)) but its validity would have been in doubt because of the confounding effect of age.

The third case, of two ordinal factors, leads (Mantel, 1963) to a generalization of the correlation-type statistic (12.11) distributed approximately as $\chi^2_{(1)}$:

$$X^2 = \frac{(\sum_h S_{xyh})^2}{\sum_h [S_{xxh} S_{yyh}/(N_h - 1)]}. \qquad (12.21)$$

Finally, it is useful to note the stratified version of the test for trends in counts given in §12.4. Again using the subscript h to denote a particular stratum, the

$\chi^2_{(1)}$ statistic is

$$X^2_{1P} = \frac{\left\{ \sum_h \left[\sum_i x_{hi}(r_{hi} - e_{hi}) \right] \right\}^2}{\sum_h \left[\sum_i e_{hi}x^2_{hi} - \left(\sum_i e_{hi}x_{hi} \right)^2 / R_h \right]}. \tag{12.22}$$

This formula is derived from (12.12) by summing over the strata before the numerator is squared, and by summing also in the denominator. Extensive use is made of this statistic by Darby and Reissland (1981) in comparing the numbers of deaths from various causes amongst workers exposed to different doses of radiation (the x variable) with the numbers expected from the person-years at risk in the different categories (see §14.9). The strata were defined by various personal characteristics, including age and length of time since start of employment.

12.8 Generalized linear models

In Chapter 10 we considered multiple linear regression and noted that in this method the mean value of the dependent variable is expressed as a linear function of a set of explanatory variables and that for an observed value of the dependent variable there would be an error term (10.1). The classical method applies to the case where the error terms are independently and normally distributed with zero mean and constant variance. Thus the method is not strictly applicable to the case where the dependent variable is qualitative. Yet the concept of a relationship between the distribution of a dependent variable and a number of explanatory variables is just as valid when the dependent variable is qualitative as when it is continuous. For example, consider a binomial variable representing presence or absence of disease. For a homogeneous group of individuals the number with disease would be distributed according to the binomial distribution with a constant probability of disease (§2.5). Often the individuals will not come from a homogeneous group but will differ on a number of variables associated with the probability of having the disease. That is, there would be a relationship between probability of disease and a set of explanatory variables. This relationship would not usually be linear since a straight-line relationship would imply probabilities outside the legitimate range of 0 to 1 for some values of the explanatory variables. In order to fit the relationship into the framework of linear regression it is necessary to apply a transformation and this leads to the methods of *logistic regression* and *probit analysis* discussed below. A second example is when the dependent variable is distributed according to the Poisson distribution (§2.6) and the expectation of the Poisson process is related to a number of explanatory variables. Although regression methods to analyse qualitative variables have been known for several decades—for example, the first edition of Finney's book *Probit Analysis* was published in 1947—it is only in the last two decades that the methods have been used widely in a variety of situations. An important paper by

Nelder and Wedderburn (1972) developed the concept of *generalized linear models*, which placed all the commonly used models into a unified framework. This in turn led to the introduction of computer software to carry out the calculations.

In this section we consider some of the properties of generalized linear models and illustrate their application with examples. Readers interested in a more detailed exposition are referred to the books by McCullagh and Nelder (1989) and Dobson (1990). Cox and Snell (1989) and Hosmer and Lemeshow (1989) give details of logistic regression.

General theory

Consider a random variable y distributed according to the probability density $f(y; \mu)$, where μ is the expected value of y; that is,

$$E(y) = \mu. \tag{12.23}$$

Suppose that for each observation y there is a set of explanatory variables $x_1, x_2, \ldots, x_p$ and that μ depends on the values of these variables. Suppose further that after some transformation of μ, $g(\mu)$, the relationship is linear; that is,

$$\eta = g(\mu) = \alpha + \beta_1 x_1 + \beta_2 x_2 + \ldots + \beta_p x_p. \tag{12.24}$$

Then the relationship between y and the explanatory variables is a *generalized linear model*. The transformation, $g(\mu)$, is termed the *link function*, since it provides the link between the linear part of the model, η, and the random part represented by μ. The linear function, η, is termed the *linear predictor* and the distribution of y, $f(y; \mu)$, is the *error distribution*.

Normal distribution

When the error distribution is normal, the classic linear regression model is:

$$E(y) = \alpha + \beta_1 x_1 + \beta_2 x_2 + \ldots + \beta_p x_p.$$

Thus from (12.23) and (12.24), $\eta = \mu$, and the link function is the identity, $g(\mu) = \mu$. Thus the familiar multiple linear regression is a member of the family of generalized linear models.

Binomial distribution

Since the linear predictor of (12.24) covers an unlimited range, the link function should transform μ, the binomial probability, from the range 0 to 1 to $-\infty$ to ∞.

Two commonly used transformations that achieve this are the probit transformation (11.5)

$$g(\mu) = \Phi^{-1}(\mu),$$

where Φ is the cumulative distribution function of a standardized normal variable, and the logit transformation (11.7)

$$g(\mu) = \ln[\mu/(1 - \mu)].$$

This transformation gives the method of *logistic regression*:

$$\ln\left(\frac{\mu}{1 - \mu}\right) = \alpha + \beta_1 x_1 + \beta_2 x_2 + \ldots + \beta_p x_p. \tag{12.25}$$

The probit transformation is reasonable on biological grounds in some circumstances and is used in biological assay (see Chapter 17). The logit transformation is similar to the probit but on biological grounds is more arbitrary. The logit transformation has important advantages, however. First, it is easier to calculate since it requires only the log function rather than tables of the normal distribution. Secondly, and more importantly, the logit is the logarithm of the odds, and logit differences are logarithms of odds ratios. The odds ratio is important in the analysis of epidemiological studies and logistic regression can be used for a variety of epidemiological study designs (§16.2); this is not possible with the probit transformation.

Poisson distribution

The expectation of a Poisson variable is positive and so limited to the range 0 to ∞. A link function is required to transform this to the unlimited range $-\infty$ to ∞. The usual transformation is the logarithmic transformation

$$g(\mu) = \ln \mu,$$

leading to the log-linear model

$$\ln \mu = \alpha + \beta_1 x_1 + \beta_2 x_2 + \ldots + \beta_p x_p. \tag{12.26}$$

Fitting a model

We shall discuss two approaches: first an approximate method using *empirical weights* and secondly the theoretically more satisfactory maximum likelihood solution.

Approximate solution with empirical weights

This method will be considered in the context of logistic regression. Suppose that in a sample of n individuals there are r positives and $n - r$ negatives, with $p = r/n$, and that the expected proportion of positives is π. Define $q = 1 - p$. The logit of p is defined as

$$y = \ln \frac{p}{q};$$
(12.27)

(see (11.7)). A difficulty arises if $r = 0$ or n, for then $p = 0$ or 1 and $y = -\infty$ or ∞ respectively. A modified definition,

$$y = \ln \left(\frac{r + \frac{1}{2}}{n - r + \frac{1}{2}} \right),$$
(12.28)

is useful. If more than the occasional values of p are 0 or 1, it is probably wise to use (12.28) throughout but preferable to use the method of maximum likelihood. Use of (12.28) also reduces bias for small values of n.

From (2.13) and (3.17), an approximate formula for var(y) is

$$\text{var}(y) \simeq \frac{1}{n\pi(1 - \pi)},$$
(12.29)

which may be estimated by

$$\frac{1}{npq}.$$
(12.30)

Defining a weighting coefficient

$$w = pq,$$
(12.31)

we could attach a weight nw to the logit, y, and thereby weight each value of y in inverse proportion to its variance. This is the general approach adopted in a weighted analysis (§7.2), and we may expect the general method of weighted regression (p. 334) to provide an approximate solution.

The model here would be of the form given in (12.25). The proposed method is not exact; first because the ys are not normally distributed about their population values; and secondly because the weight now used for any y is not exactly in inverse proportion to var(y), being expressed in terms of the estimated proportion p. For this reason the weights are often called *empirical*.

In problems requiring an analysis of variance approach, the empirical weight now takes the place of the number of observations in a particular subgroup. Since the various values of nw will in general be different, the situation is analogous to an unbalanced experimental design, and the methods of non-orthogonal analysis (§10.4) may often be used.

Example 12.9

Table 12.9 shows some data reported by Lombard and Doering (1947) from a survey of knowledge about cancer. These data have been used by several other authors (Dyke and

Table 12.9 A 2^4 factorial set of proportions (Lombard and Doering, 1947)

Factor combination	(1) Number of individuals n	(2) Number with good score r	(3) Proportion (2)/(1) p	(4) Logit (p) y	(5) Weighting coefficient $w = pq$	(6) Weight $(1) \times (5)$ nw	(7) Variance $1/(6)$ $1/nw$
(1)	477	84	0·176	− 1·54	0·1450	69·16	0·014
(a)	231	75	0·325	− 0·73	0·2194	50·68	0·020
(b)	63	13	0·206	− 1·35	0·1636	10·31	0·097
(ab)	94	35	0·372	− 0·52	0·2336	21·96	0·046
(c)	150	67	0·447	− 0·21	0·2472	37·08	0·027
(ac)	378	201	0·532	0·13	0·2490	94·12	0·011
(bc)	32	16	0·500	0·00	0·2500	8·00	0·125
(abc)	169	102	0·604	0·42	0·2392	40·42	0·025
(d)	12	2	0·167	− 1·61	0·1391	1·67	0·600
(ad)	13	7	0·538	0·15	0·2486	3·23	0·310
(bd)	7	4	0·571	0·29	0·2450	1·72	0·581
(abd)	12	8	0·667	0·69	0·2222	2·67	0·375
(cd)	11	3	0·273	− 0·98	0·1985	2·18	0·459
(acd)	45	27	0·600	0·41	0·2400	10·80	0·093
(bcd)	4	1	0·250	− 1·10	0·1875	0·75	1·333
(abcd)	31	23	0·742	1·06	0·1914	5·93	0·169

Patterson, 1952; Naylor, 1964). Each line of the table corresponds to a particular combination of factors in a 2^4 factorial arrangement, n being the number of individuals in this category and r the number who gave a good score in response to questions about cancer knowledge. The four factors are: A, newspaper reading; B, listening to radio; C, solid reading; D, attendance at lectures.

Although the data are obtained from a survey rather than from a randomized experiment, we can usefully study the effect on cancer knowledge of the four main effects and their interactions. In a 2^p factorial design with disproportionate numbers the usual analysis of variance is inappropriate, but the main effects and interactions, although no longer orthogonal, can be estimated. For the main effect of A, for example, the other three factors form eight strata. The effect of A can be estimated in each stratum and these estimates combined appropriately. The approach is essentially the same as that used in (8.25) for the estimation of a row effect in a non-orthogonal $2 \times c$ table. Each stratum provides a difference, $d = y_1 - y_2$, an estimated $\mathrm{var}(d)$, obtained from the sum of the two entries in column (7) of Table 12.9, and a weight equal to the reciprocal of $\mathrm{var}(d)$. These are as follows:

	d	$\mathrm{var}(d)$	w
$(a)-(1)$	0·81	0·034	29·2
$(ab)-(b)$	0·83	0·143	7·0
$(ac)-(c)$	0·34	0·038	26·6
$(abc)-(bc)$	0·42	0·150	6·7
$(ad)-(d)$	1·76	0·910	1·1
$(abd)-(bd)$	0·40	0·956	1·0
$(acd)-(cd)$	1·39	0·552	1·8
$(abcd)-(bcd)$	2·16	1·502	0·7
			74·1

These values of d may be combined in a weighted mean, as in (8.25), giving

$$\bar{d} = 47{\cdot}67/74{\cdot}1 = 0{\cdot}643,$$

$$\mathrm{var}(\bar{d}) = 1/\textstyle\sum w = 0{\cdot}0135$$

and

$$\mathrm{SE}(\bar{d}) = 0{\cdot}116.$$

A test of the effect is provided by $\bar{d}/\mathrm{SE}(\bar{d})$, assessed as a standardized normal deviate, or its square as a $\chi^2_{(1)}$ variate. The estimates of the four main effects, with standard errors and test statistics, are:

	$\bar{d}$	$\mathrm{SE}(\bar{d})$	z	P
A	0·643	0·116	5·54	< 0·001
B	0·292	0·124	2·35	0·019
C	0·997	0·111	8·98	< 0·001
D	0·441	0·196	2·25	0·024

The approximate method is adequate if most of the sample sizes are reasonably large and few of the ps are close to 0 or 1. If the observed proportions p are based on $n = 1$ observation only, their values will be either 0 or 1, and the empirical method cannot be used. This situation occurs in the analysis of prognostic data, where an individual patient is classified as 'success' or 'failure', several explanatory variables x_j are observed, and the object is to predict the probability of success in terms of the xs.

Maximum likelihood

A general method of estimation, that of *maximum likelihood*, has certain desirable theoretical properties and can be applied in those circumstances discussed above where the empirical method is unsatisfactory. The likelihood of the data is proportional to the probability of obtaining the data (§2.8). For data of known distributional form, and where the mean value is given in terms of a generalized linear model, the probability of the observed data can be written down using the appropriate probability distributions. For example, with logistic regression the probability for each group or individual can be calculated using the binomial probability from (12.25) in (2.9) and the likelihood of the whole data is the product of these probabilities over all groups or individuals. This likelihood depends on the values of the regression coefficients and the maximum likelihood estimates of these regression coefficients are those values that maximize the likelihood—that is, the values for which the data are most likely to occur. For theoretical reasons, and also for practical convenience, it is preferable to work in terms of the logarithm of the likelihood. Thus it is the log-likelihood, L, that is maximized. The method also gives standard errors of the estimated regression coefficients and significance tests of specific hypotheses.

By analogy with the analysis of variance for a continuous variable the *analysis of deviance* is used in generalized linear models. The *deviance* is defined as twice the difference between the log-likelihood of a perfectly fitting model and the current model, and has associated degrees of freedom equal to the difference in the number of parameters between these two models. Where the error distribution is completely defined by the link between the random and linear parts of the model, and this will be the case for binomial and Poisson variables but not for a normal variable for which the size of the variance is also required, then deviances follow approximately the χ^2 distribution and can be used for the testing of significance. In particular, reductions in deviance due to adding extra terms into the model can be used to assess whether the inclusion of the extra terms had resulted in a significant improvement to the model. This is analogous to the procedure described in §10.4 for a continuous variable.

The procedure for fitting a model using the maximum likelihood method usually involves iteration—that is, repeating a sequence of calculations until a stable solution is reached. Fitted weights are used and, since these depend on the parameter estimates, they change from cycle to cycle of the iteration. The approximate solution using empirical weights could be the first cycle in this iterative procedure, and the whole procedure is sometimes called *iterative weighted least squares.* The technical details of the procedure will not be given since the process is obviously rather tedious; for further details of the maximum likelihood method see Wetherill (1981). A general computer program is essential, e.g. PROC LOGISTIC in the SAS program, LOGISTIC REGRESSION in SPSS, or GLIM.

Example 12.10

The data considered in Example 12.9 will now be analysed by maximum likelihood. There are 16 groups of individuals and a model containing all main effects and all interactions would fit the data perfectly. Thus by definition it would have a deviance of zero and serves as the reference point in assessing the fit of simpler models.

The first logistic regression model fitted was that containing only the main effects. This gave a model in which the logit of the probability of a good score was estimated as

$$-1{\cdot}460 \quad + \quad 0{\cdot}650A \quad + \quad 0{\cdot}310B \quad + \quad 0{\cdot}981C \quad + \quad 0{\cdot}420D$$

SE:	0·115	0·122	0·111	0·191
z:	5·65	2·54	8·84	2·20
P:	< 0·001	0·011	< 0·001	0·028

Here the terms involving A, B, C and D are included when these factors are present and omitted otherwise.

The estimates of the main effects and their standard errors are close to the weighted estimates given in Example 12.9. The significance of the main effects may be tested by the ratio of its estimate to its standard error assessed as a standardized normal deviate. This is known as the *Wald* test, and its square as the *Wald* χ^2. Alternatively the significance may be established by analysis of deviance by fitting the model containing only the main effects of B, C and D, which gives a deviance of 45·47 with 12 DF. Adding the main effect of A to the model reduces the deviance to 13·59 with 11 DF, so that the deviance test for the effect of A, after allowing for B, C and D, is $45{\cdot}47 - 13{\cdot}59 = 31{\cdot}88$ as an approximate $\chi^2_{(1)}$. This test is numerically equivalent to the z test, since $\sqrt{31{\cdot}88} = 5{\cdot}65$, but in general such exact agreement would not be expected. Although the deviance tests of main effects are not necessary here, in general they are needed. For example, if a factor with more than two levels were fitted, using dummy variables (§10.2), a deviance test with the appropriate degrees of freedom would be required.

The deviance associated with the model including all the main effects is 13·59 with 11 DF, and this represents the 11 interactions not included in the model. Taking the deviance as a $\chi^2_{(11)}$ there is no evidence that the interactions are significant and the model with just main effects is a good fit. There is still scope for one of the two-factor interactions to be significant. It is therefore prudent to try including each of the six two-factor interactions in turn to the model. As an example, when the interaction of the two kinds of reading, AC, is included, the deviance reduces to 10·72 with 10 DF. Thus this interaction has an approximate $\chi^2_{(1)}$ of 2·87, which is not significant ($P = 0{\cdot}091$). Similarly none of the other interactions is significant.

Example 12.11

Consider the data in Table 8.14, which have been analysed in Examples 8.9 and 10.5. The data consist of 41 men, classified by three age groups and two treatment groups, and the variable to be analysed is the number of cerebrovascular accidents. This variable takes integral values and the highest value observed is 3. If the number of accidents is taken as having a Poisson distribution with expectation dependent on age and treatment group, then a log-linear model (12.26) would be appropriate.

Several log-linear models have been fitted and the following analysis of deviance constructed:

Analysis of deviance

Fitting	Deviance	DF	Effect	Deviance difference	DF
Constant term	40·54	40			
Treatment, T	31·54	39	T (unadj.)	9·00	1
Age, A	37·63	38	A (unadj.)	2·91	2
T + A	28·84	37	T (adj.)	8·79	1
			A (adj.)	2·70	2
T + A + T × A	27·04	35	T × A	1·80	2

The test of the treatment effect after allowing for age is obtained from the deviance difference after adding in a treatment effect to a model already containing age; that is, $37·63 - 28·84 = 8·79$ (1 DF). Similarly, the effect of age adjusted for treatment has a test statistic of 2·70 (2 DF). As previously, there is no evidence of an interaction between treatment and age, or of a main effect of age.

The log-linear model fitting just treatment is

$$\ln \mu = 0·00 - 1·386 \text{ (treated group)},$$

$$\text{SE: } 0·536$$

giving fitted expectations of $\exp(0·00) = 1·00$ for the control group and $\exp(-1·386) = 0·25$ for the treated group. These values are identical with the observed values—25 accidents in 25 men in the control group and four accidents in 16 men in the treated group—although if it had proved necessary to adjust for age this would not have been so.

The deviance of 27·04 with 35 DF after fitting all effects is a measure of how well the Poisson model fits the data. However, it would not be valid to assess this deviance as an approximate $\chi^2_{(35)}$ because of the low counts on which it is based. Note that this restriction does not apply to the tests of main effects and interactions since these comparisons are based on amalgamated data, as illustrated above for the effect of treatment.

The data of Example 10.7 could be analysed using logistic regression. In this case the observed proportions are each based on one observation only. As a model we could suppose that the logit of the population probability of survival, Y, was related to haemoglobin, x_1, and bilirubin, x_2, by the linear logistic regression formula (12.25)

$$Y = \alpha + \beta_1 x_1 + \beta_2 x_2.$$

Application of the maximum likelihood method gave the following estimates of α, β_1 and β_2 with their standard errors:

$$\hat{a} = -2\cdot354 \pm 2\cdot416,$$
$$\hat{\beta}_1 = 0\cdot5324 \pm 0\cdot1487, \qquad (12.32)$$
$$\hat{\beta}_2 = -0\cdot4892 \pm 0\cdot3448.$$

The picture is similar to that presented by the discriminant analysis of Example 10.7. Haemoglobin is an important predictor; bilirubin is not. An interesting point is that, if the distributions of the xs are multivariate normal, with the same variances and covariances for both successes and failures (the basic model for discriminant analysis), the discriminant function (10.42) can also be used to predict Y. The formula is:

$$Y = \alpha' + \beta'_1 x_1 + \beta'_2 x_2 + \ldots + \beta'_m x_m,$$

where

$$\beta'_j = b_j$$

and

$$\alpha' = -\tfrac{1}{2}[\beta'_1(\bar{x}_{A1} + \bar{x}_{B1}) + \ldots + \beta'_m(\bar{x}_{Am} + \bar{x}_{Bm})] + \ln(n_A/n_B). \qquad (12.33)$$

In Example 10.7, using the discriminant function coefficients b_1 and b_2 given there, we find

$$\left.\begin{array}{l} \alpha' = -4\cdot135 \\ \beta'_1 = 0\cdot6541 \\ \beta'_2 = -0\cdot3978 \end{array}\right\}$$

which lead to values of Y not differing greatly from those obtained from (12.32), except for extreme values of x_1 and x_2.

An example of the use of the linear discriminant function to predict the probability of coronary heart disease is given by Truett et al. (1967). The point should be emphasized that in situations in which the distributions of xs are far from multivariate normal this method may be unreliable, and the maximum likelihood solution will be preferable.

To test the adequacy of the generalized linear model (12.24), after fitting by maximum likelihood, an approximate χ^2 test statistic is given by the deviance. This was the approach in Example 12.10, where the deviance after fitting the four main effects was 13·59 with 11 DF (since four main effects and a constant term had been estimated from 16 groups). The fit is clearly adequate, suggesting that there is no need to postulate interactions, although, as was done in the example, a further refinement to testing the goodness of fit is to try interactions since a single effect with 1 DF could be undetected when tested with other effects contributing 10 DF.

In general terms the adequacy of the model (12.24) can be assessed by including terms such as x_i^2, to test for linearity in x_i, and $x_i x_j$, to test for an interaction between x_i and x_j.

The approximation to the distribution of the deviance by χ^2 is unreliable if a high proportion of the observations are based on small values of n, and is particularly useless in the case discussed above, where all values of n are 1, or in Example 12.11. In such cases tests based on grouping the data may be constructed. For a logistic regression, grouping could be by the estimated probabilities and a χ^2 test produced by comparing observed and expected frequencies (Lemeshow and Hosmer, 1982).

Diagnostic methods based on residuals similar to those used in classical regression (§10.1) can be applied. If the data are already grouped, as in Example 12.9, then standardized residuals can be produced and assessed, where each residual is standardized by its estimated standard error. For example, in logistic regression the standardized residual is

$$\frac{r - n\hat{\mu}}{\sqrt{[n\hat{\mu}\,(1 - \hat{\mu})]}}$$

where there are r events out of n. For individual data the residual may be defined using the above expression, with r either 0 or 1, but the individual residuals are of little use since they are not distributed normally and cannot be assessed individually. For example, if $\hat{\mu} = 0.01$, the only possible values of the standardized residual are 9·9 and -0.1; the occurrence of the larger residual does not necessarily indicate an outlying point, and if accompanied by 99 of the smaller residuals the fit would be perfect. It is, therefore, necessary to group the residuals, defining groups as individuals with similar values of the x_i.

Alternative definitions of the residual include correcting for the leverage of the point in the space of the explanatory variables to produce a residual equivalent to the studentized residual (10.18). Another definition is the *deviance residual*, defined as the square root of the contribution of the point to the deviance. Cox and Snell (1989, §2.7) give a good description of the use of residuals in logistic regression.

Cox and Snell (1989) also discuss the use of influence diagnostics. The concept of Cook's distance can be used in logistic regression and (10.23) applies, although in this case only approximately (Pregibon, 1981).

The model might be inadequate because of an inappropriate choice of the link function. An approach to this problem is to extend the link function into a family indexed by one or more parameters. Tests can then be derived to determine if there is evidence against the particular member of the family originally used (Pregibon, 1980; Brown, 1982; McCullagh and Nelder, 1989).

We conclude our discussion of the generalized linear model (12.24) with an example of a log-linear model applied to Poisson counts.

Example 12.12

Table 12.10 gives data on the number of incident cases of cancer in a large group of ex-servicemen, who had been followed up over a 20-year period. The servicemen are in two groups according to whether they served in a combat zone (veterans) or not, and the experience of each serviceman is classified into subject-years at risk in 5-year age groups. The study is described in Australian Institute of Health and Welfare (1992), where the analysis was also controlled for calender year. Each serviceman passed through several of these groups during the period of follow-up. The study was carried out in order to assess if there was a difference in cancer risk between veterans and non-veterans. The model used was a variant on (12.26). If y_{ij} is the number of cases of cancer in group i and age-group j, and N_{ij} is the corresponding number of subject-years then y_{ij}/N_{ij} is the incidence rate. The log-linear model is that the logarithm of incidence will follow a linear model on variables representing the group and age. Thus if μ_{ij} is the expectation of y_{ij} then

$$\ln \mu_{ij} = \ln N_{ij} + \alpha + \beta_i x_i + \gamma_j z_j,$$

where x_i and z_j are dummy variables representing the veteran groups and the age groups respectively (the dummy variables were defined as in §10.2, with $x_1 = 1$ for the veterans group, and $z_1, z_2, \ldots, z_{10} = 1$ for age groups 25–29, 30–34, ..., 70–; no dummy variable was required for the non-veterans or the youngest age group as their effects are included within the coefficient α). This model differs from (12.26) in the inclusion of the first term on the right-hand side, which ensures that the number of years at risk is taken into account (see (14.25)).

Table 12.10 Number of incident cases of cancer and subject-years at risk in a group of ex-servicemen

Age	Veterans		Non-veterans	
	Number of cancers	Subject-years	Number of cancers	Subject-years
–24	6	60 840	18	208 487
25–29	21	157 175	60	303 832
30–34	54	176 134	122	325 421
35–39	118	186 514	191	312 242
40–44	97	135 475	108	165 597
45–49	58	42 620	74	54 396
50–54	56	25 001	88	40 716
55–59	54	13 710	120	33 801
60–64	34	6163	141	26 618
65–69	9	1575	108	17 404
70–	2	273	99	14 146
Total	509	805 480	1129	1502 660

The model was fitted by maximum likelihood using GLIM with $\ln N_{ij}$ included as an OFFSET. The estimates of the regression coefficients were:

	Estimate	SE
a	-9.324	
b_1 (veterans)	-0.0035	0.0555
c_1 (25–29)	0.679	0.232
c_2 (30–34)	1.371	0.218
c_3 (35–39)	1.940	0.212
c_4 (40–44)	2.034	0.216
c_5 (45–49)	2.727	0.222
c_6 (50–54)	3.203	0.221
c_7 (55–59)	3.716	0.218
c_8 (60–64)	4.093	0.218
c_9 (65–69)	4.236	0.224
c_{10} (70–)	4.364	0.227

The estimate of the veterans effect is not significant, Wald $z = -0.0035/0.0555 = 0.06$ ($P = 0.95$). Converting back from the log scale, the estimate of the relative risk of cancer in veterans compared with non-veterans, after controlling for age, is $\exp(-0.0035) = 1.00$. The 95% confidence limits are $\exp(-0.0035 \pm 1.96 \times 0.0555) = 0.89$ and 1.11.

Polytomous regression

The procedures described in earlier sections of this chapter for the analysis of ordered categorical data are limited in two respects: they are appropriate for relatively simple data structures, where the factors to be studied are few in number; and the emphasis has so far been mainly on significance tests, with little discussion of the need to describe the nature of any associations revealed by the tests. Both of these limitations are overcome by generalized linear models, which relate the distribution of the ordered categorical response to a number of explanatory variables. Because response variables of this type have more than two categories they are often referred to as *polytomous responses* and the corresponding procedures as *polytomous regression*.

Three approaches are described very briefly here. The first two are generalizations of logistic regression, and the third is related to the earlier discussions (see (12.7)) about comparisons of mean scores.

The cumulative logits model

Denote the polytomous response variable by Y, and a particular category of Y by j. The set of explanatory variables, $x_1, x_2, \ldots, x_p$, will be denoted by the vector x.

Let

$$F_j(x) = P(Y \le j, \text{ given } x)$$

and

$$L_j(x) = \text{logit } F_j(x)$$

$$= \ln\left[\frac{F_j(x)}{1 - F_j(x)}\right].$$

The model is described by the equation

$$L_j(x) = \alpha_j - \beta'x, \tag{12.34}$$

where $\beta'x$ represents the usual linear function of the explanatory variables, $\beta_1 x_1 + \beta_2 x_2 + \dots + \beta_p x_p$.

This model effectively gives a logistic regression, as in (12.25), for each of the binary variables produced by drawing boundaries between two adjacent categories. For instance, if there are four categories numbered 1 to 4, there are three binary variables representing the splits between 1 and 2–4, 1–2 and 3–4, and 1–3 and 4. Moreover, the regression coefficients β for the explanatory variables are the same for all the splits, although the intercept term α_j varies with the split.

Although a standard logistic regression could be carried out for any one of the splits, a rather more complex analysis is needed to take account of the inter-relations between the data for different splits. Computer programs are available (for instance, in SAS) to estimate the coefficients in the model and their precision, either by maximum likelihood (as in SAS LOGIST) or weighted least squares (as in SAS CATMOD), the latter being less reliable when many of the frequencies in the original data are low.

The adjacent categories model

Here we define logits in terms of the probabilities for adjacent categories. Define

$$L_j = \ln\left(\frac{\pi_j}{\pi_{j+1}}\right),$$

where π_j is the probability of falling into the jth response category. The model is described by the equation

$$L_j = \alpha_j - \beta'x. \tag{12.35}$$

When there are only two response categories, (12.34) and (12.35) are entirely equivalent, and both the cumulative logits model and the adjacent categories model reduce to ordinary logistic regression. In the more general case, with more than two categories, computer programs are available for estimation of the coefficients. For example, SAS CATMOD uses weighted least squares.

The mean response model

Suppose that scores x are assigned to the categories, as in §12.2, and denote by $M(x)$ the mean score for individuals with explanatory variables x. The model specifies the same linear relation as in multiple regression:

$$M(x) = \alpha + \beta' x. \tag{12.36}$$

The approach is thus a generalization of that underlying the comparison of mean scores by (12.7) in the simple two-group case. In the general case the regression coefficients cannot accurately be estimated by standard multiple regression methods, because there may be large departures from normality and disparities in variance. Nor can exact variances such as (12.5) be easily exploited. Computer programs are available for estimation by weighted least squares (e.g. SAS CATMOD).

Choice of model

The choice between the models described briefly above, or any others, is largely empirical: which is the most convenient to use, and which best describes the data? There is no universally best choice. The two logistic models attempt to describe the relative frequencies of observations in the various categories, and their adequacy for any particular data set may be checked by comparing observed and expected frequencies. The mean response model is less searching, since it aims to describe only the mean values. It may therefore be a little more flexible in fitting data, and particularly appropriate where there is a natural underlying continuous response variate or scoring system, but less appropriate when the fine structure of the categorical response is under study.

   Further descriptions of these models are given in Agresti (1990, Chapter 9), and an application to repeated measures data is described in Agresti (1989).

12.9 Standardization

Problems similar to those discussed in §§12.6–12.8 arise frequently in vital statistics and have given rise to a group of methods called standardization. We shall describe briefly one or two of the most well-known methods, and discuss their relationship to the methods described above.

   Mortality in a population is usually measured by an annual death rate, for example, the number of individuals dying during a certain calendar year divided by the estimated population size midway through the year. Frequently this ratio is multiplied by a convenient base, such as 1000, to avoid small decimal fractions; it is then called the annual death rate per 1000 population. If the death rate is calculated for a population covering a wide age range, it is called a *crude death rate*.

In a comparison of the mortality of two populations, say those of two different countries, the crude rates may be misleading. Mortality depends strongly on age. If the two countries have different age structures, this contrast alone may explain a difference in crude rates (just as, in Table 12.6, the contrast between the 'crude' proportions with factor A was strongly affected by the different sex distributions in the disease and control groups). An example is given in Table 12.11 on p. 440, which shows the numbers of individuals and numbers of deaths separately in different groups, for two countries: A, typical of highly industrialized countries, with a rather high proportion of individuals at the older ages; and B, a developing country with a small proportion of old people. The death rates at each age (which are called, *age-specific death rates*) are substantially higher for B than for A, and yet the crude death rate is higher for A than for B.

The situation here is precisely the same as that discussed at the beginning of §12.6, in connection with Example 12.6. Sometimes, however, mortality has to be compared for a large number of different populations, and some form of adjustment for age differences is required. For example, the mortality in one country may have to be compared over several different years; different regions of the same country may be under study; or one may wish to compare the mortality for a large number of different occupations. Two obvious generalizations are (i) in standardizing for factors other than, or in addition to, age—for example, sex, as in Table 12.6; and (ii) in morbidity studies where the criterion studied is the occurrence of a certain illness rather than of death. We shall discuss the usual situation—the standardization of mortality rates for age.

The basic idea in standardization is that we introduce a *standard population* with a fixed age structure. The mortality for any *special population* is then adjusted to allow for discrepancies in age structure between the standard and special populations. There are two main approaches: *direct* and *indirect* methods of standardization. The following brief account may be supplemented by reference to Hill and Hill (1991), Liddell (1960) or Kalton (1968).

The following notation will be used.

Age group	Standard			Special		
	(1) Population	(2) Deaths	(3) Death rate (2)/(1)	(4) Population	(5) Deaths	(6) Death rate (5)/(4)
1	N_1	R_1	P_1	n_1	r_1	p_1
$\vdots$						
i	N_i	R_i	P_i	n_i	r_i	p_i
$\vdots$						
k	N_k	R_k	P_k	n_k	r_k	p_k

Direct method

The standardized death rate for the special population, by the direct method, is

$$p' = \frac{\sum N_i p_i}{\sum N_i}. \tag{12.37}$$

It is obtained by applying the special death rates, p_i, to the standard population sizes, N_i. Alternatively, p' can be regarded as a weighted mean of the p_i, using the N_i as weights. The variance of p' may be estimated as

$$\text{var}(p') = \frac{\sum (N_i^2 p_i q_i / n_i)}{(\sum N_i)^2}, \tag{12.38}$$

where $q_i = 1 - p_i$; if, as is often the case, the p_i are all small, the binomial variance of p_i, $p_i q_i / n_i$, may be replaced by the Poisson term p_i / n_i ($= r_i / n_i^2$), giving

$$\text{var}(p') \simeq \frac{\sum (N_i^2 p_i / n_i)}{(\sum N_i)^2}. \tag{12.39}$$

To compare two special populations, A and B, we could calculate a standardized rate for each (p_A' and p_B'), and consider

$$\bar{d} = p_A' - p_B'.$$

From (12.37),

$$\bar{d} = \frac{\sum N_i (p_{Ai} - p_{Bi})}{\sum N_i},$$

which has exactly the same form as (12.14), with $w_i = N_i$, and $d_i = p_{Ai} - p_{Bi}$ as in (12.13). The method differs from that of Cochran's test only in using a different system of weights. The variance of $\bar{d}$ is given by

$$\text{var}(\bar{d}) = \frac{\sum N_i^2 \; \text{var}(d_i)}{(\sum N_i)^2}, \tag{12.40}$$

with $\text{var}(d_i)$ given by (12.16). Again, when the p_{0i} are small, q_{0i} can be put approximately equal to 1 in (12.16).

The variance given by (12.39) may be unsatisfactory for the construction of confidence limits if the numbers of deaths in the separate age groups are small, since the normal approximation is then unsatisfactory and the Poisson limits are asymmetric (§4.10). The standardized rate (12.37) is a weighted sum of the Poisson counts, r_i. Dobson *et al.* (1991) gave a method of calculating an approximate confidence interval based on the confidence interval of the total number of deaths.

Example 12.13

In Table 12.11 a standardized rate p' could be calculated for each population. What should be taken as the standard population? There is no unique answer to this question. The choice may not greatly affect the comparison of two populations, although it will certainly affect the absolute values of the standardized rates. If the contrast between the age-specific rates is very different at different age groups, we may have to consider whether we wish the standardized rates to reflect particularly the position at certain parts of the age scale; for example, it might be desirable to give less weight to the higher age groups because the purpose of the study is mainly to compare mortality at younger ages, or because the information at higher ages is less reliable, or because the death rates at high ages are more affected by sampling error.

At the foot of Table 12.11 we give standardized rates with three choices of standard population: (a) population A, (b) population B, and (c) a hypothetical population, C, whose *proportionate* distribution is midway between A and B, i.e.

$$N_{Ci} \propto \frac{1}{2}\left(\frac{n_{Ai}}{\sum n_{Ai}} + \frac{n_{Bi}}{\sum n_{Bi}} \right).$$

Note that for method (a) the standardized rate for A is the same as the crude rate; similarly for (b) the standardized rate for B is the same as the crude rate. Although the absolute values of the standardized rates are different for the three choices of standard population, the contrast is broadly the same in each case.

Indirect method

This method is more easily thought of as a comparison of observed and expected deaths than in terms of standardized rates. In the special population the total number of deaths observed is $\sum r_i$. The number of deaths expected if the age-specific death rates were the same as in the standard population is $\sum n_i P_i$. The overall mortality experience of the special population may be expressed in terms of that of the standard population by the ratio of observed to expected deaths:

$$M = \frac{\sum r_i}{\sum n_i P_i}. \tag{12.41}$$

When multiplied by 100 and expressed as a percentage, (12.41) is known as the *standardized mortality ratio* (SMR).

To obtain the variance of M we can use the result $\mathrm{var}(r_i) = n_i p_i q_i$, and regard the P_i as constants without any sampling fluctuation (since we shall often want to compare one SMR with another using the same standard population; in any case the standard population will often be much larger than the special population, and var (P_i) will be much smaller than $\mathrm{var}(p_i)$). This gives

$$\mathrm{var}(M) = \frac{\sum n_i p_i q_i}{(\sum n_i P_i)^2}. \tag{12.42}$$

Table 12.11 Death rates for two populations, A and B, with direct standardization using A, B and a midway population C

Age (years)	A Population 1000s	A Population %	A Deaths	A Age-specific DR per 1000	B Population 1000s	B Population %	B Deaths	B Age-specific DR per 1000	C Population 1000s	C Population %
0–	2100	8·97	10 000	4·76	185	14·51	4100	22·16	1174	11·74
5–	1900	8·12	800	0·42	170	13·33	100	0·59	1072	10·72
10–	1700	7·26	700	0·41	160	12·55	100	0·62	990	9·90
15–	1900	8·12	2000	1·05	120	9·41	180	1·50	876	8·76
20–	1700	7·26	1700	1·00	100	7·84	190	1·90	755	7·55
25–	1500	6·41	1400	0·93	80	6·27	160	2·00	634	6·34
30–	1500	6·41	1700	1·13	70	5·49	170	2·43	595	5·95
35–	1500	6·41	2700	1·80	65	5·10	200	3·08	576	5·76
40–	1600	6·84	4800	3·00	65	5·10	270	4·15	597	5·97
45–	1500	6·41	7800	5·20	60	4·71	370	6·17	556	5·56
50–	1500	6·41	14 200	9·47	55	4·31	530	9·64	536	5·36
55–	1500	6·41	23 800	15·87	40	3·14	690	17·25	478	4·78
60–	1300	5·56	34 900	26·85	30	2·35	880	29·33	396	3·96
65–	900	3·85	40 700	45·22	30	2·35	1500	50·00	310	3·10
70–	600	2·56	42 000	70·00	20	1·57	1520	76·00	207	2·07
75–	700	2·99	98 100	140·14	25	1·96	4100	164·00	248	2·48
Total	23 400	99·99	287 300		1275	99·99	15 060		10 000	100·00

Crude rate   A: 12·28   B: 11·81

(a) *Standardization by population A*
Expected deaths   A: 287 300   B: 365 815
Standardized rate   A: 12·28   B: 15·63

(b) *Standardization by population B*
Expected deaths   A: 10 242   B: 15 060
Standardized rate   A: 8·03   B: 11·81

(c) *Standardization by population C*
Expected deaths   A: 101 657   B: 137 338
Standardized rate   A: 10·17   B: 13·73

As usual, if the p_i are small, $q_i \simeq 1$ and

$$\text{var}(M) \simeq \frac{\sum r_i}{\left(\sum n_i P_i\right)^2}. \tag{12.43}$$

Confidence limits for M constructed using (12.43) are equivalent to method **3** of §4.10 (p. 142). Where the total number of deaths, $\sum r_i$, is small this is unsatisfactory and either the better approximations of methods **1** or **2** or exact limits should be used (see Example 4.16).

If the purpose of calculating $\text{var}(M)$ is to see whether M differs significantly from unity, $\text{var}(r_i)$ could be taken as $n_i P_i Q_i$, on the assumption that p_i differs from a population value P_i by sampling fluctuations. If again the P_i are small, $Q_i \simeq 1$, we have

$$\text{var}(M) = \frac{\sum n_i P_i}{\left(\sum n_i P_i\right)^2} = \frac{1}{\sum n_i P_i}, \tag{12.44}$$

the reciprocal of the total expected deaths. Denoting the numerator and denominator of (12.41) by O and E (for 'observed' and 'expected'), an approximate significance test would be to regard O as following a Poisson distribution with mean E. If E is not too small, the normal approximation to the Poisson leads to the use of $(O - E)/\sqrt{E}$ as a standardized normal deviate, or, equivalently, $(O - E)^2/E$ as a $\chi^2_{(1)}$ variate. This is, of course, the familiar formula for a $\chi^2_{(1)}$ variate.

Example 12.14

Table 12.12 shows some occupational mortality data, a field in which the SMR is traditionally used. The special population is that of farmers in 1951, aged 20 to 65 years. The standard population is that of all males in these age groups, whether occupied or retired. Deaths of farmers over a 5-year period are used to help reduce the sampling errors, and the observed and expected numbers are expressed on a 5-year basis.

The SMR is

$$100\,M = \frac{(100)(7678)}{11\,005} = 69 \cdot 8\%$$

and

$$\text{var(SMR)} = 10^4\,\text{var}(M)$$

$$= \frac{(10^4)\,(7678)}{(11\,005)^2} \quad \text{from (12.43)}$$

$$= 0 \cdot 634,$$

and

$$\text{SE(SMR)} = 0 \cdot 80\%.$$

Table 12.12 Mortality of farmers in England and Wales, 1949–53, in comparison with that of the male population

Age i	(1) Annual death rate per 100 000, all males (1949–53) $\frac{1}{5}P_i \times 10^5$	(2) Farmers, 1951 census population n_i	(3) Deaths of farmers 1949–53 r_i	(4) Deaths expected in 5 years $5 \times (1) \times (2) \times 10^{-5}$ $n_i P_i$
20–	129·8	8 481	87	55
25–	152·5	39 729	289	303
35–	280·4	65 700	733	921
45–	816·2	73 376	1998	2 994
55–64	2312·4	58 226	4571	6 732
			7678	11 005

Source: Registrar General of England and Wales (1958).

The smallness of the standard error of the SMR in Example 12.14 is typical of much vital statistical data, and is the reason why sampling errors are often ignored in this type of work. Indeed, there are problems in the interpretation of occupational mortality statistics which often overshadow sampling errors. For example, occupations may be less reliably stated in censuses than in the registration of deaths, and this may lead to biases in the estimated death rates for certain occupations. Even if the data are wholly reliable, it is not clear whether a particularly high or low SMR for a certain occupation reflects a health risk in that occupation or a tendency for selective groups of people to enter it. In Example 12.14, for example, the SMR for farmers may be low because farming is healthy, or because unhealthy people are unlikely to enter farming or are more likely to leave it. Note also that in the lowest age group there is an *excess* of deaths among farmers (87 observed, 55 expected). Any method of standardization carries the risk of oversimplification, and the investigator should always compare age-specifc rates to see whether the contrasts between populations vary greatly with age.

The method of indirect standardization is very similar to that described as the comparison of observed and expected frequencies on p. 418. Indeed if, in the comparison of two groups, A and B, the standard population were defined as the pooled population A + B, the method would be precisely the same as used in the Cochran–Mantel–Haenszel method (p. 419). We have seen (p. 438) that Cochran's test is equivalent to a comparison of two *direct*-standardized rates. There is thus a very close relationship between the direct and indirect methods when the standard population is chosen to be the sum of the two special populations.

The SMR is a weighted mean, over the separate age groups, of the ratios of the observed death rates in the special population to those in the standard population, with weights that depend on the age distribution of the special population. This means that SMRs calculated for several special populations are not strictly comparable (Yule, 1934), since they have been calculated with different weights. The SMRs will be comparable under the hypothesis that the ratio of the death rates in the special and standard populations is independent of age, that is, in a proportional-hazards situation (§14.8).

The relationship between standardization and generalized linear models is discussed by Little and Pullum (1979) and Freeman and Holford (1980).

12.10 Kappa measure of agreement

When a categorical variable is difficult to record objectively, it is common practice to use more than one rater to assess the variable, and to use the mean, or median, values in the main data analysis. It is, however, prudent to confirm before the calculation of any sort of average value that the raters are using the categories similarly since otherwise it would be unclear what the average values represented. Examples are the assessment of classification of a condition on a scale with two or more categories based on an assessment of presenting signs and symptoms, and the reading of chest radiographs.

Consider first the case where there are just two categories, presence or absence of some condition and suppose that two raters assess n subjects independently. Then the results can be set out in a 2×2 table as follows:

	Rater 2		
Rater 1	Present	Absent	
Present	a	b	$a + b$
Absent	c	d	$c + d$
	$a + c$	$b + d$	n

A natural way of assessing agreement between the raters would be to note that the raters agree on $a + d$ of the subjects and to express this in terms of the number of patients as the ratio $(a + d)/n$. Two examples illustrate the disadvantage of this simple approach:

A

	Rater 2		
Rater 1	Present	Absent	
Present	5	5	10
Absent	5	85	90
	10	90	100

B

	Rater 2		
Rater 1	Present	Absent	
Present	35	5	40
Absent	5	55	60
	40	60	100

In both of these examples the raters agree on 90% of the subjects, but the disagreement appears greater in example A than in example B since, in the former there is agreement that the condition is present for only five subjects out of the 15 assessed by at least one of the raters as having the condition, whilst in the latter it is agreed that the condition is present in 35 out of 45 subjects assessed as having the condition by at least one of the raters.

The difficulty has arisen because no account has been taken of agreements that could occur due to chance. If there was no real agreement between the raters, then the expected frequencies in the cells of the 2×2 table would be determined by chance. For example A it would be expected that there would be 81 subjects rated negative by both raters and one subject rated positive by both raters, where these expected numbers have been calculated by exactly the same methods as used to calculate expected frequencies in a χ^2 test (§4.9). The observed agreement for 90 subjects does not appear so impressive when contrasted with an expected agreement for 82 patients. In example B the expected number of agreements is only 52 and the observed number is much greater than this.

The above rationale is the basis for the *kappa* measure of agreement, introduced by Cohen (1960). The method is as follows. First, define I_o as the observed measure of agreement, and I_e as the corresponding expected measure. Then

$$I_o = \frac{a + d}{n}$$

$$I_e = \frac{(a + c)(a + b) + (b + d)(c + d)}{n^2}.$$

Secondly, kappa is defined as the difference between observed and expected agreement expressed as a fraction of the maximum difference. Since the maximum value of I_o is 1 this gives

$$\kappa = \frac{I_o - I_e}{1 - I_e}. \tag{12.45}$$

For examples A and B the values of kappa are 0·44 and 0·79 respectively. The maximum value of kappa is 1, which represents perfect agreement, and kappa will take the value zero if there is only chance agreement. Although negative values are mathematically possible, representing an agreement to disagree, these are unlikely to occur in practice.

Example 12.15

In a study by Bergen *et al.* (1992), tardive dyskinesia was assessed by two raters by scoring seven items on a five-point scale, coded 0 to 4. One definition of tardive dyskinesia is that there should be either two scores of at least 2 or one of at least 3. For one series of assessments there were 168 subjects and the agreement was as follows:

	Rater a		
Rater b	Present	Absent	
Present	123	10	133
Absent	6	29	35
	129	39	168

Then

$$I_o = \frac{152}{168} = 0\text{·}905$$

$$I_e = \frac{129 \times 133 + 39 \times 35}{168^2} = 0\text{·}656$$

$$\kappa = \frac{0\text{·}905 - 0\text{·}656}{1 - 0\text{·}656} = 0\text{·}72.$$

The agreement between the two raters was good, and so the two assessments were combined and tardive dyskinesia was recorded for those patients who were diagnosed by both raters.

Weighted kappa

Where there are more than two categories and the categories are ordered, a difference between raters of just one category is less disagreement than a difference of two categories, and a difference of three categories would indicate even more disagreement, etc. It is clearly desirable to incorporate this in a measure of agreement and this is done using the *weighted kappa* (Cohen, 1968). This measure is calculated by assigning a weight, w_i, to subjects for whom the raters differ by i categories. When the raters agree, the weight is unity, that is, $w_o = 1$. If there are k categories then the maximum disagreement is of $k - 1$ categories and this is given weight zero. The most common set of weights for the intermediate values is that they are equally spaced, and this gives

$$w_i = 1 - \frac{i}{k-1}.$$

Then the observed index of agreement is defined as

$$I_o = \frac{\sum w_i r_i}{n},$$

where r_i is the number of subjects for whom the raters differ by i categories. The expected value is calculated similarly using expected frequencies and the weighted kappa evaluated using (12.45).

Example 12.16

In a study by Cookson *et al.* (1986), chest radiographs were classified by two readers according to the 1980 ILO Classification of Radiographs of Pneumoconiosis. The readings are given in Table 12.13.

Table 12.13 Readings of chest radiographs by two readers (Cookson *et al.*, 1986)

Reader 1	Reader 2								
	0/0	0/1	1/0	1/1	1/2	2/1	2/2	2/3	Total
0/0	626	32	26	3					687
0/1	53	20	17	3					93
1/0	22	3	21	8		1	1		56
1/1	2	2	6	1	2	1			14
1/2	3		1	3		4			11
2/1									0
2/2									0
2/3								1	1
Total	706	57	71	18	2	6	1	1	862

The observed number of exact agreements is obtained by summing the frequencies in the diagonal extending from the top left cell to the bottom right cell of the table. Observed numbers of disagreements are obtained similarly by summing the frequencies in parallel lines displaced either side of the main diagonal. The expected numbers are obtained from the marginal totals, and summed in the same way. This gives:

Number of categories of disagreement	obs	exp	w	$w \times$ obs	$w \times$ exp
0 (agreement)	669	573·8	1	669·0	573·8
1	128	135·6	0·86	109·7	116·2
2	55	106·5	0·71	39·3	76·1
3	6	27·2	0·57	3·4	15·5
4	4	11·4	0·43	1·7	4·9
5	0	5·0	0·29	0	1·4
6	0	1·0	0·14	0	0·1
7	0	1·6	0	0	0
	862	862·0		823·1	788·0

Summarizing we have

$$I_o = 823·1/862 = 0·955$$

$$I_e = 788·0/862 = 0·914$$

$$\kappa = \frac{0·955 - 0·914}{1 - 0·914} = 0·48.$$

There is fair agreement.

The weighted kappa and the intraclass correlation coefficient are related, and if the weights were taken as $w_i = 1 - i^2/(k-1)^2$ then the weighted kappa and the intraclass correlation coefficient would be equal except for terms in $1/n$. In Example 12.16 the weighted kappa using these weights was 0·620 and the intraclass correlation coefficient, using the categories values, 0, 1, . . . , 7, was 0·621. It follows that the value of kappa is influenced by the selection of subjects over which it is defined, as well as by the underlying agreement between observers. As for the intraclass correlation coefficient, this may not matter if the only purpose is to assess agreement between raters within a particular study, but comparisons of kappa between studies are difficult to interpret.

The standard error of a kappa may be evaluated but is seldom needed since the estimation of agreement is not usually an end in itself. Also agreement is usually better than chance and a significance test of the null hypothesis that there is no agreement is unnecessary. For fuller details see Chapter 13 of Fleiss (1981). Fleiss recommends that values of kappa exceeding 0·75 represent excellent agreement, values between 0·4 and 0·75 fair to good agreement, and values less than 0·4 poor agreement. There would be little purpose in using a measure with such poor agreement since it would be unclear what the measure represented.

13: Distribution-Free Methods

13.1 Introduction

Some of the statistical methods described earlier in connection with categorical data have involved rather simple assumptions: for example, χ^2 methods often test simple hypotheses about the probabilities for various categories—that they are equal, or that they are proportional to certain marginal probabilities. The methods used for quantitative data, in contrast, have relied on relatively complex assumptions about distributional forms—that the random variation is normal, Poisson, etc. These assumptions are often likely to be clearly untrue; to overcome this problem we sometimes argue that methods are *robust*—that is, not very sensitive to non-normality. At other times we may use transformations to make the assumptions more plausible.

Clearly, there would be something to be said for methods which avoided unnecessary distributional assumptions. Such methods, called *distribution-free methods*, exist and are widely used by some statisticians. Standard statistical methods frequently use statistics which in a fairly obvious way estimate certain population parameters; the sample estimate of variance s^2, for example, estimates the population parameter σ^2. In distribution-free methods there is little emphasis on population parameters, since the whole object is to avoid a particular functional form for a population distribution. The hypotheses to be tested usually relate to the nature of the distribution as a whole rather than to the values assumed by some of its parameters. For this reason they are often called *non-parametric hypotheses* and the appropriate techniques are often called *non-parametric tests* or *methods*.

The justification for the use of distribution-free methods will usually be along one of the following lines.

1   There may be obvious non-normality.

2   There may be possible non-normality, perhaps to a very marked extent, but the sample sizes may be too small to establish whether or not this is so.

3   One may seek a rapid statistical technique, perhaps involving little or simple calculation. Many distribution-free methods have this property: J. W. Tukey's epithet 'quick and dirty methods' is often used to describe them.

4   A measurement to be analysed may consist of a number of ordered categories, such as $--$, $-$, 0, $+$ and $++$ for degrees of clinical improvement; or a number of observations may form a rank order—for example, patients may be asked to classify six pharmaceutical formulations in order of palatability. In such cases the investigator may be unwilling to allot a numerical scale, but would wish to use methods which took account of the rank order of the observations. Many distribution-free methods are of this type. The first type of data referred to here, namely ordered categorical data, has already been discussed at some length in Chapter 12. There is, in fact, a close relation between some of the methods described there and those to be discussed in the present chapter.

The methods described in the following sections are merely a few of the most useful distribution-free techniques. These methods have been developed primarily as significance tests and are not always easily adapted for purposes of estimation. Nevertheless, the statistics used in the tests can often be said to estimate something, even though the parameter estimated may be of limited interest. Some estimation procedures are therefore described briefly, although the emphasis will be on significance tests. Some of the general issues about the use of distribution-free methods are discussed in §13.6.

Fuller accounts of distribution-free methods are given by Siegel and Castellan (1988), who concentrate on significance tests, Lehmann (1975) and Conover (1980).

13.2 One-sample tests for location

In this section we consider tests of the null hypothesis that the distribution of a random variable x is symmetric about zero. If, in some problem, the natural hypothesis to test is that of symmetry about some other value, μ, all that need be done is to subtract μ from each observation; the test for symmetry about zero can then be used. The need to test for symmetry about zero commonly arises with paired comparisons of two treatments, when the variable x is the difference between two paired readings.

The normal-theory test for this hypothesis is, of course, the one-sample t test, and we shall illustrate the present methods by reference to Table 4.1, the data of which were analysed by a paired t test in Example 4.3.

The sign test

Suppose the observations in a sample of size n are $x_1, x_2, \ldots, x_n$, and that of these r are positive and s negative. Some values of x may be exactly zero, and these would not be counted with either the positives or the negatives. The sum $r + s$ may therefore be less than n, and will be denoted by n'.

On the null hypothesis positive and negative values of x are equally likely. Both r and s therefore follow a binomial distribution with parameters n' (instead of the n of §2.5) and $\frac{1}{2}$ (for the parameter π of §2.5). Excessively high or low values of r (or, equivalently, of s) can be tested exactly from tables of the binomial distribution. For large enough samples, any of the normal approximations (4.11), (4.12), (4.28) or (4.29) may be used (with r and s replacing x_1 and x_2 in (4.28) and (4.29)).

Example 13.1

Consider the differences in the final column of Table 4.1. Here $n' = n = 10$ (since there are no zero values), $r = 4$ and $s = 6$. For a two-sided significance test the probability level is twice the probability of $r \leq 4$, which from tables of the binomial distribution is 0·75. The normal approximation, with continuity correction, would give, for a $\chi^2_{(1)}$ test,

$$X^2 = \frac{(|6 - 4| - 1)^2}{6 + 4} = 0\cdot10 \quad (P = 0\cdot75).$$

The verdict agrees with that of the t test in Example 4.3: there is no evidence that differences in anxiety score tend to be positive more (or less) often than they are negative.

The mid-P value (see §4.7) from the binomial distribution is 0·55, and this corresponds to the uncorrected $\chi^2_{(1)}$ value of 0·40 ($P = 0\cdot53$). Note that these mid-P values approximate more closely to the result of the t test in Example 4.3, where, with $t = -0\cdot90$ on 9 DF, $P = 0\cdot39$.

The signed rank sum test

The sign test clearly loses something by ignoring all information about the numerical magnitudes of the observations other than their sign. If a high proportion of the numerically large observations were positive this would strengthen the evidence that the distribution was asymmetric about zero, and it seems reasonable to try to take this evidence into account. Wilcoxon's (1945) signed rank sum test works as follows. The observations are put in ascending order of magnitude, ignoring the sign, and given the ranks 1 to n' (zero values being ignored as in the sign test). Let T_+ be the sum of the ranks of the positive values and T_- that of the negative. On the null hypothesis T_+ and T_- would not be expected to differ greatly; their sum $T_+ + T_-$ is $\frac{1}{2}n'(n' + 1)$, so an appropriate test would consist in evaluating the probability of a value of, say, T_+ equal to or more extreme than that observed. Table A7 gives critical values for the *smaller* of T_+ and T_-, for two-sided tests at the 5% and 1% levels, for n' up to 25. The distribution is tabulated fully for n' up to 20 by Lehmann (1975, Table H), and other percentiles are given in the Geigy Scientific Tables (1982, p. 163). For larger values of n', T_+ and T_- are approximately normally distributed with variance $n'(n' + 1)(2n' + 1)/24$, and a standardized normal deviate, with continuity correction, is given by

$$\frac{|T_+ - \frac{1}{4}n'(n' + 1)| - \frac{1}{2}}{\sqrt{[n'(n' + 1)(2n' + 1)/24]}}. \tag{13.1}$$

If some of the observations are numerically equal they are given tied ranks equal to the mean of the ranks which would otherwise have been used. This feature reduces the variance of T_+ by $(t^3 - t)/48$ for each group of t tied ranks, and the critical values shown in Table A7 are somewhat conservative (i.e. the result is somewhat more significant than the table suggests).

Example 13.2

The 10 differences in Table 4.1 may be ranked numerically as follows:

	1	2	3	4		6	7		9	10
Rank		Equal $2\frac{1}{2}$			5	$6\frac{1}{2}$		8	$9\frac{1}{2}$	
Numerical value	1	1	1	1	2	3	3	7	8	8
Sign	+	+	+	−	−	−	−	−	+	−

$$T_+ = 2\tfrac{1}{2} + 2\tfrac{1}{2} + 2\tfrac{1}{2} + 9\tfrac{1}{2} = 17,$$
$$T_- = 2\tfrac{1}{2} + 5 + 6\tfrac{1}{2} + 6\tfrac{1}{2} + 8 + 9\tfrac{1}{2} = 38.$$

From Table A7, for $n' = 10$, the 5% point for the minimum of T_+ and T_- is 8. Both T_+ and T_- exceed this critical value, and the effect is clearly non-significant.

For the large-sample test, we calculate

$$E(T_+) = \tfrac{1}{4}(10)(11) = 27\cdot5,$$

$$\text{var}(T_+) = \frac{10(11)(21)}{24} - \frac{1}{48}[(4^3 - 4) + (2^3 - 2) + (2^3 - 2)]$$

$$= 96\cdot25 - 1\cdot50$$

$$= 94\cdot75,$$

$$\text{SE}(T_+) = \sqrt{94\cdot75} = 9\cdot73,$$

and the standardized normal deviate is $(10\cdot5 - 0\cdot5)/9\cdot73 = 1\cdot03$, clearly non-significant (from Table A1, $P = 0\cdot303$). From Lehmann's table, ignoring the ties, the probability of the observed result or one more extreme is $0\cdot322$. Both the P values quoted here are approximate (one because of the normal approximation, the other because of the ties), but they agree reasonably well.

Estimation

Suppose the observations (or differences, in the case of a paired comparison as in Example 13.2) are distributed symmetrically not about zero, as specified by the null hypothesis, but about some other value, μ. How can we best estimate μ? One obvious suggestion is the sample mean. Another is the sample median, which, if subtracted from each observation, would give the null expectation in the sign test, since there would be equal numbers of positive and negative differences. A somewhat better suggestion is related to the signed rank test. We could choose that value $\hat{\mu}$ which, if subtracted from each observation, would give the null expectation in the signed rank test. It is not difficult to see that the test statistic T_+ is the number of positive values amongst the 'pair means', which are formed by taking the mean of each pair of observations (including each observation with itself). The estimate $\hat{\mu}$ is then the median of these pair means.

Confidence limits for μ are the values which, if subtracted from each observation, just give a significantly high or low test result. For this purpose all n readings may be used. The limits may be obtained by ranking the $\frac{1}{2}n(n + 1)$ pair means, and taking the values whose ranks are one greater than the appropriate entry in Table A7 (p. 577), and the symmetric rank obtained by subtracting this from $\frac{1}{2}n(n + 1) + 1$. That is, one excludes the tabulated number of observations from each end of the ranked series. For values of n beyond the range of Table A7 the number of values to be excluded is the integer part of

$$\tfrac{1}{4}n(n + 1) - z \sqrt{\left[\frac{n(n + 1)(2n + 1)}{24}\right]},$$

where $z = 1.96$ for 95% confidence limits and 2·58 for 99% limits.

The procedure is illustrated below. Because of the discreteness of the ranking, the confidence coefficient is somewhat greater than the nominal value (e.g. greater than 95% for the limits obtained from the entries for 0·05 in Table A7). If there are substantial ties in the data, as in the example below, a further widening of the confidence coefficient takes place.

Example 13.2, continued

The 10 differences from Table 4.1, used earlier in this example for the signed rank sum test, are shown in the following table, arranged in ascending order in both rows and columns. They give the following 55 ($= \frac{1}{2} \times 10 \times 11$) pair means:

	− 8	− 7	− 3	− 3	− 2	− 1	+ 1	+ 1	+ 1	+ 8
− 8	− 8	− 7·5	− 5·5	− 5·5	− 5	− 4·5	− 3·5	− 3·5	− 3·5	0
− 7		− 7	− 5	− 5	− 4·5	− 4	− 3	− 3	− 3	+ 0·5
− 3			− 3	− 3	− 2·5	− 2	− 1	− 1	− 1	+ 2·5
− 3				− 3	− 2·5	− 2	− 1	− 1	− 1	+ 2·5
− 2					− 2	− 1·5	− 0·5	− 0·5	− 0·5	+ 3
− 1						− 1	0	0	0	+ 3·5
+ 1							+ 1	+ 1	+ 1	+ 4·5
+ 1								+ 1	+ 1	+ 4·5
+ 1									+ 1	+ 4·5
+ 8										+ 8

Note that the numbers of positive and negative pair means (counting zero values as contributing $\frac{1}{2}$ to each sum) are 17 and 38, respectively, agreeing with the values of T_+ and

T_- obtained earlier. The estimate $\hat{\mu}$ is the median value of the pair means, namely -1. For 95% confidence limits, note that the entry in Table A7 for $n = 10$ and $P = 0.05$ is 8. $T = 56 - 9$). From the display above, these values are -4.5 and $+1.0$. For comparison, the t distribution used for these data in Example 4.3 gave limits of -4.55 and $+1.95$, not too dissimilar from the present values.

13.3   Comparison of two independent groups

Suppose we have two groups of observations: a random sample of n_1 observations, x_i, from population X and a random sample of n_2 observations, y_j, from population Y. The null hypothesis to be tested is that the distribution of x in population X is exactly the same as that of y in population Y. We should like the test to be sensitive to situations in which the two distributions differ primarily in location, so that x tends to be greater (or less) than y.

The normal-theory test is the two-sample (unpaired) t test described in §4.4. Three distribution-free tests in common usage are all essentially equivalent to each other. They are described briefly here.

The Mann–Whitney U test

The observations are ranked together in order of increasing magnitude. There are $n_1 n_2$ pairs (x_i, y_j); of these,

$$U_{XY} \text{ is the number of pairs for which } x_i < y_j,$$
$$\text{and } U_{YX} \text{ is the number of pairs for which } x_i > y_j.$$

Any pairs for which $x_i = y_j$ count $\frac{1}{2}$ a unit towards both U_{XY} and U_{YX}.

Either of these statistics may be used for a test, with exactly equivalent results. Using U_{YX}, for instance, the statistic must lie between 0 and $n_1 n_2$. On the null hypothesis its expectation is $\frac{1}{2}n_1 n_2$. High values will suggest a difference between the distributions, with x tending to take higher values than y. Conversely, low values of U_{YX} suggest that x tends to be less than y.

Wilcoxon's rank sum test

Again there are two equivalent statistics:

$$T_1 \text{ is the sum of the ranks of the } x_i\text{s;}$$
$$T_2 \text{ is the sum of the ranks of the } y_j\text{s.}$$

Low values assume low ranks (i.e. rank 1 is allotted to the smallest value). Any group of tied ranks is allotted the midrank of the group.

The smallest value which T_1 can take arises when all the xs are less than all the ys; then $T_1 = \frac{1}{2}n_1(n_1 + 1)$. The maximum value possible for T_1 arises when all xs are greater than all ys; then $T_1 = n_1 n_2 + \frac{1}{2}n_1(n_1 + 1)$. The null expectation of T_1 is $\frac{1}{2}n_1(n_1 + n_2 + 1)$.

Kendall's S

This is defined in terms of the two Mann–Whitney statistics:

$$S = U_{XY} - U_{YX}. \tag{13.2}$$

Its minimum value (when all ys are less than all xs) is $-n_1 n_2$; its maximum value (when all xs are less than all ys) is $n_1 n_2$. The null expectation is 0.

Interrelationships between tests

There are, first, two relationships between the two Mann–Whitney statistics and between the two Wilcoxon statistics:

$$U_{XY} + U_{YX} = n_1 n_2, \tag{13.3}$$

$$T_1 + T_2 = \frac{1}{2}(n_1 + n_2)(n_1 + n_2 + 1). \tag{13.4}$$

These show that tests based on either of two statistics in each pair are equivalent; given T_1 and the two sample sizes, for example, T_2 can immediately be calculated from (13.4).

Secondly, the three tests are interrelated by the following formulae:

$$U_{YX} = T_1 - \frac{1}{2}n_1(n_1 + 1), \tag{13.5}$$

$$U_{XY} = T_2 - \frac{1}{2}n_2(n_2 + 1) \tag{13.6}$$

and

$$S = U_{XY} - U_{YX},$$

as already given in (13.2).

The three tests are exactly equivalent. From (13.5) for instance, the probability of observing a value of T_1 greater than or equal to that observed is exactly equal to the probability of a value of U_{YX} greater than or equal to that observed. Significance tests based on T_1 and U_{YX} will therefore yield exactly the same significance level. The choice between these tests depends purely on familiarity with a particular form of computation and accessibility of tables.

The probability distributions of the various statistics are independent of the distributions of x and y. They have been tabulated for small and moderate sample sizes, for situations in which there are no ties. Table A8 gives critical values for T_1 (the samples being labelled so that $n_1 \leqslant n_2$). The table provides for two-sided tests at the 5% and 1% levels, for n_1 and n_2 up to 15. More extensive tables are given in the Geigy Scientific Tables (1982, pp. 156–162), and the exact distribution (in terms of U_{XY}) is given by Lehmann (1975, Table B) for some smaller values of n_1 and n_2. Beyond the range of Table A8, the normal approximation based on the variance formulae of Table 13.1 is adequate unless the smaller of n_1 and n_2 is less than 4.

When there are ties the variance formulae are modified as shown in Table 13.1. The summations in the formulae are taken over all groups of tied observations, t being the number of observations in a particular group. As with the signed rank sum test, the tables of critical values are somewhat conservative in the presence of ties.

Example 13.3

We illustrate the use of Kendall's S, and the equivalent Mann–Whitney U test, in a set of data shown in Table 13.2. The observations are measurements of the percentage change in area of gastric ulcers after 3 months' treatment, the comparison being between 32 inpatients and 32 outpatients. A percentage change is an awkward measurement; its minimum value is -100 (when the ulcer has disappeared); each group contains several readings bunched at or near this lower limit. In the other direction very large values may be recorded (when the ulcer was initially very small and increased greatly during the period of observation).

A point which may be noted in the calculation of S when there are ties is that there is no need to count $\frac{1}{2}$ for each (x, y) tie, for these contributions form part of both U_{XY} and U_{YX} and therefore cancel out in S because of (13.2). We can therefore calculate S as $P - Q$, where P and Q are calculated like U_{XY} and U_{YX} except that nothing is added for (x, y) ties.

In this example, denote the inpatients by x and the outpatients by y. To calculate P, take each member of the x sample in turn and count the number of members of the y sample greater than this value. For the first few values of x, we find:

x_i	$-100^{(12)}$	-93	-92	$-91^{(2)}$	-90	$-85\ldots$
Number of $y_j > x_i$	27	26	26	26	26	$25\ldots$

Thus,

$$P = 12(27) + 5(26) + 3(25) + 24 + 23 + 17 + 2(16) + 11 + 9 + 7 + 2(4) + 2 + 0$$
$$= 662$$

$$Q = 5(20) + 19 + 15 + 11 + 7(10) + 9 + 5(7) + 2(6) + 2(5) + 2(4) + 3 + 2(2) + 2(1)$$
$$= 298,$$

and

$$S = 662 - 298 = 364.$$

From Table 13.1,

$$\mathrm{var}(S) = \frac{(32)(32)}{3(64)(63)}[64^3 - 64 - (17^3 - 17) - \cdots],$$

Table 13.1. Some properties of three equivalent two-sample distribution-free tests

	Bounds		Mean	Sampling distribution	
	All $x_i <$ all y_j	All $y_j <$ all x_i		No ties	Variance — Ties
Mann–Whitney U test					
U_{XY} = No. of pairs with $x_i < y_j$	$n_1 n_2$	$\left.\begin{array}{c}0\\ n_1 n_2\end{array}\right\}$	$\frac{1}{2}n_1 n_2$	$\dfrac{n_1 n_2(n+1)}{12}$	$\dfrac{n_1 n_2}{12n(n-1)}\left[n^3 - n - \sum_t(t^3 - t)\right]$
U_{YX} = No. of pairs with $y_j < x_i$	0				
Wilcoxon rank sum test					
T_1 = Sum of ranks for x_is	$\frac{1}{2}n_1(n_1 + 1)$	$n_1 n_2 + \frac{1}{2}n_1(n_1 + 1)$	$\frac{1}{2}n_1(n_1 + n_2 + 1)$	as above	
T_2 = Sum of ranks for y_js	$n_1 n_2 + \frac{1}{2}n_2(n_2 + 1)$	$\frac{1}{2}n_2(n_2 + 1)$	$\frac{1}{2}n_2(n_1 + n_2 + 1)$		
Kendall's S test					
$S = U_{XY} - U_{YX}$	$n_1 n_2$	$-n_1 n_2$	0	$\dfrac{n_1 n_2(n+1)}{3}$	$\dfrac{n_1 n_2}{3n(n-1)}\left[n^3 - n - \sum_t(t^3 - t)\right]$

Notation: n_1 = Sample size of x_is.
$\quad\quad\quad\; n_2$ = Sample size of y_js.
$\quad\quad\quad\; n = n_1 + n_2$.

Table 13.2. Percentage change in area of gastric ulcer after 3 months' treatment (Doll and Pygott, 1952)

	Number	
X: Inpatients	32	$-100^{(12)}$, -93, -92, $-91^{(2)}$, -90, -85, -83, -81, -80, -78, -46, -40, -34, 0, 29, 62, 75, 106, 147, 1321
Y: Outpatients	32	$-100^{(5)}$, -93, -89, -80, -78, -75, -74, -72, -71, -66, -59, -41, -30, -29, -26, -20, -15, 20, 25, 37, 55, 68, 73, 75, 145, 146, 220, 1044

Notation: $-100^{(5)}$ indicates 5 observations at -100, etc.

where the terms arising from the small groups of ties (like the two observations at -93) have been omitted as they can easily be seen to be very much smaller than the other terms.

$$\text{var}(S) = (0.084656)(257\,184)$$

$$= 21\,772,$$

$$\text{SE}(S) = \sqrt{21\,772} = 147.5.$$

Using the normal approximation, the standardized normal deviate is $364/147.5 = 2.47$ ($P = 0.014$).

For the Mann–Whitney version, each tie contributes $\frac{1}{2}$ to U_{XY} and U_{YX}. Thus, for example,

$$U_{YX} = 5(26) + 19\tfrac{1}{2} + 15 + 11\tfrac{1}{2} + \cdots$$

$$= 330,$$

$$E(U_{YX}) = \tfrac{1}{2}(32)(32) = 512,$$

$$U_{YX} - E(U_{YX}) = -182 \; (= \tfrac{1}{2}S),$$

$$\text{var}(U_{YX}) = 5443 \; (= \tfrac{1}{4}\text{var}(S)),$$

and the standardized deviate is -2.47, as before apart from the sign.

This is an example in which the difference between the x and y samples would not have been detected by a t test. The distributions are exceedingly non-normal, and the two-sample t test gives $t = 0.51$—clearly non-significant.

The ability of these two-sample tests to handle ties provides an interesting link with some tests already described for contingency tables. In Example 12.1, for instance, illustrating the test for a trend in proportions, we could ask whether the distribution of time since last visit is the same for the attenders and non-attenders. Taking the four time periods as the values of a heavily grouped variate, the distribution-free tests just described could be applied. It can be shown (Armitage, 1955) that the resulting normal deviate is exactly the same as X_{1a}, the square root of the statistic given by (12.6), provided that in the latter test the x scores are chosen in a particular way. The scores must be equal to the midranks of the different groups; in Example 12.1, for instance, they would be 78·5, 177·0, 221·5 and 262·0. When these scores, which are referred to as *modified ridits*, are used, the Wilcoxon/Mann–Whitney test and the test for trend in proportions given by (12.6) are entirely equivalent. In this example the $\chi^2_{(1)}$ statistics, X^2_{1a} is 8·48 ($P = 0.003$).

A 2×2 contingency table is an extreme case of this situation, and here the normal deviate from the distribution-free test (making due allowance for the ties) is the same as that for the usual normal approximation of §4.8 and §4.9, apart from a factor of $\sqrt{[(n-1)/n]}$.

Estimation

Suppose the two distributions have the same shape, but differ in their location by a displacement δ along the scale of measurement, this being positive when the xs tend to exceed the ys. The parameter δ, with confidence limits, may be estimated as follows. First note that U_{YX} is the number of pairs for which $x_i > y_j$. Therefore, if all the $n_1 n_2$ differences $x_i - y_j$ are formed, then U_{YX} is the number of positive values (assuming no ties); so U_{YX} is a test statistic for the hypothesis that the median difference is zero. If a constant quantity δ were subtracted from all the xs, and therefore from all the differences, the two samples would be effectively drawn from the same distribution and the null hypothesis would be true. If U_{YX} were recalculated after the subtraction, it would provide a test of the hypothesis that the displacement, or median difference, is in fact δ. Confidence limits for the displacement are thus obtained by finding those values, which, if subtracted from all the differences, give a result on the borderline of significance. If the differences are ranked, then the confidence interval is the middle part of the distribution, with a number of differences excluded from both ends according to the critical value of the test of U_{YX}. The number of values to be excluded can be evaluated by using Table A8 and (13.5), as illustrated in the following example. A point estimate of the parameter δ is given by the median of the differences, since this is the value which, if subtracted from all the differences, would make the test statistic equal to its expectation.

Example 13.4

The data of Table 4.2 may be ranked as follows, denoting the low and high protein as groups 1 and 2 respectively, so that $n_1 = 7$ and $n_2 = 12$.

Values		Ranks	
High protein	Low protein	High protein	Low protein
	70		1
83		2	
	85		3
	94		4
97		5	
	101		6
104		7	
107		8·5	
	107		8·5
113		10	
	118		11
119		12	
123		13	
124		14	
129		15	
	132		16
134		17	
146		18	
161		19	
Sum of ranks		$T_2 = 140·5$	$T_1 = 49·5$
		$n_2 = 12$	$n_1 = 7$

From Table A8 there would be a significant difference at the 5% level if $T_1 \leq 46$; using (13.5), that is if $U_{YX} \leq 18$. Therefore 18 of the differences are eliminated from each end of the set of ordered differences to give the 95% confidence interval. The 84 differences, high protein minus low protein, are tabulated below.

Low protein	High protein											
	83	97	104	107	113	119	123	124	129	134	146	161
70	13	27	34	37	43	49	53	54	59	64	76	91
85	− 2	12	19	22	28	34	38	39	44	49	61	76
94	− 11	3	10	13	19	25	29	30	35	40	52	67
101	− 18	− 4	3	6	12	18	22	23	28	33	45	60
107	− 24	− 10	− 3	0	6	12	16	17	22	27	39	54
118	− 35	− 21	− 14	− 11	− 5	1	5	6	11	16	28	43
132	− 49	− 35	− 28	− 25	− 19	− 13	− 9	− 8	− 3	2	14	29

The median of these 84 differences is 18·5 and excluding the 18 highest and the 18 lowest differences gives a 95% confidence interval from − 3 to 40. These values are in close agreement with those found using the t distribution in Example 4.4, as would be expected since the data satisfy the conditions for this analysis.

For values outside the range of Table A8 an approximation to the number of differences to be excluded from each end of the ordered set is given by the integral part of

$$\frac{1}{2}n_1 n_2 - z \sqrt{\left[\frac{n_1 n_2 (n_1 + n_2 + 1)}{12}\right]}.$$

The methods of estimation described above could be applied to the data of Example 13.3. The 95% confidence limits are calculated as -66 and -2, in the units of percentage change used in Table 13.2. However, the method is inappropriate here, since the hypothesis of a constant displacement in the distributions is quite unrealistic in view of the bunching of observations at the lower bound of -100%. Other parameters need to be used to describe the difference between the groups. For instance, one might report the difference in the proportions of observations at the lower bound, or less than -90%. An alternative approach, which is available for any application of the Wilcoxon/Mann–Whitney test, is to note that the statistic $U_{XY}/n_1 n_2$ is clearly an estimate of the probability that a randomly chosen value of x is less than a randomly chosen value of y. However, the variance of this statistic is difficult to evaluate since it depends on the precise way in which the two distributions differ; it is important to realize that the usual binomial variance for a proportion with $n_1 n_2$ observations is wholly inappropriate here since the $n_1 n_2$ differences are not independent.

Normal scores

An alternative approach to the two-sample distribution-free problem is provided by the Fisher–Yates *normal scores*. Instead of using ranks, the observations are transformed to a different set of scores which depend purely on the ranks in the combined sample of size n. The score for the observation of rank number r is, in fact, numerically equal to the mean value of the rth smallest observation in a sample of n from a standardized normal distribution, $N(0, 1)$. The scores are tabulated for various sample sizes by Fisher and Yates (1963, Table XX).

Now, these scores can be regarded as a method of transforming to normality as a preliminary step to the use of standard normal methods, and this is usually a perfectly adequate use of the method. However, normal methods inevitably introduce an approximation, since the transformed data cannot be regarded as randomly drawn from a normal distribution. If one wished to have an exact distribution-free test, one could calculate the difference between the means of the two sets of scores and use the fact that its sampling distribution does not depend on the distribution of the original observations. Tables are given by Klotz (1964).

An incidental use of normal scores is to provide a graphical test of normality (see §11.5). Given sample observations $z_1, z_2, \ldots, z_n$, ranked in order, z_i can be plotted against the ith normal score for a sample of n. If the sample is from a normal distribution, the points should lie fairly close to a straight line (the closeness being better for large samples than for small ones). Systematic departures from normality will tend to produce non-linearity in very much the same way as in the use of the probit transformation or probability paper (§11.4).

Some further general comments about the value of two-sample distribution-free tests are made in §13.6.

13.4 Comparison of several groups

Related groups: *Friedman's test*

Suppose we have more than two groups of observations and the data are also classified by a block structure so that the data form a two-way classification of the type considered in §8.1, where the two-way analysis of variance of a randomized block design was described. Suppose that there are t treatments and b blocks. A distribution-free test for such a situation was given by Friedman (1937) and this test is a generalization of the sign test to more than two groups. The test is based on ranking the values within each block.

The test procedure can best be explained by considering a two-way analysis of variance of the ranks, using the formulae of §8.1. In such an analysis the sums of squares and their degrees of freedom, may be written as follows:

	SSq	DF
Blocks	0	0
Treatments	S_{tr}	$t - 1$
Residual	S_{res}	$(b - 1)(t - 1)$
Total	S_{tot}	$b(t - 1)$

Both the sum of squares and the degrees of freedom for blocks are zero because the sum of the ranks is the same for every block, namely $\frac{1}{2}t(t + 1)$. In the calculation of the sums of squares the correction term (T^2/N in Table 8.2) is $\frac{1}{4}bt(t + 1)^2$. The usual form of the Friedman test statistic is

$$T_1 = \frac{b(t - 1)S_{tr}}{S_{tot}}, \tag{13.7}$$

which is distributed approximately as χ^2_{t-1}. This statistic is the ratio of the Treatment SSq to the Total MSq in the analysis of variance. A somewhat preferable test statistic is analogous to the usual variance ratio in the analysis of variance, i.e. the ratio of the Treatment MSq to the Residual MSq:

$$T_2 = \frac{(b-1)S_{tr}}{S_{tot} - S_{tr}},\qquad(13.8)$$

which is distributed approximately as F, with $t-1$ and $(t-1)(b-1)$ DF.

When there are no ties the Total SSq, S_{tot} can be calculated directly as $bt(t+1)(2t+1)/6$, and the formulae for the test statistics are often written in forms that make use of this expression. When $t = 2$ the test statistic T_1 is identical to the sign test statistic without a continuity correction.

Example 13.5

Table 13.3 shows the data given in Table 8.3 with the values within each block ranked.

The effect of treatments is highly significant by either test, in agreement with the analysis of Example 8.1. Note that T_2 is more significant than T_1; this will generally be true when the effect is in any case highly significant, because the Residual MSq used as the basis for T_2 will then be substantially smaller than the Total MSq used in T_1. This is the reason for the general preference for the second of the two tests.

Table 13.3. Clotting times of plasma from eight subjects, treated by four methods, after ranking the four values within each subject

	Treatment				
Subject	1	2	3	4	Total
1	1	2	3	4	10
2	1	4	2	3	10
3	2	1	4	3	10
4	2	1	3	4	10
5	2	1	3·5	3·5	10
6	1	3	2	4	10
7	1	2	3	4	10
8	1	2	3	4	10
Total	11.0	16.0	23.5	29.5	80

Correction term $= 80^2/32 = 200$,
Between-Treatments SSq, $S_{tr} = (11 \cdot 0^2 + 16 \cdot 0^2 + 23 \cdot 5^2 + 29 \cdot 5^2)/8$
$$- 200$$
$$= 24 \cdot 9375,$$
Total SSq, $S_{tot} = 1^2 + 2^2 + \ldots + 4^2 - 200 = 39 \cdot 5$,
$T_1 = 8 \times 3 \times 24 \cdot 9375/39 \cdot 5 = 15 \cdot 15$ (as $\chi^2_{(3)}$; $P = 0 \cdot 002$),
$T_2 = 7 \times 24 \cdot 9375/14 \cdot 5625 = 11 \cdot 99$ (as $F_{3, 21}$; $P < 0 \cdot 001$).

In some studies treatments may be compared within strata or blocks, but with more than one observation per treatment in each stratum, and the numbers of replicates may be unbalanced, as in Example 8.9. This situation is referred to later in this section.

Independent groups: the Kruskal–Wallis test

Suppose we have more than two groups of observations and the data form a one-way classification of the type considered in §7.1, where the one-way analysis of variance was described. Suppose that there are t groups. A distribution-free test for such a situation would be a generalization of the Mann–Whitney or Wilcoxon rank sum test to more than two groups. A generalization was given by Kruskal and Wallis (1952). This test is based on ranking all the values and then the test proceeds by a method which has similarities with a one-way analysis of variance on the ranks.

Suppose that there are n_i observations for group i, and let $N = \sum n_i$. The observations are ranked from 1 to N, and the ranks are subjected to a one-way analysis of variance. Let T_i be the sum of the ranks in group i. Denote the corrected sum of squares for groups by S_{tr}, and the corrected total sum of squares by S_{tot}. In these calculations the correction term is given by $\frac{1}{4}N(N + 1)^2$. The test statistic is then calculated as

$$T = \frac{(N - 1)S_{tr}}{S_{tot}}, \qquad (13.9)$$

distributed approximately as $\chi^2_{(t-1)}$. If there are no ties, S_{tot} can be evaluated directly and the formula for the test statistic simplifies to

$$T = \frac{12}{N(N + 1)} \sum T_i^2/n_i - 3(N + 1). \qquad (13.10)$$

Example 13.6

Table 13.4 shows the data from Table 7.1, ranked from 1 to 20. From (13.9), $T = 19 \times 217/664 \cdot 5 = 6 \cdot 20$ (as $\chi^2_{(3)}$; $P = 0 \cdot 10$). If (13.10) is used in spite of the single pair of tied ranks, $T = 12 \times 2422/(20 \times 21) - 3 \times 21 = 6 \cdot 20$ again; the effect of this small degree of tying in the ranks is negligible. The conclusions from the analysis are very similar to those from the analysis of variance in Example 7.1: the differences are non-significant.

When the data are stratified by one or more factors (e.g. if data like those in Table 13.4 are obtained on each of several days) the Kruskal–Wallis test needs to be adapted to take account of the stratification. We shall not attempt a full discussion here, partly because the methods become more arduous and partly because for complex sets of data it may be advisable to consider a multiple regression approach to the original data or a transformed data set.

Table 13.4 Counts of adult worms in four groups each of five rats, after ranking

	Experiment			
	1	2	3	4
	6	17	1	18
	14	5	12·5	16
	11	19	12·5	15
	2	4	7	20
	9	8	3	10
Total	42	53	36	79

Correction term $= \frac{1}{4} \times 20 \times 441 = 2205$,

Between-Treatments SSq, $S_{tr} = (42^2 + 53^2 + 36^2 + 79^2)/5$
$$- 2205$$
$$= 217,$$

Total SSq, $S_{tot} = 6^2 + 17^2 + \ldots + 10^2 - 2205 = 664\cdot5$.

Two points may be noted, however. First, if there are two treatments, so that the solution required is a stratified version of the Wilcoxon/Mann–Whitney test, van Elteren (1960) has described a test based on a weighted sum of the Wilcoxon rank sum statistics T_{1h} (where the subscript h refers to a particular stratum). Secondly, data of this sort often arise in situations where the observations are heavily grouped, so that the groups may be regarded as categories in an ordinal categorical variable. The analysis of this type of data has already been discussed briefly on p. 420 (above (12.20)).

13.5 Rank correlation

Suppose that, in a group of n individuals, each individual provides observations on two variables, x and y. The closeness of the association between x and y is usually measured by the product–moment correlation coefficient r (§5.3). The use of this statistic might be thought objectionable on one of the following grounds: (i) it is based on the concept of closeness to linear regression, and its value may be affected drastically by a non-linear transformation; (ii) the measurements to be analysed may be qualitative, although ordered, and the investigator may not wish to assume any particular numerical scale; (iii) the sampling variation of r depends on the distribution of the variables, normality being usually assumed—a distribution-free approach may be desired.

These objections would be overcome by a correlation coefficient dependent only on the ranks of the observations. To preserve comparability with the product–moment correlation coefficient, r, a rank correlation coefficient should have at least the following properties.

1 It should lie between -1 and $+1$, taking the value $+1$ when the individuals are ranked in exactly the same order by x as by y, and -1 when the order is reversed.

2 For large samples in which the distribution of x is independent of y (and conversely), the value should be zero.

A satisfactory rank correlation coefficient can be obtained from Kendall's S statistic described in §13.3, with a generalization of the definition used there. The total number of pairs of individuals is $\frac{1}{2}n(n-1)$. Let P be the number of pairs which are ranked in the same order by x and by y, and Q the number of pairs in which the rankings are in the opposite order. Then

$$S = P - Q.$$

(The previous definition is a particular case of this in which one variable represents a dichotomy into the two groups, with group X being ranked before group Y; and the other variable represents the measurement under test, both x_i and y_i as previously defined being values of this second variable.)

The rank correlation coefficient, τ, is now defined by

$$\tau = \frac{S}{\frac{1}{2}n(n-1)}. \tag{13.11}$$

It is fairly easy to see that for complete agreement of rankings $\tau = 1$, and for complete reversal $\tau = -1$. A significance test of the null hypothesis that the x ranking is independent of the y ranking can conveniently be done on S. The null expectation of S (as of τ) is zero, and, in the absence of ties,

$$\mathrm{var}(S) = n(n-1)(2n+5)/18. \tag{13.12}$$

If there are ties, (13.12) is modified to give

$$\mathrm{var}(S) = \frac{1}{18}\left[n(n-1)(2n+5) - \sum_t t(t-1)(2t+5) - \sum_u u(u-1)(2u+5) \right]$$

$$+ \frac{1}{9n(n-1)(n-2)}\left[\sum_t t(t-1)(t-2) \right]\left[\sum_u u(u-1)(u-2) \right]$$

$$+ \frac{1}{2n(n-1)}\left[\sum_t t(t-1) \right]\left[\sum_u u(u-1) \right],$$

where the summations are over groups of ties, t being the number of tied individuals in a group of x values and u the number of a group of tied y values.

For further discussion of rank correlation, including tables for the significance of S, see Kendall and Gibbons (1990).

An alternative, and earlier, method of rank correlation, due to Spearman, uses the product–moment correlation of the ranks. In the absence of ties the formula for the Spearman coefficient may be simplified by the fact that the ranked observations in each group are the integers from 1 to n, to give

$$r_s = 1 - \frac{6 \sum d^2}{n^3 - n},$$ (13.13)

where the ds are the differences in the paired ranks. Significance may be tested approximately by the usual formula (5.21) for testing product–moment correlation coefficients.

Example 13.7

A sample of 10 students training as clinical psychologists are ranked by a tutor at the end of the course according to (a) suitability for their career, and (b) knowledge of psychology.

Student	A	B	C	D	E	F	G	H	I	J
Rank on (a)	4	10	3	1	9	2	6	7	8	5
Rank on (b)	5	8	6	2	10	3	9	4	7	1

Rearranging according to the (a) ranking, we have:

(a)	1	2	3	4	5	6	7	8	9	10
(b)	2	3	6	5	1	9	4	7	10	8

To calculate P take each of the (b) rankings in turn and count how many individuals to the right of this position have a higher ranking. These counts are then added. Thus, starting with the first individual, with rank 2, there are eight ranks greater than 2 to the right of this; for the next individual with rank 3 there are seven ranks greater than 3 to the right of this; and so on. Similarly, Q is defined by counting lower rather than higher ranks.

$$P = 8 + 7 + 4 + 4 + 5 + 1 + 3 + 2 + 0 + 0 = 34,$$

$$Q = 1 + 1 + 3 + 2 + 0 + 3 + 0 + 0 + 1 + 0 = 11.$$

As a check, $P + Q = \frac{1}{2}n(n-1)$ in the absence of ties; here $P + Q = 45 = \frac{1}{2}(10)(9)$.

$$S = P - Q = 23.$$

From Appendix Table 1 of Kendall and Gibbons (1990), the null probability of a value of S equal to 23 or more is 0·023. A one-sided test is perhaps appropriate here. For a two-sided test, the significance probability would be $2 \times 0·023 = 0·046$, still rather low. There is therefore a definite suggestion of an association between the two rankings.

The rank correlation coefficient is, by (13.11),

$$\tau = \frac{23}{\frac{1}{2}(10)(9)} = \frac{23}{45} = 0·51.$$

For the normal approximation to the significance test, from (13.12),

$$\mathrm{var}(S) = 10(9)(25)/18 = 125,$$

$$\mathrm{SE}(S) = 11·18.$$

It is useful to apply a continuity correction of 1 unit, since the possible values of S turn out to be separated by an interval of 2 units. The standardized normal deviate is $22/11\cdot18 = 1\cdot97$, for which $P = 0\cdot049$, rather close to the exact value.

For this set of data Spearman's rank correlation coefficient is $0\cdot68$. The approximate t test from (5.21) gives $t = 2\cdot66$ on 8 DF ($P = 0\cdot029$). A more exact significance level, allowing for the discreteness of the distribution, is $0\cdot031$. Both these values are smaller, indicating a more significant result, than for Kendall's test. However, different measures of association which are not logically equivalent will necessarily achieve different levels of significance, and the reader will hardly need to be reminded that the method chosen for final presentation should not be selected merely as the one showing the most significance.

13.6 General comments

Distribution-free tests are supported by remarkably strong theoretical arguments. Suppose that, in the two-sample problem of §13.3, one wished to test the null hypothesis that the two samples were drawn from the same distribution, and that one wished the test to have high power against alternative hypotheses specifying that the distributions differed only in their location, i.e. one distribution could be changed into the other by a simple shift along the scale of the measurement.

If the distributions are normal with the same variance, the t test is the most efficient test, but the rank test (Wilcoxon, Mann–Whitney, or Kendall) has a relative efficiency* of $0\cdot96$. If the distributions are not normal, the relative efficiency of the rank test is never less than $0\cdot86$ and may be infinitely high. For detecting a shift in location, therefore, the rank test is never much worse than the t test, and can be very much better.

Furthermore, the distribution-free test based on normal scores has a relative efficiency against the t test which is never less than unity and may be infinite. Why, then, should one not always use either the rank test or the normal score test in preference to the t test? The first point to make is that significance tests form only a part of the apparatus of statistical analysis. The main purpose of an analysis is usually to provide as much information as possible about the nature of the random variation affecting a set of observations. This can usually be done only by specifying a model for that variation, estimating the parameters of the model in a reasonably efficient way and informing oneself about the precision of these estimates.

Distribution-free methods were devised initially as significance tests, and they are not always easily adapted for purposes of estimation. We have described a number of estimation methods. None of these is particularly difficult, and the computational effort, which may be substantial in all but quite small samples, is alleviated by computer programs, which are readily available. However, as noted

*This measure of efficiency can be interpreted as the ratio of sample sizes needed to provide a certain power of detecting a given small shift in location.

earlier, the methods tend to assume a particular model for the contrasts between samples; for example the model used in conjunction with the Wilcoxon/Mann–Whitney test assumes a constant displacement in location between the two distributions. If the model is judged to be inappropriate, it may be difficult to find a satisfactory alternative, and hence to decide what should be estimated. A related point is that the theoretical results on power also refer to a particular form of difference between two distributions. In other situations the relative merits of different tests are less clear.

Another point to bear in mind is that distribution-free methods are at their best for relatively simple data structures. For complex data sets, perhaps with many factors and covariates, it will usually be best to aim for a parametric model such as the linear model underlying multiple regression.

In general, then, distribution-free methods are perhaps best regarded as a set of techniques to fall back on when standard assumptions have particularly doubtful validity; it is often useful to be able to confirm the results of a normal-theory significance test by also performing an appropriate distribution-free test.

14: Survival Analysis

14.1 Introduction

In many studies the variable of direct interest is the length of time that elapses before some event occurs. This event may be death, or death due to a particular disease, and for this reason the analysis of such data is often referred to as *survival analysis*.

An example of such a study is a clinical trial for the treatment of a malignant tumour where the prognosis is poor; death or remission of the tumour would be the end-point. Such studies usually include individuals for whom the event has not occurred at the time of the analysis. Although the time to the event for such a patient is unknown, there is some information on its value since it is known that it must exceed the current survival time; an observation of this type is referred to as a *censored* value. Methods of analysis must be able to cope with censored values. Often a number of variables are observed at the commencement of a trial, and survival is related to the values of these variables; that is, the variables are prognostic. Methods of analysis must be able to take account of the distribution of prognostic variables in the groups under study.

The number of studies of the above type has increased during the last two decades and statistical methods have been developed to analyse them; many of these methods were developed during the 1970s. Some of the methods will be described in this chapter; readers interested in more details are referred to the books by Kalbfleisch and Prentice (1980), Lawless (1982), and Cox and Oakes (1984), and to the two papers by Peto *et al.* (1976, 1977).

A second situation where survival analysis has been used occurs in the study of occupational mortality where it is required to assess if a group of workers who are exposed to a pollutant are experiencing excess mortality. Subjects enter the study when healthy, in contrast to a clinical trial where subjects are suffering from a disease. For this reason a common method of analysis has been the comparison of observed mortality, both in timing and cause, with what would be expected if the study group were subject to a similar mortality to that of the population of which it is a part.

Many of the methods of analysis are based on a life-table approach and in the next section the life table is described.

14.2 Life tables

The *life table*, first developed adequately by E. Halley (1656–1742), is one of the basic tools of vital statistics and actuarial science. Standardization was introduced in §12.9 as a method of summarizing a set of age-specific death rates, thus providing a composite measure of the mortality experience of a community at all ages and permitting useful comparison with the experience of other groups of people. The life table is an alternative summarizing procedure with rather similar attributes. Its purpose is to exhibit the pattern of survival of a group of individuals subject, throughout life, to the age-specific rates in question.

There are two distinct ways in which a life table may be constructed from mortality data for a large community; the two forms are usually called the *current life table* and the *cohort* or *generation life table*. The current life table describes the survival pattern of a group of individuals subject throughout life to the age-specific death rates currently observed in a particular community. This group is necessarily hypothetical. A group of individuals now aged 60 years will next year experience approximately the current mortality rate specific to ages 60–61; but those who survive another 10 years will, in the 11th year, experience not the *current* rate for ages 70–71 but the rate prevailing 10 years hence. The current life table, then, is a convenient summary of current mortality rather than a description of the actual mortality experience of any group.

The method of constructing the current life tables published in national sources of vital statistics or in those used in life assurance offices is rather complex (Chiang, 1984). A simplified approach is described by Hill and Hill (1991). The main features of the life table can be seen from Table 14.1, the left side of which summarizes the English Life Table No. 10 based on the mortality of males in England and Wales in 1930–32. The second column gives q_x, the probability that an individual, alive at age x years exactly, will die before his next birthday. The third column shows l_x, the number of individuals out of an arbitrary 1000 born alive who would survive to their xth birthday. To survive for this period an individual must survive the first year, then the second, and so on. Consequently,

$$l_x = l_0 p_0 p_1 \cdots p_{x-1}, \tag{14.1}$$

where $p_x = 1 - q_x$. This formula can be checked from Table 14.1 for $x = 1$, but not subsequently because values of q_x are given here only for selected values of x; such a table is called an *abridged life table*.

The fourth column shows $\overset{\circ}{e}_x$, the expectation of life at age x. This is the mean length of additional life beyond age x of all the l_x people alive at age x. In a complete table $\overset{\circ}{e}_x$ can be calculated approximately as

$$\overset{\circ}{e}_x = (l_{x+1} + l_{x+2} + \cdots)/l_x + \tfrac{1}{2}, \tag{14.2}$$

Table 14.1 Current and cohort life tables for men in England and Wales born around 1931

| Age (years) x | Current life tables 1930–32 | | | Cohort life table, 1931 cohort |
	Probability of death between age x and $x + 1$ q_x	Life-table survivors l_x	Expectation of life $\mathring{e}_x$	Life-table survivors l_x
0	0·0719	1000	58·7	1000
1	0·0153	928·1	62·2	927·8
5	0·0034	900·7	60·1	903·6
10	0·0015	890·2	55·8	894·8
20	0·0032	872·4	46·8	884·2
30	0·0034	844·2	38·2	874·1
40	0·0056	809·4	29·6	861·8
50	0·0113	747·9	21·6	829·7
60	0·0242	636·2	14·4	—
70	0·0604	433·6	8·6	—
80	0·1450	162·0	4·7	—

since the term in brackets is the total number of years lived beyond age x by the l_x individuals if those dying between age y and age $y + 1$ did so immediately after the yth birthday, and the $\frac{1}{2}$ is a correction to allow for the fact that deaths take place throughout each year of age, which very roughly adds half a year to the mean survival time.

The cohort life table describes the actual survival experience of a group, or 'cohort', of individuals born at about the same time. Those born in 1900, for instance, are subject during their first year to the mortality under 1 year of age prevailing in 1900–01; if they survive to 10 years of age they are subject to the mortality at that age in 1910–11; and so on. Cohort life tables summarize the mortality at different ages at the times when the cohort would have been at these ages. The right-hand side of Table 14.1 summarizes the l_x column from the cohort life table for men in England and Wales born in the five years centred around 1931. As would be expected, the values of l_1 in the two life tables are very similar, being dependent on infant mortality in about the same calendar years. At higher ages the values of l_x are greater for the cohort table because this is based on mortality rates at the higher ages which were experienced since 1931 and which are lower than the 1931 rates.

Both forms of life table are useful for vital statistical and epidemiological studies. Current life tables summarize current mortality and may be used as an alternative to methods of standardization for comparisons between the mortality patterns of different communities. Cohort life tables are particularly useful in studies of occupational mortality, where a group may be followed up over a long period of time (§14.9).

14.3 Follow-up studies

Many medical investigations are concerned with the survival pattern of special groups of patients—for example, those suffering from a particular form of malignant disease. Survival may be on average much shorter than for members of the general population. Since age is likely to be a less important factor than the progress of the disease, it is natural to measure survival from a particular stage in the history of the disease, such as the date when symptoms were first reported or the date on which a particular operation took place.

The application of life-table methods to data from follow-up studies of this kind will now be considered in some detail. In principle the methods are applicable to situations in which the critical end-point is not death, but some non-fatal event such as the recurrence of symptoms and signs after a remission, although it may not be possible to determine the precise time of recurrence whereas the time of death can usually be determined accurately. Indeed, the event may be favourable rather than unfavourable; the disappearance of symptoms after the start of treatment is an example. The discussion below is in terms of survival after an operation.

At the time of analysis of such a follow-up study patients are likely to have been observed for varying lengths of time, some having had the operation a long time before, others having been operated on recently. Some patients will have died, at times which can usually be ascertained relatively accurately; others are known to be alive at the time of analysis; others may have been lost to follow-up for various reasons between one examination and the next; others may have had to be withdrawn from the study for medical reasons—perhaps by the intervention of some other disease or an accidental death.

If there were no complications like those just referred to, and if every patient was followed until the time of death, the construction of a life table in terms of time after operation would be a simple matter. The life-table survival rate, l_x, is l_0 times the proportion of survival times greater than x. The problem would be merely that of obtaining the distribution of survival time—a very elementary task. To overcome the complications of incomplete data, a table like Table 14.2 is constructed.

This table is adapted from that given by Berkson and Gage (1950) in one of the first papers describing the method. In the original data the time intervals were measured from the time of hospital discharge, but for purposes of exposition we have changed these to intervals following operation. The columns (1)–(8) are formed as follows.

Table 14.2 Life-table calculations for patients with a particular form of malignant disease, adapted from Berkson and Gage (1950)

(1)	(2)	(3)	(4)	(5)	(6)	(7)	(8)
Interval since operation (years) x to $x + 1$	Last reported during this interval		Living at start of interval	Adjusted number at risk	Estimated probability of death	Estimated probability of survival	Percentage of survivors after x years
	Died d_x	Withdrawn w_x	n_x	n'_x	q_x	p_x	l_x
0–1	90	0	374	374·0	0·2406	0·7594	100
1–2	76	0	284	284·0	0·2676	0·7324	75·9
2–3	51	0	208	208·0	0·2452	0·7548	55·6
3–4	25	12	157	151·0	0·1656	0·8344	42·0
4–5	20	5	120	117·5	0·1702	0·8298	35·0
5–6	7	9	95	90·5	0·0773	0·9227	29·1
6–7	4	9	79	74·5	0·0537	0·9463	26·8
7–8	1	3	66	64·5	0·0155	0·9845	25·4
8–9	3	5	62	59·5	0·0504	0·9496	25·0
9–10	2	5	54	51·5	0·0388	0·9612	23·7
10–	21	26	47	—	—	—	22·8

(1) The choice of time intervals will depend on the nature of the data. In the present study estimates were needed of survival rates for integral numbers of years, to 10, after operation. If survival after 10 years had been of particular interest, the intervals could easily have been extended beyond 10 years. In that case, to avoid the table becoming too cumbersome it might have been useful to use 2-year intervals for at least some of the groups. Unequal intervals cause no problem; for an example see Merrell and Shulman (1955).

(2) and (3) The patients in the study are now classified according to the time interval during which their condition was last reported. If the report was of a death, the patient is counted in Column (2); patients who were alive at the last report are counted in Column (3). The term 'withdrawn' thus includes patients recently reported as alive, who would continue to be observed at future follow-up examinations, and those who have been lost to follow-up for some reason.

(4) The numbers of patients living at the start of the intervals are obtained by cumulating columns (2) and (3) from the foot. Thus, the number alive at 10 years is $21 + 26 = 47$. The number alive at 9 years includes these 47 and also the $2 + 5 = 7$ died or withdrawn in the interval 9–10 years; the entry is therefore $47 + 7 = 54$.

(5) The adjusted number at risk during the interval x to $x + 1$ is

$$n'_x = n_x - \tfrac{1}{2}w_x. \tag{14.3}$$

The purpose of this formula is to provide a denominator for the next column. The rationale is discussed below.

(6) The estimated probability of death during the interval x to $x + 1$ is

$$q_x = d_x/n'_x. \tag{14.4}$$

For example, in the first line,

$$q_0 = 90/374 \cdot 0 = 0 \cdot 2406.$$

The adjustment from n_x to n'_x is needed because the w_x withdrawals are necessarily at risk for only part of the interval. It is possible to make rather more sophisticated allowance for the withdrawals, particularly if the point of withdrawal during the interval is known. However, it is usually quite adequate to assume that the withdrawals have the same effect as if half of them were at risk for the whole period; hence the adjustment (14.3). An alternative argument is that, if the w_x patients had *not* withdrawn, we might have expected about $\frac{1}{2}q_x w_x$ extra deaths. The total number of deaths would then have been $d_x + \frac{1}{2}q_x w_x$, and we should have had an estimated death rate

$$q_x = \frac{d_x + \frac{1}{2}q_x w_x}{n_x}. \tag{14.5}$$

(14.5) can easily be seen to be equivalent to (14.3) and (14.4).

(7) $p_x = 1 - q_x$.

(8) The estimated probability of survival to, say, 3 years after the operation is $p_0 p_1 p_2$. The entries in the last column, often called the *life-table survival rates*, are thus obtained by successive multiplication of those in column (7), with an arbitrary multiplier $l_0 = 100$. Formally,

$$l_x = l_0 p_0 p_1 \dots p_{x-1}, \tag{14.6}$$

as in (14.1).

Two important assumptions underlie these calculations. First, it is assumed that the withdrawals are subject to the same probabilities of death as the non-withdrawals. This is a reasonable assumption for withdrawals who are still in the study and will be available for future follow-up. It may be a dangerous assumption for patients who were lost to follow-up, since failure to examine a patient for any reason may be related to the patient's health. Secondly, the various values of p_x are obtained from patients who entered the study at different points of time. It must be assumed that these probabilities remain reasonably constant over time; otherwise the life-table calculations represent quantities with no simple interpretation.

In Table 14.2 the calculations could have been continued beyond 10 years. Suppose, however, that d_{10} and w_{10} had both been zero, as they would have been if no patients had been observed for more than 10 years. Then n_{10} would have been zero, no values of q_{10} and p_{10} could have been calculated and in general no value of l_{11} would have been available, unless l_{10} were zero (as it would be if any one of $p_0, p_1, \ldots, p_9$ were zero), in which case l_{11} would also be zero. This point can be put more obviously by saying that no survival information is available for periods of follow-up longer than the maximum observed in the study. This means that the expectation of life (which implies an indefinitely long follow-up) cannot be calculated from follow-up studies unless the period of follow-up, at least for some patients, is sufficiently long to cover virtually the complete span of survival. For this reason the life-table survival rate (column (8) of Table 14.2) is a more generally useful measure of survival. Note that the value of x for which $l_x = 50\%$ is the *median* survival time; for a symmetric distribution this would be equal to the expectation of life.

For further discussion of life-table methods in follow-up studies, see Berkson and Gage (1950), Merrell and Shulman (1955), Cutler and Ederer (1958) and Newell *et al.* (1961).

14.4 Sampling errors in the life table

Each of the values of p_x in a life-table calculation is subject to sampling variation. Were it not for the withdrawals the variation could be regarded as binomial, with a sample size n_x. The effect of withdrawals is approximately the same as that of reducing the sample size to n'_x. The variance of l_x is given approximately by the following formula due to Greenwood (1926), which can be obtained by taking logarithms in (14.6) and using an extension of (3.18).

$$\text{var}(l_x) = l_x^2 \sum_{i=0}^{x-1} \frac{d_i}{n'_i(n'_i - d_i)}. \tag{14.7}$$

In Table 14.2, for instance, where $l_4 = 35 \cdot 0\%$,

$$\text{var}(l_4) = (35 \cdot 0)^2 \left[\frac{90}{(374)(284)} + \frac{76}{(284)(208)} + \frac{51}{(208)(157)} + \frac{25}{(151)(126)} \right]$$

$$= 6 \cdot 14$$

and

$$\text{SE}(l_4) = \sqrt{6 \cdot 14} = 2 \cdot 48.$$

Approximate 95% confidence limits for l_4 are

$$35 \cdot 0 \pm (1 \cdot 96)(2 \cdot 48) = 30 \cdot 1 \text{ and } 39 \cdot 9.$$

Application of (14.7) can lead to impossible values for confidence limits outside the range 0 to 100%. An alternative that avoids this is to apply the double-log transformation, $\ln(-\ln l_x)$, to (14·6), with $l_0 = 1$ so that l_x is a proportion with permissible range 0 to 1 (Kalbfleisch and Prentice, 1980). Then Greenwood's formula is modified to give 95% confidence limits for l_x of

$$l_x^{\exp(\pm 1·96s)}, \tag{14.8}$$

where

$$s = SE(l_x)/(-l_x \ln l_x).$$

For the above example, $l_4 = 0·35$, $SE(l_4) = 0·0248$, $s = 0·0675$, $\exp(1·96s) = 1·14$, $\exp(-1·96s) = 0·876$, and the limits are $0·35^{1·14}$ and $0·35^{0·876}$, which equal 0·302 and 0·399. In this case, where the limits using (14.7) are not near either end of the permissible range, (14.8) gives almost identical values to (14.7).

Peto *et al.* (1977) give a formula for $SE(l_x)$ that is easier to calculate than (14.7),

$$SE(l_x) = l_x \sqrt{[(1 - l_x)/n'_x]}. \tag{14.9}$$

As in (14.8), it is essential to work with l_x as a proportion. In the example, (14.9) gives $SE(l_4) = 0·0258$. Formula (14.9) is conservative but may be more appropriate for the period of increasing uncertainty at the end of life tables when there are few survivors still being followed.

Methods for calculating the sampling variance of the various entries in the life table, including the expectation of life, are given by Chiang (1984, Chapter 8).

14.5 The product-limit estimate of survival

The estimated life table given in Table 14.2 was calculated after dividing the period of follow-up into time intervals. In some cases the data may only be available in group form and often it is convenient to summarize the data into groups. Forming groups does, however, involve an arbitrary choice of time intervals and this can be avoided by using a method due to Kaplan and Meier (1958). In this method the data are, effectively, regarded as grouped into a large number of short time intervals, with each interval as short as the accuracy of recording permits. Thus if survival is recorded to an accuracy of 1 day then time intervals of 1-day width would be used. Suppose that at time t_j there are d_j deaths and that just before the deaths occurred there were n'_j subjects surviving. Then the estimated probability of death at time t_j is

$$q_{t_j} = d_j/n'_j. \tag{14.10}$$

This is equivalent to (14.4). By convention, if any subjects are censored at time t_j, then they are considered to have survived for longer than the deaths at time t_j and adjustments of the form of (14.3) are not applied. For most of the time intervals $d_j = 0$ and hence $q_{t_j} = 0$ and the survival probability $p_{t_j}(= 1 - q_{t_j}) = 1$. These intervals may be ignored in calculating the life-table survival as the product of survivals, as in (14.6). The survival at time t, l_t, is then estimated by

$$l_t = \prod_j p_{t_j} = \prod_j \frac{n'_j - d_j}{n'_j},\qquad(14.11)$$

where the product is taken over all time intervals in which a death occurred, up to and including t. This estimator is termed the *product-limit* estimator because it is the limiting form of the product in (14.6) as the time intervals are reduced towards zero. The estimator is also the maximum likelihood estimator. The estimates obtained are invariably expressed in graphical form. The survival curve consists of horizontal lines with vertical steps each time a death occurred (see Fig. 14.1 on p. 480). The calculations are illustrated in Table 14.4.

14.6 The logrank test

The test described in this section is used for the comparison of two or more groups of survival data. The first step is to arrange the survival times, both observed and censored, in rank order. Suppose, for illustration, that there are two groups, A and B. If at time t_j there were d_j deaths and there were n'_{jA} and n'_{jB} subjects alive just before t_j in groups A and B respectively, then the data can be arranged in a 2×2 table:

	Died	Survived	Total
Group A	d_{jA}	$n'_{jA} - d_{jA}$	n'_{jA}
Group B	d_{jB}	$n'_{jB} - d_{jB}$	n'_{jB}
Total	d_j	$n'_j - d_j$	n'_j

Except for tied survival times, $d_j = 1$ and each of d_{jA} and d_{jB} is 0 or 1. Note also that if a subject is censored at t_j then that subject is considered at risk at that time and so included in n'_j.

On the null hypothesis that the risk of death is the same in the two groups, then we would expect the number of deaths at any time to be distributed between the two groups in proportion to the numbers at risk. That is,

$$\left.\begin{aligned}\mathrm{E}(d_{jA}) &= n'_{jA} d_j / n'_j,\\[4pt]\mathrm{var}(d_{jA}) &= \frac{d_j(n'_j - d_j)n'_{jA}n'_{jB}}{n'^2_j(n'_j - 1)}.\end{aligned}\right\}\qquad(14.12)$$

In the case of $d_j = 1$, (14.12) simplifies to

$$\mathrm{E}(d_{jA}) = p'_{jA},$$

$$\mathrm{var}(d_{jA}) = p'_{jA}(1 - p'_{jA}),$$

where $p'_{jA} = n'_{jA}/n'_j$, the proportion of survivors who are in group A.

The difference between d_{jA} and $E(d_{jA})$ is evidence against the null hypothesis. The logrank test is the combination of these differences over all the times at which deaths occurred. It is analogous to the Mantel–Haenszel test for combining data over strata (see §12.6) and was first introduced in this way (Mantel, 1966).

Summing over all times of death, j, gives

$$O_A = \sum d_{jA}$$
$$E_A = \sum E(d_{jA})$$
$$V_A = \sum \text{var}(d_{jA}).$$

E_A may be referred to as the 'expected' number of deaths in group A but since, in some circumstances, E_A may exceed the number of individuals starting in the group a more accurate description is the *extent of exposure to risk of death* (Peto *et al.*, 1977). A test statistic for the equivalence of the death rates in the two groups is

$$X_1^2 = \frac{(O_A - E_A)^2}{V_A}, \tag{14.13}$$

which is approximately a $\chi_{(1)}^2$. An alternative and simpler test statistic, which does not require the calculation of the variance terms, is

$$X_2^2 = \frac{(O_A - E_A)^2}{E_A} + \frac{(O_B - E_B)^2}{E_B}. \tag{14.14}$$

This statistic is also approximately a $\chi_{(1)}^2$. In practice (14.14) is usually adequate, but errs on the conservative side (Peto and Pike, 1973).

The logrank test may be generalized to more than two groups. The summation in (14.14) is extended to cover all the groups and O_A and E_A, etc., are calculated in the same way as for two groups. The test statistic would have $k - 1$ DF if there were k groups.

The ratios O_A/E_A and O_B/E_B are referred to as the relative death rates and estimate the ratio of the death rate in each group to the death rate amongst both groups combined. The ratio of these two relative rates estimates the death rate in group A relative to that in group B, sometimes referred to as the *hazard ratio*. The hazard ratio and sampling variability are given by

$$\left. \begin{array}{c} h = \dfrac{O_A/E_A}{O_B/E_B} \\[4mm] \text{SE}[\ln(h)] = \sqrt{\left(\dfrac{1}{E_A} + \dfrac{1}{E_B}\right)}. \end{array} \right\} \tag{14.15}$$

An alternative estimate is

$$h = \exp\!\left(\frac{O_A - E_A}{V_A}\right) \left.\vphantom{\sqrt{\dfrac{1}{V_A}}}\right\}$$

$$SE[\ln(h)] = \sqrt{\frac{1}{V_A}} \qquad (14.16)$$

(Machin and Gardner, 1989). Formula (14.16) is similar to (4.23). Both (14.15) and (14.16) are biased and confidence intervals based on the standard errors will have less than the nominal coverage, when the hazard ratio is not close to unity. Formula (14.15) is less biased and adequate for h less than 3, but for larger hazard ratios an adjusted standard error may be calculated (Berry *et al.*, 1991) or a more complex analysis is advisable (§14.8).

Example 14.1

In Table 14.3 data are given of the survival of patients with diffuse histiocytic lymphoma according to stage of tumour (data abstracted from McKelvey *et al.*, 1976). Survival is measured in days after entry to a clinical trial. There was little difference in survival between the two treatment groups, which are not considered in this example.

The calculations of the product-limit estimate of the life table are given in Table 14.4 for the stage-3 group and the comparison of the survival for the two stages is shown in Fig. 14.1. It is apparent that survival is longer, on average, for patients with a stage-3 tumour than for those with stage 4. This difference may be formally tested using the logrank test.

The basic calculations necessary for the logrank test are given in Table 14.5. For brevity only deaths occurring at the beginning and end of the observation period are shown. The

Table 14.3 Survival of patients with diffuse hystiocytic lymphoma according to stage of tumour

	Survival (days)							
Stage 3	6	19	32	42	42	43*	94	126*
	169*	207	211*	227*	253	255*	270*	310*
	316*	335*	346*					
Stage 4	4	6	10	11	11	11	13	17
	20	20	21	22	24	24	29	30
	30	31	33	34	35	39	40	41*
	43*	45	46	50	56	61*	61*	63
	68	82	85	88	89	90	93	104
	110	134	137	160*	169	171	173	175
	184	201	222	235*	247*	260*	284*	290*
	291*	302*	304*	341*	345*			

*Still alive (censored value).

Table 14.4 Calculation of product-limit estimate of life table for stage-3 tumour data of Table 14.3

Time (days) t_j	Died d_j	Living at start of day n'_j	Estimated probability of: Death q_{t_j}	Survival p_{t_j}	Percentage of survivors at end of day l_{t_j}
0	—	19	—	—	100
6	1	19	0·0526	0·9474	94·7
19	1	18	0·0556	0·9444	89·5
32	1	17	0·0588	0·9412	84·2
42	2	16	0·1250	0·8750	73·7
94	1	13	0·0769	0·9231	68·0
207	1	10	0·1000	0·9000	61·2
253	1	7	0·1429	0·8571	52·5

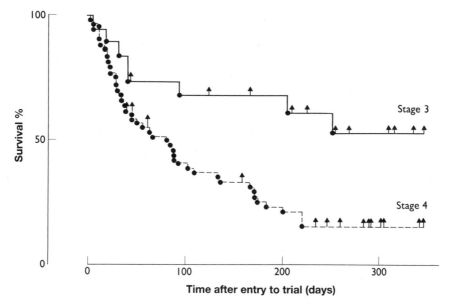

Fig. 14.1 Life tables for patients with stage-3 or stage-4 lymphoma. Circles = times of death, arrows = censored times of survivors.

two groups are indicated by subscripts 3 and 4, instead of A and B as used in the general description.

Applying (14.13) gives

$$X_1^2 = (8 - 16·6870)^2/11·2471$$
$$= 8·6870^2/11·2471$$
$$= 6·71 \quad (P = 0·010).$$

Table 14.5 Calculations for logrank test (data of Table 14.3) to compare survival of patients with tumours of stages 3 and 4

Days when deaths occurred	Numbers at risk		Deaths		$E(d_3)$	$\mathrm{var}(d_3)$
	n'_3	n'_4	d_3	d_4		
4	19	61	0	1	0·2375	0·1811
6	19	60	1	1	0·4810	0·3606
10	18	59	0	1	0·2338	0·1791
11	18	58	0	3	0·7105	0·5278
13	18	55	0	1	0·2466	0·1858
17	18	54	0	1	0·2500	0·1875
19	18	53	1	0	0·2535	0·1892
20	17	53	0	2	0·4857	0·3624
⋮						
201	10	12	0	1	0·4545	0·2479
207	10	11	1	0	0·4762	0·2494
222	8	11	0	1	0·4211	0·2438
253	7	8	1	0	0·4667	0·2489
Total			8	46	16·6870	11·2471
			O_3	O_4	E_3	V_3

To calculate (14.14) we first calculate E_4 using the relationship $O_3 + O_4 = E_3 + E_4$. Thus $E_4 = 37\cdot3130$ and

$$X^2_2 = 8\cdot6870^2(1/16\cdot6870 + 1/37\cdot3130)$$

$$= 6\cdot54 \quad (P = 0\cdot010).$$

Thus it is demonstrated that the difference shown in Fig. 14.1 is unlikely to be due to chance.

The relative death rates are $8/16\cdot6870 = 0\cdot48$ for the stage-3 group and $46/37\cdot3130 = 1\cdot23$ for the stage-4 group. The ratio of these rates estimates the death rate of stage 4 relative to that of stage 3 as $1\cdot23/0\cdot48 = 2\cdot57$. Using (14.15), $SE[\ln(h)] = 0\cdot2945$ and the 95% confidence interval for the hazard ratio is $\exp[\ln(2\cdot57) \pm 1\cdot96 \times 0\cdot2945] = 1\cdot44$ to $4\cdot58$. Using (14.16) the hazard ratio is $2\cdot16$ (95% confidence interval $1\cdot21$ to $3\cdot88$).

The logrank test is a non-parametric test. Other tests can be obtained by modifying Wilcoxon's rank sum test (§13.3) so that it can be applied to compare survival times for two groups in the case where some survival times are censored values (Cox and Oakes, 1984, p. 124). These tend to be more sensitive than the logrank test to situations where the ratio of hazards is higher at early survival times than at late ones.

14.7 Parametric models

In mortality studies the variable of interest is the survival time. A possible approach to the analysis is to postulate a distribution for survival time and to estimate the parameters of this distribution from the data. This approach is usually applied by starting with a model for the death rate and determining the form of the resulting survival time distribution.

The death rate will usually vary with time since entry to the study, t, and will be denoted by $\lambda(t)$; sometimes $\lambda(t)$ is referred to as the *hazard function*. Suppose the probability density of survival time is $f(t)$ and the corresponding distribution function is $F(t)$. Then since the death rate is the rate at which deaths occur divided by the proportion of the population surviving we have

$$\left. \begin{aligned} \lambda(t) &= \frac{f(t)}{1 - F(t)} \\[2mm] &= f(t)/S(t), \end{aligned} \right\} \qquad (14.17)$$

where $S(t) = 1 - F(t)$ is the proportion surviving and is referred to as the *survivor function*.

Equation (14.17) enables $f(t)$ and $S(t)$ to be specified in terms of $\lambda(t)$. Rather than consider the general solution we will consider certain cases. The simplest form is that the death rate is a constant, i.e. $\lambda(t) = \lambda$ for all t. Then integrating (14.17) with respect to t and noting that $f(t)$ is the derivative of $F(t)$ (§2.3) give

$$\lambda t = - \ln[S(t)]. \qquad (14.18)$$

That is,

$$S(t) = \exp(- \lambda t).$$

The survival time has an exponential distribution with mean $1/\lambda$. If this distribution is appropriate, then, from (14.18), a plot of the logarithm of the survivor function against time should give a straight line through the origin.

Data from a group of subjects consist of a number of deaths with known survival times and a number of survivors for whom the censored length of survival is known. These data can be used to estimate λ, using the method of maximum likelihood (§12.8). For a particular value of λ the likelihood consists of the product of terms $f(t)$ for the deaths and $S(t)$ for the survivors. The maximum likelihood estimate of λ, the standard error of the estimate and a significance test against any hypothesized value are obtained using the general method of maximum likelihood, although, in this simple case, the solution can be obtained directly without iteration.

The main restriction of the exponential model is the assumption that the death rate is independent of time. It would usually be unreasonable to expect this assumption to hold except over short time intervals. One way of overcoming this restriction is to divide the period of follow-up into a number of shorter intervals, and assume that the hazard rate is constant within each interval but that it is different for the different intervals (Holford, 1976).

Another method of avoiding the assumption that the hazard is constant is to use a different parametric model of the hazard rate. One model is the *Weibull*, defined by

$$\lambda(t) = \alpha\gamma t^{\gamma-1}, \tag{14.19}$$

where γ is greater than 1. This model has proved applicable to the incidence of cancer by age in humans (Cook *et al.*, 1969) and by time after exposure to a carcinogen in animal experiments (Pike, 1966). A second model is that the hazard increases exponentially with age, that is,

$$\lambda(t) = \alpha\exp(\beta t).$$

This is the *Gompertz* hazard and describes the death rate from all causes in adults fairly well. A model in which the times of death are lognormally distributed has also been used but has the disadvantage that the associated hazard rate starts to decrease at some time.

14.8 Regression and proportional-hazards models

It would be unusual to analyse a single group of homogeneous subjects but the basic method may be extended to cope with more realistic situations by modelling the hazard rate to represent dependence on variables recorded for each subject as well as on time. For example, in a clinical trial it would be postulated that the hazard rate was dependent on treatment, which could be represented by one or more dummy variables (§10.2). Again, if a number of prognostic variables were known, then the hazard rate could be expressed as a function of these variables. In general the hazard rate could be written as a function of both time and the covariates, that is as $\lambda(t, x)$ where x represents the set of covariates $(x_1, x_2, \ldots, x_k)$.

Zippin and Armitage (1966) considered one prognostic variable, x, the logarithm of white blood count, and an exponential survival distribution, with

$$\lambda(t, x) = (\alpha + \beta x)^{-1};$$

the mean survival time was thus linear in x. Analysis consisted of the estimation of α and β. A disadvantage of this representation is that the hazard rate becomes negative for high values of x (since β was negative). An alternative model avoiding this disadvantage, proposed by Glasser (1967), is

$$\lambda(t, x) = \alpha\exp(\beta x);$$

the logarithm of the mean survival time was thus linear in x.

Generally the hazard would depend on time and could be written as

$$\lambda(t, x) = \lambda_0(t)\exp(\boldsymbol{\beta}x) \qquad (14.20)$$

where $\boldsymbol{\beta}x$ represents the regression function, $\beta_1 x_1 + \beta_2 x_2 + \ldots + \beta_p x_p$, and $\lambda_0(t)$ is the time-dependent part of the hazard. The term $\lambda_0(t)$ could represent any of the models considered in the previous section or other parametric functions of t. Equation (14.20) is a regression model in terms of the covariates. It is also referred to as a *proportional-hazards* model since the hazards for different sets of covariates remain in the same proportion for all t. Data can be analysed parametrically using (14.20) provided that some particular form of $\lambda_0(t)$ is assumed. The parameters of $\lambda_0(t)$ and also the regression coefficients, $\boldsymbol{\beta}$, would be estimated. Inference would be in terms of the estimate $\mathbf{b}$ of $\boldsymbol{\beta}$, and the parameters of $\lambda_0(t)$ would have no direct interest.

Another way of representing the effect of the covariates is to suppose that the distribution of survival time is changed by multiplying the time-scale by $\exp(\boldsymbol{\beta}'x)$, that is that the logarithm of survival time is increased by $\boldsymbol{\beta}'x$. The hazard could then be written

$$\lambda(t, x) = \lambda_0(t\exp(-\boldsymbol{\beta}'x))\exp(-\boldsymbol{\beta}'x). \qquad (14.21)$$

This is referred to as an *accelerated failure time model*. For the exponential distribution, $\lambda_0(t) = \lambda$, (14.20) and (14.21) are equivalent, with $\boldsymbol{\beta}' = -\boldsymbol{\beta}$, so the accelerated failure time model is also a proportional-hazards model. The same is true for the Weibull (14.19), with $\boldsymbol{\beta}' = -\boldsymbol{\beta}/\gamma$, but in general the accelerated failure time model would not be a proportional-hazards model.

Procedures for fitting models of the type discussed above are available in a number of statistical computing packages; for example, a range of parametric models, including the exponential, Weibull and lognormal, may be fitted using PROC LIFEREG in the SAS program.

Cox's proportional-hazards model

Since often an appropriate parametric form of $\lambda_0(t)$ is unknown and, in any case, not of primary interest, it would be more convenient if it was unnecessary to substitute any particular form for $\lambda_0(t)$ in (14.20). This was the approach introduced by Cox (1972). The model is then non-parametric with respect to time but parametric in terms of the covariates. Estimation of $\boldsymbol{\beta}$ and inferences are developed by considering the information supplied at each time that a death occurred. Consider a death occurring at time t_j, and suppose that there were n_j' subjects alive just before t_j, that the values of x for these subjects are $x_1, x_2, \ldots, x_{n_j}$, and that the subject that died is denoted, with no loss of generality, by the subscript 1. The set of n_j' subjects at risk is referred to as the *risk set*. The risk of death at time t_j for each subject in the risk set is given by (14.20).

This does not supply absolute measures of risk, but does supply the relative risks for each subject, since although $\lambda_0(t_j)$ is unknown it is the same for each subject. Thus the probability that the death observed at t_j was of the subject who did die at that time is

$$p_j = \exp(\boldsymbol{\beta}\boldsymbol{x}_1)/\sum \exp(\boldsymbol{\beta}\boldsymbol{x}_i), \tag{14.22}$$

where summation is over all members of the risk set. Similar terms are derived for each time that a death occurred and are combined to form a likelihood. Technically this is called a *partial likelihood* since the component terms are derived conditionally on the times that deaths occurred and the composition of the risk sets at these times. The actual times at which deaths occurred are not used but the order of the times of death and of censoring, that is the ranks, determine the risk sets. Thus the method has, as far as the treatment of time is concerned, similarities with non-parametric rank tests (Chapter 13). It also has similarities with the logrank test, which is also conditional on the risk sets.

As time is used non-parametrically, the occurrence of ties, either of times of death or involving a time of death and a time of censoring, causes some complications. As with the non-parametric tests discussed in Chapter 13, this is not a serious problem unless ties are extensive. The simplest procedure is to use the full risk set, of all the individuals alive just before the tied time, for all the tied individuals (Breslow, 1974).

The model is fitted by the method of maximum likelihood and this is usually done using specific statistical software, such as **PROC PHREG** in the **SAS** program. In Example 14.2 some of the steps in the fitting process are detailed to illustrate the rationale of the method.

Example 14.2

The data given in Table 14.3 and Example 14.1 may be analysed using Cox's approach. Define a dummy variable that takes the value zero for stage 3 and unity for stage 4. Then the death rates, from (14.20), are $\lambda_0(t)$ for stage 3 and $\lambda_0(t)\exp(\beta)$ for stage 4, and $\exp(\beta)$ is the death rate of stage 4 relative to stage 3. The first death occurred after 4 days (Table 14.5) when the risk set consisted of 19 stage-3 subjects and 61 stage-4 subjects. The death was of a stage-4 subject and the probability that the one death known to occur at this time was the particular stage-4 subject who did die is, from (14.22).

$$p_1 = \exp(\beta)/[19 + 61 \exp(\beta)].$$

The second time when deaths occurred was at 6 days. There were two deaths on this day and this tie is handled approximately by assuming that they occurred simultaneously so that the same risk set, 19 stage-3 and 60 stage-4 subjects, applied for each death. The probability that a particular stage-3 subject died is $1/[19 + 60 \exp(\beta)]$ and that a particular stage-4 subject died is $\exp(\beta)/[19 + 60\exp(\beta)]$ and these two probabilities are combined, using the multiplication rule, to give the probability that the two deaths consist of the one subject from each stage,

$$p_2 = \exp(\beta)/[19 + 60\exp(\beta)]^2.$$

Strictly this expression should contain a binomial factor of 2 (§2.5) but, since a constant factor does not influence the estimation of β, it is convenient to omit it. Working through Table 14.5, similar terms can be written down and the log likelihood is equal to the sum of the logarithms of the p_j. Using a computer the maximum likelihood estimate of β, b, is obtained with its standard error:

$$b = 0{\cdot}9610,$$

$$\mathrm{SE}(b) = 0{\cdot}3856.$$

To test the hypothesis that $\beta = 0$, that is $\exp(\beta) = 1$, we have the following as an approximate standardized normal deviate:

$$z = 0{\cdot}9610/0{\cdot}3856 = 2{\cdot}49 \quad (P = 0{\cdot}013).$$

Approximate 95% confidence limits for b are

$$0{\cdot}9610 \pm 1{\cdot}96 \times 0{\cdot}3856$$

$$= 0{\cdot}2052 \quad \text{and} \quad 1{\cdot}7168.$$

Taking exponentials gives, as an estimate of the death rate of stage 4 relative to stage 3, 2·61 with 95% confidence limits of 1·23 and 5·57.

The estimate and the statistical significance of the relative death rate using Cox's approach (Example 14.2) are similar to those obtained using the logrank test (Example 14.1). The confidence interval is wider, in accord with the earlier remark that the confidence interval calculated using (14.15) has less than the required coverage when the hazard ratio is not near to unity.

The full power of the proportional-hazards model comes into play when there are several covariates and (14.20) represents a multiple regression model. For example, Kalbfleisch and Prentice (1980) discuss data from a trial of treatment of tumours of any of four sites in the head and neck. There were many covariates that might be expected to relate to survival. Four of these were shown to be prognostic: sex, the patient's general condition, extent of primary tumour (T classification), and extent of lymph-node metastasis (N classification). All of these were related to survival when included multivariately in (14.20). Terms for treatment were also included but, unfortunately, the treatment effects were not statistically significant.

With multiple covariates the rationale for selecting the variables to include in the regression is similar to that employed in multiple regression of a normally distributed response variable (§10.1). Corresponding to the analysis of variance test for the deletion of a set of variables is the *Wald test*, which gives a statistic approximately distributed as χ^2 on q DF, to test the deletion of q covariates. For

$q = 1$, the Wald χ^2 on 1 DF is equivalent to the standardized normal deviate as used in Example 14.2.

Diagnostic methods

Plots of the survival against time, usually with some transformation of one or both of these items, are useful for checking on the distribution of the hazard. The *integrated* or *cumulative hazard*, defined as

$$H(t) = \int_0^t \lambda(u)\mathrm{d}u = -\ln[S(t)], \tag{14.23}$$

is often used for this purpose. The integrated hazard may be obtained from the Kaplan–Meier estimate of $S(t)$ using (14.23), or from the cumulative hazard, evaluated as the sum of the estimated discrete hazards at all the event times up to t. A plot of $\ln H(t)$ against $\ln t$ is linear with a slope of γ for the Weibull, or slope 1 for the exponential. The same plot for different subgroups of individuals defined by different covariate values may give guidance on whether a proportional-hazards or accelerated failure time model is the more appropriate choice for the effect of the covariates. For a proportional-hazards model the curves are separated by constant vertical distances, and for an accelerated failure time model by constant horizontal distances. Both of these conditions are met if the plots are linear, reflecting the fact that the Weibull and exponential are both proportional-hazards and accelerated failure time models. Otherwise it may be difficult to distinguish between the two possibilities against the background of chance variability, but then the two models may give similar inferences of the effects of the covariates (Solomon, 1984). The choice of a particular distributional form can be avoided by using the Cox semiparametric model, and inferences on the effects of the covariates will be similar with the Cox model to the inferences with an appropriate distributional form (Kay, 1977; Byar, 1983), but the use of a distributional form will tend to give slightly more precise estimates of the regression coefficients.

As discussed in §10.1, residual plots are often useful as a check on the assumptions of the model and for determining if extra covariates should be included. With survival data, what is meant by a residual is not as clear as it is for a continuous outcome variable. One approach is the *martingale residual*, defined in terms of the outcome and the cumulative hazard up to either the occurrence of the event or censoring; for an event the martingale residual is $1 - H(t)$, and for a censored individual the residual is $-H(t)$. These residuals have approximately zero mean and unit standard deviation but are distributed asymmetrically, with large negative values for long-term survivors and a maximum of 1 for a short-term survivor. This skewness makes these residuals difficult to interpret.

An alternative is the *deviance residual* (Therneau *et al.*, 1990). It is defined as the square root of the contribution to the deviance (§12.8) between a model maximizing the contribution of the point in question to the likelihood and the fitted model. These residuals have approximately a standard normal distribution and are available in the SAS program PROC PHREG.

Chen and Wang (1991) discuss some diagnostic plots that are useful for assessing the effect of adding a covariate, detecting non-linearity or identifying influential points in Cox's proportional-hazards model.

Extensions to more complicated situations

The above discussion has been in terms of data from a sample of independent individuals, with constant covariates, and where the survival time is either known fairly precisely or is known to be larger than the current period of observation, that is, it is *right-censored*. In some situations not all of these conditions apply.

If the values of the covariates for an individual are not constant throughout the period of follow-up, then the method needs to be adjusted to take account of this. In principle this causes no problem when using Cox's regression model, although the complexity of setting up the calculations is increased. For each time of death the appropriate values of the covariates are used in (14.22). A time-dependent covariate may be created to give a diagnostic test of the proportional-hazards assumption. In an analysis with one explanatory variable x, suppose that a time-dependent variable z is defined as $x \ln t$, and that in a regression of the log hazard on x and z the regression coefficients are, respectively, β and γ. Then the relative hazard for an increase of 1 unit in x is $t^\gamma \exp(\beta)$. The proportional-hazards assumption holds if $\gamma = 0$, and a test of this assumption is provided by the test of the regression coefficient γ against the null hypothesis that $\gamma = 0$.

In some situations the time of failure may not be known precisely. For example, individuals may be examined at intervals, say a year apart, and it is observed that the event has occurred between examinations but there is no information on when the change occurred within the interval. Such observations are referred to as *interval-censored*. If the lengths of interval are short compared with the total length of the study, it would be adequate to analyse the data as if each event occurred at the midpoint of its interval, but otherwise a more exact treatment would be necessary. This situation is discussed by Finkelstein (1986).

McGilchrist and Aisbett (1991) considered recurrence times to infection in patients on kidney dialysis. Following an infection a patient is treated and, when the infection is cleared, is put back on dialysis. Thus a patient may have more than one infection, so the events are not independent; some patients may be more likely to have an infection than others and in general it is useful to consider that, in addition to the covariates that may influence the hazard rate, each individual has an unknown tendency to become infected, referred to as the *frailty*. There will usually be insufficient data from each individual to estimate the frailties for each individual separately and the approach is to assume a distributional form for the frailties and use the whole data set to estimate the parameters of this distribution as well as the regression coefficients for the covariates. The situation is similar to those where empirical Bayesian methods may be employed (§4.13) and the frailty estimates are shrunk towards the mean. This approach is similar to that given by Clayton and Cuzick (1985), and Clayton (1991) discusses the problem in terms of Bayesian inference.

14.9 Subject-years methods

A commonly used research method is the *cohort study*, in which a group is classified by exposure to some substance and is followed over time, with the vital status of each member determined up to the time at which the analysis is being conducted. A review of methods of cohort study design and application is given by Liddell (1988). It may be possible to use existing records to determine exposure in the past, and this gives the *historical prospective cohort* study, used particularly in occupational health research. Such studies often cover periods of over 20 years. The aim is to compare the mortality experience of subgroups, such as high exposure with low exposure, in order to establish whether exposure to the agent might be contributing to mortality. As such studies cover a long period of time individuals will be ageing and their mortality risk will be changing. In addition there may be period effects on the mortality rate. Both the age and period effects will need to be taken into account. One approach is the *subject-years method*, sometimes referred to as the *modified life-table approach*; an early use of this method was by Doll (1952). In this approach the number of deaths in the group, or in the subgroups, is expressed in terms of the number of deaths expected if the individuals had experienced the same death rates as the population of which the group is a part.

The expected mortality is calculated using published national or regional death rates. The age of each subject, both at entry to the study and as it changes through the period of follow-up, has to be taken into account. Also, since age-specific death rates depend on the period of time at which the risk occurs, the cohort of each subject must be considered. Official death rates are usually published in 5-year intervals of age and period and may be arranged as a rectangular array consisting of cells, such as the age group 45–49 during the period 1976–80. Each subject passes through several of these cells during the period of follow-up and experiences a risk of dying according to the years of risk in each cell and the death rate. This risk is accumulated so long as a subject is at risk of dying in the study, that is until the date of death or until the end of the follow-up period for the survivors. This accumulated risk is the same as the cumulative hazard (14.23). The expected number of deaths is obtained by adding over all subjects in the group, and it is computationally convenient to add the years at risk in each cell over subjects before multiplying by the death rates. This is the origin of the name of the method since subject-years at risk are calculated.

The method can be applied for total deaths and also for deaths from specific causes. The same table of subject-years at risk is used for each cause with different tables of death rates, and when a particular cause of death is being considered deaths from any other cause are effectively treated as censored survivals. For any cause of death the observed number is treated as a Poisson variable with expectation equal to the expected number (Example 4.15). The method is similar to indirect standardization of death rates (§12.9) and the ratio of observed to expected deaths is often referred to as the standardized mortality ratio (SMR).

Example 14.3

A group of 512 men working in an asbestos factory was followed up (Newhouse *et al.*, 1985). All men who started work in particular jobs at any time after 1933 were included and mortality was assessed over the period from 10 years after start of employment in the factory for each man up to the end of 1980. Mortality from lung cancer was of particular relevance. The subject-years at risk and the death rates for lung cancer in England and Wales are shown in Table 14.6 in 5-year age groups and 10-year periods (in the original application 5-year periods were used).

The expected number of deaths due to lung cancer is

$$(82 \times 2 + 62 \times 1 + 13 \times 1 + \ldots + 72 \times 756) \times 10^{-5} = 13\cdot8.$$

Table 14.6 Subject-years at risk (y) of asbestos workers and death rates (d) per 100 000 for lung cancer in men in England and Wales

	Period							
	1941–50		1951–60		1961–70		1971–80	
Age group	y	d	y	d	y	d	y	d
25–29	82	2	62	1	13	1	3	1
30–34	148	3	273	4	156	3	43	2
35–39	74	9	446	10	435	8	141	6
40–44	41	21	395	25	677	22	290	16
45–49	33	46	229	58	749	54	485	46
50–54	23	78	172	124	590	119	642	106
55–59	14	112	158	216	399	226	621	201
60–64	11	137	109	294	288	370	479	346
65–69	4	137	78	343	185	508	273	530
70–74	0	107	47	325	124	562	151	651
75 +	0	86	16	270	58	518	72	756

The observed number was 67, so the SMR is $67/13\cdot8 = 4\cdot9$. Using the methods given in §4.10, a test of the null hypothesis that the asbestos workers experienced national death rates is

$$z = (67 - 13\cdot8)/\sqrt{13\cdot8} = 14\cdot3 \quad (P < 0\cdot001),$$

and approximate 95% confidence limits for the SMR are $3\cdot8$ and $6\cdot2$.

The method has usually been applied to compare observed and expected mortality within single groups but may be extended to compare the SMR between different subgroups, or more generally to take account of covariates recorded for each individual, by expressing the SMR as a proportional-hazards regression model (Berry, 1983), that is, by the use of a generalized linear model (§12.8). For subgroup i, if m_i is the cumulative hazard from the reference population and γ_i the proportional-hazards multiplier, then μ_i, the expected number of deaths, is given by

$$\ln \mu_i = \ln m_i + \ln \gamma_i.$$

If γ_i is modelled in terms of a set of covariates by

$$\ln \gamma_i = \alpha + \beta_1 x_{i1} + \beta_2 x_{i2} + \ldots + \beta_p x_{ip},$$

then

$$\ln \mu_i = \ln m_i + \alpha + \beta_1 x_{i1} + \beta_2 x_{i2} + \ldots + \beta_p x_{ip}. \tag{14.24}$$

This model is similar to the generalized linear model of a Poisson variable (12.26) but contains the additional term $\ln m_i$, which ensures that age and period are both adjusted for. An example, in which the covariates are represented by a three-factor structure, is given in Berry (1983).

A disadvantage of the above approach is that it involves the assumption of proportional hazards between the study population and the external reference population across all the age–period strata, that is, that the reference death rates apply to the study population at least to a constant of proportionality. An alternative approach that does not depend on this assumption is to work entirely within the data set without any reference to an external population. The number of deaths and the subject-years at risk are accumulated for each cell of the rectangular array of age groups by period of time and, within these cells, for subgroups defined in terms of the covariates. The simplest approach is then to produce SMRs for each of the subgroups based on the observed death rates in each cell, instead of on external death rates (Breslow and Day, 1987, §3.5). If there are more than two subgroups, comparison of these internal SMRs still depends on proportional hazards of the subgroups across the age–period strata, but a proportional-hazards assumption between the study population and a reference population is no longer necessary. This approach is known to be conservative and may be improved by a Mantel–Haenszel approach (Breslow, 1984; Breslow and Day, 1987, §3.6).

The most comprehensive approach is that of Poisson modelling. For sub-group i and age–period stratum j, if n_{ij} is the number of subject-years and γ_{ij} the death rate, then μ_{ij}, the expected number of deaths, is given by

$$\ln \mu_{ij} = \ln n_{ij} + \ln \gamma_{ij}.$$

If γ_{ij} is modelled in terms of the age–period stratum and a set of covariates by

$$\ln \gamma_{ij} = \alpha_j + \beta_1 x_{ij1} + \beta_2 x_{ij2} + \ldots + \beta_p x_{ijp},$$

then

$$\ln \mu_{ij} = \ln n_{ij} + \alpha_j + \beta_1 x_{ij1} + \beta_2 x_{ij2} + \ldots + \beta_p x_{ijp}. \qquad (14.25)$$

This is a generalized linear model of a Poisson variable (12.26) with the additional term $\ln n_{ij}$. An application is given as Example 12.12 (p. 433). Breslow and Day (1987, Chapter 4) give fuller details and worked examples.

In many cases the external method (14.24) and the internal method (14.25) will give similar inferences on the effect of the covariates. The latter has the advantage that there is no assumption that the death rates in all the age–period strata follow a proportional-hazards model with respect to the reference population, but the precision of the comparisons is slightly poorer than with the external method. A combination of the two approaches, using (14.24) for the overall group and main subgroups and (14.25) for regression modelling, has the advantage of estimating the effects of the covariates and also estimating how the mortality in the overall group compares with that in the population of which it is a part. An example where this was done is given by Checkoway *et al.* (1993).

15: Sequential Methods

15.1 General

In most of the examples described in earlier chapters the number of observations could reasonably be assumed to be determined quite independently of the numerical values of the observations. In controlled laboratory experiments the number of observations will usually be decided in advance. In many other medical studies, such as clinical trials or epidemiological surveys, the ultimate sample size may depend on the ease with which observations can be made or on the rate at which suitable patients become available. Even here, though, the sample size is not necessarily affected by the observed values of the random variables on which the analysis is performed.

In these circumstances it seems reasonable to regard the sample size as a variable whose main importance lies in its effect on precision, giving in itself no information about the contrasts which are under study. In assessing the effect of random variation it is usual to imagine the sample size to be fixed; that is, one enquires about the random variation which would be observed in hypothetical repetitions of the investigation with the same sample size.

Some other types of investigation are rather different in that the ultimate size of the study not only may be unpredictable before its start but may depend on the numerical values of the observations. Certain classes of observation may, for instance, lead to a relatively early closure of the study; others may lead to a long investigation. A study of this type is called *sequential*. If the sequential aspect of the design is sufficiently formal, it will be described by a *stopping rule*, which defines the way in which the decision to stop the investigation at some stage depends on the results obtained. The stopping rule is thus a special feature of sequential design, supplementing the more familiar features of randomization and blocking (in experiments) and random selection (in surveys).

The methods of analysis of data collected sequentially form a subject called *sequential analysis*, the classical work on which is due to Wald (1947).

Before even a brief consideration of detailed methods of sequential design and analysis it is useful to note a few possible reasons for using sequential methods.

(a) *Economy*

In industrial sampling inspection there may be a large number of materials to be classified as being of good or bad quality on the basis of tests whose outcomes are subject to random variation. In the pharmaceutical industry, for example, drugs may be screened for specific activity by their performance in a particular biological test. Instead of a constant amount of experimentation with each drug, it may be more efficient to experiment sequentially so that most drugs are quickly rejected but a minority of drugs with initially promising results are allowed more observations before a decision is reached (Armitage and Schneiderman, 1958; King, 1963). Such sequential procedures usually reduce the total amount of experimentation, and perhaps the cost of the whole operation, whilst achieving a given level of discrimination between good and bad quality.

(b) To achieve specified precision

In §6.6 it was noted that the size of a random sample required to reduce the standard error of a mean to some specified level depends on the residual standard deviation, σ. If σ is initially unknown, it can be estimated from a pilot study. Alternatively one could merge the pilot study into the definitive sampling by maintaining a sequence of estimates of σ, using all observations made so far, and stopping the survey when the estimated standard error reached its required level.

Suppose that, in a random sample of size n from a distribution with mean μ and variance σ^2, the estimated mean is $\bar{x}_n$ and the estimated standard deviation is s_n. The subscripts here emphasize the fact that both these statistics will change randomly as n increases. The estimated standard error of $\bar{x}_n$ is

$$\text{SE}(\bar{x}_n) = s_n/\sqrt{n}, \tag{15.1}$$

and, although s_n will fluctuate randomly, this standard error will tend to decrease as n increases.

Suppose the purpose of the investigation is to estimate μ with specified precision, as in §6.6, criterion **1** (p. 196); specifically, suppose we require $\text{SE}(\bar{x}_n) < \varepsilon$. Then an appropriate stopping rule will be: continue sampling until $s_n/\sqrt{n}$ first falls below ε.

The question arises whether the formula (15.1) for the standard error is valid with this form of sequential sampling; its original interpretation was in terms of repeated sampling with a fixed sample size. The answer is, broadly, that the method is valid. First, if we choose to interpret the standard error as measuring the dispersion of the likelihood function, or as the standard deviation of the posterior distribution with dispersed prior knowledge (§4.12), we have an important result: *likelihood functions and posterior distributions are unaffected by the choice of stopping rule*. The sequential design is, from this point of view, irrelevant. Secondly, on the more traditional frequency view, the usual confidence limits are approximately valid, particularly in reasonably large samples. That is, if the sequential sampling procedure is repeated many times, the usual 95% confidence limits will include the true value μ approximately 95% of the time.

(c) Ethical considerations

Ethical considerations usually preclude random allocation in a clinical trial if there is strong prior evidence that one of the rival treatments is better than another. For the same reason it will usually be undesirable to continue a trial beyond a point at which one treatment is clearly seen to be better than a rival treatment. To find when such a situation is reached the investigator must proceed sequentially: the observations will be analysed continuously and the decision when to stop the trial will depend in some way on the results obtained. Such a sequential design is often possible in clinical trials since patients are usually entered into a trial serially, over a period of time, rather than all at the same time.

In all these different situations, one condition in particular is necessary for a sequential approach to be worth considering. Any observation must be recorded and made available for analysis relatively soon after it is planned; otherwise, it may not contribute to the decision when to stop the collection of data until much too late a stage. In a clinical trial of analgesics, for instance, observations on a particular patient may become available within a few days after the patient is treated; if the period of intake of patients into the trial is measured in months, there will be ample opportunity for a feedback of information. If, on the other hand, a trial is concerned with the effect of a 2-year period of treatment for patients with rheumatic conditions, feedback will be negligible and the trial must be designed on a non-sequential basis.

15.2 Sequential tests for binary data

Wald's original work was primarily concerned with sequential significance tests, which give rise to rather more difficult problems than does the estimation procedure described in §15.1(b).

It is useful to illustrate some of these by referring to a hypothetical, yet typical, crossover trial like that described in Example 4.7. Each patient receives two analgesic drugs, A and B, in adjacent weeks. The order of administration is random and the drugs are made so as to be indistinguishable by the patients. At the end of the 2-week period each patient gives a preference for the drug received in the first week or that received in the second week, on the basis of alleviation of pain. These are then decoded to form a series of preferences for A or B. We assume that any possible period effect (see §8.2) can be ignored.

A typical set of results might be that shown in Table 15.1. It seems reasonable to test the cumulative results at any stage to see whether there is a significant preponderance of preferences in favour of A or B. The appropriate conventional test, at the nth stage, would be that based on the binomial distribution with parameter n and with $\pi = \frac{1}{2}$ (see §4.7). The critical values for significance at the 5%

Table 15.1 Example illustrating the repeated use of significance tests on a series of preferences for one of two analgesic drugs

Patient number	Preference	(1) Cumulative number of preferences for A	Critical values for (1) at two-sided 5% level
1	B	0	—
2	A	1	—
3	A	2	—
4	A	3	—
5	A	4	—
6	A	5	0, 6
7	A	6	0, 7
8	B	6	0, 8
9	B	6	1, 8
10	A	7	1, 9
11	A	8	1, 10
12	B	8	2, 10
13	B	8	2, 11
14	A	9	2, 12
15	A	10	3, 12
16	A	11	3, 13
17	A	12	4, 13
18	A	13	4, 14
19	A	14	4, 15
20	B	14	5, 15
21	A	15	5, 16
22	B	15	5, 17
23	A	16	6, 17
24	A	17	6, 18
25	A	18	7, 18

level (using exact P values) are shown in Table 15.1. No result is significant until $n = 25$, when the number of preferences in favour of A reaches the critical level. The investigator, proceeding sequentially, might be inclined to stop the trial at this stage and publish his results claiming a significant difference at the 5% level. Indeed, this is a correct assessment of the evidence *at this particular stage*. The principle enunciated in the last section shows that the relative likelihoods of different parameters (in this example, different values of the probability π of obtaining a preference for A) are unaffected by the stopping rule. However, some selection of evidence has taken place. The investigator has had a large number of opportunities to stop at the 5% level. Even if the null hypothesis is true, there is a substantial probability that a 'significant' result will be found in due course, and this probability will clearly increase the longer the trial continues.

The position is very similar to that discussed in §7.4 in connection with multiple comparisons. The probability, on the null hypothesis, that a sequential trial will stop with a verdict in favour of one or the other treatment may be termed the *overall* significance level (a more formal term is the probability of a type I error (see §6.6)). To control the overall significance level at a low value such as 5%, a much higher significance level (that is, a *lower* probability) is required to assess the results at any one stage. This condition by itself is insufficient to determine the stopping rule: many different rules can be constructed to satisfy a specified overall significance level. Wald's (1947) theory provides one important general method. Some rather different sequential plans, designed specially for medical trials, are described in detail by Armitage (1975) and Whitehead (1992); these methods are outlined below.

Suppose that the stopping rule is to stop the trial if the cumulative results at any stage show a significant difference at the nominal two-sided $2\alpha'$ level, or to stop after N stages if the trial has not stopped earlier. To achieve an overall two-sided significance level, 2α, of 5%, what value should be chosen for $2\alpha'$, the significance level at any one stage? The answer clearly depends on N; the larger the value of N, the smaller $2\alpha'$ must be. Some results are given in Table 15.2.

The left-hand side of Table 15.2 refers to repeated significance tests based on the binomial distribution, as in the example at the beginning of this section. The right-hand side refers to repeated tests on cumulative series of observations on normally distributed random variables when the variance is known, a situation discussed more fully in §15.3. The distinction between the two sets of results in Table 15.2 arises primarily from the discreteness of the binomial distribution.

Table 15.2 Repeated significance tests on cumulative binomial and normal observations; nominal significance level to be used for individual tests for overall level $2\alpha = 0.05$

Number of stages N	Nominal significance level (two-sided), $2\alpha'$, for individual tests	
	Binomial	Normal
1	—	0·050
5	—	0·015
10	0·031	0·010
15	0·023	0·008
20	0·022	0·007
50	0·013	0·005
100	0·008	0·004
150	0·007	0·003

The choice of N, the maximum sample size in a sequential test, will depend on much the same considerations as those outlined in §6.6 (pp. 195–198). In particular, as in criterion **3** of that section, one may wish to select a sequential plan which not only controls the overall significance level, 2α, but has a specified power, say $1 - \beta$, of providing a significant result when a certain alternative to the null hypothesis is true. In the binomial test described earlier, a particular alternative hypothesis might specify that the probability of a preference for drug A, which we denote by π, is some value π_1 different from $\frac{1}{2}$. If the sequential plan is symmetrical, it will automatically provide the same power for $\pi = \pi_0$ ($= 1 - \pi_1$) as for $\pi = \pi_1$. For example, if $\pi_1 = 0.8$ and $\pi_0 = 0.2$, the hypothesis $\pi = \pi_1$ indicates a benefit from using drug A, and the hypothesis $\pi = \pi_0$ indicates an equal benefit from using drug B; each of these alternatives would have an equal chance of detection by a symmetrical sequential plan.

Table 15.3 shows the maximum sample sizes, and the significance levels for individual tests, for binomial sequential plans with the overall significance level $2\alpha = 0.05$ and a power $1 - \beta = 0.95$ against various alternative values of π. These are examples of *RST* (*repeated significance test*) *plans*. More extensive tables are given in Armitage (1975, Tables 3.9–3.12).

Any of the binomial RST plans from Table 15.3 can be represented graphically by a diagram like that in Fig. 15.1 (which depicts the plan with $\pi_1 = 0.85$). In this diagram the horizontal axis represents the number of preferences recorded at any stage. The vertical axis represents the difference between the numbers of preferences for A and B. The boundary points are obtained from the binomial distribution. The course of any trial is charted by starting a zigzag line at the origin and moving one unit to the right and upwards (i.e. in a 'north-easterly' direction) for each A preference, and one unit to the right and downwards (a 'south-easterly' direction) for each B preference. The data plotted in Fig. 15.1 are taken from a trial to assess some cough suppressants (Snell and Armitage, 1957; see also Armitage 1975, Example 3.3); A is an active drug, B is a placebo. The results are

Table 15.3 Maximum sample size, N, and nominal significance levels for individual tests, $2\alpha'$, for binomial RST plans with overall level $2\alpha = 0.05$ and power $1 - \beta = 0.95$ against various values of π differing from the null value of 0.5

π_1	$2\alpha'$	N
0.95	0.0313	10
0.90	0.0225	16
0.85	0.0193	25
0.80	0.0147	38
0.75	0.0118	61
0.70	0.0081	100

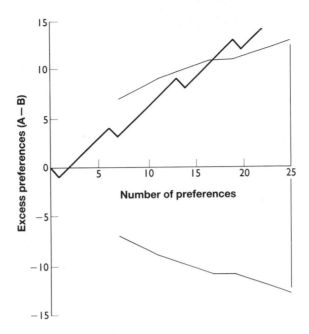

Fig. 15.1 A sequential RST plan for a series of preferences. The overall significance level is 0·05, individual tests are performed at the 0·0193 level and the plan has a power of 0·95 against a situation in which the probability of a preference for A is 0·85 or 0·15. The data are taken from a trial of cough suppressants (Table 15.4).

summarized in Table 15.4. The superiority of the active drug was demonstrated by the seventeenth preference, and it would have been reasonable to terminate the trial at or shortly after that stage. In fact, as Table 15.4 shows, a number of additional preferences were obtained (perhaps because treatment had already started for these patients), and these tended to confirm the earlier results.

This trial was originally designed by slightly different methods of sequential analysis (*restricted plans*, described on p. 52 of Armitage, 1975). A comparison of Fig. 15.1 with Fig. 3.7 of that book or the chart in the original paper shows that the two plans are extremely similar; the essential difference is that the earlier plans had approximately linear boundaries whereas the present boundaries are rather more curved. A further difference is that in the earlier plans the vertical part of the boundary was modified by stopping the trial as soon as it became clear that neither of the outer boundaries could be reached; the resulting boundary was shaped thus: < . The same device could be used here.

In any trial using a series of preferences, it is likely that some comparisons will fail to yield a definite preference in either direction. In the data of Table 15.4, for instance, some patients were unwilling to state a preference for either preparation. For the purposes of a significance test, only the definite preferences are used; the

Table 15.4 Preferences expressed by patients between an active drug, A, and a placebo, B, as cough suppressants

Patient number	Preference	Patient number	Preference
1	—	24	A
2	B	25	A
3	—	26	A
4	A	27	—
5	A	28	—
6	—	29	—
7	—	30	A
8	—	31	A
9	A	32	—
10	A	33	B
11	—	34	A
12	—	35	A
13	—	36	—
14	A	37	B
15	B	38	—
16	—	39	A
17	A	40	A
18	A	41	A
19	A	42	A
20	A	43	—
21	A	44	—
22	A	45	B
23	B		

A dash indicates that the patient stated no preference.

others may be ignored. However, in estimating the relative merits of the treatments it will be extremely important to know whether many patients were unable to make a preference, and any summary of the data must certainly contain a clear statement on this point.

15.3 Normal approximations

The example illustrated in Table 15.1 and most of the discussion in §15.2 relate to binary data, and Table 15.3 summarizes briefly the characteristics of some binomial RST plans. The types of data encountered in clinical trials are very varied, and cannot all be discussed in detail in this chapter. It is useful, however, to consider plans for testing the mean of a normal distribution with known variance—not so much because this situation arises frequently in practice (distributions are often non-normal and variances are usually unknown), but rather because it can be used as a good approximation to a wide range of situations.

Table 15.5 Maximum sample size, N, nominal significance level for individual tests, $2\alpha'$, and standardized normal deviate, k, for normal RST plans with overall level $2\alpha = 0.05$ and power $1 - \beta = 0.95$ against various values of $\delta_1 = \mu_1/\sigma$

$\delta_1 = \mu_1/\sigma$	$2\alpha'$	k	N
0·3	0·003	2·95	200
0·4	0·004	2·89	111
0·5	0·005	2·84	71
0·6	0·005	2·80	49
0·8	0·006	2·73	28
1·0	0·008	2·65	17
1·2	0·009	2·60	12
1·4	0·012	2·52	8

Suppose that, in a trial to compare two treatments, A and B, the response variable, d, is distributed as $N(\mu, \sigma^2)$, and that $\mu = 0$ under the null hypothesis that A and B have equal effects; (d might well be the difference between paired responses from A and B). We may wish to select an RST plan which (i) controls the overall significance level at 2α, and (ii) provides a power $1 - \beta$ against an alternative value $\mu = \mu_1$ or the opposite situation with $\mu = -\mu_1$. Table 15.5 summarizes the characteristics of some plans with $2\alpha = 0.05$ and $1 - \beta = 0.95$. As in §15.2, $2\alpha'$ is the nominal significance level and N is the maximum number of responses to be observed; k is the standardized normal deviate exceeded with a probability $2\alpha'$ (so in Table A1, $z = k$ and $P = 2\alpha'$). A suitable graphical procedure is to plot $y = \sum d$ against the number of observations n, with two outer boundaries representing the rejection of the null hypothesis in favour of A or B.

More extensive tables are given in Armitage (1975, Tables 5.5 and 5.6).

These RST plans for normally distributed variables can be used as approximations for more general situations, including, for example, two-sample tests. Suppose that we are interested in some parameter, θ, that the null hypothesis specifies $\theta = 0$, and that we want high power against an alternative hypothesis that $\theta = \theta_1$ or that $\theta = -\theta_1$. Let the error probabilities be 2α and β, as before.

Suppose further that:

1 at any stage in the sequential procedure we can estimate θ by its maximum likelihood estimate $\hat{\theta}$, and its variance by $\text{var}(\hat{\theta})$;

2 we inspect the accumulating data at intervals (up to a maximum of N times), in such a way that after n such inspections $\text{var}(\hat{\theta})$ is inversely proportional to n. Writing $\text{var}(\hat{\theta}) = 1/nI$, we see that $1/\text{var}(\hat{\theta})$, called the *information*, increases by an amount I between successive tests.

Then Table 15.5 may be used, with $2\alpha'$ and k retaining their original definitions, but with N now referring to the maximum number of inspections (not necessarily the same as the sample size since the data need not be inspected after every observation).

To use Table 15.5, we also need to know δ_1, which was defined as μ_1/σ in the original case of a normal response variable, d. In that situation the variance of the estimate of μ after n observations was σ^2/n. In general we can equate this with $\text{var}(\hat\theta)$, and so obtain $\delta_1 = \theta_1/\sqrt{[n\,\text{var}(\hat\theta)]}$, or $\theta_1\sqrt{I}$ in the notation introduced earlier.

In practice, it may not be feasible to arrange that $1/\text{var}(\hat\theta)$ increases by exactly the same amount I between successive tests, in which case a rough average value of I may be used.

This general approach is described in considerable detail by Whitehead (1992), with applications to a number of specialized forms of analysis such as the logrank test for survival data and the comparison of groups with ordered categorical responses. In this second edition of his book, Whitehead removes the restriction to inspections separated by constant increments of information, I. His methods are thus very widely applicable. In the present chapter we retain this restriction for simplicity of exposition.

15.4 Group sequential plans

The sequential methods described in earlier sections are appropriate for trials in which the accumulated data are examined very frequently, either after every new observation or at a large number of inspection points. A different situation often arises in which the investigator wishes to monitor the progress of a trial, but to inspect the data on only a small number of occasions. In a large multicentre trial, for example, the investigators may arrange for the accumulated data to be monitored once a year, during an intake period of 5 years. Often the responsibility for undertaking these interim analyses, and deciding whether to recommend early stopping of the trial on the basis of the current data, is delegated to an independent data-monitoring committee.

For this purpose we need to allow for the effect of repeated inspections of the data, but the number of inspections, N, will be much smaller than most of the entries in Table 15.5. As in Table 15.5, suppose that the response variable, d, is distributed as $N(\mu, \sigma^2)$, and that we require an overall significance level 2α and a power $1 - \beta$ against alternative values of μ_1 and $-\mu_1$ for μ, the null value being $\mu = 0$. Suppose that during each inspection interval m observations accumulate. Table 15.6 shows the characteristics of group sequential plans based on repeated significance tests at N inspection points, with $2\alpha = 0{\cdot}05$ and $1 - \beta = 0{\cdot}95$. Note that δ_1 is now defined as $\mu_1\sqrt{m}/\sigma$, whereas in Table 15.5 (where $m = 1$) we had $\delta_1 = \mu_1/\sigma$.

As in §15.3, the plans for normal response variables, like those in Table 15.6, may be used as approximate solutions to more general problems. Suppose, as

Table 15.6 Characteristics of group sequential plans for normal variables, with N repeated tests at nominal level $2\alpha'$, and m observations between successive inspection points, for overall level $2\alpha = 0.05$ and power $1 - \beta = 0.95$ against various values of $\delta_1 = \mu_1\sqrt{m}/\sigma$

N	$2\alpha'$	k	$\delta_1 = \mu_1\sqrt{m}/\sigma$
2	0.029	2.18	2.66
3	0.022	2.29	2.22
4	0.018	2.36	1.95
5	0.016	2.41	1.76
6	0.014	2.45	1.62
7	0.013	2.48	1.51
8	0.012	2.51	1.42
9	0.011	2.54	1.34
10	0.011	2.56	1.28

before, that we are studying a parameter θ, and wish to test the null hypothesis that $\theta = 0$ against the alternative values θ_1 and $-\theta_1$. As before, suppose that $1/\mathrm{var}(\hat{\theta})$ increases by an amount I between successive tests. Then Table 15.6 may be used, with δ_1 representing $\theta_1\sqrt{I}$, or $\theta_1/\sqrt{[n\,\mathrm{var}(\hat{\theta})]}$ where $\mathrm{var}(\hat{\theta})$ is the variance of $\hat{\theta}$ after n inspections.

Example 15.1

In a trial discussed by Pocock (1983, p. 192), Cockburn *et al.* (1980) assessed the effect of vitamin D supplementation for pregnant women in comparison with a control treatment, measuring the response by the infant's plasma calcium concentration 6 days after birth. The standard deviation of the response (mg per 100 ml) was about 1.2. Suppose that, in such a trial, it was required to detect a change in mean plasma calcium of 0.3 mg per 100 ml, and that it was intended to examine the data after three approximately equal groups of responses had been obtained. How many women should be included in each group?

Suppose that each of the three groups contains m_0 women on each of the two treatments. Using the general formulation, and the plan with $N = 3$ from Table 15.6, we can write θ for the difference in mean values between the two groups, and $\theta_1 = 0.3$. After n stages ($n = 1, 2$ and 3), $\mathrm{var}(\hat{\theta}) = 2\sigma_0^2/m_0 n$, so $\delta_1 = \theta_1/\sqrt{(2\sigma_0^2/m_0)}$, with $\sigma_0^2 = (1.2)^2 = 1.44$. From Table 15.6, we have also that $\delta_1 = 2.22$. Therefore,

$$2.22 = 0.3\sqrt{\left[\frac{m_0}{2(1.44)}\right]},$$

and

$$m_0 = \frac{2(1.44)(2.22)^2}{(0.3)^2} = 157.7,\ \text{say } 160.$$

The total number of patients would thus be $3 \times 320 = 960$, unless the trial were stopped after one of the two interim analyses. From Table 15.6, the repeated tests would each be carried out at the 2.2% level.

Example 15.2

In a trial for the secondary prevention of myocardial infarction, patients receive long-term treatment with one of two drugs, starting shortly after the first infarction. The aim is to compare the proportions of patients who experience a 'critical' event (death or reinfarction) within 12 months after start of treatment. It is required to detect a possible difference such that one drug reduces this proportion to 20% below that for the other drug. The expected proportion with either drug is about 0·15. Five inspections of the data are envisaged.

  Since the proportion of patients 'affected' (i.e. having a critical event) is low, the observed number of affected patients in each group can be regarded as approximately a Poisson variable. Denoting the probabilities of an event within 12 months on the two treatments as λ_1 and λ_2, it is natural to consider the parameter $\theta = \ln(\lambda_1/\lambda_2)$, since the power requirement is expressed in terms of a proportionate effect. A 20% reduction corresponds to $\theta_1 = \ln(0·8) = -0·223$, or (for a difference in the other direction) 0·223. Suppose that m_0 patients are assigned to each treatment in each inspection interval, and the numbers of affected patients in the two treatment groups, after n inspections, are r_1 and r_2. Then, $\hat{\lambda}_1 = r_1/nm_0$, $\hat{\lambda}_2 = r_2/nm_0$ and $\hat{\theta} = \ln(r_1/r_2)$. Since r_1 is a Poisson variable its variance is estimated by r_1, and, from (3.17), $\text{var}(\ln r_1) \simeq (1/r_1^2)r_1 = 1/r_1$. So

$$\text{var}(\hat{\theta}) = \text{var}(\ln r_1) + \text{var}(\ln r_2)$$

$$\simeq \frac{1}{r_1} + \frac{1}{r_2} = \frac{\hat{\lambda}_1^{-1} + \hat{\lambda}_2^{-1}}{nm_0}.$$

Thus,

$$\delta_1 = \theta_1/\sqrt{[n\,\text{var}(\hat{\theta})]}$$

$$= 0·223\sqrt{\left(\frac{m_0}{\hat{\lambda}_1^{-1} + \hat{\lambda}_2^{-1}}\right)};$$

and also from Table 15.6, with $N = 5$, $\delta_1 = 1·76$. Therefore,

$$0·223\sqrt{\left(\frac{m_0}{\hat{\lambda}_1^{-1} + \hat{\lambda}_2^{-1}}\right)} = 1·76.$$

Setting $\hat{\lambda}_1 = \hat{\lambda}_2 = 0·15$ approximately,

$$m_0 = \left(\frac{2}{0·15}\right)\left(\frac{1·76}{0·223}\right)^2 = 830·5, \text{ say } 830.$$

The total number of patients required would be about $5 \times 2 \times 830 = 8300$.

  The Poisson approximation used here has led to an unduly high value for m_0. The more appropriate binomial distribution would have involved a multiplying factor of $1 - 0·15 = 0·85$ for $\text{var}(\hat{\theta})$ (see the discussion on p. 65), and consequently also for m_0. The resulting value is $m_0 = 8300 \times 0·85 = 7050$, approximately.

These conclusions illustrate the need for large trials in the study of diseases with a low incidence of critical events, where only modest reductions in the event rate are likely to be achieved, but where even such modest improvements would be of considerable importance.

15.5 Concluding remarks

It is important to emphasize that sequential stopping rules should not be regarded as inviolable once they have been prescribed. There are two main reasons for this remark.

1 The considerations that lead to the selection of a particular sequential plan involve a number of rather arbitrary choices. After these choices have been made, various relevant circumstances may change: the rate of intake of patients to the trial may decline, newly published work may make it reasonable to review the objectives of the current trial, and so on. Of course, it would be wrong to change the agreed stopping rules merely because the results are unexpected and, perhaps, unwelcome.

2 The decision to stop a trial for ethical reasons must depend on a number of factors besides the sequential analysis. It will be necessary to consider side-effects of treatments, differences between treatments in the ease of administration and perhaps cost, evidence from other sources, the plausibility of the apparent findings as compared with the possibility that they are affected by random error, and so on. The sequential analysis should thus be regarded as a guide in one aspect of the decision, explicitly allowing for the effect of repeated inspections of the data, and not as the only determinant of that decision.

The plans described in this chapter have all involved repeated significance tests at some fixed nominal significance level. Many other forms of stopping rule have been proposed and examined, and the book by Whitehead (1992) should be consulted for details; see also Jennison and Turnbull (1990). In particular, group sequential designs may be constructed with nominal significance levels that vary from one stage to another. For example, Peto *et al.* (1976) and O'Brien and Fleming (1979) have suggested two quite different approaches which are less likely to lead to very early stopping than the RST plans. They are therefore arguably more appropriate in situations where only small differences are a priori at all likely.

Each of the approaches referred to in the previous paragraph requires that the stopping rule is predetermined. The schemes differ in the way in which the probability of early stopping (the overall significance level or type I error probability, when the null hypothesis is true) is distributed along the boundaries. It will, however, often be inconvenient or impracticable to fix the number and times of data inspections in advance. Lan and DeMets (1983) have described a method by which the predetermined type I error probability can be 'spent' in a flexible manner, the schedule being decided for the convenience of the data-monitoring team, although independently of the trial results (see also Kim and DeMets, 1992).

A quite different approach (Lan *et al.*, 1982, 1984) is that of *stochastic curtailment*, whereby a trial may be stopped prematurely if, at any stage, the conclusion that would have been drawn at the intended termination point is already quite clear. The proposal is usually advocated for situations where interim results for, say, two treatments are very similar, and when it can be predicted that the final difference would almost certainly be non-significant. Although this approach may be useful in enabling research efforts to be switched to more promising directions, there is a danger of placing too much importance on the results of a final significance test. Data showing non-significant treatment effects may nevertheless be valuable for estimation, especially in contributing to overviews. It may be unwise to terminate such studies prematurely, particularly when there is no treatment difference to provide an ethical reason for stopping.

The methods described in this chapter, and those outlined in the paragraphs above, have been developed from a non-Bayesian point of view. As indicated in §15.1(b), in the Bayesian approach the stopping rule is irrelevant to the inferences to be made at any stage. A trial could reasonably be stopped whenever the posterior distribution suggested strong evidence of a clear advantage for one treatment. This approach to the design and analysis of clinical trials has been strongly advocated, for instance by Berry (1987a, b) and Spiegelhalter and Freedman (1988). There are some points at which the two approaches may usefully interact. For instance, in stochastic curtailment the prediction of the future result can usefully be done by Bayesian methods, as in §4.13 (Spiegelhalter *et al.*, 1986; Armitage, 1988; Spiegelhalter and Freedman, 1988). Grossman *et al.* (1994) have discussed the design of group sequential trials which preserve type I error probabilities and yet involve boundaries determined by a Bayesian formulation, the prior distribution representing initial scepticism about the possible treatment effect.

Finally, we note that in clinical trials it may be useful to base a stopping rule on tests of a non-zero difference between treatment effects (Meier, 1975; Freedman *et al.*, 1984; also see §6.6, p. 198). All the sequential methods outlined in this chapter can readily be adapted by basing the boundaries on tests of the required non-zero value.

16: Statistical Methods in Epidemiology

16.1 Introduction

There is no standard definition of the branch of medical science called *epidemiology*. In broad terms epidemiology is concerned with the distribution of disease, or of a physiological condition, and of the factors that influence the distribution. It is now customary to include within its orbit the study of chronic diseases as well as the communicable diseases which give rise to epidemics of the classical sort. The subject overlaps to some extent with *social medicine, community medicine* or *public health*. These terms are also difficult to define precisely, but they would usually be understood to include social and administrative topics, such as the organization of health services, which might not be regarded as part of epidemiology.

Epidemiology is concerned with certain characteristics of groups of individuals rather than single subjects, and inevitably gives rise to statistical problems. Many of these are conceptually similar to statistical problems arising in other branches of medical science, and indeed in the non-medical sciences, and can be approached by the methods of analysis described earlier in this book; several examples in earlier chapters have been drawn from epidemiological studies. Other methodological problems in epidemiology, although of statistical interest, are bound up with considerations of a non-statistical nature and cannot be discussed here. Examples are the interpretation of vital and health statistical data, which requires a close knowledge of administrative procedures for the recording of such data and of the classification of diseases and causes of death (Benjamin, 1968; World Health Organization, 1978); and the proper use and potential development of medical records of various sorts (Acheson, 1967). There is also a considerable body of literature concerned with the mathematical theory of epidemic disease; the monographs by Bailey (1975) and Becker (1989) provide useful summaries of this work. For general accounts of epidemiological methods the reader may consult Alderson (1983), Elwood (1988), Hennekens *et al.* (1987), Kelsey *et al.* (1986), Kleinbaum *et al.* (1982), Miettinen (1985) and Rothman (1986).

In this chapter we consider briefly certain problems arising in epidemiological research for which special statistical methods have been developed.

Since epidemiology is concerned with the distribution of disease in populations, summary measures are required to describe the amount of disease in a population. These are two basic measures, incidence and prevalence.

Incidence is a measure of the rate at which new cases of disease occur in a population previously without disease. Thus the incidence, denoted by I, is defined as

$$I = \frac{\text{number of new cases in period of time}}{\text{population at risk}}.$$

The period of time is specified in the units in which the rate is expressed. Often the rate is multiplied by a base such as 1000 or 1 000 000 to avoid small decimal fractions. For example, there were 256 new cases of cancer of the pancreas in men in New South Wales in 1990 out of a population of 2·903 million males. The incidence was $256/2\cdot903 = 88$ per million per year.

Prevalence, denoted by P, is a measure of the frequency of existing disease at a given time, and is defined as

$$P = \frac{\text{total number of cases at given time}}{\text{total population at that time}}.$$

Both incidence and prevalence usually depend on age, and possibly sex, and sex- and age-specific figures would be calculated.

The prevalence and incidence rates are related since an incident case is, immediately on occurrence, a prevalent case and remains as such until recovery or death (disregarding emigration and immigration). Provided the situation is stable, the link between the two measures is given by

$$P = It, \tag{16.1}$$

where t is the average duration of disease. For a chronic disease from which there is no recovery, t would be the average survival after occurrence of the disease.

16.2 Relative risk

Cohort and case–control methods for studying the aetiology of disease were discussed in §6.3. In such studies it is usual to make comparisons between groups with different characteristics, in particular between a group of individuals exposed to some factor and a group not exposed. A measure of the increased risk (if any) of incurring a particular disease in the exposed compared with the non-exposed is required. The measure usually used is the ratio of the incidences in the groups being compared and is referred to as *relative risk*, ϕ. Thus

$$\phi = I_E/I_{NE}, \tag{16.2}$$

where I_E and I_{NE} are the incidence rates in the exposed and non-exposed respectively. This measure may also be referred to as the *risk ratio*.

In a cohort study the relative risk can be estimated directly, since estimates are available of both I_E and I_{NE}. In a case–control study the relative risk cannot be estimated immediately since neither I_E not I_{NE} can be estimated, and we now consider how to obtain a useful solution.

Suppose that each subject in a large population has been classified as positive or negative according to some potential aetiological factor, and positive or negative according to some disease state. The factor might be based on a current classification or (more usually in a retrospective study) on the subject's past history. The disease state may refer to the presence or absence of a certain category of disease at a particular instant, or to a certain occurrence (such as diagnosis or death) during a stated period, that is, to *prevalence* and *incidence*, respectively.

For any such categorization the population may be enumerated in a 2×2 table, as follows. The entries in the table are *proportions* of the total population.

$$
\begin{array}{c c c c c}
 & & \multicolumn{2}{c}{\text{Disease}} & \\
 & & + & - & \\
\text{Factor} & + & P_1 & P_3 & P_1 + P_3 \\
 & - & P_2 & P_4 & P_2 + P_4 \\
\hline
 & & P_1 + P_2 & P_3 + P_4 & 1
\end{array}
\tag{16.3}
$$

If these proportions were known, the association (if any) between the factor and the disease could be measured by the ratio of the risks of being disease-positive for those with and those without the factor.

$$
\begin{aligned}
\text{Risk ratio} &= \frac{P_1}{(P_1 + P_3)} \div \frac{P_2}{(P_2 + P_4)} \\
 &= \frac{P_1(P_2 + P_4)}{P_2(P_1 + P_3)}.
\end{aligned}
\tag{16.4}
$$

Where the cases are incident cases the risk ratio is the relative risk.

Now, in many (although not all) situations in which aetiological studies are done, the proportion of subjects classified as disease-positive will be small. That is, P_1 will be small in comparison with P_3, and P_2 will be small in comparison with P_4. In such a case, (16.4) will be very nearly equal to

$$
\frac{P_1 P_4}{P_2 P_3} \, (= \psi, \text{say}).
\tag{16.5}
$$

The ratio (16.5) is properly called the *odds ratio* (because it is the ratio of P_1/P_3 to P_2/P_4, and these two quantities can be thought of as odds in favour of having the disease), but it is often referred to as *approximate relative risk* (because of the approximation referred to above) or simply as *relative risk*. Another term is *cross-ratio* (because the two products $P_1 P_4$ and $P_2 P_3$ which appear in (16.5) are obtained by multiplying diagonally across the table).

The odds ratio (16.5) could be estimated from a random sample of the population, or from a sample stratified by the two levels of the factor (such as a prospective cohort study started some time before the disease assessments are made). It could also be estimated from a sample stratified by the two disease states (i.e. from a case–control study), and it is this fact which makes it such a useful measure of relative risk. Suppose a case–control study is carried out by selecting separate random samples of diseased and non-diseased individuals, and that the *frequencies* (not proportions) are as follows, using the notation of §4.8:

		Disease		
		+ (Cases)	− (Controls)	
Factor	+	a	c	$a + c$
	−	b	d	$b + d$
		$a + b$	$c + d$	n

(16.6)

Frequently, of course, the sampling plan will lead to equal numbers of cases and controls; then $a + b = c + d = \frac{1}{2}n$. Now, a/b can be regarded as a reasonable estimate of P_1/P_2, and c/d similarly estimates P_3/P_4. The observed odds ratio

$$\hat{\psi} = \frac{ad}{bc} \qquad (16.7)$$

is the ratio of a/b to c/d, and therefore can be taken as an estimate of

$$\frac{P_1}{P_2} \div \frac{P_3}{P_4} = \frac{P_1 P_4}{P_2 P_3} (= \psi),$$

the population odds ratio or approximate relative risk defined by (16.5).

The assumption that the case and control groups are random samples from the same relevant population group is difficult to satisfy in case–control studies. Nevertheless, the estimates of relative risk derived from case–control studies often agree quite well with those obtained from corroborative cohort studies, and the theory seems likely to be useful as a rough guide. In retrospective studies cases are often matched with control individuals for various factors; the effect of this matching is discussed below.

Equation (16.7) is identical to (4.18) and the sampling variation of an odds ratio is best considered on the logarithmic scale as in (4.19) so that, approximately,

$$\text{var}(\ln \hat{\psi}) = \frac{1}{a} + \frac{1}{b} + \frac{1}{c} + \frac{1}{d}. \qquad (16.8)$$

Approximate limits, known as the *logit limits*, can be obtained as in Example 4.12. If any of the cell frequencies are small, more complex methods, as discussed in §4.9, must be used. Apart from exact limits (Baptista and Pike, 1977), the limits due to Cornfield (1956) are the most satisfactory. The 95% limits are the two values of ψ for which the observed value of a has a one-sided P value of 0.025. That is, the limits are the solutions of

$$\frac{a - A(\psi)}{\sqrt{[\text{var}(a; \psi)]}} = \pm 1.96, \tag{16.9}$$

where $A(\psi)$ is the value of a which in (16.6), with the observed marginal totals, would give an odds ratio of ψ, and $\text{var}(a; \psi)$ is the variance of a for that value of ψ. That is,

$$\frac{A(d - a + A)}{(a + b - A)(a + c - A)} = \psi \tag{16.10}$$

and

$$\text{var}(a; \psi) = \left(\frac{1}{A} + \frac{1}{a + c - A} + \frac{1}{a + b - A} + \frac{1}{d - a + A} \right)^{-1}. \tag{16.11}$$

It is tedious to solve (16.9) but the calculation can readily be set up as a spreadsheet calculation and solved quickly by trial and error. Using a value for A, ψ is obtained from (16.10) and $\text{var}(a; \psi)$ from (16.11). These are then substituted in the left-hand side of (16.9). The aim is to choose values of A so that (16.9) gives ± 1.96. This is achieved by trying different values and iterating.

Example 16.1

In a case–control study of women with breast cancer (Ellery *et al.*, 1986) the data on whether oral contraceptives were used before first full-term pregnancy were:

		Cases	Controls	
	Yes	4	11	15
OC before FFTP				
	No	63	107	170
		67	118	185

Proceeding as in Example 4.12 the estimated odds ratio is 0·62 with 95% logit limits of 0·19 and 2·02. The upper Cornfield limit is for $A = 7·62$. Substituting this value in (16.10) gives $\psi_U = 1·92$, $\text{var}(a; \psi = 1·92) = 3·417$ and evaluating (16.9) gives $-1·96$. The lower limit was found for $A = 1·66$, giving $\psi_L = 0·20$. Therefore the Cornfield limits are 0·20 and 1·92.

Frequently an estimate of relative risk is made from each of a number of subsets of the data, and there is some interest in the comparison and combination of these different estimates. There may, for example, be several studies of the same aetiological problem done at different times and places; or, in any one study, the data may have been subdivided into one or more categories such as age groups, which affect the relative proportions in the rows of the 2×2 table or in the columns or in both rows and columns. One approach, illustrated in Example 16.2 below, is to take the separate estimates of $\ln \hat{\psi}$ and weight them by the reciprocal of the sampling variance (16.8). The estimates can then be combined by taking a weighted mean, and they can be tested for heterogeneity by a χ^2 index like (7.15) (Woolf, 1955). This method breaks down when the subsets contain few subjects and therefore becomes unsuitable with increasing stratification of a data set. Although in these circumstances the method may be improved by adding $\frac{1}{2}$ to each observed frequency, it is preferable to use an alternative method of combination due to Mantel and Haenszel (1959). For many situations this method gives similar results to the method of Woolf but the Mantel–Haenszel method is more robust when some of the strata contain small frequencies; in particular, it may still be used without modification when some of the frequencies are zero. The method was introduced in §12.6 as a significance test. We now give further details from the viewpoint of estimation. Denote the frequencies in the 2×2 table for the ith subdivision by the notation of (16.6) with subscript i. The Mantel–Haenszel pooled estimate of ψ is then

$$R_{MH} = \frac{\sum (a_i d_i / n_i)}{\sum (b_i c_i / n_i)}. \tag{16.12}$$

Mantel and Haenszel gave a significance test of the hypothesis that $\psi = 1$. If there were no association between the factor and the disease, the expected value and the variance of a_i would, as in (12.17) and (14.12), be given by

$$E(a_i) = \frac{(a_i + b_i)(a_i + c_i)}{n_i},$$

$$\text{var}(a_i) = \frac{(a_i + b_i)(c_i + d_i)(a_i + c_i)(b_i + d_i)}{n_i^2(n_i - 1)}.$$

The test is calculated by adding the differences between the observed and expected values of a_i over the subsets. Since these subsets are independent, the variance of the sum of differences is equal to the sum of the separate variances. This gives as a test static

$$X_{MH}^2 = \frac{\left[\sum a_i - \sum E(a_i)\right]^2}{\sum \text{var}(a_i)}, \tag{16.13}$$

which is approximately a $\chi_{(1)}^2$ (see (12.19)). If desired, a continuity correction may be included.

A number of options are now available for estimating the variance of R_{MH}, and hence constructing confidence limits. First, using the method proposed by Miettinen (1976), *test-based* confidence limits may be constructed. If the standard error of $\ln R_{MH}$ were known, then, under normal theory, a test statistic of the hypothesis $\psi = 1 (\ln \psi = 0)$ would be

$$z = \ln R_{MH}/\mathrm{SE}(\ln R_{MH}),$$

taken as an approximate standardized normal deviate. The test statistic X^2_{MH} is approximately a $\chi^2_{(1)}$ and taking the square root gives an approximate standardized normal deviate (§3.4). The test-based method consists of equating these two test statistics to give an estimate of $\mathrm{SE}(\ln R_{MH})$. That is,

$$\mathrm{SE}(\ln R_{MH}) = (\ln R_{MH})/X_{MH}. \tag{16.14}$$

This method is strictly only valid if $\psi = 1$, but in practice gives reasonable results provided R_{MH} is not extreme (see Breslow and Day (1980, §4.3), who recommend using X_{MH} calculated without the continuity correction for this purpose). Unfortunately, the method breaks down if $R_{MH} = 1$. The calculations are illustrated in Example 16.2.

Another method was given by Breslow and Liang (1982), amending an earlier result of Hauck (1979), but this method is not suitable for the case when a large data set is subdivided into many strata, some containing small frequencies. The method proposed by Robins *et al.* (1986) is satisfactory for the above case, as well as when there are only a few strata, none containing small frequencies. Using their notation,

$$P_i = (a_i + d_i)/n_i, \quad Q_i = (b_i + c_i)/n_i,$$
$$R_i = a_i d_i/n_i, \quad S_i = b_i c_i/n_i, \quad R_+ = \sum R_i$$

and

$$S_+ = \sum S_i \text{ (so that } R_{MH} = R_+/S_+);$$

then

$$\mathrm{var}(\ln R_{MH}) = \frac{\sum P_i R_i}{2R_+^2} + \frac{\sum (P_i S_i + Q_i R_i)}{2R_+ S_+} + \frac{\sum Q_i S_i}{2S_+^2}. \tag{16.15}$$

Breslow and Day (1980, §4.4) set out a method for testing the homogeneity of the odds ratio over the strata. However, like the method of Woolf discussed above, the method breaks down with increasing stratification.

A special case of subdivision occurs in case–control studies, in which each case is matched with a control subject for certain important factors, such as age, sex, residence, etc. Strictly, each pair of matched subjects should form a subdivision for the calculation of relative risk, although of course the individual estimates from such pairs would be valueless. The Mantel–Haenszel pooled estimate (16.12) can, however, be calculated, and takes a particularly simple form. Suppose there are altogether $\frac{1}{2}n$ matched pairs. These can be entered into a 2×2 table according as the two individuals are factor-positive or factor-negative, with frequencies as follows:

		Control		
		Factor +	Factor −	
Case	Factor +	t	r	a
	Factor −	s	u	b
		c	d	$\frac{1}{2}n$

$$(16.16)$$

The marginal totals in (16.16) are the cell frequencies in the earlier table (16.6). The Mantel–Haenszel estimate is then

$$R = \frac{r}{s}. \tag{16.17}$$

This can be shown to be a particularly satisfactory estimate if the true relative risk, as measured by the cross-ratio of the probabilities (16.5), is the same for every pair. The Mantel–Haenszel test statistic is identical to that of McNemar's test (4.11).

Inferences are made by treating r as a binomial variable with sample size $r + s$. The methods of §4.7 may then be applied and the confidence limits of the relative risk, ψ_L and ψ_U, obtained from those of the binomial parameter π, using the relation

$$\psi = \frac{\pi}{1 - \pi}.$$

Liddell (1983) showed that the limits given by (4.10) simplify after the above transformation to give

$$\left. \begin{array}{l} \psi_L = \dfrac{r}{(s + 1)F_{0.025,\, 2(s+1),\, 2r}}, \\[2ex] \psi_U = \dfrac{(r + 1)F_{0.025,\, 2(r+1),\, 2s}}{s}, \end{array} \right\} \tag{16.18}$$

and that an exact test of $\psi = 1$ is given by

$$F = \frac{r}{s + 1}, \tag{16.19}$$

tested against the F distribution with $2(s + 1)$ and $2r$ degrees of freedom (in this formulation, if $r < s$, r and s should be interchanged). This exact test may be used instead of the approximate McNemar's test (§4.8).

A general point is that the logarithm of ψ is, from (16.5),

$$\ln(P_1/P_3) - \ln(P_2/P_4)$$

$$= \text{logit (probability of disease when factor } +)$$
$$- \text{logit (probability of disease when factor } -).$$

The methods of analysis suggested in this section can thus be seen to be particularly appropriate if the effect of changing from factor + to factor − is to change the probability of being in the diseased state by a constant amount *on the logit scale*. It has been indicated in §12.8 that this is a reasonable general approach to a wide range of problems, but in any particular instance it may be far from true. The investigator should therefore guard against too ready an assumption that a relative risk calculated in one study is necessarily applicable under somewhat different circumstances.

Example 16.2 uses the above methods to combine a number of studies into a summary analysis. It may be regarded as a simple example of meta-analysis (§7.2).

Example 16.2

Table 16.1 summarizes results from 10 retrospective surveys in which patients with lung cancer and control subjects were classified as smokers or non-smokers. In most or all of these surveys cases and controls would have been matched, but the original data are usually not presented in sufficient detail to enable relative risks to be estimated from (16.17) and matching is ignored in the present analysis. (The effect of ignoring matching when it is present is, if anything, to underestimate the departure of the relative risk from unity.) The data were compiled by Cornfield (1956) and have been referred to also by Gart (1962).

Defining w_i as the reciprocal of $\text{var}(\ln \hat{\psi}_i)$ from (16.8), the weighted mean is

$$\frac{\sum w_i \ln \hat{\psi}_i}{\sum w_i} = \frac{161 \cdot 36}{105 \cdot 4} = 1 \cdot 531,$$

and the pooled estimate of ψ is $\exp(1 \cdot 531) = 4 \cdot 62$.

For the heterogeneity test, the $\chi^2_{(9)}$ statistic is

$$\sum w_i (\ln \hat{\psi}_i)^2 - \frac{(\sum w_i \ln \hat{\psi}_i)^2}{\sum w_i} = 253 \cdot 678 - 247 \cdot 061 = 6 \cdot 62 \quad (P = 0 \cdot 68).$$

There is evidently no strong evidence of heterogeneity between separate estimates. It is, of course, likely that the relative risk varies to some extent from study to study, particularly as the factor 'smoking' covers such a wide range of activity. However, the sampling variation of the separate estimates is evidently too large to enable such real variation to emerge. If we assume that all the variation is due to sampling error, the variance of the weighted mean of

Table 16.1 Combination of relative risks from 10 retrospective surveys on smoking and lung cancer (Cornfield, 1956; Gart, 1962)

| Study number | Lung cancer patients | | Control patients | | Woolf's method | | | | | Mantel–Haenszel | | | | |
	Smokers a_i	Non-smokers b_i	Smokers c_i	Non-smokers d_i	$\hat{\psi}_i$	$\ln\hat{\psi}_i$	(1) $1/a_i + 1/b_i + 1/c_i + 1/d_i$	$w_i = \dfrac{1}{(1)}$	$w_i \ln\hat{\psi}_i$	n_i	$a_i d_i/n_i$	$b_i c_i/n_i$	$E(a_i)$	$\text{var}(a_i)$
1	83	3	72	14	5·38	1·683	0·4307	2·3	3·87	172	6·756	1·256	77·50	3·85
2	90	3	227	43	5·68	1·737	0·3721	2·7	4·69	363	10·661	1·876	81·21	7·68
3	129	7	81	19	4·32	1·463	0·2156	4·6	6·73	236	10·386	2·403	121·02	5·67
4	412	32	299	131	5·64	1·730	0·0447	22·4	38·75	874	61·753	10·947	361·19	33·18
5	1350	7	1296	61	9·08	2·206	0·1608	6·2	13·68	2714	30·343	3·343	1323·00	16·58
6	60	3	106	27	5·09	1·627	0·3965	2·5	4·07	196	8·265	1·622	53·36	5·57
7	459	18	534	81	3·87	1·353	0·0720	13·9	18·81	1092	34·047	8·802	433·76	22·17
8	499	19	462	56	3·18	1·157	0·0747	13·4	15·50	1036	26·973	8·473	480·50	17·41
9	451	39	1729	636	4·25	1·447	0·0300	33·3	48·19	2855	100·468	23·619	374·15	73·30
10	260	5	259	28	5·62	1·726	0·2434	4·1	7·08	522	13·188	2·346	249·16	7·76
Total	3793	136	5065	1096				105·4	161·37		302·840	64·687	3554·85	193·17

$\ln \hat{\psi}_i$ can be obtained as

$$\frac{1}{\sum w_i} = 0.00949.$$

Approximate 95% confidence limits for $\ln \psi$ are

$$1.531 \pm (1.96) \sqrt{0.00949} = 1.340 \text{ and } 1.722.$$

The corresponding limits for ψ are obtained by exponentials as 3.82 and 5.60.
   The Mantel–Haenszel estimate of ψ is

$$R_{MH} = \frac{302.840}{64.687} = 4.68.$$

The statistic for testing that this estimate differs from unity is

$$X_{MH}^2 = (3793 - 3554.85)^2/193.17$$

$$= 293.60 \quad (P < 0.001).$$

The test-based method of calculating confidence limits from (16.14) gives

$$SE(\ln R_{MH}) = \ln(4.68)/\sqrt{293.60}$$

$$= 1.543/17.13$$

$$= 0.0901,$$

and approximate 95% confidence limits for $\ln \psi$ are

$$1.543 \pm 1.96 \times 0.0901$$

$$= 1.366 \text{ and } 1.720.$$

The corresponding limits for ψ are the exponentials, 3.92 and 5.58. The point estimate and the confidence limits are very similar indeed to those derived using Woolf's method. Details of the calculation are not given here but (16.15) gives $SE(\ln R_{MH}) = 0.0977$ to give 95% confidence limits of 3.86 and 5.67, similar to both sets of limits derived earlier.

   Another frequently occurring situation is when the factor, instead of having just two levels, presence or absence, has three or more levels that have a definite order. For example, instead of classifying people as non-smokers or smokers, the smokers could be divided further according to the amount smoked. Such a situation was discussed in §12.7. Mantel (1963) has extended the Mantel–Haenszel procedure to provide a test for trend and to combine a number of subsets of the data (12.20). An example of the method is given in Example 12.8.
   The methods discussed above are powerful in the commonly occurring situation where it is required to analyse the association between a disease and a single exposure factor, making allowance for one, or at most a few, other factors, and where the effect of the other factors may be adequately represented by subdivision of the data into strata. The methods are inconvenient where several exposure factors are of interest and for each factor allowance must be made for the others,

as was the case in Example 12.9. Also, where several factors are to be adjusted for, stratification would involve a large number of strata; in the limit each stratum would contain only one subject, so that comparisons within strata would be impossible. In these cases more general methods must be used and the generalized linear models (§12.8) are appropriate. It was observed above that the odds ratio can be estimated from a case–control study and that the logarithm of the odds ratio is a difference of logits. These two features combine to make the method of logistic regression applicable to data from a case–control study. All the coefficients of (12.25) may be estimated except for the constant term α, which is distorted by the investigator's choice of the size of the case and control groups. The estimate of a regression coefficient measures the logarithm of the odds ratio for a change of unity in the corresponding variable, and so the exponentials of the regression coefficients give estimated odds ratios or approximate relative risks.

It was observed above that, for a case–control study where a matched control is chosen for each case, the Mantel–Haenszel method may be applied, and leads to McNemar's test. When the number of cases available is limited, the precision of a study may be increased, to some extent, by choosing more than one matched control per case. The Mantel–Haenszel method can be applied, treating each set of a case and its controls as a subset. The analysis may be simplified by grouping together sets providing identical information; for example, with three controls per case those sets where the case and just two of the three controls are positive for the exposure factor all provide identical information. This is an extension of (16.16). For further details of the analysis see Pike and Morrow (1970) and Miettinen (1969, 1970).

In a matched case–control study there may be covariates recorded on each individual and it may be necessary to take account of the possible influence of the covariates on the probability of disease. The covariates may be included in a logistic regression model but account also has to be taken of the matching. This is done by working conditionally within each set. Suppose that x represents the set of covariates, including the exposure factor of principal interest, and use a subscript of zero for the case and 1 to c for the c controls. Then, using the logistic regression model (12.25) and assuming that the probability of disease is small, so that the logit is approximately equal to the logarithm of the probability of disease, the probability of disease of each member of the set is $\exp(\alpha_s + \boldsymbol{\beta}\boldsymbol{x}_i)$, $i = 0, 1, \ldots, c$. The parameter α has a subscript s to indicate that it depends on the particular set. Now each set has been chosen to include exactly one case of disease. Arguing conditionally that there is just one individual with disease in the set, the probability that it is the observed case is

$$\exp(\alpha_s + \boldsymbol{\beta}\boldsymbol{x}_0)/\sum \exp(\alpha_s + \boldsymbol{\beta}\boldsymbol{x}_i),$$

where summation is over all members of the set, $i = 0, 1, \ldots, c$. The numerator and denominator contain the common factor $\exp(\alpha_s)$ and so the probability may be expressed as

$$\exp(\boldsymbol{\beta x}_0)/\sum \exp(\boldsymbol{\beta x}_i), \qquad (16.20)$$

a result first given by Thomas in Liddell *et al.* (1977). An expression of the form of (16.20) is obtained for each case and combined to form a likelihood; then β is estimated by the method of maximum likelihood (§12.8). By working conditionally within sets the large number of parameters α_s (one per case) have been eliminated. This exposition has been relatively brief and readers interested in further details of the analysis of case–control studies are referred to the monographs by Breslow and Day (1980) and Schlesselman (1982).

In §14.6 it was observed that the logrank test for analysing survival data was similar to the Mantel–Haenszel test. Comparing (16.20) with (14.22) shows that the method of logistic regression in a matched case–control study is similar to the proportional-hazards model for survival analysis. A case–control study may be considered as a sample from a hypothetical cohort study; indeed, for validity it should be just that. It is, therefore, no coincidence that methods originally derived for the analysis of cohort studies should also be applicable to case–control studies. An analysis based on (16.20) can be carried out using PROC PHREG in the SAS program, with each case–control set defining a stratum.

16.3 Attributable risk

The full implications of an excess risk depend not only on the size of the relative risk but also on the proportion of the population positive for the aetiological factor. A moderate relative risk applicable to a high proportion of the population would produce more cases of disease than a high relative risk applicable to just a small proportion of the population. A measure of association, due to Levin (1953), that takes account of the proportion of the population at risk is the *attributable risk*. Terminology is not completely standard and other names for this measure are *aetiological fraction, population attributable risk* and *attributable fraction*. The attributable risk is defined as the proportion of cases in the total population that are attributable to the risk factor. It is usually calculated in circumstances in which it is considered justifiable to infer causation from an observed association. Then it may be interpreted as the proportion of cases in the population that are due to the factor, and hence as a measure of the importance of eliminating the factor as part of a disease-prevention strategy.

Suppose I_p is the incidence of the disease in the population and, as earlier, I_E and I_{NE} are the incidences in the exposed and non-exposed respectively. Then the excess incidence attributable to the factor is $I_p - I_{NE}$ and dividing by the population incidence gives the attributable risk,

$$\lambda = \frac{I_p - I_{NE}}{I_p}. \qquad (16.21)$$

Now suppose a proportion θ_E of the population are exposed to the factor, then

$$I_p = \theta_E I_E + (1 - \theta_E) I_{NE}$$
$$= \theta_E \phi I_{NE} + (1 - \theta_E) I_{NE}$$
$$= I_{NE}[1 + \theta_E(\phi - 1)], \tag{16.22}$$

where ϕ is the relative risk and the second line is obtained using (16.2). Substituting in (16.21) gives

$$\lambda = \frac{\theta_E(\phi - 1)}{1 + \theta_E(\phi - 1)}, \tag{16.23}$$

and the attributable risk can be estimated from the relative risk and the proportion of the population exposed. Often the attributable proportion is multiplied by 100 to give a result in percentage terms and this gives rise to the terms *attributable risk per cent* and *population attributable risk per cent*.

An alternative expression may be derived using the notation of (16.3). If the probability of disease in those positive for the factor were the same as for those negative, then the proportion of the population positive for both factor and disease would be

$$(P_1 + P_3) \times \frac{P_2}{P_2 + P_4}.$$

Subtracting this from the actual proportion, P_1, gives the excess proportion related to the factor, and, dividing by the proportion with disease, the attributable risk is given by

$$\lambda = \left[P_1 - \frac{P_2(P_1 + P_3)}{P_2 + P_4} \right] \div (P_1 + P_2)$$
$$= \frac{P_1}{P_1 + P_2} \left[1 - \frac{P_2(P_1 + P_3)}{P_1(P_2 + P_4)} \right]$$
$$= \frac{P_1}{P_1 + P_2} \left(1 - \frac{I_{NE}}{I_E} \right)$$
$$= \theta_1 \frac{\phi - 1}{\phi}, \tag{16.24}$$

where θ_1 is the proportion of cases exposed to the factor.

It follows from (16.23) that the attributable risk can be estimated from any study that provides estimates both of relative risk and the proportion of the population exposed to the factor. Thus, it may be estimated from a case–control study since the relative risk can be estimated approximately and the proportion of the population exposed can be estimated from the controls (again assuming that the disease is rare). Alternatively, (16.24) could be used, since θ_1 can be estimated in a case–control study. Clearly, attributable risk may be estimated from a cohort study of a random sample of the total population, but only from a sample stratified by the two levels of exposure if the proportion of the population exposed is known.

The attributable risk may be defined specifically for the exposed group as the proportion of exposed cases attributable to the factor. This measure is

$$\frac{I_E - I_{NE}}{I_E} = \frac{\phi - 1}{\phi}.$$

This measure is properly called the *attributable risk among the exposed*, but because of the possibility of confusion with the attributable risk in the population as a whole it is preferable to specify that the attributable risk defined by (16.23) and (16.24) is the *population* attributable risk.

The above formulation has been in terms of a factor which increases risk, i.e. relative risk greater than unity. For a factor which is protective, i.e. relative risk less than unity, a slightly different formulation is necessary; this is discussed by Kleinbaum *et al.* (1982; Chapter 9).

We now consider the sampling variation of an estimate of population attributable risk from a case–control study, and give an example.

Consider data of the form (16.6) from a case–control study. Since $a/(a + b)$ estimates $P_1/(P_1 + P_2)$ or θ_1, and ad/bc estimates ψ, which is approximately ϕ, substitution in (16.24) gives as an estimate of λ

$$\hat{\lambda} = \frac{a}{a + b}\left(1 - \frac{bc}{ad}\right)$$

$$= \frac{ad - bc}{d(a + b)}. \qquad (16.25)$$

It is convenient to work with $\ln(1 - \hat{\lambda})$ since, as Walter (1975) showed, this variable is approximately normally distributed.

$$1 - \hat{\lambda} = \frac{bd + bc}{d(a + b)}$$

$$= \frac{b}{a + b}\bigg/\frac{d}{c + d}$$

$$= \frac{1 - \hat{\theta}_1}{1 - \hat{\theta}_2}$$

and

$$\ln(1 - \hat{\lambda}) = \ln(1 - \hat{\theta}_1) - \ln(1 - \hat{\theta}_2),$$

where $\hat{\theta}_1$ is an estimator of $P_1/(P_1 + P_2)$ and $\hat{\theta}_2$ of $P_3/(P_3 + P_4)$. $\hat{\theta}_1$ and $\hat{\theta}_2$ are independent estimators of proportions, so using (3.4) and (3.17) we obtain

$$\text{var}[\ln(1 - \hat{\lambda})] = \frac{a}{b(a + b)} + \frac{c}{d(c + d)}. \tag{16.26}$$

Example 16.3

Consider the data from study 1 of Table 16.1 in which 83 out of 86 lung cancer patients were smokers compared with 72 out of 86 controls. Then using (16.25) and (16.26),

$$\hat{\lambda} = \frac{83 \times 14 - 3 \times 72}{14 \times 86}$$

$$= 0.7857,$$

$$\ln(1 - \hat{\lambda}) = -1.540,$$

$$\text{var}[\ln(1 - \hat{\lambda})] = \frac{83}{3 \times 86} + \frac{72}{14 \times 86}$$

$$= 0.3815.$$

Therefore approximate 95% limits for $\ln(1 - \hat{\lambda})$ are

$$-1.540 \pm (1.96)\sqrt{0.3815}$$

$$= -2.751 \text{ and } -0.329.$$

The corresponding limits for $\hat{\lambda}$ are 0.281 and 0.936.

Whittemore (1983) extended Levin's measure to account for confounding variables. Where the confounders are accounted for by a stratified analysis, then the relative risk is often estimated using the Mantel–Haenszel approach, and this method can be used to estimate the attributable risk using (16.24). Kuritz and Landis (1988) used this approach for a matched case–control study and proposed a method of calculating the confidence interval. Greenland (1987) gave variance estimators for the attributable risk based on the sampling variability of R_{MH} (16.15); these estimators are satisfactory for both large strata and sparse data, that is, data divided into a large number of strata with small numbers within each stratum.

16.4 Diagnostic tests and screening procedures

In epidemiological studies much use is made of diagnostic tests, based either on clinical observations or on laboratory techniques, by means of which individuals are classified as healthy or as falling into one of a number of disease categories. Such tests are, of course, important throughout the whole of medicine, and in particular form the basis of screening programmes for the early diagnosis of disease. Most such tests are imperfect instruments, in the sense that healthy individuals will occasionally be classified wrongly as being ill, while some individuals who are really ill may fail to be detected. How should we measure the ability of a particular diagnostic test to give the correct diagnosis both for healthy and for ill subjects?

The reliability of diagnostic tests

Suppose that each individual in a large population can be classified as truly positive or negative for a particular diagnosis. This true diagnosis may be based on more refined methods than are used in the test; or it may be based on evidence which emerges after the passage of time, for instance at autopsy. For each class of individual, true positive and true negative, we can consider the probabilities that the test gives a positive or negative verdict, as in the table below.

		Test		
		$+$	$-$	Total
True	$+$	$1 - \beta$	β	1
	$-$	α	$1 - \alpha$	1

$$(16.27)$$

An individual in the top right corner of this 2×2 table is called a *false negative*; β is the probability of a false negative, and $1 - \beta$ is called the *sensitivity* of the test. Those in the lower left corner are called *false positives*; α is the probability of a false positive, and $1 - \alpha$ is the *specificity* of the test. There is an analogy here with significance tests. If the null hypothesis is that an individual is a true negative, and a positive test result is regarded as 'significant', then α is analogous to the significance level and $1 - \beta$ is analogous to the power of detecting the alternative hypothesis that the individual is a true positive (p. 197).

Clearly it is desirable that a test should have small values of α and β, although other considerations such as cost and ease of application are highly relevant. Other things being equal, if test A has smaller values of both α and β than test B it can be regarded as a better test. Suppose, though, that A has a smaller value of α but a larger value of β. Unless some relative weight can be attached to the two forms of error—false positives and false negatives—no clear judgement is possible. If the two errors are judged to be of approximately equal importance, a natural method of combination is by the sum of two error probabilities, $\alpha + \beta$. Youden (1950) proposed an essentially equivalent index,

$$J = 1 - (\alpha + \beta). \tag{16.28}$$

If the test has no diagnostic value, $\alpha = 1 - \beta$ and $J = 0$. If the test is invariably correct, $\alpha = \beta = 0$ and $J = 1$. Values of J between -1 and 0 could arise if the test result were negatively associated with the true diagnosis, but this situation is unlikely to arise in practice.

The use of Youden's index implicitly assumes that the sensitivity and specificity have equal importance, since α and β are given equal weight in (16.28). There may be good reasons against this view. First, the two types of error will have very different consequences, and it will often be reasonable to attach much more weight to a false negative than a false positive; this consideration would suggest giving more weight to β than to α, and would lead to the choice of a procedure with a relatively small value of β/α. On the other hand, if the disease is rare, the false negatives will be numerically few, and the number of individuals wrongly diagnosed would be minimized by choosing $\beta > \alpha$. These two considerations clearly conflict, and a resolution must be achieved in the light of the consequences of diagnostic errors for the disease in question.

The discussion so far has been in terms of probabilities. In practice these could be estimated from surveys. Suppose a special survey of a random sample of the population gave the following frequencies:

$$
\begin{array}{ccccc}
 & & & \text{Test} & \\
 & & + & - & \\
 & + & a & b & \qquad(16.29) \\
\text{True} & & & & \\
 & - & c & d &
\end{array}
$$

The probability of a false negative would be estimated by $\hat{\beta} = b/(a + b)$; the probability of a false positive by $\hat{\alpha} = c/(c + d)$. Youden's index J would be estimated by $\hat{J} = 1 - (\hat{\alpha} + \hat{\beta})$. The sampling errors of these estimates follow from standard binomial expressions.

An important point to note is that the expected proportions of misdiagnoses amongst the *apparent* positives and negatives depend not only on α and β but on the true prevalence of the disease. This may be seen from the following two sets of frequencies. In each case the sensitivity and specificity are both 0.9.

Case (a)

		Test			
		+	−		
	+	450	50	500	
True					
	−	50	450	500	
		500	500	1000	

Case (b)

		Test			
		+	−		
	+	90	10	100	
True					
	−	90	810	900	
		180	820	1000	

(16.30)

Proportion of
true +ves   0·90   0·10   0·50   0·01

The proportion of true positives amongst the apparent positives is sometimes called the *predictive value of a positive test*; the proportion of true negatives amongst the apparent negatives is the *predictive value of a negative test*. In case (a), the true prevalence is $500/1000 = 0.5$; the predictive value of a positive test is high (0.9). In case (b), however, where the true prevalence is $100/1000 = 0.1$, the same predictive value is only 0.5. The predictive values are conditional probabilities of the test results and may be calculated using Bayes' theorem (§2.8) with the prevalences of disease and non-disease as the prior probabilities, and the likelihoods of the test results obtained from the sensitivity and specificity.

Case (b) illustrates the position in many presymptomatic screening procedures where the true prevalence is low. Of the subjects found positive by the screening test a rather high proportion may be false positives. To avoid this situation the test may sometimes be modified to reduce α, but such a step often results in an increased value of β and hence a reduced value of $1 - \beta$; the number of false positives amongst the apparent positives will have reduced, but so will the number of true positives detected.

The sort of modification referred to in the last sentence is particularly relevant when the test, although dichotomous, is based on a continuous measurement. Examples are the diagnosis of diabetes by blood-sugar level, or of glaucoma by intraocular pressure. Any change in the critical level of the measurement will affect α and β. One very simple model for this situation would be to assume that the variable, x, on which the test is based is normally distributed with the same variance σ^2 for the normal and diseased populations, but with different means, μ_N and μ_D (Fig. 16.1). For any given α, the value of β depends solely on the standardized distance between the means,

$$\Delta = \frac{\mu_D - \mu_N}{\sigma}.$$

If the critical value for the test is the midpoint between the means, $\frac{1}{2}(\mu_N + \mu_D)$, α and β will both be equal to the single-tail area of the normal distribution beyond a standardized deviate of $\frac{1}{2}\Delta$. To compare the merits of different tests one could, therefore, compare their values of Δ; tests with high values of Δ will differentiate between normal and diseased groups better than those with low values. There is a clear analogy here with the generalized distance as a measure of the effectiveness of a discriminant function (p. 360); the discrimination is performed here by the single variable x.

Instead of an all-or-none classification as healthy or diseased, it may sometimes be useful to express the strength of the evidence for any individual falling into each of the two groups. For the model described above, the logarithm of the likelihood ratio is linearly related to x, as shown in the lower part of Fig. 16.1. (This is a particular case of the more general result for discriminant functions referred to on p. 361.) The likelihood ratio may, from Bayes' theorem (§2.8), be

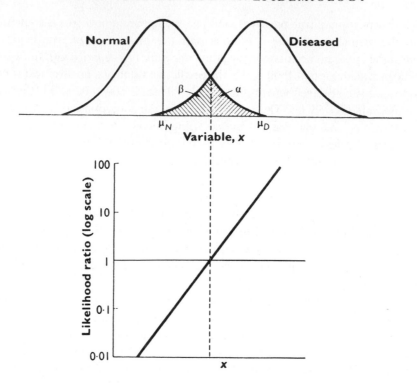

Fig. 16.1 The performance of a diagnostic test based on a normally distributed variable when the normal and diseased groups differ in the mean but have the same variance. The lower diagram shows on a log scale the ratio of the likelihood that an observation comes from the diseased group to that of its coming from the normal group.

combined with the ratio of prior probabilities to give the ratio of posterior probabilities. Suppose, for example, that a particular value of x corresponds to a likelihood ratio of 10, and that the prior probability of a diseased individual (i.e. the population prevalence) is 0·01. The posterior odds that the individual is diseased are then

$$\frac{10}{1} \times \frac{0·01}{0·99} = 0·10 \text{ to } 1.$$

It is thus much more likely that the individual is healthy than that he or she is diseased; as in case (b) of (16.30) where the prevalence was low, a high proportion of apparent positives are in fact false positives.

　　The assumptions underlying the above discussion are unlikely to be closely fulfilled in practice. Distributions may be non-normal and have different variances; there may be various categories of disease, each with a different distribution of x. Nevertheless, the concepts introduced here usually provide a good basis

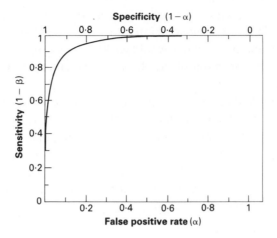

Fig. 16.2 Receiver operating characteristic curve corresponding to Fig. 16.1.

for discussing the performance of a diagnostic test. For further discussion see Greenhouse and Mantel (1950).

Another way of expressing the situation shown in Fig. 16.1 is the *receiver operating characteristic (ROC) curve*. This is a line diagram with the sensitivity, $1 - \beta$, plotted vertically and the false positive rate, α, on the horizontal axis. The horizontal axis may also be shown by a reversed scale of the specificity, $1 - \alpha$. The ROC curve is constructed by finding the sensitivity and specificity for a range of values of x. Figure 16.2 shows the ROC curve corresponding to Fig. 16.1. The possible combinations of sensitivity and specificity that may be chosen by varying the critical values of the test may be read off the curve. Tests with the ROC curves furthest into the top left corner are the better tests.

Misclassification errors are not restricted to the classification of disease. In a retrospective case–control study, for example, the disease classification is likely to be based on highly accurate diagnostic methods, but the factor classification often depends on personal recollection and will not, therefore, be completely accurate. False positives and false negatives can be defined in terms of the factor classification in an obvious way. If the specificity and sensitivity are the same for the disease group as for the control group, the effect is to reduce any measures of association between factor and disease; for instance the relative risk is brought nearer to unity than it would be if the errors were not present, and the difference between the two proportions of positives is reduced numerically.

If either the specificity or sensitivity (or both) differ between groups, the bias in risk estimate may be in either direction (Diamond and Lilienfeld, 1962a, b; Newell, 1962). A particular danger in a case–control study where classification of the exposure factor depends on recollection and the disease is traumatic is that the cases may be likely to recall events that the controls either might not recall or might dismiss as unimportant; this would lead to an exaggeration of the estimate of risk. For a fuller discussion of the effects of misclassification, see Kleinbaum *et al.* (1982, Chapter 12).

Our discussion of diagnostic tests has been restricted to a comparison of the result of a single test with the true diagnosis. In many situations the true diagnosis cannot conveniently be established in a large survey population but there may be an opportunity to compare a new test against a reference test. Buck and Gart (1966) (also Gart and Buck, 1966) discuss the rather complicated analysis of data of this type. Under certain assumptions about the reference test it may be possible to infer something about the sensitivity and specificity of the new test.

The assessment of screening procedures

The effectiveness of a programme for the early screening of disease depends not only on the reliability of the tests used, but even more on the availability of treatment capable of improving the prognosis for an individual in whom the early stages of disease have been detected.

If the disease is commonly fatal, the primary aim of screening will be to reduce the risk of death or at least to increase survival time. The effectiveness of a screening programme may therefore sometimes be assessed by observing any trend in the cause-specific mortality rate for the community in which the programme is introduced. However, trends in mortality rates occur for various reasons, and cannot unambiguously be attributed to the screening programme. In a few instances it has been possible to carry out randomized trials, in which volunteers are assigned to receive or not to receive screening. After an appropriate follow-up period the mortality experiences of the two groups can be compared.

It is often useful to study the time periods between certain stages in the development of a disease. The following comments indicate briefly some of the basic concepts. Figure 16.3 shows the principal events.

The sojourn time, y, is the period during which the disease is asymptomatic but detectable by screening, and will vary between individuals, with a mean value m. The lead time, x, is of interest because (i) it measures the time gained for potentially effective treatment; and (ii) in comparing duration of survival between screened and unscreened groups, it would be misleading to measure survival from T_3 for the unscreened group but from t for the screened group. The lead time provides a correction for this bias.

The estimation of lead time is somewhat complex (Walter and Day, 1983; Day and Walter, 1984). The following points should be noted, for the situation where there is a single screening.

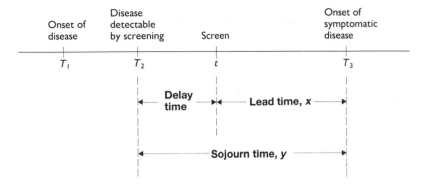

Fig. 16.3 Schematic representation of events in the development of a chronic disease, with a screening procedure during the asymptomatic phase.

1   Lead time is a random variable, partly because y varies between individuals, but also because t can occur at any point between T_2 and T_3 (or indeed outside that range, in which case the disease will be undetected by the screen). If y were constant, the mean lead time, L, for those individuals whose disease was detected by the screen, would be $\frac{1}{2}m$. However, since y varies, the longer sojourn times will be more likely to contain a screening point, and are correspondingly more highly represented in the 'detected' group than in the whole group of cases. (This is an example of 'length-biased sampling'.) A consequence is that $L = \frac{1}{2}[m + (\sigma^2/m)]$, where σ^2 is the variance of y.

2   We shall be interested in the mean lead time for the whole group of cases, including those in whom the disease is not detected. This is called the programme lead time, and is equal to $(1 - \beta)L$, where β is the proportion of false negatives (i.e. cases missed).

3   To estimate m, use may be made of the relation (16.1),

$$P = Im, \tag{16.31}$$

where P is the prevalence of presymptomatic disease (which can be estimated from the results of the screen, allowing for the false negatives), and I is the incidence of symptomatic disease (which might be estimated from a control series).

4   The estimation of σ^2, which is needed for the calculation of L, is more troublesome than that of m, and may require a further assumption about the functional form of the distribution of y.

The discussion so far has been in terms of a single screening occasion. In practice it will be preferable to consider a series of screening occasions, so that each individual who develops the disease at some time has a reasonable chance of being screened whilst the disease is presymptomatic (see Walter and Day, 1983; Day and Walter, 1984).

16.5 Disease clustering

Many epidemiological investigations are concerned with the detection of some form of clustering of cases of a certain disease—clustering in time, in space, or in both time and space. For example, one might enquire whether cases of a certain congenital malformation (which might normally occur at a fairly constant rate in a community) appear with unduly high frequency in certain years. Such a tendency towards clustering in time might indicate aetiological factors, such as maternal virus infections, which were particularly severe in certain years. Again, one might suspect that certain forms of illness are more common amongst people who work or live in certain areas, perhaps because of environmental factors peculiar to these places. The groups in which cases tend to be clustered may be families or households; such familial aggregation might again be caused by environmental factors, but it might be due also to intrafamilial infection or to genetic predisposition to disease. In the study of the possible infectious aetiology of rare diseases such as leukaemia or certain congenital malformations, clustering in either space or time will be less interesting than a space–time association. By this we mean a tendency for those cases which are relatively close together in space also to be relatively close together in time.

Many such problems give rise to quite complicated considerations; it is not possible to explore the subject fully here. This section contains a brief account of some of these considerations. Further details may be obtained from the references.

A general warning should be issued against the overinterpretation of striking instances of clustering. Epidemiological studies are often carried out after some unusual coincidences have been noticed. The degree of clustering may well be 'significant' when taken in isolation, and yet it may nevertheless be a purely random phenomenon. Many other possible opportunities for clustering, in other places or at other times, might have been put under scrutiny; if they had been studied, perhaps nothing remarkable would have been found except in the original instance which caused the enquiry. Our attention may, therefore, have been focused on merely the most extreme of a large number of random fluctuations. Similarly, in any one study there are often many ways of examining the data for possible clusters. To report only that method of analysis that gives the most significant finding is to provide a misleading interpretation of the true situation. The problem is similar to that of multiple comparisons (§7.4), but in the present context the number of possible comparisons is likely to be so large, and so difficult to define, that no satisfactory method of adjustment is available.

Clustering in time

A rather simple approach to many problems of this sort is to divide the time period into equal intervals, to express the incidence rate in each interval as a proportion and to test the significance of differences between these proportions by standard $2 \times k$ contingency table methods. If the population at risk is almost constant and the incidence rate is low, the number of cases appearing in the different intervals will, on the null hypothesis of constant risk, follow a Poisson distribution; the usual heterogeneity test (§7.8) may be used. A test, due to Edwards (1961) that is particularly sensitive to seasonal clustering of cases is described in §10.3 (p. 347).

It may be sensible to concentrate attention on the maximum of the various numbers of cases, on the grounds that occasional clustering may affect only one or two of the time intervals. Ederer *et al.* (1964) describe some methods for doing this.

Clustering in space

Rather similar methods can be applied to detect clustering in space which may result in differences in incidence between different groups of people. It will usually be convenient to subdivide the total population into administrative areas containing quite different numbers of individuals; the Poisson distribution is not then applicable, but contingency table methods can be used.

If the geographical distribution of the population is unknown, it is sometimes useful to carry out a case–control study to show whether the cases are in some sense closer together than a comparable group of controls. Lloyd and Roberts (1973), for example, applied this method to the study of spatial clustering of congenital limb defects in Cardiff. The distribution of differences between all pairs of cases can be compared with that of distances between pairs of controls, to see whether small distances occur more frequently for cases than for controls. Suppose there are n cases and m controls. A *permutation test* may be carried out by computer, by making repeated random selections of n individuals from the total of $m + n$, and counting the number of close pairs, Z, within each set of n. The significance of the *observed* value of Z can then be adjudged by seeing whether it falls in the tails of the distribution of Z formed by the random permutations. Alternatively, the values of $E(Z)$ and $var(Z)$ in the permutation distribution can be calculated by an adaptation of exact formulae derived for Knox's test for space–time clustering described on p. 352 (David and Barton, 1966; Mantel, 1967; Smith and Pike, 1974). Cuzick and Edwards (1990) proposed a test based on the distribution of cases and controls in space. For each case the nearest k neighbours are found and the number of these that are cases forms the basis of a test. The test is carried out for different values of k and the results are combined into an overall test.

The question sometimes arises whether cases of a particular disease occurring within a certain time period tend to cluster near a well-defined location, such as an industrial plant suspected of emitting toxic material. Here, the population could be divided into subgroups according to distance from the focus, and a test performed to show whether the incidence of the disease was particularly high in the subgroup nearest to the focus, or perhaps whether it declined with distance from the focus. If the spatial distribution of the population is unknown, a case–control study may provide evidence as to whether cases within a certain region are more likely to be close to the focus than are a comparable group of controls. Gardner (1989) considered the problems involved in establishing whether there was an association between childhood cancers and proximity to nuclear installations.

Clustering in time and space

Knox (1964) pointed out that if a relatively rare condition was in part caused by an infectious agent one would expect to find a space–time interaction in the sense that cases which occurred close together in space would tend also to be close in time. In a study of childhood leukaemia in north-east England he obtained information about 96 cases occurring in a certain area during a particular period of time, and tabulated each pair of cases in a 2×2 table according to certain 'closeness' criteria. A pair of cases was called 'adjacent' in time if the interval between times of onset was less than 60 days, and 'adjacent' in space if the distance was less than 1 km. The results are shown in Table 16.2. The total frequency, 4560, is the number of pairs formed from 96 cases, $96 \times 95/2$.

If there were no relationship between the time at which a case occurred and the spatial position, the cell frequencies in Table 16.2 would have been expected to be proportional to the marginal totals. In particular the expected value for the smallest frequency, is $(152)(25)/4560 = 0.83$. The deviations of observed from expected frequencies cannot be tested by the usual methods for 2×2 tables since the entries are not independent (if cases A and B form an adjacent pair, and so do B and C, it is rather likely that A and C will also do so). However, it can be shown that when the proportions of both types of adjacency are small, a good approximation to the correct significance test is to test the observed frequency as a

Table 16.2 Pairs of cases of childhood leukaemia tabulated according to adjacency in time and space (Knox, 1964)

| Time | Space | | |
	Adjacent	Not adjacent	Total
Adjacent	5	147	152
Not adjacent	20	4388	4408
	25	4535	4560

possible observation from a Poisson distribution with mean equal to the expected frequency. In a Poisson distribution with mean 0·83 the probability of observing five or more events is 0·0017, so the excess must be judged highly significant.

A number of developments have been made since Knox's paper was published. In particular, account can be taken of the actual distances in time and space, rather than the dichotomies used in Knox's test (Mantel, 1967); and allowance can be made for known periods of time, or spatial distances, within which infection could have taken place (Pike and Smith, 1968). For a general review, see Smith (1982). Raubertas (1988) proposed a method of analysis which separates the effects of clustering in space, clustering in time, and space–time clustering. The method involves estimating main effects associated with regions, main effects of the time intervals, and their interaction. Then for each region a weighted average is formed consisting of the effects of nearby regions with each region weighted by a measure of closeness in space. These weighted averages are combined into a test statistic that is sensitive to space clustering. A test for time clustering is produced in a similar manner, and the test for space–time clustering is based on weighted averages of the interaction terms with weights taken as the product of the weights used for space and time. The method was applied to the 329 cases of Creutzfeldt–Jakob disease identified in France over the period 1968–82 with space defined in terms of 94 departments.

Clustering in families

Clustering of disease in families may be due to an infective agent or to a genetic cause. These are the main reasons for studying familial aggregation, but other possible causes often complicate the issue. Members of the same family or household share the same natural environment and social conditions, all of which may affect the incidence of a particular disease. Age is a further complication, particularly in sibling studies, since siblings tend to be more similar in age than are members of different sibships.

If we ignore these complications, the testing of heterogeneity of disease incidence between families seems a similar problem to that of testing heterogeneity between any other groups of individuals. There is, however, a special problem of *ascertainment*. Family data may be collected by several different methods, as indicated below. The reader should be warned that nomenclature, particularly as regards the words 'selection' and 'ascertainment', is far from standard. Here we follow Bailey (1961).

1 *Ascertainment through families.* Here the family is selected as a unit, either from a sampling frame of families (perhaps identified by their parents), or by inclusion of all the families in a region.

2 *Ascertainment through cases.* In this method families are obtained through affected individuals. (This is a natural method if one wishes to estimate the

proportion of affected individuals amongst close relatives of affected individuals; the original cases are then called *probands* or *propositi*.) An immediate consequence is that families with no affected individuals are not included; the frequency of these is therefore not observed directly. There are important subdivisions of ascertainment through cases.

(a) *Complete ascertainment*, in which all the affected individuals are probands and families with more than one proband are counted only once; or where they are obtained from a register of probands in which each family could appear only once (e.g. from a register of births during a period of 6 months).

(b) *Single ascertainment*, in which the sampling fraction is so small that only a small fraction of families are included and the chance of a family being ascertained more than once is ignored.

(c) *Incomplete multiple ascertainment*, in which families may be ascertained through any of the affected individuals, with a certain probability (normally unknown) of ascertainment through each affected individual.

The importance of these distinctions is the following. Suppose we are studying families of size n, and that the risk is constant for each person (as in traits governed by recessive Mendelian inheritance, where the risk in offspring of parents who both carry the gene is $\frac{1}{4}$). In **1** and **2**(a) the expected frequencies of families with r affected individuals, on the null hypothesis of a constant risk for each person, will be given by a binomial distribution, the term for $r = 0$ being missing in **2**(a). In **2**(b), however, the probability of a family with r affected individuals being ascertained is proportional to r; the expected frequencies will therefore be proportional to the binomial probabilities multiplied by r. In **2**(c), the situation is intermediate: families with more affected individuals have a higher chance of being selected, but to an extent which depends on the unknown probability of ascertainment through any one individual.

These distinctions have been much considered in genetic research (Bailey, 1961) and have given rise to a number of methods of estimating the mean risk per individual and of testing for heterogeneity. A useful simple method for case **2**(a) has, for instance, been published by Gart (1968). Haenszel (1959) discusses the problem particularly in relation to chronic disease studies. Here, the assumption of a uniform risk is not normally appropriate, and the proportion of affected individuals amongst relatives of cases may have to be compared with that amongst a sample of control individuals, perhaps obtained by method **1**. Care must be taken to allow for the effects of age, and any other factors of known importance, in comparing the prevalence of disease in the two groups.

17: Biological Assay

17.1 Introduction

Biological assay, or *bioassay*, is an important, although specialized, area of application of statistical methods. The general principles were established mainly during the 1930s and 1940s, and were rapidly developed in detail to an extent which cannot be adequately covered here. The interested reader will find a comprehensive account in Finney (1978).

A biological assay is an experiment to determine the concentration of a key substance $\mathscr{S}$ in a preparation $\mathscr{P}$ by measuring the activity of $\mathscr{P}$ in a biological system $\mathscr{B}$. There are three important items in this definition.

$\mathscr{S}$, the substance under investigation, may be a pharmaceutical preparation like digitalis or penicillin, a steroid like gonadotrophin, or an ill-defined material like the protective antigen in a certain vaccine.

$\mathscr{P}$, the preparation, is usually some quantity of a naturally occurring diluent or of a product of a manufacturing process, containing an unknown concentration of $\mathscr{S}$.

$\mathscr{B}$, the biological system, is usually a response in experimental animals which should as far as possible be specific to $\mathscr{S}$. For example, vitamin D can be assayed by its antirachitic activity in rats. The biological material may, however, be humans, plants or microorganisms. The important point is that the system is purely a measuring device; the effect of $\mathscr{S}$ on $\mathscr{B}$ is of interest only in so far as it permits one to measure the concentration of $\mathscr{S}$ in $\mathscr{P}$.

The strength of $\mathscr{S}$ in $\mathscr{P}$ cannot usually be measured directly as a function of the specific response, since this is likely to vary according to experimental conditions and the nature of the biological material $\mathscr{B}$. This difficulty is overcome by the use of a standard preparation which contains $\mathscr{S}$ at constant concentration in an inert diluent and is maintained under conditions which so far as possible preserve its activity. The institution of a standard preparation usually leads to the definition of the *standard unit* as the activity of a certain amount of the standard. Any test preparation, T, can now be assayed against the standard, S, by simultaneous experimentation. If, say, S is defined to contain 1000 units per g and T happens to contain 100 units per g, a dose $10X$ g of T should give the same response as X g of S. The *relative potency* or *potency ratio* of T in terms of S is then said to be 1/10, or equivalently T may be said to have a potency of 100 units per g.

In the ideal situation described above we have assumed that S and T both contain different concentrations of exactly the same substance $\mathscr{S}$ in inert diluents, and any assay with a response specific to $\mathscr{S}$ will measure the unique potency ratio. Such an assay is called an *analytical dilution assay*; it perhaps rarely exists in the real world. In practice most biological responses are specific to a range of substances, perhaps closely related chemically like the various penicillins. In such cases the potency may depend to some extent on the assay system, because the different varieties of the active substances may have differential effects in different biological systems. An assay which for a particular biological system behaves *as though* the ideal situation were true is called a *comparative dilution assay*.

The term 'bioassay' is often used in a more general sense, to denote any experiment in which specific responses to externally applied agents are observed in animals or some other biological system. The emphasis in such experiments is often to measure the effects of various agents on the response variable, and no attempt is made to estimate relative potency. This usage is, for example, common in the extensive programmes for the testing of new drugs, pesticides, food additives, etc. for potential carcinogenic effects. It is usual to include, in a set of experiments on various test preparations, observations on control preparations. These may include both 'negative' controls (inert materials) and 'positive' controls (known carcinogens). The objective is to detect test preparations showing any carcinogenic effect rather than to estimate relative potencies. In this chapter we are concerned solely with bioassays in the more specific sense described earlier in this section, in which the central purpose is the estimation of relative potency.

The simplest form of assay is the *direct assay*, in which increasing doses of S and T can be administered to an experimental unit until a certain critical event takes place. This situation is rare; an example is the assay of prepared digitalis in the guinea-pig, in which the critical event is arrest of heart beat. The dose given to any one animal is a measure of the individual tolerance of that animal, which can be expected to vary between animals through biological and environmental causes. On any one occasion for a particular animal, suppose that the tolerance dose of S is X_S and that of T is X_T (in practice, of course, only one of these can be observed). Then the potency, ρ, of T in terms of S is given by X_S/X_T. If S and T were each administered to large random samples from a population of animals, the tolerance doses X_S and X_T would form two distributions related to each other, as in Fig. 17.1(a); the distribution of X_S would differ from that of X_T by a multiplying factor ρ, exactly as if the scale were extended or contracted by this factor. From random samples on T and S, ρ could be estimated from the distributions of X_T and X_S. The estimation problem becomes much simpler, though, if the doses are recorded logarithmically, as in Fig. 17.1(b). If $x_S = \log X_S$ and $x_T = \log X_T$, we can estimate $\log \rho$ from the two sample means $\bar{x}_S$ and $\bar{x}_T$ by

$$M = \bar{x}_S - \bar{x}_T.$$

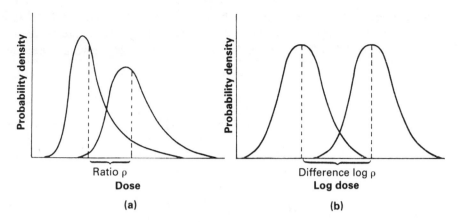

Fig. 17.1 Direct assay. Distributions of tolerance doses and their logarithms for standard and test preparations.

The distributions of x_S and x_T are automatically guaranteed to be the same shape, and in practice they are likely to be reasonably normal. The standard theory of the t distribution in the two-sample case thus provides confidence limits for $\log \rho$, centred about M, and (by taking antilogs) the corresponding limits for ρ. Unfortunately, the continuous administration of doses and the immediate response needed for direct assays are rarely feasible. Instead, the assayer has to rely on *indirect assays*, in which predetermined doses of T and S are given to groups of experimental units and the resulting responses are observed. Two different models for this situation are considered in the next two sections.

17.2 Parallel-line assays

Suppose that, for a particular assay system, the mean response, y, is linearly related to log dose, x. That is, for a log dose x_S of S, the expected response is

$$E(y) = \alpha + \beta x_S. \tag{17.1}$$

Now, the same expected response would be obtained by a log dose x_T of T, where $x_S - x_T = \log \rho$, the log potency-ratio of T in terms of S. Consequently the equation of the regression line for T is

$$\left. \begin{aligned} E(y) &= \alpha + \beta(x_T + \log \rho) \\ &= (\alpha + \beta \log \rho) + \beta x_T. \end{aligned} \right\} \tag{17.2}$$

The regression lines (17.1) and (17.2) for S and T respectively are parallel, but differ in position if $\log \rho$ is different from zero (i.e. if ρ is different from 1). The horizontal distance between the two lines is $\log \rho$.

In any one assay, values of y will be observed at various values of x_S for S and at values of x_T for T. The regression relationships (17.1) and (17.2) are estimated by fitting two parallel lines exactly as in §9.4 (equation (9.24)), giving equations

$$Y_S = \bar{y}_S + b(x_S - \bar{x}_S) \tag{17.3}$$

and

$$Y_T = \bar{y}_T + b(x_T - \bar{x}_T). \tag{17.4}$$

The estimate, M, of the log potency-ratio is the difference $x_S - x_T$ when $Y_S = Y_T$; from (17.3) and (17.4), this gives

$$M = \bar{x}_S - \bar{x}_T - \frac{\bar{y}_S - \bar{y}_T}{b}. \tag{17.5}$$

The position is indicated in Fig. 17.2. The only difference in emphasis from the treatment of the problem in §9.4 is that in the earlier discussion we were interested in estimating the vertical distance between the parallel lines, whereas now we estimate, from (17.5), the horizontal distance.

Note that, if the regression is not linear, the two regression curves will still be 'parallel' in the sense that their *horizontal* distance on the log-dose scale will be constant. In general, though, the *vertical* distance will not be constant unless the regression is linear. To achieve linear regression some transformation of the response variable may be necessary. For the analysis described below we also assume that the residual variance about the line is normal and has constant variance. These conditions may be difficult to fulfil simultaneously.

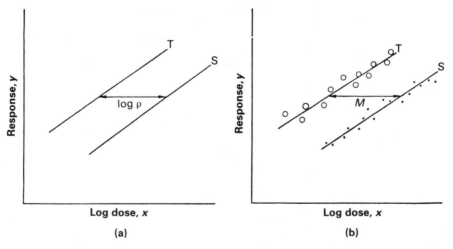

Fig. 17.2 Parallel-line assay. True (a) and fitted (b) regression lines for standard and test preparations.

Suppose that there are n_S and n_T observations on S and T respectively, and that the residual MSq about parallel lines (the s_c^2 of (9.34)) is s^2. An approximate formula for $\mathrm{var}(M)$ is, from (3.15),

$$\mathrm{var}(M) \simeq \frac{s^2}{b^2}\left[\frac{1}{n_S} + \frac{1}{n_T} + \frac{(\bar{y}_S - \bar{y}_T)^2}{b^2\sum(S_{xx})}\right], \tag{17.6}$$

where $\sum(S_{xx})$ is the pooled Within-Preparations SSq of x. The last term in the square brackets can also be written, from (17.5), as

$$\frac{(M - \bar{x}_S + \bar{x}_T)^2}{\sum(S_{xx})}.$$

It will be relatively small if the doses of T and S are chosen so that the mean responses $\bar{y}_S$ and $\bar{y}_T$ are nearly equal. (To achieve this one needs either luck or some preliminary estimate of the potency.) To a further degree of approximation, then,

$$\mathrm{var}(M) \simeq \frac{s^2}{b^2}\left(\frac{1}{n_S} + \frac{1}{n_T}\right). \tag{17.7}$$

This formula shows that the precision of the estimate of potency depends mainly on (i) the numbers n_S and n_T, which are at the experimenter's disposal, and (ii) the value of $\lambda = s/b$. The latter quantity is sometimes called the *index of precision* (although 'imprecision' would be a better description); it represents the inherent imprecision of the assay method. To improve the precision of the assay per unit observation it would be useful to modify the experimental method so that s decreases, b increases, or both. Unfortunately, s and b often tend to increase and decrease together and improvement may be difficult. Furthermore, reductions in λ may be attainable only by increased cost and the question then arises whether it is more economical to improve precision by increasing the number of observations made rather than to modify the technique.

Approximate confidence limits for $\log \rho$ may be obtained by setting limits around M, using the t distribution on the DF appropriate for s^2, $n_S + n_T - 3$. Corresponding limits for ρ are then obtained by taking antilogs. A more exact expression for confidence limits uses a result known as *Fieller's theorem*. Suppose $100(1 - 2\alpha)\%$ limits are required. Let $t_{v,2\alpha}$ be the percentage point of the t distribution on $v = n_S + n_T - 3$ DF and corresponding to a two-sided probability of 2α. The limits for $\log \rho$ are then

$$\bar{x}_S - \bar{x}_T + \frac{M - \bar{x}_S + \bar{x}_T \pm \dfrac{t_{v,2\alpha}s}{b}\left[(1 - g)\left(\dfrac{1}{n_S} + \dfrac{1}{n_T}\right) + \dfrac{(M - \bar{x}_S + \bar{x}_T)^2}{\sum(S_{xx})}\right]^{1/2}}{1 - g}, \tag{17.8}$$

where

$$g = \frac{t_{v,\,2\alpha}^2 s^2}{b^2 \sum(S_{xx})} \tag{17.9}$$

and $[\ ]^{1/2}$ indicates a square root.

The quantity g depends on the significance level of the departure of b from zero. If b is just significant at the 2α level, $g = 1$; more highly significant values of b give values of $g < 1$. If g is very small, (17.8) becomes close to the limits given by (17.6), using $t_{v,\,2\alpha}$ times the standard error of M. A safe rule is to use (17.6) whenever $g < 0.1$, and otherwise to check the adequacy of the approximation by calculating (17.8). If $g > 1$, the quantity in square brackets may be negative and therefore have no real square root; or the limits may not include the estimate M. The method is therefore useful only when the slope of the parallel lines is significant at the level required for the confidence limits.

Example 17.1

Table 17.1 shows results from an assay of vitamin D, using a standard vitamin D preparation, S, and a test preparation, I. The data for S have already been given in Table 9.3, and the assay method is described in more detail in Example 9.2. The mean values of the response variable y for the various doses of each preparation are plotted against the log dose, x, in Fig. 17.3.

A preliminary calculation of the two separate slopes gives $b_1 = 2.6166$ for S, and $b_2 = 2.7962$ for I. The test for $b_1 - b_2$, as on p. 295, gives $t = -0.20$ on 57 DF, clearly not significant. We therefore proceed with the potency calculations. The relevant basic statistics are as follows:

Group	n	$\bar{x}$	$\bar{y}$	S_{xx}	S_{xy}	S_{yy}	Within-doses S_{yy}
S	31	0·8741	2·8710	2·0576	5·3840	58·7339	41·7418
I	30	1·0000	1·8833	5·4361	15·2005	63·8417	20·9583
				7·4937	20·5845	122·5756	62·7001

The within-doses S_{yy} was obtained for the standard on p. 288; that for I is obtained likewise.

It is instructive at this stage to derive the analysis of variance shown in Table 17.2. The SSq for items (1), (2), (6) and (7) are all straightforward. Those for (3) and (4) are obtained using the method of the latter part of Example 9.3, and that for (5) follows by subtraction. The variance ratio between slopes confirms the result of the t test reported above (the 57 DF used there corresponding to a pooling of items (5) and (6) in Table 17.2), and supports the assumption of parallel linear regression.

Proceeding with the analysis, the common slope is estimated as

$$b = \frac{20.5845}{7.4937} = 2.7469.$$

Table 17.1 Radiographic assessment of bone healing for various doses of two preparations.

Standard preparation of vitamin D

Dose (i.u.)	3·5	7	14		Total
Log dose, x	0·544	0·845	1·146		
	0	1·50	2·00		
	0	2·50	2·50		
	1·00	5·00	5·00		
	2·75	6·00	4·00		
	2·75	4·25	5·00		
	1·75	2·75	4·00		
	2·75	1·50	2·50		
	2·25	3·00	3·50		
	2·25		3·00		
	2·50		2·00		
			3·00		
			4·00		
			4·00		
Number	10	8	13		31
Mean	1·8000	3·3125	3·4231		

Preparation I

Dose (mg)	2·5	5	10	20	40	
Log dose, x	0·398	0·699	1·000	1·301	1·602	
	0	1·00	1·50	3·00	3·50	
	1·00	1·50	1·00	3·00	3·50	
	0	1·50	2·00	5·50	4·50	
	0	1·00	3·50	2·50	3·50	
	0	1·00	2·00	1·00	3·50	
	0·50	0·50	0	2·00	3·00	
Number	6	6	6	6	6	30
Mean	0·2500	1·0833	1·6667	2·8333	3·5833	

From (17.5),

$$M = 0.8741 - 1.0000 - \frac{2.8710 - 1.8833}{2.7469}$$

$$= -0.1259 - 0.3596$$

$$= -0.4855.$$

The estimate of potency is

$$\text{antilog } M = 0.327,$$

measured in international units per mg (these being the scales on which doses of S and I are measured). As a rough check we note from Table 17.1 that the doses of 3·5, 7 and 10 i.u. of S give about the same mean responses as 10, 20 and 40 mg of I, which suggests that I has a potency of about 0·35 i.u. per mg.

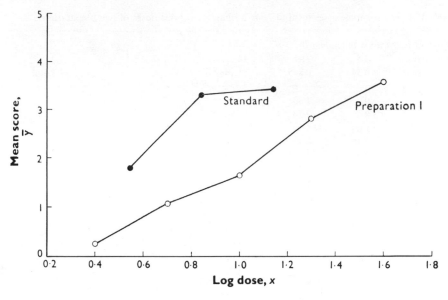

Fig. 17.3 Scores for bone healing in an assay of vitamin D (Table 17.1).

Table 17.2 Analysis of variance for vitamin D assay, using standard preparation and preparation I (data from Table 17.1)

	DF	SSq	MSq	VR
(1) *Between doses*	7	74.7467		
(2) Between preparations	1		14·8712	14·8712
(3) Common slope	1		56·5437	56·5437 47·80 (P < 0·001)
(4) Between slopes	1		0·0481	0·0481 0·04
(5) Non-linearity	4		3·2837	0·8209 0·69
(6) *Within doses*	53	62·7001		1·1830 1·00
(7) Total	60	137·4468		

In considering the sampling variation of M we need the residual MSq about parallel lines. This is obtained from Table 17.2 as

$$s^2 = \frac{62 \cdot 7001 + 3 \cdot 2837 + 0 \cdot 0481}{53 + 4 + 1}$$

$$= 66 \cdot 0319 / 58$$

$$= 1 \cdot 1385,$$

very little different from the Within-Doses MSq in Table 17.2. From (17.9), noting that $t_{58,0\cdot05} = 2\cdot002$,

$$g = \frac{(2\cdot002)^2 (1\cdot1385)}{(2\cdot7469)^2 (7\cdot4937)}$$

$$= 0\cdot081.$$

This is sufficiently small to permit the use of the approximate formula (17.6).

$$\mathrm{var}(M) = \frac{1\cdot1385}{(2\cdot7469)^2}\left[\frac{1}{31} + \frac{1}{30} + \frac{(0\cdot3596)^2}{7\cdot4937}\right]$$

$$= (0\cdot15089)(0\cdot03226 + 0\cdot03333 + 0\cdot01726)$$

$$= (0\cdot15089)(0\cdot08285)$$

$$= 0\cdot012501,$$

$$\mathrm{SE}(M) = \sqrt{0\cdot012501} = 0\cdot1118.$$

Approximate 95% confidence limits for $\log \rho$ are

$$-0\cdot4855 \pm (2\cdot002)(0\cdot1118)$$

$$= -0\cdot7093 \text{ and } -0\cdot2617.$$

Taking antilogs, the limits for ρ are 0·195 and 0·547 i.u. per mg.

The design used for the assay analysed in Example 17.1, which may be called a 3 + 5 design since there were three doses of the standard and five doses of the test preparation, allowed the possibility of testing for departures from parallelism and linearity. Non-linearity can often be corrected by a transformation of the response scale. Non-parallelism when the regressions are apparently linear is more troublesome, and may indicate a basically invalid assay system. Both these types of departure from the model can be tested provided there are sufficient dose levels; a 2 + 2 design is too small for this purpose, since non-parallelism and non-linearity both affect the same SSq in the analysis. A 2 + 3 design or a 3 + 3 design allows the effects to be separated. There is considerable advantage in the use of a completely symmetric design, with the same number of doses in each preparation, the same number of observations at each dose level, and a constant log dose interval throughout. The component parts of the SSq between dose groups, and many of the quantities entering into the calculation of M and its confidence limits, can then be expressed in terms of simple linear contrasts. Examples will be found in Finney (1978), where there is a very detailed account of experimental design in biological assays.

Radioimmunoassays

Potency estimations of hormones and certain other substances are now commonly performed by radioimmunoassays (RIAs) or other forms of radioligand assays. In RIAs, the system $\mathscr{B}$ is an antigen–antibody reaction, in which a quantity of antigen is initially labelled with a radioisotope, a known dose of the test or standard preparation is added, and the response is measured by a radiation count of antibody-bound labelled antigen. The bound count is affected by the dose of the substance under assay, and the dose–response curve is typically sigmoid in shape, with an upper asymptote, D, to the mean response, at zero dose, and a lower asymptote, C, at very high doses. If the mean bound count at log dose x is U, the quantity

$$Y = \ln\left(\frac{U - C}{D - U}\right)$$

is analogous to the logit transformation for proportions, (11.7), and it is often (although not always) found that Y is approximately linearly related to x.

The precision of RIAs is relatively high, and potency estimates, particularly for routine clinical use, are often made by eye. If responses are obtained for a series of doses of the standard preparation, the asymptotes C and D may be estimated roughly and values of y obtained from the observed counts u. A regression of y on x may then be fitted by eye. If a response is obtained at a single dose of a test preparation, the log potency can be estimated by measuring the horizontal distance between the test point and the standard line. However, a formal approach, providing estimates of error and validity tests, is preferable. Finney (1978) gives details of such an approach, and also (Finney, 1979) describes the desiderata for computer programs intended for the routine analysis of RIAs. The statistical methodology is a direct extension of that described earlier in this section, with some additional features. In particular, (i) the lower and upper asymptotes, C and D, need to be estimated from the data (counts will usually have been observed at each of the extremes of dose level); (ii) the variance of the observed count u is likely to increase with the mean U; the way in which it does so needs to be assessed from the data so that an appropriate form of weighting can be used in the analysis.

17.3 Slope-ratio assays

In some assay systems the response, y, can conveniently be related linearly to the dose, rather than to the log dose, the residual variation being approximately normal and having approximately constant variance. This situation arises particularly in microbiological assays where the response is a turbidometric measure of growth of microorganisms. If the potency of T in terms of S is ρ, the same expected response will be given by doses X_T of T and X_S of S, where $X_S = \rho X_T$. If, therefore, the regression equation for S is

$$\mathrm{E}(y) = \alpha + \beta_S X_S, \tag{17.10}$$

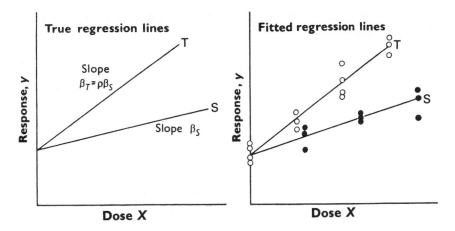

Fig. 17.4 Slope-ratio assay. True and fitted regression lines for standard and test preparations.

that for T will be

$$E(y) = \alpha + \beta_S(\rho X_T)$$

$$= \alpha + \beta_T X_T, \tag{17.11}$$

where $\beta_T = \rho\beta_S$. Equations (17.10) and (17.11) represent two straight lines with the same intercept, α, on the vertical axis and with slopes in the ratio $1:\rho$. Hence the term *slope ratio*. The intercept α is the expected response at zero dose, whether of T or of S. The position is shown in Fig. 17.4.

In the analysis of results from a slope-ratio assay the observed responses at various doses X_S of S and at doses X_T of T must be fitted by two lines of the form

$$Y = a + b_S X_S \tag{17.12}$$

and

$$Y = a + b_T X_T, \tag{17.13}$$

which are, like the true regression lines, constrained to pass through the same intercept on the vertical axis (Fig. 17.4). This is a form of regression analysis not previously considered in this book. The problem can be conveniently regarded as one of multiple regression. For each observation we consider the values of three variables, y, X_S and X_T, of which y is the dependent variable and X_S and X_T are predictor variables. For any observation on S, X_S is non-zero and $X_T = 0$; for an observation on T, $X_S = 0$ and X_T is non-zero. The assay may include control observations (so-called *blanks*) without either S or T; for these, $X_S = X_T = 0$. The true regression equations (17.10) and (17.11) can now be combined into one multiple regression equation

$$E(y) = \alpha + \beta_S X_S + \beta_T X_T, \tag{17.14}$$

and the estimated regressions (17.12) and (17.13) are combined in the estimated multiple regression:

$$Y = a + b_S X_S + b_T X_T. \tag{17.15}$$

This relationship can be fitted by standard multiple regression methods, and the potency $\rho(= \beta_T/\beta_S)$ estimated by

$$R = b_T/b_S. \tag{17.16}$$

The residual variance of y is estimated by the usual residual MSq, s^2, and the variances and covariance of b_S and b_T are obtained from (10.16) and (10.17). Write v_{jh} instead of the c_{jh} of (10.16) and (10.17), so that

$$\mathrm{var}(b_S) = v_{11}s^2, \quad \mathrm{var}(b_T) = v_{22}s^2, \quad \mathrm{cov}(b_S, b_T) = v_{12}s^2.$$

Approximate confidence limits for ρ are obtained by the following formula derived from (3.18):

$$\mathrm{var}(R) = \frac{s^2}{b_S^2}(v_{22} - 2Rv_{12} + R^2 v_{11}). \tag{17.17}$$

A more exact solution, using Fieller's theorem, is available (see Finney, 1978, §7.6) by analogy with (17.8), but is not normally required in assays of this type.

For numerical examples of the calculations see Finney (1978, Chapter 7).

The adequacy of the model in a slope-ratio assay can be tested by a rather elegant analysis of variance procedure. Suppose the design is of a $1 + k_S + k_T$ type; that is, there is one group of 'blanks' and there are k_S dose groups of S and k_T dose groups of T. Suppose also that there is replication at some or all of the dose levels, giving n observations in all. A standard analysis (as described on p. 324) leads to the following subdivision of DF:

Between doses	$k_S + k_T$	
Regression		2
Deviations from model		$k_S + k_T - 2$
Within doses	$n - k_S - k_T - 1$	
Total	$n - 1$	

The SSq for deviations from the model can be subdivided into the following parts:

Blanks	1
Intersection	1
Non-linearity for non-zero doses	$k_S + k_T - 4$
	$k_S + k_T - 2$

The SSq for 'blanks' indicates whether the 'blanks' observations are sufficiently consistent with the remainder. It can be obtained by refitting the multiple regression with an extra dummy variable (1 for 'blanks', 0 otherwise), and noting the reduction in the deviations SSq. A significant variance-ratio test for 'blanks' might indicate non-linearity for very low doses; if the remaining tests were satisfactory, the assay could still be analysed adequately by omitting the 'blanks'.

The SSq for 'intersection' shows whether the data can justifiably be fitted by two lines intersecting on the vertical axis. Significance here is more serious and usually indicates invalidity of the assay system. It can be obtained by fitting two separate lines to the observations at non-zero doses of S and to those at non-zero doses of T. The difference in residual between this analysis and that referred to above (for the 'blanks' test) gives the required SSq.

The third component, due to non-linearity at non-zero doses, can be obtained either by subtraction or directly from the two separate regressions ($k_S - 2$ DF for S and $k_T - 2$ for T add to the required $k_S + k_T - 4$).

Further details, with examples, are given by Finney (1978, Chapter 7), who also discusses the use of symmetric designs which permit simplification of the analysis by the use of linear contrasts.

17.4 Quantal-response assays

Frequently the response is quantal, as in direct assays, and yet the assay has to be done indirectly by selection of doses and observation of the responses elicited. If a particular dose of one preparation is applied to n_i experimental units, the investigator observes that a certain number of responses, say r_i, are positive and $n_i - r_i$ are negative. Examples of assays yielding this type of response are as follows.

1   Pyrethrin, the response being death in houseflies.
2   Insulin, the response being presence of convulsions in mice.
3   Virus preparations, the response being presence of viral growth in egg membranes.

For any one preparation the response curve relating the expected response (expressed as the probability of a positive response) to the dose or to the log dose is likely to be sigmoid in shape, as described in §11.4. Indeed, the fitting of the response curve for one preparation presents precisely the sort of problem considered in §12.8 and, as we shall see, the methods described there are immediately applicable.

A further point is worth noting. The response curve, rising from 0 to 1 on the vertical scale, may be regarded as the cumulative distribution function of a random variable which can be called the *tolerance* of experimental units to the agent under test. The tolerances are precisely the critical doses which would be observed in a direct assay. If, for example, a dose X corresponds to a response P, we can

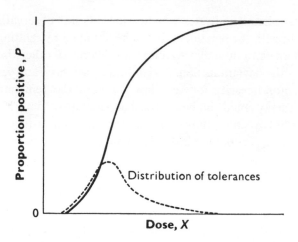

Fig. 17.5 Quantal-response curve with the corresponding tolerance distribution.

interpret this as showing that a proportion P of the animals have a tolerance less than X (and therefore succumb to X), and $1 - P$ have a tolerance greater than X. The response function P is thus the distribution function of tolerance; the corresponding density function is called the *tolerance distribution* (see Fig. 17.5). A very similar situation holds in psychological tests of the stimulus–response type. An individual given a stimulus X will respond if the threshold (corresponding to the tolerance in biological assay) is less than X. Neither in the psychological example nor in biological assay is there any need to suppose that X is a constant quantity for any individual; it may vary considerably from occasion to occasion in the same individual.

In an assay of T and S, the response curves, plotted against $x = \log X$, will be parallel in the sense that they differ by a constant horizontal distance, $\log \rho$, and a full analysis requires that the data be fitted by two parallel curves of this sort (Fig. 17.6). A natural approach is to linearize the response curves by applying to the response one of the transformations described in §11.4 and §12.8. Using the logit transformation, for example, one could suppose that Y, the logit of P, is linearly related to the log dose, x, by the equations

and
$$\left. \begin{array}{ll} Y = \alpha_S + \beta x & \text{for S} \\ Y = \alpha_T + \beta x & \text{for T.} \end{array} \right\} \qquad (17.18)$$

The relationships (17.18) could be fitted iteratively by the maximum likelihood procedure described in §12.8, using a dummy variable to distinguish between S and T, as in §10.4. Writing $\alpha_T = \alpha_S + \delta$, the log potency-ratio is given by $\log \rho = \delta/\beta$. A computer program for generalized linear models may be used to

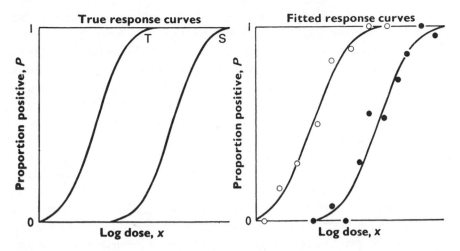

Fig. 17.6 Quantal-response assay. True and fitted response curves for standard and test preparations.

obtain the estimates a_S, d and b of α_S, δ and β, respectively, and hence $\log \rho$ is estimated by $M = d/b$. From (3.18), an approximate formula for $\text{var}(M)$ is

$$\text{var}(M) \simeq \frac{V_d}{b^2} - \frac{2dC_{db}}{b^3} + \frac{d^2 V_b}{b^4},$$

where $V_d = \text{var}(d)$, $C_{db} = \text{cov}(d, b)$ and $V_b = \text{var}(b)$. These variances and the covariance may be obtainable from the computer output. Approximate $100(1 - 2\alpha)\%$ confidence limits for $\log \rho$ are then

$$M \pm z_{2\alpha}\sqrt{\text{var}(M)},$$

where $z_{2\alpha}$ is the usual standardized normal deviate. Limits for ρ are obtained by taking antilogs.

By analogy with (17.8), Fieller's theorem can be used to give more reliable approximations. The limits for $\log \rho$ then become

$$\frac{M - \dfrac{gC_{db}}{V_b} \pm \dfrac{z_{2\alpha}}{b}\left[V_d - 2MC_{db} + M^2 V_b - g\left(V_d - \dfrac{C_{db}^2}{V_b}\right)\right]^{\frac{1}{2}}}{1 - g},$$

where

$$g = \frac{z_{2\alpha}^2 V_b}{b^2}.$$

Approximate χ^2 tests for (i) parallelism and (ii) linearity may be obtained by the analysis of deviance, by taking (i) the difference between the deviances of the fitted model and a model with separate slopes for S and T, and (ii) the deviance of the latter model.

The use of the logistic transformation in biological assay was strongly advocated by J. Berkson, who favoured non-iterative curve-fitting by the use of empirical weights (Berkson, 1944). The maximum likelihood calculations for the *probit* transformation are fully described, with examples, by Finney (1971), and this method, called *probit analysis*, is perhaps more widely used in biological assay than the corresponding logit method. There is no evidence to suggest that either model is more consistent with real data than the other, and curves fitted by the two methods are invariably very similar indeed.

Another group of short-cut methods for the analysis of quantal-response assays relies effectively on attempts to measure the horizontal distance between the two log dose–response curves without estimating the entire curves. The position of either of the curves in the first diagram of Fig. 17.6 can be summarized by the dose at which $P = 0.5$. This is called the *ED50* (ED standing for 'effective dose') or *median effective dose*; it is clearly the median of the underlying tolerance distribution. Now the ED50s for T and S are in the ratio $1 : \rho$. If they were estimated by X_{0T} and X_{0S}, the ratio X_{0S}/X_{0T} would provide an estimate of ρ; equivalently, the quantity

$$M = \log X_{0S} - \log X_{0T}$$

would estimate $\log \rho$.

The ED50 is sometimes given slightly different names according to the type of response: LD50 or median lethal dose if the response is lethal; ImD50 if the response is the proportion of animals protected by an immunizing agent from a challenge dose of virulent organisms, and so on. It can often be estimated roughly by eye from a plot of the observed responses, but a subjective estimation of this sort suffers from its lack of reproducibility, even on the same data, and has the further disadvantage that an adequate estimate of sampling error is virtually unobtainable. Several simple objective methods of estimating the ED50 were in common use until recently, but the wide availability of computer programs for the efficient analysis of quantal-response data has made these methods largely obsolete. A full account is given by Finney (1978, §§18.6–18.8).

18: Statistical Computation

18.1 Introduction

All statistical analyses involve some calculation. These calculations range from a simple formula which could be calculated in one's head (4.12) to complex calculations, such as multiple logistic regression (§12.8), which one would not normally contemplate doing without a computer.

In one sense it is legitimate to consider an electronic computer as a large, fast, programmable calculator. It is certainly that, since it can perform all the operations that can be carried out on a calculator at a faster rate (although this is not the same as saying it will always be quicker as far as the investigator is concerned), on large sets of data, and it can store all the steps of a calculation in a program. However, this view is restrictive since it ignores the operations a computer can do that cannot be carried out at all on a calculator. Such operations include the storage, checking and sorting of data, the counting of individuals and the categorization of variables. If *computation* encompasses all the operations that can be carried out on a computer, then computation is a much wider term than *calculation* and the extra features form a considerable part of many statistical analyses. Many examples could be given but two should suffice to make this point clear.

First, suppose it is required to analyse an association that may be set out in a two-way contingency table; then the first stage would involve setting up the frequencies in the contingency table. This may be far from trivial. It involves extracting the values of both classifying factors from a collection of many more variables on each individual and then counting the number of individuals in each cell of the table. Moreover, the variables may not be already categorized; it may be necessary to form categories from data recorded on a continuous scale, e.g. to divide age into 10-year age groups. None of this process can conveniently be carried out on a calculator. The counting to form frequencies would be done by tallying (see Table 1.5). As a second example, suppose it has been decided to carry out an analysis using a distribution-free method such as one of the rank tests discussed in Chapter 13. Then the first stage is to rank the data—that is, to sort the values into ascending order of magnitude. Again this cannot be done on a calculator. Both these examples involve operations which cannot be carried out on a calculator but which are, except for small data sets, tedious, time-consuming and prone to error if done by hand. Most research workers with access to

Table 18.1 Stages in the data-handling process

Stage	Operations
Data processing	
Collecting	Recording of observations
Transferring	Coding; transfer of data to computer for storage
Cleaning	Checking; correcting
Statistical analysis	
Organizing	Categorization; derivation of new variables; tabulating; sorting
Calculating	Application of statistical methods involving calculation of standard formulae

a computer prefer such tedious categorizations, tabulations, and sorting operations to be carried out on a computer from the point of view of both saving time and improving accuracy.

Most descriptions of statistical analysis—and on the whole this book is no exception—start from the assumption that the data are available in some standard format. For example, the calculation of a χ^2 test statistic for a 2×2 table (4.21) is almost a trivial calculation which can be performed in less than a minute on the simplest of electronic calculators. But, as discussed above, setting up the frequencies in the contingency table may be far from trivial. When considering the role of computers it is advantageous to think of the whole process that involves the data, from the collection of the data through to the completed analysis. It is convenient for discussion to divide the process into five stages (Table 18.1); the first three stages would often be labelled as data processing and the last two stages as the statistical analysis. To a first approximation the five stages are gone through in sequence but there are interactions between them in a 'backward' as well as in a 'forward' sense.

18.2 Data processing

Data collection

This stage is discussed in Chapter 1 (pp. 9–10). Often computers are not used but, in some cases the data may be recorded directly onto a computer. In any case the design of the data-collection stage should facilitate, as far as possible, the transfer of the data to a computer.

Data transfer

This stage is also discussed in Chapter 1 (pp. 11–13). It often involves coding of all data to numerical form (see Fig. 1.4). The data format must be compatible with the statistical package it is intended to use. It will often be useful to punch the data in the way that leads to the fewest mistakes, and then to use a special editing program to get the data into the form needed for the package. When data are expressed in numerical form in a strictly defined format, there is unlikely to be any problem, but care must be taken over missing information. One option is to leave the corresponding entries blank, but as there is no uniformity on how blanks are interpreted by programs this should be avoided. It is better to have a code for 'missing'. Thus, if the marital status could not be determined for a subject responding to the questionnaire in Fig. 1.4, then column 8 could be coded as a '9'. Some programs allow the use of alphabetic characters and this would enable sex to be coded as 'M' or 'F' instead of '1' or '2'. This would be preferable to the use of an artificial numerical code and may reduce the error rate, but the possibility that a different program may be used, which may not accept alphabetic codes, should be borne in mind (although powerful editing facilities on a computer may enable the codes to be transferred to numerical format very easily).

Data cleaning

The use of logical and statistical checks to detect impossible or implausible values is discussed in §11.6. Such checks may reveal errors that can be corrected by reference back to the source of the data. Some errors may only be detected by sophisticated checks based on preliminary analysis, e.g. a check of weights in relation to height (§11.6), or only become apparent when a two-way table is constructed.

These three stages are sometimes combined in part by the use of interactive data entry, as discussed in Chapter 1, but the aim is to produce a 'clean' set of data for statistical analysis.

18.3 Statistical analysis

The subdivision into two stages is somewhat arbitrary since often the two will be combined into a single computer run. Nevertheless, the distinction serves some purpose since, particularly with large data sets that may be analysed in several ways, it is more efficient to go through a stage of organizing the data into a new data file for the future analysis. This new data file will contain categorized variables and variables derived from the recorded data. As an example of a derived variable, age might be calculated from the dates of birth and interview.

After derivation and categorization of variables, many of the original recorded variables might no longer be needed and thus the new data file is usually more compact than the original. In other cases the data might be reduced to a multiway table, which is then analysed in detail. An example of this is given by Example 12.9 (p. 425), in which data on five variables for 1729 individuals have been reduced to a 2×2^4 contingency table, without any loss of information.

The stage of applying statistical methods and formulae to data arranged for this purpose is what is often regarded as the statistical analysis. It is, of course, important since it leads to the interpretation; but it is no more important than the earlier stages. Indeed, it could be argued that the earlier stages are more important since without adequate data checking and cleaning the results of the analysis may be misleading.

As well as the formal statistical methods, Tukey (1977) advocates exploratory data analysis, many of the methods of which are graphical. The task of producing graphs is greatly eased by the availability of graphical facilities within modern statistical packages.

18.4 Statistical packages

In order to be able to carry out a particular method of statistical analysis on a computer, a *program* setting out the statistical method, step by step, is required. Thus to cover all the different methods discussed in this book a set of programs would be required. A set of programs integrated together into a single piece of software is called a *package* and such packages are the most convenient software to use for statistical analysis. They are each supplied by an organization, which provides documentation and regularly produces revised versions adding new statistical methods, improving ease of use and making the output clearer. Because of their widespread use they are practically error-free. A package includes procedures for the organization of the data, prior to application of the method proper, and most allow a new file of reorganized data to be saved and used as input for future runs. Graphical procedures are also included.

The most tedious and lengthy part of preparing a program to run in any package is the definition of the variables, which includes specifying the names of variables, specifying labels describing each level of a categorical variable, deriving new variables, and categorizing variables. It is tempting to take short cuts in this and end up with an output that is not properly labelled. This may be perfectly intelligible at the time but, when referring back months later, there are likely to be regrets that the program was not properly set up originally. The results of this process can be saved in a system file, which can then be used as input for future runs. This is useful for large data sets, but is less critical for smaller data sets since computer time is becoming less critical. In contrast to this part of the program the application of a particular statistical method can often be defined by just a few lines.

Personal computers (PCs), or *microcomputers* are now the most common form of computer used for analysing data, and *mainframe computers* are only necessary for large data sets. PCs are often in a network and a wide range of software may be available from the network server.

Only a few of the statistical packages available will be considered in this chapter and only brief details of each discussed. Three packages that were originally produced for mainframe computers, SPSS, BMDP and SAS, and proved very popular in that environment, are now available for PCs. Other packages, also originally developed in the mainframe era but now translated into the PC age, are Minitab, Genstat and GLIM. Some packages come in a range of versions suitable for different computing configurations.

SPSS

The first manual for the *Statistical Package for the Social Sciences* (*SPSS*) was published in 1970. The latest edition (SPSS Inc., 1990) describes an enhanced version of SPSS. A wide range of statistical methods is available, including multivariate methods, time series, logistic regression and survival analysis. All the procedures in the package are available within a single run. Some of the procedures have a number of options available and it is important to check the manual carefully to ensure that the required option is selected. Also a number of statistics are available for some procedures and it is necessary to select those required. Some users are tempted to select all statistics and then try to find a meaning for those that are not really relevant to the particular job.

SAS

The *Statistical Analysis System* (*SAS*) was first introduced in 1972 and has become very popular; the most recent manual was produced in 1989 (SAS Institute Inc., 1989). An introduction to the use of SAS is given by Cody and Smith (1991). SAS contains a full range of statistical procedures including multiple regression with diagnostic facilities, multivariate methods, survival analysis including proportional hazards, and logistic regression, and all can be accessed within a single run. Results can be kept in files and used as input in future runs. SAS is particularly useful in data management and report writing, and contains powerful graphical facilities. As with SPSS, the user must choose options and statistics with care.

BMDP

This is the oldest of the packages and the manual for the original *BMD Biomedical Computer Programs* was published in 1961. The package was renamed BMDP in 1975 and the most recent version (Dixon, 1990) describes the current capabilities. This package covers a wide range of statistical methods, including logistic regression, and survival analysis including proportional hazards. A disadvantage is that the package consists of separate routines, only one of which can be accessed in a single run. However, the results from one program can be saved in a BMDP file and used as input for other programs.

Minitab

This package was developed originally at Pennsylvania State University in 1972; details are available in the latest manual (Minitab Inc., 1991) and Ryan *et al.* (1985) give a description of how to use the package. Its coverage of methods is not as wide as the packages discussed above but multiple regression is included. It is suitable for small data sets, permits interactive use and has proved popular with students and non-specialist users.

Genstat

This *General Statistical Program* was first introduced in 1972 and the latest manual published in 1987 (Genstat 5 Committee, 1987). It is generally regarded as one the more difficult packages to learn to use; an introductory text is by Alvey *et al.* (1982). Genstat is a language, as well as a package, because it is written so that the type of algebraic operations commonly used in statistics can be programmed easily and this enables new methods to be carried out. This facility of Genstat makes it popular with statisticians developing new methodology or wishing to try variants of existing methods. Genstat has particularly good facilities for the analysis of designed experiments.

GLIM

The *Generalized Linear Interactive Modelling* system was first introduced in 1974. It was written to fit generalized linear models and to be operated in interactive mode. This allows an investigator to try different models, progressing according to the results of each fit. Thus variables can be added in or dropped out and the effect of such a change on the model assessed before deciding on the next step. It is most suitable for small to moderately sized data sets. A recent manual is edited by Francis *et al.* (1993), and Aitken *et al.* (1989) give a description and examples of its use.

Other packages have been produced specifically for PCs without going through the mainframe stage. Statistical software reviews are published regularly in the *American Statistician* and *Applied Statistics*. Some of the popular packages used for statistical analysis are SYSTAT (Wilkinson, 1990), STATA (Computing

Resource Center, 1992) and SPIDA (Gebski *et al.*, 1992). EGRET (Statistics and Epidemiology Research Corporation, 1988) is popular for the analysis of epidemiological data and Epi Info (Dean *et al.*, 1990) is useful in the design of epidemiological questionnaires.

A recent exciting development is StatXact (CYTEL Software Corporation, 1991). This makes available for the first time in convenient form a number of exact calculations for discrete data. These include the exact test of an $r \times c$ table (§7.6), which is also available in SAS, an exact trend test for an $r \times 2$ table with ordered rows (§12.2), and the exact test for the combination of 2×2 tables, suitable for situations when the Mantel–Haenszel test breaks down (§12.6). It also enables the calculation of mid-P significance levels, which we recommend should be used for discrete data (§§4.7, 4.9). A lot of research has been needed to produce a package that makes these calculations feasible, even on today's fast computers. Related packages are LogXact for logistic regression, and EaSt for group sequential trials with survival data.

The various packages have been presented as distinct entities. Whilst they may be viewed as such and a user with a good working knowledge of just one of the general statistical packages, such as SAS, SPSS or BMDP, will be able to perform most required analyses, some users prefer to use different packages for different parts of an analysis. This may be facilitated by using output files from a run of one package as input to another package. The transfer of an analysis from package to package is facilitated by utility programs, such as dmbs/copy and Stat/Transfer, which allow a two-way conversion of system files between a plethora of statistical packages and spreadsheet programs. Spreadsheet programs are particularly useful for tabular calculations such as standardization (§12.9).

18.5 General remarks

Although the above packages cover most statistical methods, they can never be completely up to date with new developments or include very specialized methods. For this reason some writers make available their own software. For example, the book by Breslow and Day (1980) includes programs for the analysis of case–control studies, which served as a useful source for many years until the methods were included in standard packages, for instance PROC PHREG in SAS. Coleman *et al.* (1986) describe a program suitable for the analysis of mortality by the subject-years method (§14.9).

The increasing availability of statistical software over the last 20 years has been an enormous benefit to research workers. Nevertheless, it is important not to lose sight of the fact that a computer and associated software are tools available to carry out a job. It is relatively easy to apply complex statistical methods to data but it is not so easy to interpret the results unless the method has been carefully selected as the relevant method to meet the objectives of the research study.

Although a computer might be used to carry out the bulk of an analysis, the calculator still has a role to play. It is often required to carry out subsidiary calculations on computer output or to examine tabular output produced by a computer in detail. Where such subsidiary analyses require the input of just a few items of data, a calculator is suitable. Programmable calculators allow quite sophisticated calculations to be carried out, for example, calculation of an exact test of a 2×2 table (see Example 4.14, p. 138) or a Mantel–Haenszel calculation ((16.12)–(16.15)), but the use of programmable calculators for complex analysis has declined in importance over the last few years.

The last few years have also seen quite marked changes in the use of computers for statistical analysis and this is likely to continue. The use of exact methods may become more widespread; there is little point in worrying about whether the conditions for the validity of an approximate test hold in marginal cases when the exact analysis can be carried out readily. Some of the Bayesian methods are computer-intensive and the use of these methods is likely to become more popular as appropriate software is developed.

Appendix Tables

Table A1 Areas in tail of the normal distribution

Single-tail areas in terms of standardized deviates. The function tabulated is $\frac{1}{2}P$, the probability of obtaining a standardized normal deviate greater than z, *in one direction*. The two-tail probability, P, is twice the tabulated value

z	0·00	0·01	0·02	0·03	0·04	0·05	0·06	0·07	0·08	0·09
0·0	0·5000	0·4960	0·4920	0·4880	0·4840	0·4801	0·4761	0·4721	0·4681	0·4641
0·1	0·4602	0·4562	0·4522	0·4483	0·4443	0·4404	0·4364	0·4325	0·4286	0·4247
0·2	0·4207	0·4168	0·4129	0·4090	0·4052	0·4013	0·3974	0·3936	0·3897	0·3859
0·3	0·3821	0·3783	0·3745	0·3707	0·3669	0·3632	0·3594	0·3557	0·3520	0·3483
0·4	0·3446	0·3409	0·3372	0·3336	0·3300	0·3264	0·3228	0·3192	0·3156	0·3121
0·5	0·3085	0·3050	0·3015	0·2981	0·2946	0·2912	0·2877	0·2843	0·2810	0·2776
0·6	0·2743	0·2709	0·2676	0·2643	0·2611	0·2578	0·2546	0·2514	0·2483	0·2451
0·7	0·2420	0·2389	0·2358	0·2327	0·2296	0·2266	0·2236	0·2206	0·2177	0·2148
0·8	0·2119	0·2090	0·2061	0·2033	0·2005	0·1977	0·1949	0·1922	0·1894	0·1867
0·9	0·1841	0·1814	0·1788	0·1762	0·1736	0·1711	0·1685	0·1660	0·1635	0·1611
1·0	0·1587	0·1562	0·1539	0·1515	0·1492	0·1469	0·1446	0·1423	0·1401	0·1379
1·1	0·1357	0·1335	0·1314	0·1292	0·1271	0·1251	0·1230	0·1210	0·1190	0·1170
1·2	0·1151	0·1131	0·1112	0·1093	0·1075	0·1056	0·1038	0·1020	0·1003	0·0985
1·3	0·0968	0·0951	0·0934	0·0918	0·0901	0·0885	0·0869	0·0853	0·0838	0·0823
1·4	0·0808	0·0793	0·0778	0·0764	0·0749	0·0735	0·0721	0·0708	0·0694	0·0681

z										
1·5	0·0668	0·0655	0·0643	0·0630	0·0618	0·0606	0·0594	0·0582	0·0571	0·0559
1·6	0·0548	0·0537	0·0526	0·0516	0·0505	0·0495	0·0485	0·0475	0·0465	0·0455
1·7	0·0446	0·0436	0·0427	0·0418	0·0409	0·0401	0·0392	0·0384	0·0375	0·0367
1·8	0·0359	0·0351	0·0344	0·0336	0·0329	0·0322	0·0314	0·0307	0·0301	0·0294
1·9	0·0287	0·0281	0·0274	0·0268	0·0262	0·0256	0·0250	0·0244	0·0239	0·0233
2·0	0·02275	0·02222	0·02169	0·02118	0·02068	0·02018	0·01970	0·01923	0·01876	0·01831
2·1	0·01786	0·01743	0·01700	0·01659	0·01618	0·01578	0·01539	0·01500	0·01463	0·01426
2·2	0·01390	0·01355	0·01321	0·01287	0·01255	0·01222	0·01191	0·01160	0·01130	0·01101
2·3	0·01072	0·01044	0·01017	0·00990	0·00964	0·00939	0·00914	0·00889	0·00866	0·00842
2·4	0·00820	0·00798	0·00776	0·00755	0·00734	0·00714	0·00695	0·00676	0·00657	0·00639
2·5	0·00621	0·00604	0·00587	0·00570	0·00554	0·00539	0·00523	0·00508	0·00494	0·00480
2·6	0·00466	0·00453	0·00440	0·00427	0·00415	0·00402	0·00391	0·00379	0·00368	0·00357
2·7	0·00347	0·00336	0·00326	0·00317	0·00307	0·00298	0·00289	0·00280	0·00272	0·00264
2·8	0·00256	0·00248	0·00240	0·00233	0·00226	0·00219	0·00212	0·00205	0·00199	0·00193
2·9	0·00187	0·00181	0·00175	0·00169	0·00164	0·00159	0·00154	0·00149	0·00144	0·00139
3·0	0·00135									
3·1	0·00097									
3·2	0·00069									
3·3	0·00048									
3·4	0·00034									
3·5	0·00023									
3·6	0·00016									
3·7	0·00011									
3·8	0·00007									
3·9	0·00005									
4·0	0·00003									

Standardized deviates in terms of two-tail areas

P	1·0	0·9	0·8	0·7	0·6	0·5	0·4
z	0	0·126	0·253	0·385	0·524	0·674	0·842

P	0·3	0·2	0·1	0·05	0·02	0·01	0·001
z	1·036	1·282	1·645	1·960	2·326	2·576	3·291

Reproduced in part from Table 3 of Murdoch and Barnes (1968) by permission of the authors and publishers.

Table A2 Percentage points of the χ^2 distribution

The function tabulated is $\chi^2_{\nu, P}$, the value exceeded with probability P in a χ^2 distribution with ν degrees of freedom (the $100P$ percentage point)

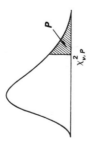

Degrees of freedom, ν	Probability of greater value, P									
	0·975	0·900	0·750	0·500	0·250	0·100	0·050	0·025	0·010	0·001
1	—	0·02	0·10	0·45	1·32	2·71	3·84	5·02	6·63	10·83
2	0·05	0·21	0·58	1·39	2·77	4·61	5·99	7·38	9·21	13·82
3	0·22	0·58	1·21	2·37	4·11	6·25	7·81	9·35	11·34	16·27
4	0·48	1·06	1·92	3·36	5·39	7·78	9·49	11·14	13·28	18·47
5	0·83	1·61	2·67	4·35	6·63	9·24	11·07	12·83	15·09	20·52
6	1·24	2·20	3·45	5·35	7·84	10·64	12·59	14·45	16·81	22·46
7	1·69	2·83	4·25	6·35	9·04	12·02	14·07	16·01	18·48	24·32
8	2·18	3·49	5·07	7·34	10·22	13·36	15·51	17·53	20·09	26·12
9	2·70	4·17	5·90	8·34	11·39	14·68	16·92	19·02	21·67	27·88
10	3·25	4·87	6·74	9·34	12·55	15·99	18·31	20·48	23·21	29·59
11	3·82	5·58	7·58	10·34	13·70	17·28	19·68	21·92	24·72	31·26
12	4·40	6·30	8·44	11·34	14·85	18·55	21·03	23·34	26·22	32·91
13	5·01	7·04	9·30	12·34	15·98	19·81	22·36	24·74	27·69	34·53
14	5·63	7·79	10·17	13·34	17·12	21·06	23·68	26·12	29·14	36·12
15	6·27	8·55	11·04	14·34	18·25	22·31	25·00	27·49	30·58	37·70

16	6·91	9·31	11·91	15·34	19·37	23·54	26·30	28·85	32·00	39·25
17	7·56	10·09	12·79	16·34	20·49	24·77	27·59	30·19	33·41	40·79
18	8·23	10·86	13·68	17·34	21·60	25·99	28·87	31·53	34·81	42·31
19	8·91	11·65	14·56	18·34	22·72	27·20	30·14	32·85	36·19	43·82
20	9·59	12·44	15·45	19·34	23·83	28·41	31·41	34·17	37·57	45·32
21	10·28	13·24	16·34	20·34	24·93	29·62	32·67	35·48	38·93	46·80
22	10·98	14·04	17·24	21·34	26·04	30·81	33·92	36·78	40·29	48·27
23	11·69	14·85	18·14	22·34	27·14	32·01	35·17	38·08	41·64	49·73
24	12·40	15·66	19·04	23·34	28·24	33·20	36·42	39·36	42·98	51·18
25	13·12	16·47	19·94	24·34	29·34	34·38	37·65	40·65	44·31	52·62
26	13·84	17·29	20·84	25·34	30·43	35·56	38·89	41·92	45·64	54·05
27	14·57	18·11	21·75	26·34	31·53	36·74	40·11	43·19	46·96	55·48
28	15·31	18·94	22·66	27·34	32·62	37·92	41·34	44·46	48·28	56·89
29	16·05	19·77	23·57	28·34	33·71	39·09	42·56	45·72	49·59	58·30
30	16·79	20·60	24·48	29·34	34·80	40·26	43·77	46·98	50·89	59·70
40	24·43	29·05	33·66	39·34	45·62	51·80	55·76	59·34	63·69	73·40
50	32·36	37·69	42·94	49·33	56·33	63·17	67·50	71·42	76·15	86·66
60	40·48	46·46	52·29	59·33	66·98	74·40	79·08	83·30	88·38	99·61
70	48·76	55·33	61·70	69·33	77·58	85·53	90·53	95·02	100·42	112·32
80	57·15	64·28	71·14	79·33	88·13	96·58	101·88	106·63	112·33	124·84
90	65·65	73·29	80·62	89·33	98·64	107·56	113·14	118·14	124·12	137·21
100	74·22	82·36	90·13	99·33	109·14	118·50	124·34	129·56	135·81	149·45

Condensed from Table 8 of Pearson and Hartley (1966) by permission of the authors and publishers.

Table A3 Percentage points of the *t* distribution

The function tabulated is $t_{\nu, P}$, the value exceeded in both directions with probability P in a t distribution with ν degrees of freedom (the $100P$ percentage point)

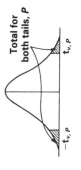

Total for both tails, P

$-t_{\nu, P}$ $t_{\nu, P}$

Degrees of freedom, ν	\multicolumn{13}{c}{Probability of greater value, P}
	0·9	0·8	0·7	0·6	0·5	0·4	0·3	0·2	0·1	0·05	0·02	0·01	0·001
1	0·158	0·325	0·510	0·727	1·000	1·376	1·963	3·078	6·314	12·706	31·821	63·657	636·619
2	0·142	0·289	0·445	0·617	0·816	1·061	1·386	1·886	2·920	4·303	6·965	9·925	31·598
3	0·137	0·277	0·424	0·584	0·765	0·978	1·250	1·638	2·353	3·182	4·541	5·841	12·924
4	0·134	0·271	0·414	0·569	0·741	0·941	1·190	1·533	2·132	2·776	3·747	4·604	8·610
5	0·132	0·267	0·408	0·559	0·727	0·920	1·156	1·476	2·015	2·571	3·365	4·032	6·869
6	0·131	0·265	0·404	0·553	0·718	0·906	1·134	1·440	1·943	2·447	3·143	3·707	5·959
7	0·130	0·263	0·402	0·549	0·711	0·896	1·119	1·415	1·895	2·365	2·998	3·499	5·408
8	0·130	0·262	0·399	0·546	0·706	0·889	1·108	1·397	1·860	2·306	2·896	3·355	5·041
9	0·129	0·261	0·398	0·543	0·703	0·883	1·100	1·383	1·833	2·262	2·821	3·250	4·781
10	0·129	0·260	0·397	0·542	0·700	0·879	1·093	1·372	1·812	2·228	2·764	3·169	4·587
11	0·129	0·260	0·396	0·540	0·697	0·876	1·088	1·363	1·796	2·201	2·718	3·106	4·437
12	0·128	0·259	0·395	0·539	0·695	0·873	1·083	1·356	1·782	2·179	2·681	3·055	4·318
13	0·128	0·259	0·394	0·538	0·694	0·870	1·079	1·350	1·771	2·160	2·650	3·012	4·221
14	0·128	0·258	0·393	0·537	0·692	0·868	1·076	1·345	1·761	2·145	2·624	2·977	4·140
15	0·128	0·258	0·393	0·536	0·691	0·866	1·074	1·341	1·753	2·131	2·602	2·947	4·073

df													
16	0·128	0·258	0·392	0·535	0·690	0·865	1·071	1·337	1·746	2·120	2·583	2·921	4·015
17	0·128	0·257	0·392	0·534	0·689	0·863	1·069	1·333	1·740	2·110	2·567	2·898	3·965
18	0·127	0·257	0·392	0·534	0·688	0·862	1·067	1·330	1·734	2·101	2·552	2·878	3·922
19	0·127	0·257	0·391	0·533	0·688	0·861	1·066	1·328	1·729	2·093	2·539	2·861	3·883
20	0·127	0·257	0·391	0·533	0·687	0·860	1·064	1·325	1·725	2·086	2·528	2·845	3·850
21	0·127	0·257	0·391	0·532	0·686	0·859	1·063	1·323	1·721	2·080	2·518	2·831	3·819
22	0·127	0·256	0·390	0·532	0·686	0·858	1·061	1·321	1·717	2·074	2·508	2·819	3·792
23	0·127	0·256	0·390	0·532	0·685	0·858	1·060	1·319	1·714	2·069	2·500	2·807	3·767
24	0·127	0·256	0·390	0·531	0·685	0·857	1·059	1·318	1·711	2·064	2·492	2·797	3·745
25	0·127	0·256	0·390	0·531	0·684	0·856	1·058	1·316	1·708	2·060	2·485	2·787	3·725
26	0·127	0·256	0·390	0·531	0·684	0·856	1·058	1·315	1·706	2·056	2·479	2·779	3·707
27	0·127	0·256	0·389	0·531	0·684	0·855	1·057	1·314	1·703	2·052	2·473	2·771	3·690
28	0·127	0·256	0·389	0·530	0·683	0·855	1·056	1·313	1·701	2·048	2·467	2·763	3·674
29	0·127	0·256	0·389	0·530	0·683	0·854	1·055	1·311	1·699	2·045	2·462	2·756	3·659
30	0·127	0·256	0·389	0·530	0·683	0·854	1·055	1·310	1·697	2·042	2·457	2·750	3·646
40	0·126	0·255	0·388	0·529	0·681	0·851	1·050	1·303	1·684	2·021	2·423	2·704	3·551
60	0·126	0·254	0·387	0·527	0·679	0·848	1·046	1·296	1·671	2·000	2·390	2·660	3·460
120	0·126	0·254	0·386	0·526	0·677	0·845	1·041	1·289	1·658	1·980	2·358	2·617	3·373
∞	0·126	0·253	0·385	0·524	0·674	0·842	1·036	1·282	1·645	1·960	2·326	2·576	3·291

Reproduced from Table III of Fisher and Yates (1963) by permission of the authors and publishers.

Table A4 Percentage points of the F distribution:
$P = 0.05, 0.025, 0.01, 0.005$

The function tabulated is F_{P, v_1, v_2}, the value exceeded with probability P in the F distribution with v_1 degrees of freedom for the numerator and v_2 degrees of freedom for the denominator (the $100P$ percentage point). The values for $P = 0.05$ and 0.01 are shown in bold type

F_{P, v_1, v_2}

		DF for numerator, v_1										
DF for denominator, v_2	P	1	2	3	4	5	6	7	8	12	24	∞
1	0·05	**161·4**	**199·5**	**215·7**	**224·6**	**230·2**	**234·0**	**236·8**	**238·9**	**243·9**	**249·1**	**254·3**
	0·025	647·8	799·5	864·2	899·6	921·8	937·1	948·2	956·7	976·7	997·2	1018
	0·01	**4052**	**5000**	**5403**	**5625**	**5764**	**5859**	**5928**	**5981**	**6106**	**6235**	**6366**
	0·005	16211	20000	21615	22500	23056	23437	23715	23925	24426	24940	25465
2	0·05	**18·51**	**19·00**	**19·16**	**19·25**	**19·30**	**19·33**	**19·35**	**19·37**	**19·41**	**19·45**	**19·50**
	0·025	38·51	39·00	39·17	39·25	39·30	39·33	39·36	39·37	39·41	39·46	39·50
	0·01	**98·50**	**99·00**	**99·17**	**99·25**	**99·30**	**99·33**	**99·36**	**99·37**	**99·42**	**99·46**	**99·50**
	0·005	198·5	199·0	199·2	199·2	199·3	199·3	199·4	199·4	199·4	199·5	199·5
3	0·05	**10·13**	**9·55**	**9·28**	**9·12**	**9·01**	**8·94**	**8·89**	**8·85**	**8·74**	**8·64**	**8·53**
	0·025	17·44	16·04	15·44	15·10	14·88	14·73	14·62	14·54	14·34	14·12	13·90
	0·01	**34·12**	**30·82**	**29·46**	**28·71**	**28·24**	**27·91**	**27·67**	**27·49**	**27·05**	**26·60**	**26·13**
	0·005	55·55	49·80	47·47	46·19	45·39	44·84	44·43	44·13	43·39	42·62	41·83
4	0·05	**7·71**	**6·94**	**6·59**	**6·39**	**6·26**	**6·16**	**6·09**	**6·04**	**5·91**	**5·77**	**5·63**
	0·025	12·22	10·65	9·98	9·60	9·36	9·20	9·07	8·98	8·75	8·51	8·26
	0·01	**21·20**	**18·00**	**16·69**	**15·98**	**15·52**	**15·21**	**14·98**	**14·80**	**14·37**	**13·93**	**13·46**
	0·005	31·33	26·28	24·26	23·15	22·46	21·97	21·62	21·35	20·70	20·03	19·32

5	0·05	6·61	5·79	5·41	5·19	5·05	4·95	4·88	4·82	4·68	4·53	4·36
	0·025	10·01	8·43	7·76	7·39	7·15	6·98	6·85	6·76	6·52	6·28	6·02
	0·01	16·26	13·27	12·06	11·39	10·97	10·67	10·46	10·29	9·89	9·47	9·02
	0·005	22·78	18·31	16·53	15·56	14·94	14·51	14·20	13·96	13·38	12·78	12·14
6	0·05	5·99	5·14	4·76	4·53	4·39	4·28	4·21	4·15	4·00	3·84	3·67
	0·025	8·81	7·26	6·60	6·23	5·99	5·82	5·70	5·60	5·37	5·12	4·85
	0·01	13·75	10·92	9·78	9·15	8·75	8·47	8·26	8·10	7·72	7·31	6·88
	0·005	18·63	14·54	12·92	12·03	11·46	11·07	10·79	10·57	10·03	9·47	8·88
7	0·05	5·59	4·74	4·35	4·12	3·97	3·87	3·79	3·73	3·57	3·41	3·23
	0·025	8·07	6·54	5·89	5·52	5·29	5·12	4·99	4·90	4·67	4·42	4·14
	0·01	12·25	9·55	8·45	7·85	7·46	7·19	6·99	6·84	6·47	6·07	5·65
	0·005	16·24	12·40	10·88	10·05	9·52	9·16	8·89	8·68	8·18	7·65	7·08
8	0·05	5·32	4·46	4·07	3·84	3·69	3·58	3·50	3·44	3·28	3·12	2·93
	0·025	7·57	6·06	5·42	5·05	4·82	4·65	4·53	4·43	4·20	3·95	3·67
	0·01	11·26	8·65	7·59	7·01	6·63	6·37	6·18	6·03	5·67	5·28	4·86
	0·005	14·69	11·04	9·60	8·81	8·30	7·95	7·69	7·50	7·01	6·50	5·95
9	0·05	5·12	4·26	3·86	3·63	3·48	3·37	3·29	3·23	3·07	2·90	2·71
	0·025	7·21	5·71	5·08	4·72	4·48	4·32	4·20	4·10	3·87	3·61	3·33
	0·01	10·56	8·02	6·99	6·42	6·06	5·80	5·61	5·47	5·11	4·73	4·31
	0·005	13·61	10·11	8·72	7·96	7·47	7·13	6·88	6·69	6·23	5·73	5·19
10	0·05	4·96	4·10	3·71	3·48	3·33	3·22	3·14	3·07	2·91	2·74	2·54
	0·025	6·94	5·46	4·83	4·47	4·24	4·07	3·95	3·85	3·62	3·37	3·08
	0·01	10·04	7·56	6·55	5·99	5·64	5·39	5·20	5·06	4·71	4·33	3·91
	0·005	12·83	9·43	8·08	7·34	6·87	6·54	6·30	6·12	5·66	5·17	4·64
12	0·05	4·75	3·89	3·49	3·26	3·11	3·00	2·91	2·85	2·69	2·51	2·30
	0·025	6·55	5·10	4·47	4·12	3·89	3·73	3·61	3·51	3·28	3·02	2·72
	0·01	9·33	6·93	5·95	5·41	5·06	4·82	4·64	4·50	4·16	3·78	3·36
	0·005	11·75	8·51	7·23	6·52	6·07	5·76	5·52	5·35	4·91	4·43	3·90

Contd on p. 568.

Table A4 (continued)

DF for denominator, v_2	P	DF for numerator, v_1										
		1	2	3	4	5	6	7	8	12	24	∞
14	0·05	4·60	3·74	3·34	3·11	2·96	2·85	2·76	2·70	2·53	2·35	2·13
	0·025	6·30	4·86	4·24	3·89	3·66	3·50	3·38	3·29	3·05	2·79	2·49
	0·01	8·86	6·51	5·56	5·04	4·69	4·46	4·28	4·14	3·80	3·43	3·00
	0·005	11·06	7·92	6·68	6·00	5·56	5·26	5·03	4·86	4·43	3·96	3·44
16	0·05	4·49	3·63	3·24	3·01	2·85	2·74	2·66	2·59	2·42	2·24	2·01
	0·025	6·12	4·69	4·08	3·73	3·50	3·34	3·22	3·12	2·89	2·63	2·32
	0·01	8·53	6·23	5·29	4·77	4·44	4·20	4·03	3·89	3·55	3·18	2·75
	0·005	10·58	7·51	6·30	5·64	5·21	4·91	4·69	4·52	4·10	3·64	3·11
18	0·05	4·41	3·55	3·16	2·93	2·77	2·66	2·58	2·51	2·34	2·15	1·92
	0·025	5·98	4·56	3·95	3·61	3·38	3·22	3·10	3·01	2·77	2·50	2·19
	0·01	8·29	6·01	5·09	4·58	4·25	4·01	3·84	3·71	3·37	3·00	2·57
	0·005	10·22	7·21	6·03	5·37	4·96	4·66	4·44	4·28	3·86	3·40	2·87
20	0·05	4·35	3·49	3·10	2·87	2·71	2·60	2·51	2·45	2·28	2·08	1·84
	0·025	5·87	4·46	3·86	3·51	3·29	3·13	3·01	2·91	2·68	2·41	2·09
	0·01	8·10	5·85	4·94	4·43	4·10	3·87	3·70	3·56	3·23	2·86	2·42
	0·005	9·94	6·99	5·82	5·17	4·76	4·47	4·26	4·09	3·68	3·22	2·69

v_2	α											
30	0·05	4·17	3·32	2·92	2·69	2·53	2·42	2·33	2·27	2·09	1·89	1·62
	0·025	5·57	4·18	3·59	3·25	3·03	2·87	2·75	2·65	2·41	2·14	1·79
	0·01	7·56	5·39	4·51	4·02	3·70	3·47	3·30	3·17	2·84	2·47	2·01
	0·005	9·18	6·35	5·24	4·62	4·23	3·95	3·74	3·58	3·18	2·73	2·18
40	0·05	4·08	3·23	2·84	2·61	2·45	2·34	2·25	2·18	2·00	1·79	1·51
	0·025	5·42	4·05	3·46	3·13	2·90	2·74	2·62	2·53	2·29	2·01	1·64
	0·01	7·31	5·18	4·31	3·83	3·51	3·29	3·12	2·99	2·66	2·29	1·80
	0·005	8·83	6·07	4·98	4·37	3·99	3·71	3·51	3·35	2·95	2·50	1·93
60	0·05	4·00	3·15	2·76	2·53	2·37	2·25	2·17	2·10	1·92	1·70	1·39
	0·025	5·29	3·93	3·34	3·01	2·79	2·63	2·51	2·41	2·17	1·88	1·48
	0·01	7·08	4·98	4·13	3·65	3·34	3·12	2·95	2·82	2·50	2·12	1·60
	0·005	8·49	5·79	4·73	4·14	3·76	3·49	3·29	3·13	2·74	2·29	1·69
120	0·05	3·92	3·07	2·68	2·45	2·29	2·17	2·09	2·02	1·83	1·61	1·25
	0·025	5·15	3·80	3·23	2·89	2·67	2·52	2·39	2·30	2·05	1·76	1·31
	0·01	6·85	4·79	3·95	3·48	3·17	2·96	2·79	2·66	2·34	1·95	1·38
	0·005	8·18	5·54	4·50	3·92	3·55	3·28	3·09	2·93	2·54	2·09	1·43
∞	0·05	3·84	3·00	2·60	2·37	2·21	2·10	2·01	1·94	1·75	1·52	1·00
	0·025	5·02	3·69	3·12	2·79	2·57	2·41	2·29	2·19	1·94	1·64	1·00
	0·01	6·63	4·61	3·78	3·32	3·02	2·80	2·64	2·51	2·18	1·79	1·00
	0·005	7·88	5·30	4·28	3·72	3·35	3·09	2·90	2·74	2·36	1·90	1·00

Condensed from Table 18 of Pearson and Hartley (1966) by permission of the authors and publishers.
For values of v_1 and v_2 not given, interpolation is approximately linear in the reciprocals of v_1 and v_2.

Table A5 Percentage points of the distribution of studentized range: $\alpha = 0.05, 0.01$

The function tabulated is $Q_{p,\alpha}$, the value exceeded with probability α in the distribution of studentized range, for p groups and f_2 DF within groups (the 100α percentage point). The values for $\alpha = 0.05$ are shown in bold type

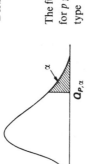

$Q_{P,\alpha}$

				Number of groups, p					
f_2	2	3	4	5	6	7	8	9	10
5	**3·64**	**4·60**	**5·22**	**5·67**	**6·03**	**6·33**	**6·58**	**6·80**	**6·99**
	5·70	6·98	7·80	8·42	8·91	9·32	9·67	9·97	10·24
6	**3·46**	**4·34**	**4·90**	**5·30**	**5·63**	**5·90**	**6·12**	**6·32**	**6·49**
	5·24	6·33	7·03	7·56	7·97	8·32	8·61	8·87	9·10
7	**3·34**	**4·16**	**4·68**	**5·06**	**5·36**	**5·61**	**5·82**	**6·00**	**6·16**
	4·95	5·92	6·54	7·01	7·37	7·68	7·94	8·17	8·37
8	**3·26**	**4·04**	**4·53**	**4·89**	**5·17**	**5·40**	**5·60**	**5·77**	**5·92**
	4·75	5·64	6·20	6·62	6·96	7·24	7·47	7·68	7·86
9	**3·20**	**3·95**	**4·41**	**4·76**	**5·02**	**5·24**	**5·43**	**5·59**	**5·74**
	4·60	5·43	5·96	6·35	6·66	6·91	7·13	7·33	7·49
10	**3·15**	**3·88**	**4·33**	**4·65**	**4·91**	**5·12**	**5·30**	**5·46**	**5·60**
	4·48	5·27	5·77	6·14	6·43	6·67	6·87	7·05	7·21
12	**3·08**	**3·77**	**4·20**	**4·51**	**4·75**	**4·95**	**5·12**	**5·27**	**5·39**
	4·32	5·05	5·50	5·84	6·10	6·32	6·51	6·67	6·81

ν									
14	**3·03** 4·21	**3·70** 4·89	**4·11** 5·32	**4·41** 5·63	**4·64** 5·88	**4·83** 6·08	**4·99** 6·26	**5·13** 6·41	**5·25** 6·54
16	**3·00** 4·13	**3·65** 4·79	**4·05** 5·19	**4·33** 5·49	**4·56** 5·72	**4·74** 5·92	**4·90** 6·08	**5·03** 6·22	**5·15** 6·35
18	**2·97** 4·07	**3·61** 4·70	**4·00** 5·09	**4·28** 5·38	**4·49** 5·60	**4·67** 5·79	**4·82** 5·94	**4·96** 6·08	**5·07** 6·20
20	**2·95** 4·02	**3·58** 4·64	**3·96** 5·02	**4·23** 5·29	**4·45** 5·51	**4·62** 5·69	**4·77** 5·84	**4·90** 5·97	**5·01** 6·09
30	**2·89** 3·89	**3·49** 4·45	**3·85** 4·80	**4·10** 5·05	**4·30** 5·24	**4·46** 5·40	**4·60** 5·54	**4·72** 5·65	**4·82** 5·76
40	**2·86** 3·82	**3·44** 4·37	**3·79** 4·70	**4·04** 4·93	**4·23** 5·11	**4·39** 5·26	**4·52** 5·39	**4·63** 5·50	**4·73** 5·60
60	**2·83** 3·76	**3·40** 4·28	**3·74** 4·59	**3·98** 4·82	**4·16** 4·99	**4·31** 5·13	**4·44** 5·25	**4·55** 5·36	**4·65** 5·45
120	**2·80** 3·70	**3·36** 4·20	**3·68** 4·50	**3·92** 4·71	**4·10** 4·87	**4·24** 5·01	**4·36** 5·12	**4·47** 5·21	**4·56** 5·30
∞	**2·77** 3·64	**3·31** 4·12	**3·63** 4·40	**3·86** 4·60	**4·03** 4·76	**4·17** 4·88	**4·29** 4·99	**4·39** 5·08	**4·47** 5·16

Condensed from Table 29 of Pearson and Hartley (1966) by permission of the authors and publishers.

Table A6 Random sampling numbers

I

03	47	43	73	86	36	96	47	36	61	46	98	63	71	62	33	26	16	80	45	60	11	14	10	95
97	74	24	67	62	42	81	14	57	20	42	53	32	37	32	27	07	36	07	51	24	51	79	89	73
16	76	62	27	66	56	50	26	71	07	32	90	79	78	53	13	55	38	58	59	88	97	54	14	10
12	56	85	99	26	96	96	68	27	31	05	03	72	93	15	57	12	10	14	21	88	26	49	81	76
55	59	56	35	64	38	54	82	46	22	31	62	43	09	90	06	18	44	32	53	23	83	01	30	30
16	22	77	94	39	49	54	43	54	82	17	37	93	23	78	87	35	20	96	43	84	26	34	91	64
84	42	17	53	31	57	24	55	06	88	77	04	74	47	67	21	76	33	50	25	83	92	12	06	76
63	01	63	78	59	16	95	55	67	19	98	10	50	71	75	12	86	73	58	07	44	39	52	38	79
33	21	12	34	29	78	64	56	07	82	52	42	07	44	38	15	51	00	13	42	99	66	02	79	54
57	60	86	32	44	09	47	27	96	54	49	17	46	09	62	90	52	84	77	27	08	02	73	43	28
18	18	07	92	46	44	17	16	58	09	79	83	86	19	62	06	76	50	03	10	55	23	64	05	05
26	62	38	97	75	84	16	07	44	99	83	11	46	32	24	20	14	85	88	45	10	93	72	88	71
23	42	40	64	74	82	97	77	77	81	07	45	32	14	08	32	98	94	07	72	93	85	79	10	75
52	36	28	19	95	50	92	26	11	97	00	56	76	31	38	80	22	02	53	53	86	60	42	04	53
37	85	94	35	12	83	39	50	08	30	42	34	07	96	88	54	42	06	87	98	35	85	29	48	39
70	29	17	12	13	40	33	20	38	26	13	89	51	03	74	17	76	37	13	04	07	74	21	19	30
56	62	18	37	35	96	83	50	87	75	97	12	25	93	47	70	33	24	03	54	97	77	46	44	80
99	49	57	22	77	88	42	95	45	72	16	64	36	16	00	04	43	18	66	79	94	77	24	21	90
16	08	15	04	72	33	27	14	34	09	45	59	34	68	49	12	72	07	34	45	99	27	72	95	14
31	16	93	32	43	50	27	89	87	19	20	15	37	00	49	52	85	66	60	44	38	68	88	11	80
68	34	30	13	70	55	74	30	77	40	44	22	78	84	26	04	33	46	09	52	68	07	97	06	57
74	57	25	65	76	59	29	97	68	60	71	91	38	67	54	13	58	18	24	76	15	54	55	95	52
27	42	37	86	53	48	55	90	65	72	96	57	69	36	10	96	46	92	42	45	97	60	49	04	91
00	39	68	29	61	66	37	32	20	30	77	84	57	03	29	10	45	65	04	26	11	04	96	67	24
29	94	98	94	24	68	49	69	10	82	53	75	91	93	30	34	25	20	57	27	40	48	73	51	92

31	38	98	32	62	66	80	59	30	33	74	51	48	94	43	83	23	17	34	60	49	47	88	87	33
03	30	95	08	89	11	95	44	13	17	70	09	29	16	39	30	70	49	72	65	66	38	94	67	76
37	94	50	84	26	00	74	38	93	74	05	77	24	67	39	74	32	14	10	54	31	13	39	61	00
02	45	75	51	55	16	52	37	95	67	91	05	56	44	29	96	99	17	99	62	07	94	80	04	89
02	38	02	48	27	57	07	49	47	02	52	58	29	94	15	02	25	97	18	82	45	53	35	16	90
68	86	16	62	85	90	08	90	36	62	83	93	16	74	50	99	07	20	60	12	04	31	60	37	32
29	30	56	91	48	37	22	43	49	89	06	16	63	85	01	36	36	89	48	29	04	46	05	70	69
21	90	53	74	43	20	12	82	16	78	78	29	92	55	27	27	18	43	12	57	80	54	44	07	30
47	70	92	01	52	83	98	33	54	78	56	51	95	17	08	95	02	41	30	35	94	31	89	48	37
60	76	16	40	00	76	22	59	39	40	59	06	44	32	13	44	07	13	24	90	74	08	72	02	94
74	02	91	41	91	68	86	55	08	06	77	15	12	42	55	26	39	88	76	09	82	28	83	49	36
71	34	04	81	53	09	14	93	31	75	59	99	11	67	06	96	18	45	03	03	19	86	24	22	38
00	37	45	66	82	65	41	62	33	10	51	62	08	50	63	94	02	48	33	59	93	46	27	82	78
19	94	78	75	86	05	27	60	02	90	03	71	32	10	78	41	93	47	81	37	77	62	03	32	85
67	02	79	87	34	11	52	07	04	01	92	61	73	42	26	12	96	10	35	45	09	33	05	39	55
12	66	38	50	13	86	90	19	02	20	13	64	54	70	41	72	12	96	68	36	91	79	21	49	90
11	74	26	01	49	95	05	75	14	93	15	99	47	80	22	50	33	69	68	41	00	94	22	42	06
64	19	51	97	33	71	88	02	40	15	85	42	66	78	36	61	23	49	73	28	33	53	97	75	03
62	09	32	38	44	05	73	96	51	06	35	98	87	37	59	41	52	04	99	58	80	81	82	95	00
83	06	33	42	96	64	75	33	97	15	22	09	54	58	87	71	23	31	31	94	98	73	73	22	39
59	06	20	38	47	14	11	00	90	79	60	23	85	53	75	71	19	69	68	90	37	43	48	14	00
66	75	16	86	91	67	45	18	73	97	70	88	85	65	68	58	21	55	81	05	74	39	77	18	70
82	94	10	16	25	40	84	51	78	58	93	10	86	61	52	77	59	52	50	38	57	04	13	80	23
90	27	24	23	96	67	90	05	46	19	26	97	71	99	65	53	26	23	20	25	50	22	79	75	96
16	11	35	38	31	66	14	68	20	64	05	07	68	26	14	17	90	41	60	91	34	85	09	88	90

Contd. on p. 574.

Table A6 (continued)

II

53	74	23	99	67	61	32	28	69	84	94	62	67	86	24	98	33	41	19	95	47	53	53	38	09
63	38	06	86	54	99	00	65	26	94	02	82	90	23	07	79	62	67	80	60	75	91	12	81	19
35	30	58	21	46	06	72	17	10	94	25	21	31	75	96	49	28	24	00	49	55	65	79	78	07
63	43	36	82	69	65	51	18	37	88	61	38	44	12	45	32	92	85	88	65	54	34	81	85	35
98	25	37	55	26	01	91	82	81	46	74	71	12	94	97	24	02	71	37	07	03	92	18	66	75
02	63	21	17	69	71	50	80	89	56	38	15	70	11	48	43	40	45	86	98	00	83	26	91	03
64	55	22	21	82	48	22	28	06	00	61	54	13	43	91	82	78	12	23	29	06	66	24	12	27
85	07	26	13	89	01	10	07	82	04	59	63	69	36	03	69	11	15	83	80	13	29	54	19	28
58	54	16	24	15	51	54	44	82	00	62	61	65	04	69	38	18	65	18	97	85	72	13	49	21
34	85	27	84	87	61	48	64	56	26	90	18	48	13	26	37	70	15	42	57	65	65	80	39	07
03	92	18	27	46	57	99	16	96	56	30	33	72	85	22	84	64	38	56	98	99	01	30	98	64
62	95	30	27	59	37	75	41	66	48	86	97	80	61	45	23	53	04	01	63	45	76	08	64	27
08	45	93	15	22	60	21	75	46	91	98	77	27	85	42	28	88	61	08	84	69	62	03	42	73
07	08	55	18	40	45	44	75	13	90	24	94	96	61	02	57	55	66	83	15	73	42	37	11	61
01	85	89	95	66	51	10	19	34	88	15	84	97	19	75	12	76	39	43	78	64	63	91	08	25
72	84	71	14	35	19	11	58	49	26	50	11	17	17	76	86	31	57	20	18	95	60	78	46	75
88	78	28	16	84	13	52	53	94	53	75	45	69	30	96	73	89	65	70	31	99	17	43	48	76
45	17	75	65	57	28	40	19	72	12	25	12	74	75	67	60	40	60	81	19	24	62	01	61	16
96	76	28	12	54	22	01	11	94	25	71	96	16	16	88	68	64	36	74	45	19	59	50	88	92
43	31	67	72	30	24	02	94	08	63	38	32	36	66	02	69	36	38	25	39	48	03	45	15	22
50	44	66	44	21	66	06	58	05	62	68	15	54	35	02	42	35	48	96	32	14	52	41	52	48
22	66	22	15	86	26	63	75	41	99	58	42	36	72	24	58	37	52	18	51	03	37	18	39	11
96	24	40	14	51	23	22	30	88	57	95	67	47	29	83	94	69	40	06	07	18	16	36	78	86
31	73	91	61	19	60	20	72	93	48	98	57	07	23	69	65	95	39	69	58	56	80	30	19	44
78	60	73	99	84	43	89	94	36	45	56	69	47	07	41	90	22	91	07	12	78	35	34	08	72

```
96 52 02 00 34   93 07 54 41 30   44 97 77 98 31   94 09 09 36 06   39 35 79 30 60
39 32 80 38 83   56 81 62 60 89   27 95 21 24 99   26 08 77 54 11   25 07 42 21 98
18 52 59 59 88   29 99 55 74 93   56 08 57 93 71   13 92 63 14 09   84 90 16 30 67
64 14 63 47 13   54 44 80 89 07   48 11 12 82 11   54 32 55 47 96   80 98 72 49 39
01 63 86 01 22   56 14 13 53 56   19 82 88 99 43   74 04 18 70 54   82 05 67 63 66

60 93 27 49 87   03 81 33 14 94   77 60 30 89 25   86 67 44 76 45   92 18 80 97 94
34 58 56 05 38   09 38 74 76 98   09 18 71 47 75   63 93 49 94 42   26 79 50 18 26
45 91 78 94 29   19 19 52 90 52   57 15 35 20 01   68 08 48 90 23   80 23 70 47 59
48 34 14 98 42   73 94 95 32 14   45 45 15 34 54   42 29 15 83 55   76 35 46 60 96
76 33 30 91 33   53 45 50 01 48   21 47 25 56 92   96 61 76 52 16   81 96 16 80 82

60 81 89 92 27   14 58 66 72 84   59 76 38 15 40   65 63 77 33 92   32 35 32 70 49
76 29 27 06 90   82 94 32 05 53   72 19 05 63 58   90 84 74 10 20   69 89 08 99 20
34 76 62 24 55   74 71 78 04 96   54 04 23 30 22   97 06 02 16 14   53 53 80 82 93
11 29 85 48 53   33 14 94 85 54   07 36 39 23 00   21 25 97 24 10   79 07 74 14 01
85 99 83 21 00   62 40 96 64 28   93 72 34 89 87   74 62 51 73 42   38 82 15 32 91

05 86 75 56 56   34 99 27 94 72   84 96 37 47 62   11 38 80 74 67   18 38 95 72 77
98 08 89 66 16   71 66 07 95 64   41 69 30 88 95   82 39 95 53 37   00 87 56 68 71
23 35 58 31 52   20 74 54 44 64   00 33 81 14 76   14 81 75 81 39   72 59 20 82 23
10 93 64 24 73   01 98 03 02 79   05 88 80 91 32   20 28 57 79 02   74 36 97 46 22
70 98 89 79 03   35 33 80 20 92   13 82 40 44 71   56 06 31 37 58   18 24 54 38 08

56 23 48 60 65   39 92 13 13 27   65 35 46 71 78   83 03 34 24 88   00 80 82 43 50
61 08 07 87 97   13 68 29 95 83   45 48 62 88 61   57 29 10 86 87   22 79 98 03 05
90 10 59 83 68   29 32 70 67 13   08 43 71 30 10   36 92 50 38 23   95 60 62 89 73
37 67 28 15 19   81 86 91 71 66   96 83 60 17 69   93 30 29 31 01   33 84 40 31 59
84 36 07 10 55   53 51 35 37 93   02 49 84 18 79   75 38 51 21 29   95 90 46 20 71
```

Reproduced from Table XXXIII of Fisher and Yates (1963) by permission of the authors and publishers.

Notes on the use of random sampling numbers (Table A6)

1 Random permutation

This is a rearrangement of the integers from 1 to n, each order being equally likely to be chosen.

Start at an arbitrary point in the table. Use as many columns in the table as there are digits in n (e.g. if $n = 16$ use two columns). Go down the columns and continue to the next group of columns, writing down the numbers from 1 to n as they occur. Count 03 as 3, etc. Ignore 00, $n + 1$, $n + 2$, . . . , 99. Ignore repetitions.

Direct tables are published, e.g. in Fisher and Yates (1963), Cochran and Cox (1957) and Cox (1958). For $n > 20$ see Moses and Oakford (1963).

2 Random selection of sample of size n from population of size N

Number the members of the population from 1 to N, start to make a random permutation of N and stop as soon as n numbers have been selected. These form the required sample.

3 Random allocation

To allocate n individuals randomly to k groups (e.g. in experimental design), form a random permutation of n and divide these from left to right into groups of the appropriate size. The permutation need not be continued beyond the stage at which $k - 1$ groups have been formed, since the remaining individuals must fall into the kth group.

4 Random allocation with serial entry

Here n may be unknown. If allocation is to two treatments with equal probability, use odd and even numbers. For three treatments use 1–3, 4–6, 7–9, ignoring 0; and so on.

5 Restricted randomization (permuted blocks) with serial entry

It may be desirable to ensure that numbers allocated to different treatments are equal at various stages; e.g. two treatments may have to be balanced after each set of 10 individuals. In this case select five individuals out of each set of 10 to be allocated to one treatment (as in §2); the other five are allocated to the other treatment.

6 Extended use of tables

The tables can be used by reading entries in different directions, e.g. along the rows. If several random selections are needed in any investigation, different parts of the table should be used. More extensive tables are given in various books, e.g. Fisher and Yates (1963).

7 Use of computers

Most microcomputers, and many calculators, have random number generators which provide random numbers in various formats (e.g. single digits or pairs of digits). These can be used as a direct substitute for the table entries.

Table A7 Percentage points for the Wilcoxon signed rank sum test

The function tabulated is the critical value for the smaller of the signed rank sums, T_+ and T_-. An observed value equal to or less than the tabulated value is significant at the two-sided significance level shown (the actual tail-area probability being less than or equal to the nominal value shown). If ties are present, the result is somewhat more significant than is indicated here

Sample size, n' (excluding zero differences)	Two-sided significance level	
	0·05	0·01
6	0	—
7	2	—
8	3	0
9	5	1
10	8	3
11	10	5
12	13	7
13	17	9
14	21	12
15	25	15
16	29	19
17	34	23
18	40	27
19	46	32
20	52	37
21	58	42
22	66	48
23	73	54
24	81	61
25	89	68

Condensed from Table H of Lehmann (1975), and the Geigy Scientific Tables (1982), by permission of the authors and publishers.

Table A8 Percentage points for the Wilcoxon two-sample rank sum test

Define n_1 as the smaller of the two sample sizes ($n_1 \le n_2$). Calculate T_1 as the sum of the ranks in sample 1, and $\mathrm{E}(T_1) = \frac{1}{2} n_1 (n_1 + n_2 + 1)$. Calculate T' as T_1 if $T_1 \le \mathrm{E}(T_1)$ and as $n_1(n_1 + n_2 + 1) - T_1$ if $T_1 > \mathrm{E}(T_1)$. The result is significant at the two-sided 5% (or 1%) level of T' is less than or equal to the upper (or lower) tabulated value (the actual tail-area probability being less than or equal to the nominal value). If ties are present, the result is somewhat more significant than is indicated here

		Smaller sample size, n_1											
n_2	P	4	5	6	7	8	9	10	11	12	13	14	15
4	0·05	10											
	0·01	—											
5	0·05	11	17										
	0·01	—	15										
6	0·05	12	18	26									
	0·01	10	16	23									
7	0·05	13	20	27	36								
	0·01	10	16	24	32								
8	0·05	14	21	29	38	49							
	0·01	11	17	25	34	43							
9	0·05	14	22	31	40	51	62						
	0·01	11	18	26	35	45	56						
10	0·05	15	23	32	42	53	65	78					
	0·01	12	19	27	37	47	58	71					
11	0·05	16	24	34	44	55	68	81	96				
	0·01	12	20	28	38	49	61	73	87				
12	0·05	17	26	35	46	58	71	84	99	115			
	0·01	13	21	30	40	51	63	76	90	105			
13	0·05	18	27	37	48	60	73	88	103	119	136		
	0·01	13	22	31	41	53	65	79	93	109	125		
14	0·05	19	28	38	50	62	76	91	106	123	141	160	
	0·01	14	22	32	43	54	67	81	96	112	129	147	
15	0·05	20	29	40	52	65	79	94	110	127	145	164	184
	0·01	15	23	33	44	56	69	84	99	115	133	151	171

Condensed from the Geigy Scientific Tables (1982) by permission of the authors and publishers.

Table A9 Sample size for comparing two proportions

This table is used to determine the sample size necessary to find a significant difference (5% two-sided significance level) between two proportions estimated from independent samples where the true proportions are π_1 and π_2 and $\delta = \pi_1 - \pi_2$ is the specified difference ($\pi_1 > \pi_2$). Sample sizes are given for 90% power (upper value of pair) and 80% power (lower value). The sample size given in the table refers to *each* of the two independent samples. The table is derived using (6.10) with a continuity correction

Note: If $\pi_2 > 0.5$, work with $\pi_1' = 1 - \pi_2$ and $\pi_2' = 1 - \pi_1$.

Smaller probability, π_2	$\delta = \pi_1 - \pi_2$									
	0·05	0·1	0·15	0·2	0·25	0·3	0·35	0·4	0·45	0·5
0·05	621	207	113	75	54	42	33	27	23	19
	475	160	88	59	43	33	27	22	19	16
0·1	958	286	146	92	65	48	38	30	25	21
	726	219	113	72	51	38	30	24	20	17
0·15	1252	354	174	106	73	54	41	33	27	22
	946	270	134	82	57	42	33	26	21	18
0·2	1504	412	198	118	80	58	44	34	28	23
	1134	313	151	91	62	45	35	27	22	18
0·25	1714	459	216	127	85	61	46	35	28	23
	1291	349	165	98	66	47	36	28	23	18
0·3	1883	496	230	134	88	62	46	36	28	23
	1417	376	176	103	68	49	36	28	23	18
0·35	2009	522	240	138	90	63	46	35	28	22
	1511	396	183	106	69	49	36	28	22	18
0·4	2093	538	244	139	90	62	46	34	27	21
	1574	407	186	107	69	49	36	27	21	17
0·45	2135	543	244	138	88	61	44	33	25	19
	1605	411	186	106	68	47	35	26	20	16
0·5	2135	538	240	134	85	58	41	30	23	18
	1605	407	183	103	66	45	33	24	19	15

Table A10 Sample size table for detecting relative risk in case–control study

This table is used to determine the sample size necessary to find the odds ratio statistically significant (5% two-sided test) in a case–control study with an equal number of cases and controls. The specified odds ratio is denoted by OR, and p is the proportion of controls that are expected to be exposed. For each pair of values the upper figure is for a power of 90% and the lower for a power of 80%. The tabulated sample size refers to the number of *cases* required. The table is derived using (6.13) and (6.10) with a continuity correction

Note: If $p > 0.5$, work with $p' = 1 - p$ and $OR' = 1/OR$.

Proportion of controls exposed, p	OR (odds ratio)							
	0·5	1·5	2·0	2·5	3·0	4·0	5·0	10·0
0·05	1369	2347	734	393	259	150	105	43
	1044	1775	560	301	200	117	82	34
0·1	701	1266	402	219	146	87	62	27
	534	958	307	168	113	68	48	22
0·15	479	913	295	163	110	67	48	23
	366	691	225	125	85	52	38	19
0·2	370	743	244	136	93	58	43	21
	282	562	187	105	72	45	34	17
0·25	306	647	216	122	85	53	40	21
	233	490	165	94	66	42	32	17
0·3	264	590	200	115	80	51	39	22
	202	447	153	88	62	40	31	18
0·35	236	556	192	111	79	51	39	23
	180	421	147	86	61	40	31	18
0·4	216	538	188	111	79	52	41	24
	165	407	144	85	61	41	32	20
0·45	203	533	189	112	81	54	43	26
	155	403	145	87	63	43	34	21
0·5	194	538	194	116	85	58	46	29
	148	407	148	90	66	45	36	23

References

Acheson E. D. (1967) *Medical Record Linkage*. London: Oxford University Press.

Agresti A. (1989) A survey of models for repeated ordered categorical response data. *Stat. Med.* **8**, 1209–1224.

Agresti A. (1990) *Categorical Data Analysis*. New York: Wiley.

AIH National Perinatal Statistics Unit and Fertility Society of Australia (1991) *Assisted Conception—Australia and New Zealand 1989*. Sydney: AIH NPSU.

Aitken M., Anderson D., Francis B. and Hinde J. (1989) *Statistical Modelling in GLIM*. Oxford: Clarendon Press.

Alderson M. (1983) *An Introduction to Epidemiology*, 2nd edn. London: Macmillan.

Altman D. G. (1991) *Practical Statistics for Medical Research*. London: Chapman and Hall.

Alvey N., Galwey N. and Lane P. (1982) *An Introduction to Genstat*. London and New York: Academic Press.

Antiplatelet Trialists' Collaboration (1988) Secondary prevention of vascular disease by prolonged antiplatelet treatment. *Br. Med. J.* **296**, 320–331.

Armitage P. (1955) Tests for linear trends in proportions and frequencies. *Biometrics* **11**, 375–386.

Armitage P. (1957) Studies in the variability of pock counts. *J. Hyg., Camb.* **55**, 564–581.

Armitage P. (1975) *Sequential Medical Trials*, 2nd edn. Oxford: Blackwell Scientific Publications.

Armitage P. (1988) Some aspects of phase-III trials. In *Clinical Trials and Related Topics*, ed T. Okuno, pp. 1–16. Amsterdam: Excerpta Medica.

Armitage P. and Hills M. (1982) The two-period crossover trial. *Statistician* **31**, 119–131.

Armitage P. and Schneiderman M. A. (1958) Statistical problems in a mass screening program. *Ann. N.Y. Acad. Sci.* **76**, 896–908.

Armitage P., McPherson C. K. and Copas J. C. (1969) Statistical studies of prognosis in advanced breast cancer. *J. Chron. Dis.* **22**, 343–360.

Atkinson A. C. (1985) *Plots, Transformations, and Regression*. Oxford: Clarendon.

Australian Institute of Health and Welfare (1992) *Dapsone Exposure, Vietnam Service and Cancer Incidence*. Canberra: Commonwealth of Australia.

Babbie E. R. (1989). *The Practice of Social Research*, 5th edn. Belmont, California: Wadsworth.

Bacharach A. L., Chance M. R. A. and Middleton T. R. (1940) The biological assay of testicular diffusing factor. *Biochem. J.* **34**, 1464–1471.

Bailar J. C. and Ederer F. (1964) Significance factors for the ratio of a Poisson variable to its expectation. *Biometrics* **20**, 639–643.

Bailey N. T. J. (1961) *The Mathematical Theory of Genetic Linkage*. Oxford: Clarendon Press.

Bailey N. T. J. (1975) *The Mathematical Theory of Infectious Diseases and its Applications*, 2nd edn. London: Griffin.

Bailey N. T. J. (1977) *Mathematics, Statistics and Systems for Health*. New York: Wiley.

Baptista J. and Pike M. C. (1977) Exact two-sided confidence limits for the odds ratio in a 2×2 table. *Appl. Stat.* **26**, 214–220.

Barnard G. A. (1989) On alleged gains in power from lower P-values. *Stat. Med.* **8**, 1469–1477.

Barnett V. and Lewis T. (1984) *Outliers in Statistical Data*, 2nd edn. Chichester: Wiley.

Bartko J. J. (1966) The intraclass correlation coefficient as a measure of reliability. *Psychol. Rep.* **19**, 3–11.

Bartlett M. S. (1937) Properties of sufficiency and statistical tests. *Proc. R. Soc. A* **160**, 268–282.

Becker N. G. (1989) *The Analysis of Infectious Disease Data*. London: Chapman and Hall.

Belsley D. A., Kuh E. and Welsch R. E. (1980) *Regression Diagnostics: Identifying Influential Data and Sources of Collinearity*. New York: Wiley.

Benjamin B. (1968) *Health and Vital Statistics*. London: Allen and Unwin.

Bergen J., Kitchin R. and Berry G. (1992) Predictors of the course of tardive dyskinesia in patients receiving neuroleptics. *Biol. Psychiatry* **32**, 580–594.

Berkson J. (1944) Application of the logistic function to bio-assay. *J. Am. Stat. Ass.* **39**, 357–365.

Berkson J. (1950) Are there two regressions? *J. Am. Stat. Ass.* **45**, 164–180.

Berkson J. and Gage R. P. (1950) Calculation of survival rates for cancer. *Proc. Staff Meet. Mayo Clin.* **25**, 270–286.

Berlin J. A., Laird N. M., Sacks H. S. and Chalmers T. C. (1989) A comparison of statistical methods for combining event rates from clinical trials. *Stat. Med.* **8**, 141–151.

Berry D. A. (1987a) Statistical inference, designing clinical trials, and pharmaceutical company decisions. *Statistician* **36**, 181–189.

Berry D. A. (1987b) Interim analysis in clinical research. *Cancer Invest.* **5**, 469–477.

Berry G. (1983) The analysis of mortality by the subject-years method. *Biometrics* **39**, 173–184.

Berry G. (1986, 1988) Statistical significance and confidence intervals. *Med. J. Aust.* **144**, 618–619; reprinted in *Br. J. Clin. Pract.* **42**, 465–468.

Berry G., Kitchin R. M. and Mock P. A. (1991) A comparison of two simple hazard ratio estimators based on the logrank test. *Stat. Med.* **10**, 749–755.

Bliss C. I. (1958) *Periodic Regression in Biology and Climatology*, Bull. No. 615. New Haven: Connecticut Agricultural Experimental Station.

Boardman T. J. (1974) Confidence intervals for variance components—a comparative Monte Carlo study. *Biometrics* **30**, 251–262.

Box G. E. P. (1954) Some theorems on quadratic forms applied in the study of analysis of variance problems. II. Effects of inequality of variance and of correlation between errors in the two-way classification. *Ann. Math. Stat.* **25**, 484–498.

Box G. E. P. and Cox D. R. (1964) An analysis of transformations (with Discussion). *J. R. Stat. Soc.* B **26**, 211–252.

Box G. E. P. and Jenkins G. M. (1976) *Time Series Analysis: Forecasting and Control*, revised edn. San Francisco: Holden-Day.

Box G. E. P. and Tiao G. C. (1973) *Bayesian Inference in Statistical Analysis*. Reading, Massachusetts: Addison-Wesley.

Bradley R. A., Katti S. K. and Coons I. J. (1962) Optimal scaling for ordered categories. *Psychometrika* **27**, 355–374.

Breslow N. E. (1974) Covariance analysis of censored survival data. *Biometrics* **30**, 89–99.

Breslow N. E. (1984) Elementary methods of cohort analysis. *Int. J. Epidemiol.* **13**, 112–115.

Breslow N. (1990) Biostatistics and Bayes (with Discussion). *Stat. Sci.* **5**, 269–298.

Breslow N. and Day N. E. (1980) *Statistical Methods in Cancer Research, Volume 1—The Analysis of Case–Control Studies*. Scientific Publications No. 32. Lyon: International Agency for Research on Cancer.

Breslow N. E. and Day N. E. (1987) *Statistical Methods in Cancer Research, Volume 2—The Design and Analysis of Cohort Studies*. Scientific Publications No. 82. Lyon: International Agency for Research on Cancer.

Breslow N. E. and Liang K. Y. (1982) The variance of the Mantel–Haenszel estimator. *Biometrics* **38**, 943–952.

Brown A., Mohamed S. D., Montgomery R. D., Armitage P. and Laurence D. R. (1960). Value of a large dose of antitoxin in clinical tetanus. *Lancet* **ii**, 227–230.

Brown C. C. (1982) On a goodness of fit test for the logistic model based on score statistics. *Commun. Stat.-Theor. Meth.* **11**, 1087–1105.

Brown M. B. (1992) A test for the difference between two treatments in a continuous measure of outcome when there are dropouts. *Cont. Clin. Trials* **13**, 213–225.

Buck A. A. and Gart J. J. (1966) Comparison of a screening test and a reference test in epidemiologic studies. I. Indices of agreement and their relation to prevalence. *Am. J. Epidemiol.* **83**, 586–592.

Bulmer M. G. (1980) *The Mathematical Theory of Quantitative Genetics.* Oxford: Oxford University Press.

Buyse M. E., Staquet M. J. and Sylvester R. J. (eds) (1984) *Cancer Clinical Trials: Methods and Practice.* Oxford: Oxford University Press.

Byar D. P. (1983) Analysis of survival data: Cox and Weibull models with covariates. In *Statistics in Medical Research: Methods and Issues with Applications in Cancer Research*, eds V. Miké and K. Stanley, pp. 365–401. New York: Wiley.

Casagrande J. T., Pike M. C. and Smith P. G. (1978) The power function of the 'exact' test for comparing two binomial distributions. *Appl. Stat.* **27**, 176–180.

Chalmers T. C., Berrier J., Sacks H. S., Levin H., Reitman D. and Nagalingan R. (1987) Meta-analysis of clinical trials as a scientific discipline. II: Replicate variability and comparison of studies that agree and disagree. *Stat. Med.* **6**, 733–744.

Chatfield, C. (1989) *The Analysis of Time Series: An Introduction*, 4th edn. London: Chapman and Hall.

Chatfield C. and Collins A. J. (1980) *Introduction to Multivariate Analysis.* London: Chapman and Hall.

Checkoway H., Heyer N. J., Demers P. A. and Breslow N. E. (1993) Mortality among workers in the diatomaceous earth industry. *Br. J. Ind. Med.* **50**, 586–597.

Chen C.-H. and Wang P. C. (1991) Diagnostic plots in Cox's regression model. *Biometrics* **47**, 841–850.

Chiang C. L. (1984) *The Life Table and its Applications.* Malabar, Florida: Krieger.

Clayton D. G. (1991) A Monte Carlo method for Bayesian inference in frailty models. *Biometrics* **47**, 467–485.

Clayton D. and Cuzick J. (1985) Multivariate generalizations of the proportional hazards model (with Discussion). *J. R. Stat. Soc. A.* **148**, 82–117.

Clayton D. and Kaldor J. (1987) Empirical Bayes estimates of age-standardized relative risks for use in disease mapping. *Biometrics* **43**, 671–681.

Cochran W. G. (1954) Some methods for strengthening the common χ^2 tests. *Biometrics* **10**, 417–451.

Cochran W. G. (1977) *Sampling Techniques*, 3rd edn. New York: Wiley.

Cochran W. G. and Cox G. M. (1957) *Experimental Designs*, 2nd edn. New York: Wiley.

Cochrane A. L. (1972) *Effectiveness and Efficiency: Random Reflections on Health Services.* London: Nuffield Provincial Hospitals Trust.

Cockburn R., Beltonn R., Purvis R. J., Giles M. M., Brown J. K., Turner T. L., Wilkinson E. M., Forfar J. O., Barrie W. J. M., McKay G. S. and Pocock S. J. (1980) Maternal vitamin D intake and mineral metabolism in mothers and their newborn infants. *Br. Med. J.* **281**, 11–14.

Cockcroft A., Edwards J., Bevan C., Campbell I., Collins G., Houston K., Jenkins D., Latham S., Saunders M. and Trotman D. (1981) An investigation of operating theatre staff exposed to humidifier fever antigens. *Br. J. Ind. Med.* **38**, 144–151.

Cockcroft A., Berry G., Brown E. B. and Exall C. (1982) Psychological changes during a controlled trial of rehabilitation in chronic respiratory disability. *Thorax* **37**, 413–416.

Cody R. P. and Smith J. K. (1991) *Applied Statistics and the SAS Programming Language*, 3rd edn. New York: North-Holland.

Cohen J. (1960) A coefficient of agreement for nominal scales. *Educ. Psychol. Meas.* **20**, 37–46.

Cohen J. (1968) Weighted kappa: nominal scale agreement with provision for scale disagreement or partial credit. *Psychol. Bull.* **70**, 213–220.

Cole T. J., Morley C. J., Thornton A. J. and Fowler M. A. (1991) A scoring system to quantify illness in babies under 6 months of age. *J. R. Stat. Soc. A* **154**, 287–304.

Coleman M., Douglas A., Hermon C. and Peto J. (1986) Cohort study analysis with a FORTRAN computer program. *Int. J. Epidemiol.* **15**, 134–137.

Collins R. L. and Meckler R. J. (1965) Histology and weight of the mouse adrenal: a diallel genetic study. *J. Endocrinol.* **31**, 95–105.

Computing Resource Center (1992) *Stata Reference Manual: Release 3*, 5th edn. Santa Monica, California: Computing Resource Center.

Connor R. J. (1987) Sample size for testing differences in proportions for the paired-sample design. *Biometrics* **43**, 207–211.

Conover W. J. (1980) *Practical Nonparametric Statistics*, 2nd edn. New York: Wiley.

Cook P., Doll R. and Fellingham S. A. (1969) A mathematical model for the age distribution of cancer in man. *Int. J. Cancer* **4**, 93–112.

Cook R. D. (1977) Detection of influential observations in linear regression. *Technometrics* **19**, 15–18.

Cook R. D. and Weisberg S. (1982) *Residuals and Influence in Regression*. New York and London: Chapman and Hall.

Cookson W. O. C. M., de Klerk N. H., Musk A. W., Armstrong B. K., Glancy J. J. and Hobbs M. S. T. (1986) Prevalence of radiographic asbestosis in crocidolite miners and millers at Wittenoom, Western Australia. *Br. J. Ind. Med.* **43**, 450–457.

Cornfield J. (1956) A statistical property arising from retrospective studies. *Proc. Third Berkeley Symp. Math. Stat. Prob.* **4**, 135–148.

Cox D. R. (1958) *Planning of Experiments*. New York: Wiley.

Cox D. R. (1972) Regression models and life-tables (with Discussion). *J. R. Stat. Soc. B* **34**, 187–220.

Cox D. R. and Oakes D. (1984) *Analysis of Survival Data*. London: Chapman and Hall.

Cox D. R. and Snell E. J. (1989) *Analysis of Binary Data*, 2nd edn. London: Chapman and Hall.

Cramér H. (1946) *Mathematical Methods of Statistics*. Princeton: Princeton University Press.

Cutler S. J. and Ederer F. (1958) Maximum utilization of the life table method in analysing survival. *J. Chron. Dis.* **8**, 699–712.

Cuzick J. and Edwards R. (1990) Spatial clustering for inhomogeneous populations (with Discussion). *J. R. Stat. Soc. B* **52**, 73–104.

CYTEL Software Corporation (1991) *StatXact—Statistical Software for Exact Nonparametric Inference, User Manual Version* 2. Cambridge, Massachusetts: CYTEL Software Corporation.

Daniel C. (1959) Use of half-normal plots in interpreting factorial two-level experiments. *Technometrics* **1**, 311–341.

Darby S. C. and Fearn T. (1979) The Chatham Blood Pressure Study. An application of Bayesian growth curve models to a longitudinal study of blood pressure in children. *Int. J. Epidemiol.* **8**, 15–21.

Darby S. C. and Reissland J. A. (1981) Low levels of ionizing radiation and cancer—are we underestimating the risk? (with Discussion). *J. R. Stat. Soc. A* **144**, 298–331.

David F. N. and Barton D. E. (1966) Two space–time interaction tests for epidemicity. *Br. J. Prev. Soc. Med.* **20**, 44–48.

Day N. E. and Walter S. D. (1984) Simplified models of screening for chronic disease: estimation procedures from mass screening programmes. *Biometrics* **40**, 1–14.

Dean A. G., Dean J. A., Burton A. H. and Dicker R. C. (1990) *Epi Info, Version 5: a Word Processing, Database, and Statistics Program for Epidemiology on Microcomputers*. Stone Mountain, Georgia: USD, Incorporated.

DerSimonian R. and Laird N. (1986) Meta-analysis in clinical trials. *Cont. Clin. Trials* **7**, 177–188.

Diamond E. L. and Lilienfeld A. M. (1962a) Effects of errors in classification and diagnosis in various types of epidemiological studies. *Am. J. Public Health* **52**, 1137–1144.

Diamond E. L. and Lilienfeld A. M. (1962b) Misclassification errors in 2×2 tables with one margin fixed: some further comments. *Am. J. Public Health* **52**, 2106–2110.

Diggle P. J. (1990) *Time Series—A Biostatistical Introduction*. Oxford: Clarendon Press.

Dixon W. J. (chief ed.) (1990) *BMDP Statistical Software Manual, Volumes 1 & 2*. Los Angeles: University of California Press.

Dobson A. J. (1990) *An Introduction to Generalized Linear Models*. London: Chapman and Hall.

Dobson A. J., Kuulasmaa K., Eberle E. and Scherer J. (1991) Confidence intervals for weighted sums of Poisson parameters. *Stat. Med.* **10**, 457–462.

Doll R. (1952) The causes of death among gas-workers with special reference to cancer of the lung. *Br. J. Ind. Med.* **9**, 180–185.

Doll R. and Hill A. Bradford (1950) Smoking and carcinoma of the lung. Preliminary report. *Br. Med. J.* **ii**, 739–748.

Doll R. and Hill A. Bradford (1954) The mortality of doctors in relation to their smoking habits. A preliminary report. *Br. Med. J.* **i**, 1451–1455.

Doll R. and Hill A. Bradford (1956) Lung cancer and other causes of death in relation to smoking. A second report on the mortality of British doctors. *Br. Med. J.* **ii**, 1071–1081.

Doll R. and Hill A. Bradford (1964) Mortality in relation to smoking: ten years' observations of British doctors. *Br. Med. J.* **i**, 1399–1410, 1460–1467.

Doll R. and Peto R. (1976) Mortality in relation to smoking: 20 years' observations on male British doctors. *Br. Med. J.* **ii**, 1525–1536.

Doll R. and Pygott F. (1952) Factors influencing the rate of healing of gastric ulcers: admission to hospital, phenobarbitone, and ascorbic acid. *Lancet* **i**, 171–175.

Donner A. (1984) Approaches to sample size estimation in the design of clinical trials—a review. *Stat. Med.* **3**, 199–214.

Draper N. R. and Smith H. (1981) *Applied Regression Analysis*, 2nd edn. New York: Wiley.

Dyke G. V. and Patterson H. D. (1952) Analysis of factorial arrangements when the data are proportions. *Biometrics* **8**, 1–12.

Early Breast Cancer Trialists' Collaborative Group (1990) *Treatment of Early Breast Cancer, Vol 1: Worldwide Evidence 1985–1990*. Oxford: Oxford University Press.

Early Breast Cancer Trialists' Collaborative Group (1992) Systemic treatment of early breast cancer by hormonal, cytotoxic, or immune therapy. *Lancet* **339**, 1–15, 71–85.

Ederer F., Myers M. H. and Mantel N. (1964) A statistical problem in space and time: do leukemia cases come in clusters? *Biometrics* **20**, 626–638.

Edwards J. H. (1961) The recognition and estimation of cyclical trends. *Ann. Hum. Genet.* **25**, 83–86.

Ehrenberg A. S. C. (1968) The elements of lawlike relationships. *J. R. Stat. Soc. A.* **131**, 280–302.

Ehrenberg A. S. C. (1975) *Data Reduction*. London: Wiley.

Ehrenberg A. S. C. (1977) Rudiments of numeracy. *J. R. Stat. Soc. A* **140**, 277–297.

Ellery C., MacLennan R., Berry G. and Shearman R. P. (1986) A case–control study of breast cancer in relation to the use of steroid contraceptive agents. *Med. J. Aust.* **144**, 173–176.

Elwood J. M. (1988) *Causal Relationships in Medicine: A Practical System for Critical Appraisal*. Oxford: Oxford University Press.

Everitt B. (1980) *Cluster Analysis*, 2nd edn. London: Heinemann.

Fienberg S. E. (1980) *The Analysis of Cross-Classified Categorical Data*, 2nd edn. Cambridge, Massachusetts: MIT Press.

Finkelstein D. M. (1986) A proportional hazards model for interval-censored failure time data. *Biometrics* **42**, 845–854.

Finney D. J. (1971) *Probit Analysis*, 3rd edn. Cambridge: Cambridge University Press.

Finney D. J. (1978) *Statistical Method in Biological Assay*, 3rd edn. London: Griffin.

Finney D. J. (1979) The computation of results from radioimmunoassays. *Meth. Inf. Med.* **18**, 164–171.

Finney D. J., Latscha R., Bennett B. M. and Hsu P. (1963) *Tables for Testing Significance in a 2 × 2 Contingency Table*. Cambridge: Cambridge University Press.

Fisher R. A. (1950, 1964) The significance of deviations from expectation in a Poisson series. *Biometrics* **6**, 17–24; reprinted in **20**, 265–272.

Fisher R. A. and Yates F. (1963) *Statistical Tables for Biological, Agricultural and Medical Research*, 6th edn. Edinburgh: Oliver and Boyd.

Fleiss J. L. (1975) Measuring agreement between two judges on the presence or absence of a trait. *Biometrics* **31**, 651–659.

Fleiss J. L. (1981) *Statistical Methods for Rates and Proportions*, 2nd edn. New York: Wiley.

Fleiss J. L., Tytun A. and Ury H. K. (1980) A simple approximation for calculating sample sizes for comparing independent proportions. *Biometrics* **36**, 343–346.

Francis B., Green M. and Payne C. (eds) (1993) *The GLIM System: Release 4 Manual*. Oxford: Oxford University Press.

Fraser P. M. and Franklin D. A. (1974) Mathematical models for the diagnosis of liver disease. Problems arising in the use of conditional probability theory. *Quart. J. Med.* **43**, 73–88.

Freedman L. S. (1982) Tables of the number of patients required in clinical trials using the logrank test. *Stat. Med.* **1**, 121–129.

Freedman L. S., Lowe D. and Macaskill P. (1984) Stopping rules for clinical trials incorporating clinical opinion. *Biometrics* **40**, 575–586.

Freeman D. H. and Holford T. R. (1980) Summary rates. *Biometrics* **36**, 195–205.

Freund R. J., Littell R. C. and Spector P. C. (1986) *SAS System for Linear Models, 1986 Edition*. Cary: SAS Institute Inc.

Friedman L. M., Furberg C. D. and DeMets D. L. (1985) *Fundamentals of Clinical Trials*, 2nd edn. Boston: Wright.

Friedman M. (1937) The use of ranks to avoid the assumption of normality implicit in the analysis of variance. *J. Am. Stat. Ass.* **32**, 675–701.

Gardner M. J. (1989) Review of reported increases of childhood cancer rates in the vicinity of nuclear installations in the UK. *J. R. Stat. Soc. A* **152**, 307–325.

Gardner M. J. and Altman D. G. (eds) (1989) *Statistics with Confidence: Confidence Intervals and Statistical Guidelines*. London: British Medical Journal.

Gardner M. J. and Heady J. A. (1973) Some effects of within-person variability in epidemiological studies. *J. Chron. Dis* **26**, 781–795.

Gart J. J. (1962) On the combination of relative risks. *Biometrics* **18**, 601–610.

Gart J. J. (1968) A simple nearly efficient alternative to the simple sib method in the complete ascertainment case. *Ann. Hum. Genet.* **31**, 283–291.

Gart J. J. and Buck A. A. (1966) Comparison of a screening test and a reference test in epidemiologic studies. II. A probabilistic model for the comparison of diagnostic tests. *Am. J. Epidemiol.* **83**, 593–602.

Gart J. J. and Nam J. (1988) Approximate interval estimation of the ratio of binomial parameters: a review and corrections for skewness. *Biometrics* **44**, 323–338.

Gart J. J. and Nam J. (1990) Approximate interval estimation of the difference in binomial parameters: correction for skewness and extension to multiple tables. *Biometrics* **46**, 637–643.

Geary D. N., Huntington E. and Gilbert R. J. (1992) Analysis of multivariate data from four dental clinical trials. *J. R. Stat. Soc. A* **155**, 77–89.

Gebski V., Leung O., McNeil D. and Lunn D. (1992) *SPIDA User's Manual, Version 6*. Eastwood, New South Wales: Statistical Computing Laboratory.

Geigy Scientific Tables (1982) *Vol. 2: Introduction to Statistics, Statistical Tables, Mathematical Formulae*, 8th edn. Basle: Ciba-Geigy.

Genstat 5 Committee (1987) *Genstat 5: Reference Manual*. Oxford: Clarendon Press.

Gevins A. S. (1980) Pattern recognition of human brain electrical potentials. *IEEE Trans. Patt. Anal. Mach. Intell.* **PAMI-2**, 383–404.

Glasser M. (1967) Exponential survival with covariance. *J. Am. Stat. Ass.* **62**, 561–568.

Glasziou P. P. and Schwartz S. (1991) Clinical decision analysis. *Med. J. Aust.* **154**, 105–110.

Goldstein H. (1979) *The Design and Analysis of Longitudinal Studies*. London: Academic Press.

Good I. J. (1950) *Probability and the Weighing of Evidence*. London: Griffin.

Greenacre M. J. (1984) *Theory and Applications of Correspondence Analysis*. London: Academic Press.

Greenhouse S. W. and Geisser S. (1959) On methods in the analysis of profile data. *Psychometrika* **24**, 95–112.

Greenhouse S. W. and Mantel N. (1950) The evaluation of diagnostic tests. *Biometrics* **6**, 399–412.

Greenland S. (1987) Variance estimators for attributable fraction estimates consistent in both large strata and sparse data. *Stat. Med.* **6**, 701–708.

Greenland S. and Salvan A. (1990) Bias in the one-step (Peto) method for pooling study results. *Stat. Med.* **9**, 247–252.

Greenwood M. (1926) *The Natural Duration of Cancer*. Rep. Publ. Hlth. Med. Subj., No. 33. London: HM Stationery Office.

Grizzle J. E. and Allen D. M. (1969) Analysis of growth and dose response curves. *Biometrics* **25**, 357–381.

Grossman J., Parmar M. K. B., Spiegelhalter D. J. and Freedman L. S. (1994) A unified method for monitoring and analysing controlled trials. *Stat. Med.* **13** (in press).

Haenszel W. (1959) Some problems in the estimation of familial risks of disease. *J. Nat. Cancer Inst.* **23**, 487–505.

Hauck W. W. (1979) The large sample variance of the Mantel–Haenszel estimator of a common odds ratio. *Biometrics* **35**, 817–819.

Hayhoe F. G. J., Quaglino D. and Doll R. (1964) *The Cytology and Cyto-chemistry of Acute Leukaemias*. Med. Res. Coun. Spec. Rep. Ser., No. 304. London: HM Stationery Office.

Healy M. J. R. (1952) Some statistical aspects of anthropometry. *J. R. Stat. Soc. B* **14**, 164–177.

Healy M. J. R. (1963) Fitting a quadratic. *Biometrics* **19**, 362–363.

Healy M. J. R. (1981) Some problems of repeated measurements (with Discussion). In *Perspectives in Medical Statistics*, eds J. F. Bithell and R. Coppi, pp. 155–171. London: Academic Press.

Healy M. J. R. (1984) The use of R^2 as a measure of goodness of fit. *J. R. Stat. Soc. A* **147**, 608–609.

Hennekens C. H., Buring J. E. and Mayrent S. L. (eds) (1987) *Epidemiology in Medicine*. Boston: Little, Brown.

Hill A. Bradford (1962) *Statistical Methods in Clinical and Preventive Medicine*. Edinburgh: Livingstone.

Hill A. Bradford and Hill I. D. (1991) *Bradford Hill's Principles of Medical Statistics*, 12th edn. London: Arnold.

Hill D. J., White V. M. and Gray N. J. (1991) Australian patterns of tobacco smoking in 1989. *Med. J. Aust.* **154**, 797–801.

Hills M. (1966) Allocation rules and their error rates. *J. R. Stat. Soc. B.* **28**, 1–20.

Hills M. (1968) A note on the analysis of growth curves. *Biometrics* **24**, 192–196.

Hills M. and Armitage P. (1979) The two-period cross-over clinical trial. *Br. J. Clin. Pharmacol.* **8**, 7–20.

Hirji K. F. (1991) A comparison of exact, mid-*P*, and score tests for matched case–control studies. *Biometrics* **47**, 487–496.

Hirji K. F., Mehta C. R. and Patel N. R. (1988) Exact inference for matched case–control studies. *Biometrics* **44**, 803–814.

Holford T. R. (1976) Life tables with concomitant information. *Biometrics* **32**, 587–597.

Hosmer D. W. and Lemeshow S. (1989) *Applied Logistic Regression*. New York: Wiley.

Ipsen J. (1955) Appropriate scores in bio-assays using death-times and survivor symptoms. *Biometrics* **11**, 465–480.

Irwig L., Turnbull D. and McMurchie M. (1990) A randomised trial of general practitioner-written invitations to encourage attendance at screening mammography. *Community Health Stud.* **14**, 357–364.

Irwig L., Glasziou P., Wilson A. and Macaskill P. (1991) Estimating an individual's true cholesterol level and response to intervention *J. Am. Med. Ass.* **266**, 1678–1685.

James G. S. (1951) The comparison of several groups of observations when the ratios of the population variances are unknown. *Biometrika* **38**, 324–329.

Jeffreys H. (1961) *Theory of Probability*, 3rd edn. Oxford: Clarendon Press.

Jennison C. and Turnbull B. W. (1990) Interim monitoring of clinical trials. *Stat. Sci.* **5**, 299–317.

Johnson W. D. and George V. T. (1991) Effect of regression to the mean in the presence of within-subject variability. *Stat. Med.* **10**, 1295–1302.

Jones B. and Kenward M. G. (1989) *Design and Analysis of Cross-Over Trials*. London: Chapman and Hall.

Kalbfleisch J. D. and Prentice R. L. (1980) *The Statistical Analysis of Failure Time Data*. New York: Wiley.

Kalton G. (1968) Standardization: a technique to control for extraneous variables. *Appl. Stat.* **17**, 118–136.

Kaplan E. L. and Meier P. (1958) Nonparametric estimation from incomplete observations. *J. Am. Stat. Ass.* **53**, 457–481.

Kay R. (1977) Proportional hazard regression models and the analysis of censored survival data. *Appl. Statist.* **26**, 227–237.

Kelsey J. L., Thompson W. D. and Evans A. S. (1986) *Methods in Observational Epidemiology*. New York: Oxford University Press.

Kendall M. G. (1951, 1952) Regression, structure and functional relationship. Part I. *Biometrika* **38**, 11–25; Part II, *Biometrika* **39**, 96–108.

Kendall M. G. (1980) *Multivariate Analysis*, 2nd edn. London: Griffin.

Kendall M. G. and Gibbons J. D. (1990) *Rank Correlation Methods*, 5th edn. London: Arnold.

Keuls M. (1952) The use of 'Studentized range' in connection with an analysis of variance. *Euphytica* **1**, 112–122.

Kim K. and DeMets D. L. (1992) Sample size determination for group sequential clinical trials with immediate response. *Stat. Med.* **11**, 1391–1399.

King E. P. (1963) A statistical design for drug screening. *Biometrics* **19**, 429–440.

Kleinbaum D. G., Kupper L. L. and Morgenstern H. (1982) *Epidemiologic Research—Principles and Quantitative Methods*. Belmont, California: Lifetime Learning Publications.

Kleinbaum D. G., Kupper L. L. and Muller K. E. (1988) *Applied Regression Analysis and Other Multivariable Methods*, 2nd edn. Boston: PWS-Kent.

Klotz J. H. (1964) On the normal scores two-sample rank test. *J. Am. Stat. Ass.* **59**, 652–664.

Knox E. G. (1964) Epidemiology of childhood leukaemia in Northumberland and Durham. *Br. J. Prev. Soc. Med.* **18**, 17–24.

Koopman P. A. R. (1984) Confidence intervals for the ratio of two binomial proportions. *Biometrics* **40**, 513–517.

Kruskal W. H. and Wallis W. A. (1952) Use of ranks in one-criterion variance analysis. *J. Am. Stat. Ass.* **47**, 583–621.

Krzanowski W. J. (1988) *Principles of Multivariate Analysis: A User's Perspective*. Oxford: Clarendon Press.

Kuritz S. J. and Landis J. R. (1988) Attributable risk estimation from matched case–control data. *Biometrics* **44**, 355–367.

Kuritz S. J., Landis J. R. and Koch G. G. (1988) A general overview of Mantel–Haenszel methods: applications and recent developments. *Ann. Rev. Public Health* **9**, 123–160.

Lan K. K. G. and DeMets D. L. (1983) Discrete sequential boundaries for clinical trials. *Biometrika* **70**, 659–663.

Lan K. K. G., Simon R. and Halperin M. (1982) Stochastically curtailed tests in long-term clinical trials. *Commun. Stat. C* **1**, 207–219.

Lan K. K. G., DeMets D. L. and Halperin M. (1984) More flexible sequential and non-sequential designs in long-term clinical trials. *Commun. Stat.-Theor. Meth.* **13**, 2339–2353.

Lancaster H. O. (1950) Statistical control in haematology. *J. Hyg., Camb.* **48**, 402–417.

Lancaster H. O. (1952) Statistical control of counting experiments. *Biometrika* **39**, 419–422.

Lancaster H. O. (1961) Significance tests in discrete distributions. *J. Am. Stat. Ass.* **56**, 223–234.

Lancaster H. O. (1965) Symmetry in multivariate distributions. *Aust. J. Stat.* **7**, 115–126.

Lawless J. F. (1982) *Statistical Models and Methods for Lifetime Data.* New York: Wiley.

Lawley D. N. and Maxwell A. E. (1971) *Factor Analysis as a Statistical Method*, 2nd edn. London: Butterworths.

Lee P. M. (1989) *Bayesian Statistics: an Introduction.* London: Arnold.

Lehmann E. L. (1975) *Nonparametrics: Statistical Methods Based on Ranks.* San Francisco: Holden-Day.

Lemeshow S. and Hosmer D. W. (1982) A review of goodness of fit statistics for use in the development of logistic regression models. *Am. J. Epidemiol.* **115**, 92–106.

Lemeshow S., Hosmer D. W., Klar J. and Lwanga S. K. (1990) *Adequacy of Sample Size in Health Studies.* Chichester: Wiley.

Levin M. L. (1953) The occurrence of lung cancer in man. *Acta Un. Int. Cancer* **9**, 531–541.

Liddell F. D. K. (1960) The measurement of occupational mortality. *Br. J. Ind. Med.* **17**, 228–233.

Liddell F. D. K. (1983) Simplified exact analysis of case–referent studies: matched pairs; dichotomous exposure. *J. Epidemiol. Community Health* **37**, 82–84.

Liddell F. D. K. (1984) Simple exact analysis of the standardized mortality ratio. *J. Epidemiol. Community Health* **38**, 85–88.

Liddell F. D. K. (1988) The development of cohort studies in epidemiology: a review. *J. Clin. Epidemiol.* **41**, 1217–1237.

Liddell F. D. K., McDonald J. C. and Thomas D. C. (1977) Methods of cohort analysis: appraisal by application to asbestos mining (with Discussion). *J. R. Stat. Soc. A* **140**, 469–491.

Liddell F. D. K., Thomas D. C., Gibbs G. W. and McDonald J. C. (1984) Fibre exposure and mortality from pneumoconiosis, respiratory and abdominal malignancies in chrysotile production in Quebec, 1926–75. *Ann. Acad. Med.* **13** (Suppl), 340–342.

Lin L. I.-K. (1992) Assay validation using the concordance correlation coefficient. *Biometrics* **48**, 599–604.

Lindley D. V. (1965) *Introduction to Probability and Statistics from a Bayesian Viewpoint. Part 1, Probability. Part 2, Inference.* Cambridge: Cambridge University Press.

Little R. J. and Pullum T. W. (1979) The general linear model and direct standardization—a comparison. *Sociol. Meth. Res.* **7**, 475–501.

Lloyd S. and Roberts C. J. (1973) A test for space clustering and its application to congenital limb defects in Cardiff. *Br. J. Prev. Soc. Med.* **27**, 188–191.

Lombard H. L. and Doering C. R. (1947) Treatment of the four-fold table by partial correlation as it relates to public health problems. *Biometrics* **3**, 123–128.

McCullagh P. and Nelder J. A. (1989) *Generalized Linear Models*, 2nd edn. London: Chapman and Hall.

McGilchrist C. A. and Aisbett C. W. (1991) Regression with frailty in survival analysis. *Biometrics* **47**, 461–466.

McKelvey M., Gottlieb J. A., Wilson H. E., Haut, A., Talley R., Stephens R., Lane M., Gamble J., Jones S. E., Grozea P., Gutterman J., Coltman C. and Moon T. E. (1976) Hydroxyldaunomycin (Adriamycin) combination chemotherapy in malignant lymphoma. *Cancer* **38**, 1484–1493.

MacKie R., Hunter J. A. A., Aitchison T. C., Hole D., McLaren K., Rankin R., Blessing K., Evans A. T., Hutcheon A. W., Jones D. H., Soutar D. S., Watson A. C. H., Cornbleet M. A. and Smyth J. F. for the Scottish Melanoma Group (1992) Cutaneous malignant melanoma, Scotland, 1979–89. *Lancet* **339**, 971–975.

Machin D. and Campbell M. J. (1987) *Statistical Tables for the Design of Clinical Trials.* Oxford: Blackwell Scientific Publications.

Machin D. and Gardner M. J. (1989) Calculating confidence intervals for survival time analyses. In *Statistics with Confidence—Confidence Intervals and Statistical Guidelines*, eds M. J. Gardner and D. G. Altman, pp. 64–70. London: British Medical Journal.

Macklin J. (1990) *Setting the Agenda for Change*. Background Paper, 1. Melbourne: National Health Strategy.

Makuch R. and Simon R. (1978) Sample size requirements for evaluating a conservative therapy. *Cancer Treat. Rep.* **62**, 1037–1040.

Mantel N. (1963) Chi-square tests with one degree of freedom: extensions of the Mantel–Haenszel procedure. *J. Am. Stat. Ass.* **58**, 690–700.

Mantel N. (1966) Evaluation of survival data and two new rank order statistics arising in its consideration. *Cancer Chemother. Rep.* **50**, 163–170.

Mantel N. (1967) The detection of disease clustering and a generalized regression approach. *Cancer Res.* **27**, 209–220.

Mantel N. (1973) Synthetic retrospective studies and related topics. *Biometrics* **29**, 479–486.

Mantel N. and Haenszel W. (1959) Statistical aspects of the analysis of data from retrospective studies of disease. *J. Nat. Cancer Inst.* **22**, 719–748.

Mardia K. V., Kent J. T. and Bibby J. M. (1979) *Multivariate Analysis*. London: Academic Press.

Marks R. G. (1982) Measuring the correlation between time series of hormonal data. *Stat. Med.* **1**, 49–57.

Marriott F. H. C. (1974) *The Interpretation of Multiple Observations*. London: Academic Press.

Marshall J. (1964) A trial of long-term hypotensive therapy in cerebrovascular disease. *Lancet* **i**, 10–12.

Marshall R. J. (1991) Mapping disease and mortality rates using empirical Bayes estimators. *Appl. Stat.* **40**, 283–294.

Martin W. J. (1949) *The Physique of Young Adult Males*. Med. Res. Coun. Mem., No. 20. London: HM Stationery Office.

Matthews J. N. S., Altman D. G., Campbell M. J. and Royston P. (1990) Analysis of serial measurements in medical research. *Br. Med. J.* **300**, 230–235.

Medical Research Council (1950) Treatment of pulmonary tuberculosis with streptomycin and para-amino-salicylic acid. *Br. Med. J.* **ii**, 1073–1085.

Mee R. W. (1984) Confidence bounds for the difference between two probabilities. *Biometrics* **40**, 1175–1176.

Mehta C. R. and Patel N. R. (1983) A network algorithm for performing Fisher's exact test in $r \times c$ contingency tables. *J. Am. Stat. Ass.* **78**, 427–434.

Mehta C. R., Patel N. R. and Gray R. (1985) Computing an exact confidence interval for the common odds ratio in several 2 by 2 contingency tables. *J. Am. Stat. Ass.* **80**, 969–973.

Meier P. (1975) Statistics and medical experimentation. *Biometrics* **31**, 511–529.

Merrell M. and Shulman L. E. (1955) Determination of prognosis in chronic disease, illustrated by systemic lupus erythematosus. *J. Chron. Dis.* **1**, 12–32.

Miettinen O. S. (1969) Individual matching with multiple controls in the case of all-or-none responses. *Biometrics* **25**, 339–355.

Miettinen O. S. (1970) Estimation of relative risk from individually matched series. *Biometrics* **26**, 75–86.

Miettinen O. S. (1976) Estimability and estimation in case–referent studies. *Am. J. Epidemiol.* **103**, 226–235.

Miettinen O. S. (1985) *Theoretical Epidemiology: Principles of Occurrence Research in Medicine*. New York: Wiley.

Miettinen O. and Nurminen M. (1985) Comparative analysis of two rates. *Stat. Med.* **4**, 213–226.

Miller R. G., Jr. (1981) *Simultaneous Statistical Inference*, 2nd edn. New York: Springer-Verlag.

Minitab Inc. (1991) *Minitab Reference Manual, PC Version, Release 8*. State College, Pennsylvania: Minitab Inc.

Morrison D. F. (1976) *Multivariate Statistical Methods*, 2nd edn. New York: McGraw-Hill.

Moser C. A. and Kalton G. (1971) *Survey Methods in Social Investigation*, 2nd edn. London: Heinemann.

Moses L. E. and Oakford R. V. (1963) *Tables of Random Permutations*. London: Allen and Unwin.

MRC Vitamin Study Group (1991) Prevention of neural tube defects: results of the Medical Research Council Vitamin Study. *Lancet* **338**, 131–137.

Murdoch J. and Barnes J. A. (1968) *Statistical Tables for Science, Engineering and Management.* London: Macmillan.

Nam J. (1987) A simple approximation for calculating sample sizes for detecting linear trend in proportions. *Biometrics* **43**, 701–705.

National Bureau of Standards (1950) *Tables of the Binomial Probability Distribution.* Applied Mathematics Series No. 7. Washington: US Dept of Commerce.

Naylor A. F. (1964) Comparisons of regression constants fitted by maximum likelihood to four common transformations of binomial data. *Ann. Hum. Genet.* **27**, 241–246.

Nelder J. A. and Wedderburn R. W. M. (1972) Generalized linear models. *J. R. Stat. Soc. A* **135**, 370–384.

Newell D. J. (1962) Errors in the interpretation of errors in epidemiology. *Am. J. Public Health* **52**, 1925–1928.

Newell D. J., Greenberg B. G., Williams T. F. and Veazey P. B. (1961) Use of cohort life tables in family studies of disease. *J. Chron. Dis.* **13**, 439–452.

Newhouse M. L., Berry G. and Wagner J. C. (1985) Mortality of factory workers in east London 1933–80. *Br. J. Ind. Med.* **42**, 4–11.

Newman D. (1939) The distribution of range in samples from a normal population, expressed in terms of an independent estimate of standard deviation. *Biometrika* **31**, 20–30.

O'Brien P. C. and Fleming T. R. (1979) A multiple testing procedure for clinical trials. *Biometrics* **35**, 549–556.

Oldham P. D. (1968) *Measurement in Medicine: the Interpretation of Numerical Data.* London: English Universities Press.

Owen D. B. (1962) *Handbook of Statistical Tables.* London: Pergamon.

Parker R. A. and Bregman D. J. (1986) Sample size for individually matched case–control studies. *Biometrics* **42**, 919–926.

Pauker S. G. and Kassirer J. P. (1992) Decision analysis. In *Medical Uses of Statistics*, 2nd edn., eds J. C. Bailar III and F. Mosteller, pp. 159–179. Boston: NEJM Books.

Pearce S. C. (1965) *Biological Statistics: an Introduction.* New York: McGraw-Hill.

Pearson E. S. and Hartley H. O. (1966) *Biometrika Tables for Statisticians, Vol. 1*, 3rd edn. Cambridge: Cambridge University Press.

Peto R. and Pike M. C. (1973) Conservatism of the approximation $\sum (O - E)^2/E$ in the logrank test for survival data or tumor incidence data. *Biometrics* **29**, 579–584.

Peto R., Pike M. C., Armitage P., Breslow N. E., Cox D. R., Howard S. V., Mantel N., McPherson K., Peto J. and Smith P. G. (1976, 1977) Design and analysis of randomized clinical trials requiring prolonged observation of each patient. I. Introduction and design. *Br. J. Cancer* **34**, 585–612; II. Analysis and examples. *Br. J. Cancer* **35**, 1–39.

Pike M. C. (1966) A method of analysis of a certain class of experiments in carcinogenesis. *Biometrics* **22**, 142–161.

Pike M. C. and Morrow R. H. (1970) Statistical analysis of patient–control studies in epidemiology—factor under investigation an all-or-none variable. *Br. J. Prev. Soc. Med.* **24**, 42–44.

Pike M. C. and Smith P. G. (1968) Disease clustering: a generalization of Knox's approach to the detection of space–time interactions. *Biometrics* **24**, 541–556.

Pocock S. J. (1974) Harmonic analysis applied to seasonal variations in sickness absence. *Appl. Stat.* **23**, 103–120.

Pocock S. J. (1983) *Clinical Trials: A Practical Approach.* Chichester: Wiley.

Pocock S. J. and Hughes M. D. (1990) Estimation issues in clinical trials and overviews. *Stat. Med.* **9**, 657–671.

Pregibon D. (1980) Goodness of link tests for generalized linear models. *Appl. Stat.* **29**, 15–24.

Pregibon D. (1981) Logistic regression diagnostics. *Ann. Stat.* **9**, 705–724.

Radhakrishna S. (1965) Combination of results from several 2×2 contingency tables. *Biometrics* **21**, 86–98.

Räisänen M. J., Virkkunen M., Huttunen M. O., Furman B. and Kärkkäinen J. (1984) Letter to the Editor. *Lancet* **ii**, 700–701.

Raubertas R. F. (1988) Spatial and temporal analysis of disease occurrence for detection of clustering. *Biometrics* **44**, 1121–1129.

Registrar General of England and Wales (1958) *Decennial Supplement, England and Wales 1951, Occupational Mortality.* Part II, Vol 2. Tables. London: HM Stationery Office.

Roberts E., Dawson W. M. and Madden M. (1939) Observed and theoretical ratios in Mendelian inheritance. *Biometrika* **31**, 56–66.

Robertson A. (1962) Weighting in the estimation of variance components in the unbalanced single classification. *Biometrics* **18**, 413–417.

Robertson J. D. and Armitage P. (1959) Comparison of two hypotensive agents. *Anaesthesia* **14**, 53–64.

Robins J. M., Breslow N. E. and Greenland S. (1986) Estimators of the Mantel–Haenszel variance consistent in both sparse data and large-strata limiting models. *Biometrics* **42**, 311–323.

Robins J. M., Prentice R. L. and Blevins D. (1989) Designs for synthetic case–control studies in open cohorts. *Biometrics* **45**, 1103–1116.

Romig H. G. (1947) *50-100 Binomial Tables.* New York: Wiley.

Rose G. A. (1962) A study of blood pressure among Negro school-children. *J. Chron. Dis.* **15**, 373–380.

Rosner B. and Muñoz A. (1988) Autoregressive modelling for the analysis of longitudinal data with unequally spaced examinations. *Stat. Med.* **7**, 59–71.

Rothman K. (1978) A show of confidence. *N. Engl. J. Med.* **299**, 1362–1363.

Rothman K. J. (1986) *Modern Epidemiology.* Boston: Little, Brown.

Rowlands R. J., Griffiths K., Kemp K.W., Nix A. B. J., Richards G. and Wilson D. W. (1983) Application of cusum techniques to the routine monitoring of analytical performance in clinical laboratories. *Stat. Med.* **2**, 141–145.

Ryan B. F., Joiner B. L. and Ryan T. A., Jr (1985) *Minitab Handbook*, 2nd edn. Boston: Duxbury Press.

St Leger A. S. (1976) Comparison of two tests for seasonality in epidemiological data. *Appl. Stat.* **25**, 280–286.

SAS Institute Inc. (1989) *SAS/STAT User's Guide, Version 6*, 4th edn., Volumes 1 & 2. Cary, North Carolina: SAS Institute Inc.

Satterthwaite F. E. (1946) An approximate distribution of estimates of variance components. *Biometrics Bull.* **2**, 110–114.

Savage L. J. (1954) *The Foundations of Statistics.* New York: Wiley.

Scheffé H. (1959) *The Analysis of Variance.* New York: Wiley.

Schlesselman J. J. (1982) *Case–Control Studies: Design, Conduct, Analysis.* New York: Wiley.

Schwartz D. and Lellouch J. (1967) Explanatory and pragmatic attitudes in therapeutic trials. *J. Chron. Dis.* **20**, 637–648.

Schwartz D., Flamant R. and Lellouch J. (1980) *Clinical Trials* (trans. M. J. R. Healy). London: Academic Press.

Shapiro S. H. and Louis T. A. (eds) (1983) *Clinical Trials: Issues and Approaches.* New York: Dekker.

Siegel S. and Castellan N. J. Jr (1988) *Nonparametric Statistics for the Behavioral Sciences*, 2nd edn. New York: McGraw-Hill.

Simons L. A., Friedlander Y., McCallum J., Simons J., Powell I., Heller R. and Berry G. (1991) The Dubbo study of the health of elderly: correlates of coronary heart disease at study entry. *J. Am. Geriatr. Soc.* **39**, 584–590.

Smith A. F. M., West M., Gordon K., Knapp M. S. and Trimble I. M. G. (1983) Monitoring kidney transplant patients. *Statistician* **32**, 46–54.

Smith C. A. B. (1961) Note on the error variance. *Ann. Hum. Genet.* **25**, 86–87.

Smith C. E. Gordon and Westgarth D. R. (1957) The use of survival time in the analysis of neutralization tests for serum antibody surveys. *J. Hyg., Camb.* **55**, 224–238.

Smith C. E. Gordon, Turner L. H. and Armitage P. (1962) Yellow fever vaccination in Malaya by subcutaneous injection and multiple puncture. *Bull. World Health Org.* **27**, 717–727.

Smith P. G. (1982) Spatial and temporal clustering. In *Cancer Epidemiology and Prevention*, eds D. Schottenfeld and J. F. Fraumeni, Chap. 22, pp. 391–407. Philadelphia: Saunders.

Smith P. G. and Pike M. C. (1974) A note on a 'close pairs' test for space clustering. *Br. J. Prev. Soc. Med.* **28**, 63–64.

Sneath P. H. A. and Sokal R. R. (1973) *Numerical Taxonomy*. San Francisco: Freeman.

Snedecor G. W. and Cochran W. G. (1989) *Statistical Methods*, 8th edn. Ames: Iowa State University Press.

Snell E. S. and Armitage P. (1957) Clinical comparison of diamorphine and pholcodine as cough suppressants, by a new method of sequential analysis. *Lancet* **i**, 860–862.

Solomon P. J. (1984) Effect of misspecification of regression models in the analysis of survival data. *Biometrika* **71**, 291–298.

Spiegelhalter D. J. and Freedman L. S. (1988) Bayesian approaches to clinical trials (with Discussion). In *Bayesian Statistics, 3,* eds J. M. Bernado, M. H. DeGroot, D. V. Lindley and A. F. M. Smith, pp. 453–477. Oxford: Oxford University Press.

Spiegelhalter D. J. and Knill-Jones R. P. (1984) Statistical and knowledge-based approaches to clinical decision-support systems, with an application to gastroenterology (with Discussion). *J. R. Stat. Soc. A* **147**, 35–76.

Spiegelhalter D. J., Freedman L. S. and Blackburn P. R. (1986) Monitoring clinical trials; conditional or predictive power? *Cont. Clin. Trials* **7**, 8–17.

Sprent P. (1969) *Models in Regression and Related Topics*. London: Methuen.

SPSS Inc. (1990) *SPSS Reference Guide*. Chicago: SPSS.

Statistics and Epidemiology Research Corporation (1988) *EGRET—Users' Manual*. Seattle: Statistics and Epidemiology Research Corporation.

Stuart A. and Ord J. K. (1983) *Kendall's Advanced Theory of Statistics*, Vol. 3. London: Arnold.

'Student' (W. S. Gosset) (1907) On the error of counting with a haemocytometer. *Biometrika* **5**, 351–360.

Sutherland I. (1946) The stillbirth-rate in England and Wales in relation to social influences. *Lancet* **ii**, 953–956.

Therneau T. M., Grambsch P. M. and Fleming T. R. (1990) Martingale-based residuals for survival models. *Biometrika* **77**, 147–160.

Trimble I. M. G., West M., Knapp M. S., Pownall R. and Smith A. F. M. (1983) Detection of renal allograft rejection by computer. *Br. Med. J.* **286**, 1695–1699.

Truett J., Cornfield J. and Kannel W. (1967) A multivariate analysis of the risk of coronary heart disease in Framingham. *J. Chron. Dis.* **20**, 511–524.

Tudehope D. I., Iredell J., Rodgers D. and Gunn A. (1986) Neonatal death: grieving families. *Med. J. Aust.* **144**, 290–292.

Tukey J. W. (1977) *Exploratory Data Analysis*. Reading, Massachusetts: Addison-Wesley.

Upton G. J. G. (1992) Fisher's exact test. *J. R. Stat. Soc. A* **155**, 395–402.

van Elteren P. H. (1960) On the combination of independent two-sample tests of Wilcoxon. *Bull. Inst. Int. Statist.* **37**, 351–361.

Wald A. (1947) *Sequential Analysis*. New York: Wiley.

Walter S. D. (1975) The distribution of Levin's measure of attributable risk. *Biometrika* **62**, 371–374.

Walter S. D. and Day N. E. (1983) Estimation of the duration of a preclinical state using screening data. *Am. J. Epidemiol.* **118**, 865–886.

Walter S. D. and Elwood J. M. (1975) A test for seasonality of events with a variable population at risk. *Br. J. Prev. Soc. Med.* **29**, 18–21.

Warner H. R., Toronto A. F., Veasey L. G. and Stephenson R. (1961) A mathematical approach to medical diagnosis. *J. Am. Med. Ass.* **177**, 177–183.

Weatherall J. A. C. and Haskey J. C. (1976) Surveillance of malformations. *Br. Med. Bull.* **32**, 39–44.

Weinstein M. C. and Fineberg H. V. (1980) *Clinical Decision Analysis*. Philadelphia: Saunders.

Welch B. L. (1951) On the comparison of several mean values: an alternative approach. *Biometrika* **38**, 330–336.

Wetherill G. B. (1981) *Intermediate Statistical Methods*. London: Chapman and Hall.

Wetherill G. B., Duncombe P., Kenward M., Köllerström J., Paul S. R. and Vowden B. J. (1986) *Regression Analysis with Applications*. London: Chapman and Hall.

Whitehead A. and Whitehead J. (1991) A general parametric approach to the meta-analysis of randomized clinical trials. *Stat. Med.* **10**, 1665–1677.

Whitehead J. (1992) *The Design and Analysis of Sequential Clinical Trials*, 2nd edn. Chichester: Horwood.

Whittemore A. S. (1983) Estimating attributable risk from case–control studies. *Am. J. Epidemiol.* **117**, 76–85.

WHO Collaborative Study of Neoplasia and Steroid Contraceptives (1990) Breast cancer and combined oral contraceptives: results from a multinational study. *Br. J. Cancer* **61**, 110–119.

Wilcocks W. J. and Lancaster H. O. (1951) Maternal mortality in New South Wales with special reference to age and parity. *J. Obstet. Gynaec. Br. Emp.* **58**, 945–960.

Wilcoxon F. (1945) Individual comparisons by ranking methods. *Biometrics Bull.* **1**, 80–83.

Wilkinson L. (1990) *SYSTAT: The System for Statistics*. Evanston, Illinois: SYSTAT, Inc.

Williams D. A. (1988) Tests for differences between several small proportions. *Appl. Stat.* **37**, 421–434.

Wilson P. D., Hebel J. R. and Sherwin R. (1981) Screening and diagnosis when within-individual observations are Markov-dependent. *Biometrics* **37**, 553–565.

Wilson P. W. and Kullman E. D. (1931) A statistical inquiry into methods for estimating numbers of rhizobia. *J. Bacteriol.* **22**, 71–90.

Woolf B. (1955) On estimating the relation between blood group and disease. *Ann. Hum. Genet.* **19**, 251–253.

Woolson R. F., Bean J. A. and Rojas P. B. (1986) Sample size for case–control studies using Cochran's statistic. *Biometrics* **42**, 927–932.

World Health Organization (1966) *Sampling Methods in Morbidity Surveys and Public Health Investigations*. Technical Report Series No. 336. Geneva: WHO.

World Health Organization (1978) *Manual of the International Statistical Classification of Diseases, Injuries and Causes of Death*, 9th revision, Vols 1 and 2. Geneva: WHO.

Yates F. (1934) Contingency tables involving small numbers and the χ^2 test. *J. R. Stat. Soc., Suppl.* **1**, 217–235.

Yates F. (1948) The analysis of contingency tables with groupings based on quantitative characters. *Biometrika* **35**, 176–181.

Yates F. (1981) *Sampling Methods for Censuses and Surveys*, 4th edn. London: Griffin.

Yates F. (1982) Regression models for repeated measurements. *Biometrics* **38**, 850–853.

Yates F. (1984) Tests of significance for 2×2 contingency tables (with Discussion). *J. R. Stat. Soc. A* **147**, 426–463.

Youden W. J. (1950) Index for rating diagnostic tests. *Cancer* **3**, 32–35.

Yule G. U. (1934) On some points relating to vital statistics, more especially statistics of occupational mortality. *J. R. Stat. Soc. A* **97**, 1–84.

Yule G. U. and Kendall M. G. (1950) *An Introduction to the Theory of Statistics*, 14th edn. London: Griffin.

Yusuf S., Peto R., Lewis J., Collins R. and Sleight P. (1985) Beta-blockade during and after myocardial infarction: an overview of the randomized clinical trials. *Prog. Cardiovasc. Dis.* **27**, 335–371.

Yusuf S., Simon R. and Ellenberg S. (eds) (1987) Proceedings of the Workshop on Methodologic Issues in Overviews of Randomized Clinical Trials. *Stat. Med.* **6**, 217–409.

Zeger S. L., Liang K.-Y. and Albert P. S. (1988) Models for longitudinal data: a generalized estimating equation approach. *Biometrics* **44**, 1049–1060.

Zippin C. and Armitage P. (1966) Use of concomitant variables and incomplete survival information in the estimation of an exponential survival parameter. *Biometrics* **22**, 665–672.

Author Index

(*See also* References, pp. 581–594.)

Acheson E. D.   507
Agresti A.   403, 405, 419, 436
Aisbett C. W.   488
Aitchison T. C.   3
Aitken M.   556
Albert P. S.   385
Alderson M.   507
Allen D. M.   382
Altman D. G.   98, 126, 276, 383, 384
Alvey N.   556
Anderson D.   556
Armitage P.   3, 217, 245, 249, 313, 315, 404,
    418, 458, 469, 476, 478, 483, 494, 497, 498,
    499, 501, 505, 506
Armstrong B. K.   446
Atkinson A. C.   328

Babbie E. R.   9
Bacharach A. L.   221, 263, 264
Bailar J. C.   142
Bailey N. T. J.   74, 507, 533, 534
Baptista J.   511
Barnard G. A.   123, 124, 140
Barnes J. A.   561
Barnett V.   401
Barrie W. J. M.   503
Bartko J. J.   275
Bartlett M. S.   234
Barton D. E.   531
Bean J. A.   206
Becker N. G.   507
Belsley D. A.   331
Beltonn R.   503
Benjamin B.   507
Bennett B. M.   140
Bergen J.   275, 385, 445
Berkson J.   290, 472, 473, 475, 550
Berlin J. A.   219
Berrier J.   195
Berry D. A.   506
Berry G.   24, 98, 275, 353, 385, 445, 479, 490,
    491, 511
Bevan C.   421

Bibby J. M.   350, 372
Blackburn P. R.   151, 506
Blessing K.   3
Blevins D.   185
Bliss C. I.   347
Boardman T. J.   222
Box G. E. P.   77, 378, 383, 390
Bradley R. A.   372
Bregman D. J.   206
Breslow N. E.   141, 153, 420, 469, 476, 478,
    85, 491, 492, 505, 513, 519, 557
Brown A.   418
Brown C. C.   432
Brown E. B.   353
Brown J. K.   503
Brown M. B.   194
Buck A. A.   528
Bulmer M. G.   255
Buring J. E.   507
Burton A. H.   557
Buyse M. E.   190
Byar D. P.   487

Campbell I.   421
Campbell M. J.   202, 206, 383, 384
Casagrande J. T.   200
Castellan N. J., Jr   449
Chalmers T. C.   195, 219
Chance M. R. A.   221, 263, 264
Chatfield C.   350, 372, 374, 376,
Checkoway H.   492
Chen C.-H.   488
Chiang C. L.   470, 476
Clayton D.   153, 489
Cochran W. G.   140, 172, 182, 232, 234, 259,
    261, 265, 266, 267, 275, 346, 413, 414, 417,
    576
Cochrane A. L.   189
Cockburn R.   503
Cockcroft A.   353, 421
Cody R. P.   555
Cohen J.   444, 445
Cole T. J.   4
Coleman M.   557
Collins A. J.   350, 372, 374

Collins G.　421
Collins R.　136, 195, 219
Collins R. L.　252
Coltman C.　479
Connor R. J.　205
Conover W. J.　397, 398, 399, 449
Cook P.　483
Cook R. D.　331, 332
Cookson W. O. C. M.　446
Coons I. J.　372
Copas J. C.　313
Cornbleet M. A.　3
Cornfield J.　141, 431, 511, 515, 516
Cox D. R.　265, 267, 390, 403, 423, 432, 469, 476, 478, 481, 484, 505, 576
Cox G. M.　261, 265, 266, 267, 576
Cramér H.　42
Cutler S. J.　475
Cuzick J.　489, 531

Daniel C.　397
Darby S. C.　382, 442
David F. N.　531
Dawson W. M.　59
Day N. E.　141, 420, 491, 492, 513, 519, 528, 529, 557
de Klerk N. H.　446
Dean A. G.　557
Dean J. A.　557
Demers P. A.　492
DeMets D. L.　190, 505, 506
DerSimonian R.　219
Diamond E. L.　527
Dicker R. C.　557
Diggle P. J.　376
Dixon W. J.　556
Dobson A. J.　423, 438
Doering C. R.　425, 426
Doll R.　185, 186, 373, 457, 483, 489
Donner A.　205, 206
Douglas A.　557
Draper N. R.　322, 324, 346, 401
Duncombe P.　323
Dyke G. V.　427

Eberle E.　438
Ederer F.　142, 475, 531
Edwards J.　421
Edwards J. H.　347, 531
Edwards R.　531
Ehrenberg A. S. C.　8, 311
Ellenberg S.　195
Ellery C.　511
Elwood J. M.　348, 507

Evans A. S.　507
Evans A. T.　3
Everitt B.　372
Exall C.　353

Fearn T.　382
Fellingham S. A.　483
Fienberg S. E.　403
Fineberg H. V.　74
Finkelstein D. M.　448
Finney D. J.　140, 394, 535, 544, 546, 547, 550
Fisher R. A.　112, 115, 120, 139, 142, 236, 261, 345, 392, 394, 460, 565, 575, 576
Flamant R.　190
Fleiss J. L.　141, 200, 276, 403, 447
Fleming T. R.　488, 505
Forfar J. O.　503
Fowler M. A.　4
Francis B.　556
Franklin D. A.　74
Fraser P. M.　74
Freedman L. S.　151, 198, 206, 506
Freeman D. H.　443
Freund R. J.　350
Friedlander Y.　24
Friedman L. M.　190
Friedman M.　461
Furberg C. D.　190
Furman B.　20

Gage R. P.　472, 473, 475
Galwey N.　556
Gamble J.　479
Gardner M. J.　98, 126, 173, 479, 532
Gart J. J.　141, 515, 516, 528, 534
Geary D. N.　370
Gebski V.　557
Geisser S.　383
George V. T.　173
Gevins A. S.　380
Gibbons J. D.　465, 466
Gibbs G. W.　132
Gilbert R. J.　370
Giles M. M.　503
Glancy J. J.　446
Glasser M.　483
Glasziou P. P.　74, 173
Goldstein H.　183
Good I. J.　76
Gordon K.　378
Gottlieb J. A.　479
Grambsch P. M.　488
Gray N. J.　7

Gray R.   419
Green M.   556
Greenacre M. J.   373
Greenberg B. G.   475
Greenhouse S. W.   383, 527
Greenland S.   136, 513, 522
Greenwood M.   475
Griffiths K.   378
Grizzle J. E.   382
Grossman J.   506
Grozea P.   479
Gunn A.   408
Gutterman J.   479

Haenszel W.   418, 512, 534
Halperin M.   506
Hartley H. O.   58, 66, 112, 115, 142, 563, 569, 571
Haskey J. C.   378
Hauck W. W.   513
Haut A.   479
Hayhoe F. G. J.   373
Heady J. A.   173
Healy M. J. R.   319, 345, 381, 401
Hebel J. R.   377
Heller R.   24
Hennekens C. H.   507
Hermon C.   557
Heyer N. J.   492
Hill A. Bradford   185, 186, 190, 437, 470
Hill D. J.   7
Hill I. D.   190, 437, 470
Hills M.   245, 249, 359, 382
Hinde J.   556
Hirji K. F.   123, 419
Hobbs M. S. T.   446
Hole D.   3
Holford T. R.   443, 483
Hosmer D. W.   205, 206, 423, 432
Houston K.   421
Howard S. V.   469, 476, 478, 505
Hsu P.   140
Hughes M. D.   219
Hunter J. A. A.   3
Huntington E.   370
Hutcheon A. W.   3
Huttunen M. O.   20

Ipsen J.   372
Iredell J.   408
Irwig L.   173, 405

James G. S.   217
Jeffreys H.   76

Jenkins D.   421
Jenkins G. M.   378
Jennison C.   505
Johnson W. D.   173
Joiner B. L.   556
Jones B.   249
Jones D. H.   3
Jones S. E.   479

Kalbfleisch J. D.   469, 476, 486
Kaldor J.   153
Kalton G.   182, 437
Kannel W.   431
Kaplan E. L.   476
Kärkkäinen J.   20
Kassirer J. P.   74
Katti S. K.   372
Kay R.   487
Kelsey J. L.   507
Kemp K. W.   378
Kendall M. G.   168, 290, 350, 372, 465, 466
Kent J. T.   350, 372
Kenward M. G.   249, 323
Keuls M.   227
Kim K.   506
King E. P.   494
Kitchin R.   275, 385, 445, 479
Klar J.   205, 206
Kleinbaum D. G.   323, 332, 333, 507, 521, 528
Klotz J. H.   460
Knapp M. S.   378
Knill-Jones R. P.   74
Knox E. G.   532
Koch G. G.   420
Köllerström J.   323
Koopman P. A. R.   141
Kruskal W. H.   463
Krzanowski W. J.   350, 370, 372
Kuh E.   331
Kullman E. D.   65
Kupper L. L.   323, 332, 333, 507, 521, 528
Kuritz S. J.   420, 522
Kuulasmaa K.   438

Laird N.   219
Lan K. K. G.   505, 506
Lancaster H. O.   59, 123, 236, 411
Landis J. R.   420, 522
Lane M.   479
Lane P.   556
Latham S.   421

Latscha R.   140
Laurence D. R.   418
Lawless J. F.   469
Lawley D. N.   358
Lee P. M.   77
Lehmann E. L.   449, 450, 455, 577
Lellouch J.   190, 193
Lemeshow S.   205, 206, 423, 432
Leung O.   557
Levin H.   195
Levin M. L.   519
Lewis J.   136, 195, 219
Lewis T.   401
Liang K. Y.   385, 513
Liddell F. D. K.   132, 143, 437, 489, 514,
    519
Lilienfeld A. M.   527
Lin L. I.-K.   275
Lindley D. V.   76, 77, 149
Littell R. C.   350
Little R. J.   443
Lloyd S.   531
Lombard H. L.   425, 426
Louis T. A.   190
Lowe D.   198, 506
Lunn D.   557
Lwanga S. K.   205, 206

Macaskill P.   173, 198, 506
McCallum J.   24
McCullagh P.   423, 432
McDonald J. C.   132, 519
McGilchrist C. A.   488
McKay G. S.   503
McKelvey M.   479
MacKie R.   3
McLaren K.   3
MacLennan R.   511
McMurchie M.   405
McNeil D.   557
McPherson C. K.   313, 469, 476, 478,
    505
Machin D.   202, 206, 479
Macklin J.   6
Madden M.   59
Makuch R.   201
Mantel N.   185, 418, 420, 421, 469, 476, 478,
    505, 512, 517, 527, 531, 533
Mardia K. V.   350, 372
Marks R. G.   378
Marriott F. H. C.   371
Marshall J.   281
Marshall R. J.   153
Martin W. J.   67

Matthews J. N. S.   383, 384
Maxwell A. E.   358
Mayrent S. L.   507
Meckler R. J.   252
Mee R. W.   141
Mehta C. R.   233, 419
Meier P.   198, 476, 506
Merrell M.   473, 475
Middleton T. R.   221, 263, 264
Miettinen O. S.   121, 141, 507, 513, 518
Miller R. G., Jr.   227
Mock P. A.   479
Mohamed S. D.   418
Montgomery R. D.   418
Moon T. E.   479
Morgenstern H.   507, 521, 528
Morley C. J.   4
Morrison D. F.   382, 383
Morrow R. H.   518
Moser C. A.   182
Moses L. E.   576
Muller K. E.   323, 332, 333
Muñoz A.   385
Murdoch J.   561
Musk A. W.   446
Myers M. H.   531

Nagalingan R.   195
Nam J.   141, 206
Naylor A. F.   427
Nelder J. A.   423, 432
Newell D. J.   475, 527
Newhouse M. L.   490
Newman D.   227
Nix A. B. J.   378
Nurminen M.   141

Oakes D.   469, 481
Oakford R. V.   576
O'Brien P. C.   505
Oldham P. D.   236, 381
Ord J. K.   223
Owen D. B.   58

Parker R. A.   206
Parmar M. K. B.   506
Patel N. R.   233, 419
Patterson H. D.   427
Pauker S. G.   74
Paul S. R.   323
Payne C.   556
Pearce S. C.   267, 277
Pearson E. S.   58, 66, 112, 115, 142, 563, 569,
    571

Peto J.   469, 476, 478, 505, 557
Peto R.   136, 186, 195, 219, 469, 476, 478, 505
Pike M. C.   200, 469, 476, 478, 483, 505, 511, 518, 531, 533
Pocock S. J.   190, 193, 219, 379, 380, 503
Powell I.   24
Pownall R.   378
Pregibon D.   432
Prentice R. L.   185, 469, 476, 486
Pullum T. W.   443
Purvis R. J.   503
Pygott F.   457

Quaglino D.   373

Radhakrishna S.   419
Räisänen M. J.   20
Rankin R.   3
Raubertas R. F.   533
Reissland J. A.   442
Reitman D.   195
Richards G.   378
Roberts C. J.   531
Roberts E.   59
Robertson A.   223
Robertson J. D.   315
Robins J. M.   185, 513
Rodgers D.   408
Rojas P. B.   206
Romig H. G.   58
Rose G. A.   67
Rosner B.   385
Rothman K.   98, 507
Rowlands R. J.   378
Royston P.   383, 384
Ryan B. F.   556
Ryan T. A., Jr   556

St Leger A. S.   348
Sacks H. S.   195, 219
Salvan A.   136
Satterthwaite F. E.   113
Saunders M.   421
Savage L. J.   76
Scheffé H.   222
Scherer J.   438
Schlesselman J. J.   202, 206, 519
Schneiderman M. A.   494
Schwartz D.   190, 193
Schwartz S.   74
Shapiro S. H.   190
Shearman R. P.   511
Sherwin R.   377

Shulman L. E.   473, 475
Siegel S.   449
Simon R.   195, 201, 506
Simons J.   24
Simons L. A.   24
Sleight P.   136, 195, 219
Smith A. F. M.   378
Smith C. A. B.   347
Smith C. E. Gordon   3, 391
Smith H.   322, 324, 346, 401
Smith J. K.   555
Smith P. G.   200, 469, 476, 478, 505, 531, 533
Smyth J. F.   3
Sneath P. H. A.   373
Snedecor G. W.   172, 234, 259, 275, 346, 413, 414
Snell E. J.   403, 423, 432
Snell E. S.   498
Sokal R. R.   373
Solomon P. J.   487
Soutar D. S.   3
Spector P. C.   350
Spiegelhalter D. J.   74, 151, 506
Sprent P.   290
Staquet M. J.   190
Stephens R.   479
Stephenson R.   73
Stuart A.   223
'Student' (Gosset W. S.)   235
Sutherland I.   312
Sylvester R. J.   190

Talley R.   479
Therneau T. M.   488
Thomas D. C.   132, 519
Thompson W. D.   507
Thornton A. J.   4
Tiao G. C.   77
Toronto A. F.   73
Trimble I. M. G.   378
Trotman D.   421
Truett J.   431
Tudehope D. I.   408
Tukey J. W.   24, 554
Turnbull B. W.   505
Turnbull D.   405
Turner L. H.   3
Turner T. L.   503
Tytun A.   200

Upton G. J. G.   123, 140
Ury H. K.   200

van Elteren P. H. 464
Veasey L. G. 73
Veazey P. B. 475
Virkkunen M. 20
Vowden B. J. 323

Wagner J. C. 490
Wald A. 493, 497
Wallis W. A. 463
Walter S. D. 348, 521, 528, 529
Wang P. C. 488
Warner H. R. 73
Watson A. C. H. 3
Weatherall J. A. C. 378
Wedderburn R. W. M. 423
Weinstein M. C. 74
Weisberg S. 331, 332
Welch B. L. 217
Welsch R. E. 331
West M. 378
Westgarth D. R. 391
Wetherill G. B. 323, 429
White V. M. 7
Whitehead A. 219
Whitehead J. 219, 497, 502, 505

Whittemore A. S. 522
Wilcocks W. J. 411
Wilcoxon F. 450
Wilkinson E. M. 503
Wilkinson L. 556
Williams D. A. 123
Williams T. F. 475
Wilson A. 173
Wilson D. W. 378
Wilson H. E. 479
Wilson P. D. 377
Wilson P. W. 65
Woolf B. 512
Woolson R. F. 206

Yates F. 112, 115, 120, 138, 139, 140, 142,
    182, 261, 345, 384, 392, 394, 408, 460, 565,
    575, 576
Youden W. J. 523
Yule G. U. 168, 443
Yusuf S. 136, 195, 219

Zeger S. L. 385
Zippin C. 483

Subject Index

Accelerated failure time model 484
Accidents
  cerebrovascular 280–282, 349, 430
  square-root transformation for 390
Adjacent categories model 435
Adjustment
  by analysis of covariance 301–311
  by means in incomplete block
      designs 266
  by standardization 436–443
  of number at risk in life table 473
  of sums of squares in non-orthogonal
      two-way table 280–282, 349
Adrenal weights of mice 252–255
Aetiologic fraction 519
Aetiology 2
  surveys to investigate 183–187, 508–522
Age, peculiarity of 29
Age-specific death rates 437, 470, 489
Agreement 274–276
  kappa measure 443–447
    weighted 445–447
Allocation
  by discriminant function 358–361, 364,
      365, 371, 375
  errors of 359, 364, 365
  in experimentation 187, 188
  optimal, in stratified sampling 179–181
  random 94, 188, 302, 576
Anaemia 367–369
Analgesics 119, 495, 496
Analysis of covariance 155, 301–311, 384
  as form of multiple regression 336, 337
  corrected means in 305, 308, 309
  identification of dependent variable
      in 310
  in complex data 311
  purposes of 301, 302
  several groups 305–311
  two groups 302–305
Analysis of deviance 428–430
Analysis of variance
  for factorial design 251–259
  for Latin square 261–264
  for simple crossover 245

  in multiple regression 317–322, 334–341
  in regression 283–288, 298–301
  mixed model 259
  model I (fixed effects) 219
  model II (random effects) 219
  multivariate 369–370
  one-way 207–228
  tests for contrasts 224–226
  two-way 237–245
    non-orthogonal 276–282
Antibody tests 3, 421
Array 285
Asbestos 132, 136, 142, 143, 490,
    491
Ascertainment 533, 534
  complete 534
  incomplete multiple 534
  simple 534
Assay
  analytical 536
  comparative 536
  computer programs 544, 550
  design 543
  dilution 536
  direct 536
  indirect 537
  non-linearity test 543, 546, 547, 549
  parallel line 537–544
  quantal response 424, 547–550
    median effective dose (ED50) 550
    simple methods 550
  radioimmuno- 378, 543, 544
  radioligand 543, 544
  slope-ratio 544–547
    blanks test 546, 547
    intersection test 546, 547
  see also Biological assay; Potency
Association
  between variables 154–156
  degree of 187
  in space and time 530, 532, 533
  surveys 176, 183–187
Attributable
  fraction 519
  risk 519–522

Automatic selection of variables   321, 322,
        365
Autoregressive modelling   385
Autoregressive series   377, 378
Average *see* Mean, arithmetic

Babies, illness in   4
Backward-elimination procedure   321
Bacterial counts
    Poisson distribution   62–65, 395
    ratio of concentrations   145
    square-root transformation for   391
Bar diagram   5, 6
Bartlett's test   234
Bayes' theorem   71–77, 149–153, 360, 525
Bayesian methods   71–77, 149–153, 324,
        378, 506, 558
    empirical   152, 153
Bernoulli sequence   41–43
Best-subset selection procedure   321, 322
Beta distribution   150
Bias
    due to selection   442
    in estimation   86
    in rounding   14
    in slope estimation   290
    in survival time   529
    in treatment allocation   188
    publication   195
Bimodal distribution   26
Binary data   16
    regression   387, 424
    underlying continuous distribution   402,
        525, 551
    see also Binomial; Categorical data;
        Generalized, linear models;
        Proportions; Quantal
Binomial
    coefficient   55
    distribution   55–59
        fitting   394
        in confidence limits for
            proportion   120–125, 128
        in relative risk   514
        in sequential tests   495–500
        in sign test   449, 450
        in significance test   118–125
        mean   58
        normal approximation   70, 71,
            119–127
        Poisson approximation   61, 62, 65, 66,
            504
        related to F distribution   121, 122,
            514

standard deviation   58
        tables   58
        variance   58
        with missing zero term   534
    theorem   57
Bioassay *see* Biological assay
Biological assay
    of Vitamin D   287, 288, 540–543
    see also Assay; Potency
Birth weight   34, 35, 160–163, 167, 168,
        285
Bivariate normal distribution   168, 169, 173
Blocks   189
    confounding with   268
    incomplete   266, 267
        balanced   266
    permuted   188, 192, 576
    randomized block design   189, 238, 381,
        384
    unbalanced block designs   267
Blood
    cell counts   236
    cholesterol   173, 174
    clotting   237, 241–244, 462
    groups and diseases   413–415
    pressures
        distribution of   26, 66, 67, 172
        in hypotensive drug trial   315–317, 319,
            320, 324–328
        time series of   377, 380, 382
BMDP   13, 555–557
Bonferroni's correction   331
Box-and-whisker plot   34, 35

Cadmium workers, vital capacity of   155,
        295–297, 300, 301, 304, 305, 309,
        310, 340, 341
Calculators   13, 14, 28, 124, 131, 315, 551,
        558
Cancer
    age incidence   483
    breast   4, 217, 218, 312, 313, 511
    gastric   413–415
    head and neck   486
    in ex-servicemen   433, 434
    knowledge about   425–427, 429
    lung
        age distribution   17, 18, 22, 23
        in asbestos workers   132, 136, 142, 143,
            490, 491
        smoking and   183, 185–187, 515–517,
            522
    lymphoma   479–481
    melanoma   3

pancreas 508
survival time in 100–102, 469, 472–476, 479–481, 485, 486
Canonical variates 369–372
Carcinogenesis experiments 483
Cardiovascular disease 186, 430, 504
see also Cerebrovascular disease
Carrier of gene 75, 76
Carry-over effect 245, 248, 260, 261
Case–control study 184–187, 508–522
attributable risk in 519–522
choice of controls 184–186
combination of 2×2 tables in 415, 416, 511–513
computer programs 557
for clustering 531
generalized linear models 518, 519
logistic regression in 518, 519
matched 185, 513, 514, 518, 519
relative risk in 202, 203, 508–522, 527, 528
stratification in 415, 416, 511–513, 522
synthetic retrospective study 185
Case–referent study see Case–control study
Categorical data 15, 402
Causation 155, 156, 183, 187, 312
Cell 8
frequencies
nearly proportionate 277
proportionate 244, 277
replication within 242–244
Censored observation 469, 476, 477, 481, 488, 490
Census 177
as multiphase sample 206
non-sampling errors in 182
Central limit theorem 81
Centring 323, 345
Cerebrovascular disease 280–282, 349, 430
Chest radiographs 446, 447
Chi-square(d) (χ^2)
components of 403, 411–415
in contingency tables 413–415
distribution 86–88
degrees of freedom for 86–88, 395
for heterogeneity of relative risks 512
for trend in counts 410, 411
for trend in proportions 404–406, 408–410, 420–422
in analysis of deviance 428–430
in approximate comparison of means 215–217
in approximate comparison of slopes 293, 294
in comparison of two counts 144–146, 236
in confidence limits for variance 114, 115
in general contingency tables 232, 233
in goodness-of-fit tests 395, 432
in hierarchical classification 411–413
in Poisson heterogeneity (dispersion) tests 234–236, 395, 531
in significance test of variance 114
in $2 \times k$ contingency table 228–232, 402
in 2×2 table 132–137, 146
normal approximation 88
related to F distribution 117, 216
related to Poisson distribution 143
small expected frequencies in 140, 229, 232, 395, 404, 430, 432
statistic (index) (X^2) notation 134
table 562, 563
Chronic bronchitis 186
Classification of disease 15, 373, 507
Clinical trials 189–195
assessment of response in 191, 192
carry-over effect in 245, 248, 260, 261
comparison of fatality rates in 129, 130, 132, 133
crossover 245–249, 495
data monitoring 502
data preparation 9
definition of patients 190, 191
definition of treatments 191
dental 370
double-blind 192
equivalence testing 195, 201, 202
ethical problems 190, 495, 505
in enuresis 246–248
in medical care 189
intention to treat 194
masking of treatments 192
meta-analysis (overviews) 194, 195, 218, 219
multicentre 190
of cough suppressant 498–500
of hypotensive drugs 315–317, 319, 320, 324–328, 333, 334, 338, 339
of screening procedures 528
of tetanus antitoxin 417–419
of tranquillizers 107, 108
of tuberculosis chemotherapy 16, 232, 233
of vitamins for NTD 3
phase I–IV 190
placebo in 192

Clinical trials (*continued*)
  pragmatic 193
  preferences for analgesics 119, 495, 496
  prophylactic 187, 189
  protocol 190
  protocol departures 193, 194, 204, 205
  randomization in 187–189, 192, 193
  sequential methods in 190, 495–506
  single-blind 192
  size 505
  subgroup analysis 191
  treatment allocation in 187–189, 192, 193
Cluster analysis 372–374
Clustering of disease 374, 530–534
  in families 533, 534
  in space 530–532
  in time 530, 531
  in time and space 530, 532, 533
Cochran's test 417–419, 438, 442
Coding 11–13, 552, 553
  of treatments 192
Coefficient of variation 40, 91, 92, 389
Cohort
  life table 470–472
  study (survey) 184–187, 508–510, 519
Coin tossing 41–46, 48, 49
Collinearity 322–324
  tolerance 323
  variance inflation factor 323
Combination
  by weighting 215–219
  of counts 291
  of general contingency tables 420–422
  of relative risks 217, 218, 511–513
  of 2×2 tables 217, 218, 415–419, 511–513
  of trends 420–422
Common slope of parallel lines 293, 294, 298
Communality 357
Community medicine 507
Comparison
  of means corrected by covariance 309
  of mortality rates 436–443
  of positions of regression lines *see* Analysis of covariance
  of several counts 234–236, 530, 531
  of several means 207–228
  of several proportions 228–232
  of several slopes 292–301
  of several variances 234
  of two counts 144–146, 236
  of two means
    paired 106–108, 200

    unpaired 89, 108–114, 196–200, 212, 225
  of two proportions
    combination of sets of data 217, 218, 415–419, 511–513
    paired 125–128
    sequential 504
    unpaired 89, 90, 128–132, 145, 146, 200, 201
  of two slopes 294–297
  of two variances
    paired 117, 118, 171, 172
    unpaired 115–118
Component
  correlations (loadings) 352
  scores 353
Components of variance 172, 219–223, 272–275
Computer
  data editing by 400, 553
  input 11–13
  micro- 11, 555
  packages 13, 554–557
  personal 11, 555
  programs
    analysis of experiments 556
    biological assay 544, 550
    case–control studies 557
    cluster analysis 373
    discriminant analysis 359, 362, 371
    exact probabilities 233, 405, 557
    generalized linear models 423, 429, 550, 555, 556
    latent roots 352
    multiple regression 315, 320, 322, 334, 340, 365, 555, 556
    multivariate analysis 352, 359, 362, 371, 373, 374, 555
    sequential methods 557
    subject-years method 557
    survival analysis 555, 556
    time series 555
  use in statistics 13, 551–558
Conditional
  distribution 138–140, 156
  expectation 156
  probability 45, 138, 485, 518, 525
Confidence
  coefficient 97
  interval 97
    mid-P 124
  limits 97
    distribution-free 452, 453, 458–460
    for correlation coefficient 169

for count   142–144
for difference between means
    paired   107
    unpaired   110–114
for difference between proportions
    paired   126, 127
    unpaired   129, 130
for mean   101–106
for median   451–453
for odds ratio   131, 132, 511–517
for proportion   120–125
for ratio of mean counts   145
for ratio of proportions   131
for regression coefficient   167
for relative risk   131, 132, 511–517
for variance   114, 115
for variance components   222, 223
in biological assay   537, 539, 546, 549
in prediction from regression   169–171
in sequential investigation   494
test-based   513, 517
Confounding   268
variable   206, 416
Congenital abnormalities   3, 43, 347, 348,
    378
Contingency tables
components of χ^2 in   413–415
general   232, 233, 551, 552
    combination of   420–422
    exact test   233, 557
    trend in   408–410
rank sum tests in   458
2×2 (fourfold)   132–141, 146, 552
    combination of   415–419, 511–513
    exact test   137–141
    mid-P test   140, 141
with two rows ($2 \times k$)   228–232, 403,
    531
see also Trend, in proportions
Continuity correction
for binomial distribution   70, 71,
    119–126
for Poisson distribution   70, 71
for 2×2 tables   136, 137, 140, 141, 146
in rank test   450, 467
in sign test   450
not used for larger tables   229
Continuous variable   16
related to binary data   402, 525, 551
Contrast, linear see Linear, contrast
Control group, contrast with   224
Controlled variable   290
Controls, choice of   184–186, 536
Cook's distance   332–334, 432

Coronary heart disease see Cardiovascular
    disease
Corrected
means in analysis of covariance   305, 308,
    309
sums of squares in analysis of
    covariance   307, 308
Correction term (CT)   38, 241
Correlation
coefficient (product-moment)   163–165,
    464
    effect of selection on   165
    standard error   169
    test for zero value   167
intraclass   273–276, 447
matrix   352, 357
multiple   318
of scores   410
rank   464–467
serial   376–378
Correspondence analysis   373
Cost
of misclassification   360
of patient care   312
Cough suppressants   498–500
Counts   16
bacterial see Bacterial counts
blood cell   236
combination of   291
comparison of several   234–236, 530, 531
difference between two   144–146, 236
Poisson distribution for   59–66
radioactivity see Radioactive particles
ratio of mean   145, 146
reduced variability of   236
trend in   410, 411, 421, 422
virus lesions (pocks)   17, 22–24
yeast cell   235, 236
Covariance   90, 91
analysis see Analysis of covariance
of partial regression coefficients   319
Covariate   313, 483–489
in case–control study   518
Cox's model for survival data   484–489, 519
Crossover design
analysis of variance   245
baseline data   245, 249
carry-over effect   245, 248, 260, 261
period effect   246, 495
run-in period   245
simple   245–249, 381, 384, 495
treatment effect   246
treatment × period interaction   248, 249
washout period   245

Crude death rate 436
Cubic regression 341–346
Cumulative
    frequency 16, 21
    logits model 434, 435
Curvilinear regression 341–348
Cusum charts 378

Data
    binary 16
    categorical 15, 402
    cleaning 399–401, 552, 553
    collection 8–10, 552, 553
    dredging 191, 226, 415
    editing 11, 386–401, 553
    entry 11–13, 553
    monitoring 502
    nominal 402
    ordinal 402
    processing 7–14, 552, 553
    qualitative 15, 402
    quantal 16
    quantitative 15
    sorting 551, 552
    transfer 11–13, 553
Death rate 436
    age-specific 437
    crude 436
    expected 439–442, 478, 489–491
Decimal digits 14
Decision theory 74, 151
Degrees of freedom (DF)
    chi-square (χ^2) distribution 86–88, 395
    t distribution 103, 104
    variance estimate 36
    variance-ratio (F) distribution 115–117
Deletion of variables 319–322
    automatic procedures for 321, 322,
        365
Dependent variable 310, 312, 313
    qualitative 422–436
Design
    of assays see Assay, design
    of experiments see Experiments, design of
    of surveys see Surveys
Deviance 428
    analysis of 428–430
    -residual 432, 488
Diagnosis
    Bayes' theorem in 72–76
    discriminant functions in 358
Diagnostic tests 522–528
    errors 360, 523–528
    predictive value 525

reference tests 528
    screening 43, 173, 174, 360, 523, 525, 528,
        529
Diagrams 4–7, 328, 386, 554
    bar 5, 6
        three-dimensional 24
    box-and-whisker 19, 34, 35
    dot 19, 20
    histogram see Histogram
    in multiple regression 324–328
    line 5–7
    pictogram 5
    pie 5, 6
    scatter see Scatter diagram
    stem-and-leaf 21–24
Diallel cross 255
Difference
    direction of 97
    sampling error of 88–90, 94
    see also Comparison
Diffusing factor 221, 222, 263, 264
Direct
    assay 536
    standardization 438, 439
Discrepancies (in contingency tables) 134
Discrete variable 16
Discriminant analysis
    Fisher's linear discriminant function (two
        groups) 358–365, 369–371, 375
        allocation by 358–361, 364, 365, 371,
            375
        and logistic regression 365, 375, 430,
            431
        as likelihood ratio 360, 361, 370, 371
        by dummy-variable regression 361, 362
        for maximal group separation 359, 360
        generalized distance 359, 360, 362, 525
    several groups 369–371
Dissimilarity index 373, 374
Distance
    generalized 359, 360, 362, 525
    standardized 525
Distribution
    beta 150
    binomial 55–59
    chi-square (χ^2) 86–88
    conditional 138–140, 156
    exponential 482, 483, 487
    frequency 15–26
    function 50, 51
    Gompertz 483
    normal (Gaussian) 66–71
    Poisson 59–66
    probability 48–51

Weibull 483, 487
see also specific distribution entries
Distribution-free methods 448–468
    confidence limits 452, 453, 458–460
    estimation 449, 451–453, 458–460, 467, 468
    for survival 481, 484, 485
    one-sample location tests 449–453, 577
    more than two samples
        independent 463, 464
        related 461–463
    rank correlation 464–467
    two-sample location tests 453–460, 467, 468, 481, 578
Dot diagram 19, 20
Dredging of data 191, 226, 415
Drug
    screening 152, 494
    trials *see* Clinical trials
Dummy variable 84, 337, 340, 361, 362
Duration of disease 508

EaSt 557
Economy in experimentation 493, 494
Efficiency 83, 467
EGRET 557
Eigenvalues 352, 369
Enuresis 246–248
Epidemiology 507–534
    attributable risk 519–522
    diagnostic tests 522–528
    disease clustering 374, 530–534
    mathematical 507
    relative risk 202, 203, 508–522, 527, 528
Equivalence testing 195, 201, 202
Errors
    distribution of 423
    in allocation by discriminant function 359, 364, 365
    in two variables 288–290
    of diagnosis 360, 523–528
    of factor classification 527, 528
    of recording 399–401
    rounding 13, 14, 37, 38
    type I 197, 497
    type II 197
Estimation
    distribution-free 449, 451–453, 458–460, 467, 468
    in surveys 176–183
    interval 97–99
    least squares 157–159, 278, 313
    maximum likelihood 148, 157, 428
    robust 401

sequential 494
    unbiased 86
Events 41
    independent 45
    mutually exclusive 44
Expectation 52–54
    conditional 156
    continuous variable 53
    discrete variable 52
    of life 470, 471, 476
    of mean square 211
Expected
    deaths 439–442, 478, 489–491
    frequencies
        in combination of 2×2 tables 418, 419
        in goodness-of-fit tests 394, 395
        in large tables 229, 232
        in 2×2 tables 133
        small, in χ^2 140, 229, 232, 395, 404, 430, 432
Experiments 175
    design of 187–189, 249
        confounding 268
        crossover 245–249, 381, 384, 495
        factorial 237, 249–259, 425–427
        fractional replication 267, 268
        Graeco-Latin square 265
        incomplete blocks 266, 267
        Latin square 259–264, 381, 384
        randomized block 189, 237, 381, 384
        simple randomization 188
        split-unit 268–273, 383, 384
Explanatory variables 313
    in survival data 469, 483–489
    interactions 327
    collinearity 322–324
    relationships between 313, 321
        see also Collinearity
    see also Covariate; Prognostic variable
Exploratory data analysis 5, 554
Exponential distribution 482, 483, 487
Exposure to risk 478
Extrapolation, danger of 171, 344

F distribution *see* Variance, ratio, distribution
Factor
    analysis 357, 358, 375
    levels 249
    loadings 357
Factorial 55
    design/experiment 237, 249–259
        advantages of 249, 250
        half-normal plot of residuals 397

Factorial (*continued*)
  design/experiment (*continued*)
    with proportions 425–427
    with two-level factors 255–257
    fractional 267, 268
    log 139
False negative/positive 197, 360, 523–528
Family
  clustering of disease in 533, 534
  infections 270, 271
Farmers, mortality of 441, 442
Fiducial limits 106
  see also Confidence, limits
Fieller's theorem 539, 546, 549
Finite population correction 82, 83
Fisher–Behrens test 112, 149
Fixed-effects model 219, 258
Follow-up
  studies
    life tables in 472–477
    variation in risk during 146
  see also Cohort, study; Survival analysis
Forms 9–13
Forward-entry procedure 321
Fourfold table *see* 2 ×2 table
Fractional
  factorial design 267, 268
  replication 267, 268
Frailty 488, 489
Frequency 5
  cumulative 16, 21
  curve 25
  distribution 15–26
    bimodal 26
    calculation of mean 28, 29
    calculation of median 30
    calculation of standard
      deviation 38–40
    for continuous variable 17
    for discrete variable 17
    grouping interval 17, 18, 20, 39
    mode 25
    number of groups 18
    skewness 26
    tails 26
    tallying in 18, 19
    unimodal 25
  domain 376, 379, 380
  expected *see* Expected frequencies
  pseudo- 277
  relative 15, 16
Friedman's test 461–463
Function, variance of 90–92
Functional relationship 288–290, 310

Gaussian distribution *see* Normal,
    distribution
General linear model 350
  types of sums of squares 350
Generalized
  distance 359, 360, 362, 525
  estimating equation 385
  linear models 422–436, 548–550, 556
    and standardization 443, 491
    computer programs 423, 429, 548, 556
    in case–control studies 518, 519
    in quantal assays 548–550
    see also Logistic, regression
Genetic
  causation of disease 530, 533, 534
  crosses
    at five loci 59
    two heterozygotes 48, 49, 53, 54
  studies, ascertainment in 533, 534
Genstat 555, 556
GLIM 555, 556
Gompertz distribution 483
Goodness of fit
  in generalized linear model 431, 432
  in logistic regression 431, 432
  in multiple regression 324–334
  Kolmogorov–Smirnov test 397, 398
  of distributions 394–399
  of normal distribution 394–399, 461
  see also Normal, distribution, checking
    adequacy
Graeco–Latin square 265
Graphs *see* Diagrams
Grief and degree of support 408–410
Group sequential plans 502–506
Growth curves 382, 383

Haemolytic disease of newborn 362–365,
    430, 431
Haemophilia 75, 76
Half-normal plot 258, 397
Harmonic analysis 379
Hazard function 482
  proportional 483–489
Health spending 6
Heights, distribution 67, 69, 70
Heterogeneity
  of means 215
    see also Analysis of variance, one-way
  of proportions 228–232
  of variances 234
    see also Heteroscedasticity
  test for Poisson *see* Poisson
Heteroscedasticity 156, 324

Hierarchical classification, χ^2 tests for 411–413
Histogram 20–25
  correction for unequal grouping 20
  for relative frequency 24, 25
Historical prospective study 184, 489
Homoscedasticity 156
Hotelling's T^2 test
  paired one-sample test 366–369, 383
  two-sample test 365, 366, 370, 384
Hypotensive drug trial 315–317, 319, 320, 324–328, 333, 334, 338, 339
Hypothesis
  approximately true 97
  null 95
  simplifying 97

Incidence 508, 509, 529
Incomplete
  block designs 266, 267
    balanced 266
  designs 264–268
  Latin squares 266
Independence
  in random sampling 82, 89, 90
  in variance ratio test 212
  of deviations 36
  of events 45
  of random variables 90
Independent variable 310, 313
  see also Explanatory variables
Indicator variable 337
  see also Dummy variable
Indifference rules 76
Indirect
  assay 537
  standardization 439–443
Infant mortality 6, 154, 155, 471
Information 501–503
Insecticides and houseflies 412, 413
Interaction
  definition in two-level factorial 255–257
  in factorial analysis 250–252, 257–259, 425–429
  in generalized linear model 425–429
  in multiple regression 327
  in two-way analysis 242
  incorrect negative sum of squares 244, 277
  qualitative 257
  quantitative 257
  significant, interpretation with 257–259
  space–time 532
  sum of squares, calculation 244

Intercept 313
Interquartile range 33
Intraclass correlation 273–276, 447
Inverse matrix 314, 315, 359, 367
Irradiation and leukaemia 183, 532
Ischaemic heart disease see Cardiovascular disease
Iterative weighted least squares 428, 429

Joint probability 45

Kaplan–Meier method 476, 477, 479, 480
Kappa 443–447
  weighted 445–447
Kendall's S 454–457, 465–467
Kendall's τ 465
Kolmogorov–Smirnov test 397–399
  Lilliefors modification 397–399
Kruskal–Wallis test 463, 464

Latent roots 352, 369
Latin square 259–264, 381, 384
  balanced for residual effect 261
  randomization 261, 381
  replication 263, 264
Lattice
  designs 267
  squares 267
Lead time 528, 529
Least significant difference 224
Least squares 157–159, 278, 313
  iterative weighted 428, 429
Length-biased sampling 529
Leukaemia
  and irradiation 183, 532
  clustering in 532
Levels of factors 249
Life
  expectation of 470, 471, 476
  table 470–477, 479, 480
    abridged 470
    adjustment for number at risk 474
    cohort 470–472
    current 470–472
    in follow-up studies 472–477
    modified 489
    product-limit (Kaplan–Meier) method 467, 477, 479, 480
    sampling variation in 475, 476
    survivors 470–477
    withdrawals 472–475
Likelihood 72
  function 147, 494
    independent of stopping rule 494

Likelihood (*continued*)
   maximum   148, 157, 428
   partial   485
   ratio
     in diagnosis   526
     in discrimination   360, 361, 370, 371
Line diagram   5–7
Linear
   contrast   224–226
     in biological assay   543, 547
     in two-level factorial   255–257
   discriminant function   358–365, 369–371,
     375
   predictor   423
   regression   156–163, 283–311
   transformation   386, 387
Linearity
   transformations for   387–390
   variance ratio test of   285–288
Link function   423
Liver disease   74, 75
Location, measures of   26–31
Logarithm, common and natural   131, 234
Logarithmic
   paper   388, 390
     double   390
     semi-   388, 390
   probability paper   394
   scale   390
   transformation   292, 327, 387–391
     as limiting power   390
     of dose in biological assay   536, 537,
     548
Logistic
   regression   365, 375, 422–436, 518, 519,
     551, 555–557
     diagnostic methods   431, 432
   transformation   394, 424
     and relative risk   515, 518, 519
     in biological assay   544, 548, 550
     in combination of 2×2 tables   417
     linear model with *see* Logistic,
     regression
Logit *see* Logistic, transformation
Log-linear model   424, 430, 491, 492
Logrank test   477–481, 486, 502
LogXact   557
Longitudinal surveys   183, 380–385
Lung function *see* Respiratory, function
Lymphoma *see* Cancer, lymphoma

McNemar's test   126, 514
Mahalanobis distance *see* Generalized,
   distance

Main effects   250
Malocclusion of teeth   138
Mann–Whitney U test   407, 453–460, 467,
   468
Mantel–Haenszel
   estimate of relative risk   512–514, 516,
     517, 558
   test   418–420, 478, 512–519, 557, 558
   trend test   410, 421
Markov scheme   377
Matched
   pairs   126, 185, 513, 514
   sets   518, 519
Maternal age, outcome of pregnancy   8
Maternal mortality   410, 411
Matrix   314
   inversion   314, 315, 359, 367
Maximum likelihood, method of   148, 157,
   428
   for exponential survival   482
   for generalized linear model   428–436
   for logistic regression   428–436
   for probit model   394, 422, 550
   for survival data   482–487
   in quantal-response assay   548, 550
   in sequential test   501
Mean
   arithmetic   26–29
     comparison with median   29–30
     from frequency distribution   28, 29
   confidence limits for   101–104
   corrected, in analysis of covariance   305,
     308, 309
   deviation   35
   difference between means *see* Comparison,
     of two means
   estimation from stratified
     sample   178–181
   geometric   30, 31, 390
   grand   208
   group   208
   harmonic   31, 391
   of random variable   52, 53
     see also Expectation
   response model   436
   sampling distribution of   80–84
   significance test of   99–101, 103, 104
   square (MSq)   211
     expectation   211, 221
   trimmed   401
   weighted   208, 215–217, 230, 515
   see also specific distribution entries
Median   29, 30
   comparison with mean   29, 30

confidence limits for 451–453
effective (lethal) dose (ED50) 550
from frequency distribution 30
sampling error of 83
survival time 475
Meta-analysis 194, 195, 218, 219
Microcomputers 11, 555
Mid-*P*
  confidence interval 124
  significance level 123, 140, 141, 557
Minimization 193
Minitab 555, 556
Misclassification *see* Errors
Missing readings 194, 277–279, 401, 553
  formulae for insertion 277–279
Mode 25
  of probability distribution 50
Model 94
  accelerated failure time 484
  additive 237
  fixed and random effects 219, 258, 259
  for factorial design 250
  for Latin square 261
  for linear regression 157
  for multiple regression 313
    adequacy of 324–334
  for parallel-line assay 537
  for slope-ratio assay 544, 545
  for two-way analysis of variance 237, 238
  general linear 350
  generalized linear 422–436, 548–550
  linear *see* Model, additive
    for transformed proportions *see* Model,
      generalized linear
  log-linear 424, 430, 491, 492
  mixed 259
  proportional-hazards 484–489, 519
Monitoring 378
  clinical trial data 502
Morbidity surveys 78, 182, 206, 437
Mortality rate *see* Death rate
Multicollinearity *see* Collinearity
Multidimensional scaling 374
Multiphase sampling 206
Multiple
  comparisons 213, 224–228, 497, 530
  correlation coefficient 318
  regression *see* Regression, multiple
Multistage sampling 181, 182, 189
  self-weighting in 182
Multivariate
  analysis 350–375, 555
    canonical variates 369–372
    cluster analysis 372–374

computer programs 352, 359, 362, 371,
    373, 374, 555
  discriminant analysis
    several groups 369–371
    two groups 358–365, 369–371, 375
  factor analysis 357, 358, 375
  growth curves 382, 383
  of variance (MANOVA) 369, 370
  principal components 351–357, 374
  scores 371, 372
  normal distribution 361, 431
Myocardial infarction, prevention 504

Nested design 272, 273
Neural tube defects 3, 43
Neurological episodes 347
Newman–Keuls test 227, 228
Nominal significance level 497, 498,
    500–505
Non-linearity 97
  effect on prediction 171
  in biological assay 543, 546, 547, 549
  test by quadratic 300, 327, 342
  test of departures 285–288
  transformation against 387–389
Non-normality
  distribution-free methods with 448,
    457
  effect on sampling theory 81, 88, 448
    in analysis of variance 213, 214
    in confidence interval for mean 103,
      104
    in inferences from variances 115, 117,
      234
    in multiple regression 324
    in sequential tests 500
    in test for mean 100
  transformations against 387–390
Non-orthogonal data 276, 277
  multiple regression in analysis
    of 348–350, 425
  two-way tables 279–282, 427
Non-parallelism 292–301
  in biological assay 543
Non-parametric methods 448
  see also Distribution-free methods
Non-response 182, 183, 185
Non-sampling errors 182, 185
Normal
  approximation
    in sequential tests 500–504
    to binomial 70, 71, 119–127
    to chi-square (χ^2) 88
    to Poisson 70, 71, 142

Normal (*continued*)
distribution 67–71
bivariate 168, 169, 173
checking adequacy
Kolmogorov–Smirnov test 397–399
normal plots 395–397
Shapiro–Wilk test 398, 399
cumulative distribution function 396
fitting 394
for sample mean 80–84
mean 68
multivariate 361, 431
standard deviation 68
standardized deviate (z) 69, 392, 429, 560
tables 69, 560, 561
testing fit 324, 395–399, 461
transformation to 387, 389
underlying diagnostic tests 525
equations 314
equivalent deviate 392
plot 324, 396–398
scores 396, 460, 461
Null hypothesis 95
non-zero difference 198, 506
Numerical taxonomy 373

Occupational mortality 441, 442, 469
Odds 48
ratio 130, 131, 424, 509, 510
confidence interval for 131, 132, 510, 511
Operating theatre staff 421
Oral contraceptives 4
Order of administration
in crossover trial 245, 246
in diffusing-factor experiment 263
in enuresis trial 246–248
in Latin squares 260, 261, 263, 264
Ordered categories 207, 371, 372, 402–411, 420–422, 448
see also Rank
Orthogonal
contrasts 226, 276
designs 348
polynomials 345, 346, 382
Outliers 328–334, 377, 386, 399–401
Overall significance level 497, 498, 500–505
Overviews *see* Meta-analysis

P value 95
Packages, statistical *see* Computer, packages

Pairs
distribution-free tests 449
effect on planning size 200
in comparison of means 106–108
in comparison of proportions 125–128
in comparison of variances 117, 118, 171, 172
matched, in case–control study 185, 513, 514
Parallel lines
common slope of 293, 294, 298
differences in position 301–311
horizontal distance between 538
in biological assay 537–544
Parameter 59
effect on standard error 93
specification by hypothesis 95
Partial
likelihood 485
regression coefficient 313
variance of 319
Peptic ulcer 413–415, 455, 457
Percentile (percentage point) 34, 87, 560–571, 577, 578
Periodic
components 379
regression *see* Regression, periodic
Permutation test 531
Permuted blocks 188, 192, 576
Personal computers 11, 555
Person-years 146, 489–492, 557
Pictogram 5
Pie chart 5, 6
Pilot investigation 200
Pitman's test 171, 172
Planning of investigations 175, 176
clinical trials 189–195
experiments 187–189
surveys 176–187
Plots, experimental 268
Poisson
distribution 59–66
binomial, approximation 61, 62, 65, 66, 504
fitting 394
for cardiovascular events 282, 430, 504
for congenital abnormalities 348, 378
for deaths 438, 441, 491, 492
for individual frequencies 395, 441
for radioactivity counts 61, 272, 273
for sickness absences 379
in bacteriology 62–65, 395
in disease clustering 531, 533
in periodic regression 348

mean 64
  normal approximation 70, 71, 142
  related to χ^2 distribution 143
  square-root transformation for 391
  standard deviation 64
  tables 66
  variance 64
heterogeneity (dispersion) test 234–236,
    395, 531
process 61
regression 422, 424, 430, 491, 492
Polynomial
  orthogonal 345, 346, 382
  regression see Regression, polynomial
Polytomous regression 434–436
Pooling
  for variance estimate in two-sample t
    test 109
  in comparison of proportions 129
  of frequencies in contingency table 232,
    415
  of interactions and residual 258
Population 36, 78, 79
  attributable fraction 519
  trend 343–345
Posterior probability 72–77, 147–151, 494,
    506, 526
Potency (ratio) 535
  in parallel-line assay 537
    confidence limits 539, 540
    variance (log scale) 539
  in quantal-response assay 548
  in slope-ratio assay 544
Power
  of significance test 197–204
    and sensitivity 523
    distribution-free test 467, 468
    sequential test 498, 501–503
  transformations 390
    logarithmic as limit 390
    reciprocal 391
    square 391
    square-root 390, 391
Precision
  index of, in biological assay 539
  of measurement 14
  specification of 196, 494
Prediction 154
  Bayesian 150, 151, 506
  by multiple regression 312, 313
  errors of 169–171
  from time series 375, 376
  of future population size 343–345
  of probability of success 428

Predictive value 525
Predictor
  linear 423
  variable 313
    see also Explanatory variables
Preferences 119, 495–500
Pregnancy outcome 3, 8
Prevalence 180, 508, 509, 529
Principal components 351–357, 374
Prior probability 71–77, 147–152, 494, 506,
    526
Probability 41–77
  addition rule for 44–47
  as degree of belief 44, 76, 77, 147–152,
    506
  as limiting frequency 41–44, 71
  conditional 45, 138, 485, 518, 525
  density 50, 51
  distribution 48
    mean 52, 53
    mode 50
    skewness 50
    variance 53
  joint 45
  multiplication rule for 44–47
  paper 394
  posterior 72–77, 147–151, 494, 506, 526
  prior 71–77, 147–152, 494, 506, 526
  subjective 76, 77
Proband 534
Probit
  analysis 394, 422, 550
  transformation 392–394, 424, 550
Product, mean and variance of 91
Product-limit estimate 476, 477, 479, 480
Product-moment correlation see Correlation
    coefficient
Prognosis 312, 313, 428, 469
Prognostic variable 469, 483
Programme lead time 529
Programs see Computer, programs
Proportional-hazards model 483–489, 519
  Cox's model 484, 485
  exponential 483
  in case–control study 519
  risk set 484
Proportions
  confidence limits for 120–125
  difference between see Comparison
  distribution of 58, 84, 85
  estimation in stratified
        sampling 179–181
  ratio of 130–132
  sequential test for 495–500

Proportions (*continued*)
  significance test for   118, 119
  transformations for   392–394
  trend in   231, 403–407, 420, 421, 457, 458,
    557
Prospective study   184
  historical   184, 489
  see also Cohort study
Psychological test response   548
Publication bias   195
Punch card   11
Purposive selection   79

Quadratic regression   300, 327, 341–346
Qualitative data   15, 402
Quality control   378
Quantal
  data   16
    see also Binary data
  response in biological assay   424,
    547–550
Quantitative data   16
Quartic regression   341–344
Quartiles   33
Questionnaires   9–13, 351
Quota sampling   79

Radioactive particles
  combination of counts   291
  components of variance of
    counts   272–275
  counts, in radioimmunoassays   544
  distribution of time intervals   26
  Poisson process formed by   61
Radioimmunoassays   378, 543, 544
Radioligand assays   543, 544
Random
  allocation   94, 188, 302, 576
    adjustment after   302
  -effects model   219, 259
  permutation   576
  sampling   79, 177–183, 576
    numbers   79, 81–83, 188
      generator   82, 576
      instructions   576
      table   572–575
  sequence   41
  series   41
  variable   48
Randomization
  in Latin squares   261, 381
  in treatment allocation   94, 188, 302,
    576
  restricted *see* Permuted blocks

Randomized block design   189, 237, 381,
    384
Randomized controlled trial (RCT) *see*
    Clinical trials
Range   32, 33
  studentized *see* Studentized range
Rank(ed data)
  correlation   464–467
  normal scores   396, 460, 461
  signed rank sum test   450–453
    table   577
  sorting   551, 552
  sum test (two-sample)   453–460, 467, 468,
    481
    table   578
  ties   455–458
Ratio
  cross-   510
  distribution of   91
  odds-   130, 131, 424, 509, 510
  of proportions (risks)   130–132
  of variance estimates *see* Variance,
    ratio
Receiver operating characteristic curve   527
Reciprocal transformation   391
Records, medical   184, 507
Recurrence time   472
Reduction in variability
  by analysis of covariance   302
  by blocking   189
Regression
  analysis of variance in   283–288
  asymptotic   346
  coefficient   159
    as contrast   225
    variance of   166
  comparison of several groups   292–301
  comparison of two groups   294–297
  curve   156
  curvilinear   341–348
  diagnostics
    Cook's distance   332–334, 432
    influential points   332–334, 432
    leverage   329–334, 432
    see also Collinearity; Residual
  equation   157
  function   156
  heteroscedastic   156
  homoscedastic   156
  intercept   313
  line   156–163
  linear   156–163, 283–311
  logistic *see* Logistic, regression
  multiple   312–350, 375

adequacy of model 324–334
as generalized linear model 423
computer programs for 315, 320, 322,
 334, 340, 365, 555, 556
deletion of variables 319–322, 365
in discriminant analysis 361, 362
in groups 334–341
in slope-ratio assay 545–547
with dummy variables
 for analysis of covariance 336, 337
 for non-orthogonal data 348–350
parallel lines 293, 294, 298, 301–311,
 537–544
partial regression coefficient 313
 variance of 319
periodic 347, 348, 379, 380, 531
polynomial 341–346
 cubic 341–346
 quadratic 300, 327, 341–346
 quartic 341–344
polytomous 434–436
prediction in 154, 312, 313
proportional-hazards 483–489, 519
residual about 159, 163
ridge 323, 324
robust 401
slope 159
 t test for 166, 167, 284
standard deviation about 159
through origin 291, 292
to the mean 150–153, 172–174
two lines 162, 163, 165, 310
Rejection of observations 401
Relationships between variables 7, 154–156
in multiple regression 313, 321, 322
in polynomial regression 345
Relative
death rates 478
frequency 15, 16
risk 508–522
 approximate 509, 510
 combination of 217, 218, 511–513
 from matched pairs 513, 514
 Mantel–Haenszel method 512–514,
  516, 517, 558
 relation to logit difference 515, 518
 variance of 510
Reliability 275
 see also Agreement
Repeated measurements 152, 173, 380–385,
 436
Repeated significance test (RST) plans 498,
 500–502
Replication 188, 189, 241, 242

in incomplete block design 266
nearly proportionate 277
of Latin squares 263, 264
proportionate 244, 277
Residual
deviance- 432, 488
effect 245, 248, 260, 261
examination of residuals 240–242,
 324–334, 396, 432
jackknife 330
martingale 487
mean square 159, 240, 252, 303, 334, 539,
 546
plots 324–328
standardized 328, 432
studentized 330, 396–398
sum of squares 157–159, 163, 164, 239,
 252, 313
time series analysis of residuals 377
variance 157, 199, 238, 250, 261, 267, 283,
 291, 294
zero, for missing reading insertion 278
Respiratory
disability 353–356
function 198, 199, 207
 age and exposure 155, 295–297, 301,
  302, 309, 310, 312, 340, 341
 repeated measurements 380
infections in families 269–271
Retrospective study 184
 see also Case–control study
Ridge regression 323, 324
Risk
attributable 519–522
number at, in life table 474
relative see Relative risk
set 484
Robust
estimation 401
regression 401
Robustness 104, 389, 401, 448
lack of, in inferences from variances 115,
 117, 234
of t distribution 104
Rotation of axes 353
Rounding errors 13, 14, 37, 38
Run-in period 245

Sample 36, 78, 79
size, choice of 93, 195–206, 505
 for comparing two means 196–200
 for comparing two
  proportions 200–202
 table 579

Sample (*continued*)
  size, choice of (*continued*)
    for odds ratio 202, 203
      table 580
    in equivalence testing 201, 202
    with non-zero null 198
    with protocol departures 204, 205
    with unequal-sized groups 203,
      204
    with withdrawals 204, 205
    see also Sequential
  surveys 176–187
  see also Sampling
Sampling 78, 79, 176–185
  distribution 80–82
  error 79–92
    see also Sampling variance
  fraction 82, 83, 178, 179, 184
  frame 79
  length-biased 529
  multiphase 206
  multistage 181, 182, 189
  quota 79
  random 79, 177–183, 576
    as model 94
  simple random 79
  stratified 178–181
  systematic 177, 178
  variance 81
    in life table 475, 476
    in stratified sampling 179–181
    of difference 88–90
      between means 88, 89
      between proportions 89, 90
    of general function 92
    of linear function 90, 91
    of mean 80–84, 179
    of mean corrected by covariance 308
    of median 83
    of partial regression coefficient 319
    of product 91
    of proportion 84, 85
    of ratio 91
    of regression coefficient 166
    of variance 88
    see also Standard error
  without replacement 82
SAS 13, 555, 557
Satterthwaite's test 112–114
Scatter diagram 7, 154–156, 386
  in multiple regression 324–328
Scheffé's test 228
Schistosomal infections 230–232
Scores 15

from canonical variates 371, 372
in contingency tables 403–410, 420
normal 396, 460, 461
Screening
  diagnostic 43, 173, 174, 360, 523, 525,
    528, 529
  drug 152, 494
  mammography 405
Seasonal trend 347, 379, 531
Selection
  bias 442
  effect on correlation coefficient 165
  in ascertainment 533, 534
  of variables *see* Deletion of variables
Self-weighting 182
Sensitivity 523
Sequential
  analysis 149, 493–506
  design 439–506
    for clinical trials 495–506
    reasons for 493–495
  estimation 494
  stopping rule 493, 505, 506
    stochastic curtailment 506
  survival analysis 502
  tests 495–506
    binomial preferences 495–500
    boundaries 498–506
    comparison of two proportions 504
    diagram for 498
    group sequential plans 502–506
    normal 497, 500–502
Serial correlation 376–378
Sex distribution 21, 46–48
Shapiro–Wilk test 398, 399
Sheppard's correction 39, 394
Shrinkage 150–153, 172
Sickness absence data 379, 380
Sigmoid curve 392, 544, 547
Sign test 449, 450
Signed rank sum test 450–453
Significance
  clinical and statistical 96, 98, 99, 198, 506
  level 95
    and specificity 523
    mid-P 123, 140, 141, 557
    nominal 497, 498, 500–505
    overall 497, 498, 500–505
    specification of 196, 197
  test 94–97
    distribution-free 448–468
    goodness-of-fit 394–399, 431, 432
    in contingency table *see* Contingency
      tables

in regression   166, 167
non-parametric   448–468
of correlation coefficient   167
of difference between counts   144–146
of difference between means
   paired   106–108
   unpaired   108–114
of difference between proportions
   paired   125–128
   unpaired   128–132
of heterogeneity of variance   234
of linearity   285–288
of mean   99–101, 103, 104
of proportion   118, 119
of variance   114
one-sided   96, 97
permutation   531
purposes of   97
repeated   498, 500–502
sequential   495–506
tail probability (P value) in   95
two-sided, 96, 97
see also Analysis of covariance; Analysis of
   variance; Chi-square; Comparison;
   Distribution-free methods;
   Regression; Sequential tests;
   t distribution; Variance ratio
Significant digits   14
Similarity index   373, 374
Simultaneous inference   227
Size of investigation   93, 194–206, 505
   see also Sample, size, choice of; Sequential
Skewness   26, 51, 324
   countered by logarithmic
      transformation   390
Slope
   of functional relationship   288–290
      bias in estimation   290
   of regression line   159
   t test for   166, 167, 284
   –ratio assay   544–547
Small area rates   152, 153
Smoking
   and chronic bronchitis   186
   and ischaemic heart disease   186
   and lung cancer   183, 185–187, 515–517,
      522
   sex ratio   7
Social medicine   507
Sojourn time   528, 529
Spearman, rank correlation coefficient   465,
   466
Specificity
   in assay response   535

in diagnostic tests   523
Spectral analysis   379, 380
SPIDA   557
Split-plot design   268–273, 383
Split-unit design   268–273, 383
SPSS   13, 555, 557
Sputum
   classification in trial   16, 232, 233
   culture on two media   127, 128
Square-root transformation   390, 391
Standard
   deviation   35
      about regression   159
      estimated   36
      from frequency distribution   38, 39
      see also specific distribution entries
   error (SE)   81
      need to estimate   93, 103
      of correlation coefficient   169
      of mean   81
      of median   83
      of proportion   85, 121
      of regression coefficient   166, 167
      specification of   196, 494
      see also Sampling, variance
   population   437–443
   preparation   535
   unit   535
Standardization   185, 436–443
   and generalized linear model   443
   direct   438, 439
   indirect   439–443
   of variables   352, 357
   relation between methods of   442
Standardized
   mortality ratio (SMR)   439–443, 490,
      491
   normal deviate (z)   69, 392, 429, 560
STATA   556
Statistic   93
Statistical
   computation   13, 551–558
      see also Computers
   inference   2, 76, 93–153
Statistics
   definition of   1
   descriptive   2, 15
   official   5
   vital   375, 436, 437, 470, 507
StatXact   557
Stem-and-leaf display   21–24
Step-down procedure   321
Step-up procedure   321
Stepwise procedure   321, 365

Stillbirths, aetiology of 312
Stochastic curtailment 506
Stopping rule 493, 505, 506
  no effect on likelihood or posterior
        distribution 494
Stratification
  in case–control study 415, 416, 511–513,
        522
  in contingency tables 415–422
  in distribution-free analysis 463, 464
Stratified sampling 178–181
  optimal allocation in 179–181
  with proportions 179–181
Stratum 178
Streptomycin treatment, sputum results 16,
    232, 233
Studentized range 227
  table 570, 571
Subject-years method 489–492, 557
Sum
  of products (SPr)
    about mean 159
    short-cut formula 159
  of squares (SSq)
    about mean 35
    about regression 159, 163
    between two groups 212
    corrected 38
    from frequency distribution 39
    in analysis of variance 208
    in general linear model 350
    on calculator 13
    partition between and within
        groups 209
    short-cut formula 37
Summation sign (Σ) 27, 293
Surveys 175–187
  aetiological 183–187, 508–522
  case–control 184–187, 508–522
  cohort 184–187, 508, 510, 519
  estimation in 176–183
  for associations 176, 183–187
  longitudinal 183, 380–385
  non-response in 182, 183, 185
  non-sampling errors in 182, 185
  of health or morbidity 78, 176–183, 206,
    437
  prospective 184
    see also Surveys, cohort
  retrospective 184, 508–522
Survival analysis/data 469–492
  accelerated failure time model 484
  censored observations 469, 476, 477, 481,
    488, 490

computer programs 555, 556
  Cox's model 484–489, 519
  diagnostic methods 487, 488
  expected exposure to risk 478
  expected mortality 478, 489–491
  exponential distribution 482, 483, 487
  Gompertz distribution 483
  hazard function 482
  life table *see* Life, table
  logrank test 477–481, 486, 502
  median survival time 475
  parametric models 482, 483
  product-limit (Kaplan–Meier)
    method 476, 477, 479, 480
  proportional-hazards model 484–489,
    519
  reciprocal transformation 391
  recurrence time 472
  relative death rates 478
  sequential 502
  subject-years methods 489–492, 557
  survivor function 482
  Weibull distribution 483
Survivor function 482
Synthetic retrospective study 185
SYSTAT 556
Systematic
  allocation 188
  errors 182, 183
  sampling 177, 178

t distribution 103, 104
  degrees of freedom for 103, 104
  distribution-free alternatives 453, 457,
    467
  for linear contrast 225
  in comparison of two slopes 295
  in confidence interval for mean 104
  in multiple regression 319–321
  in paired comparison of means 107
  in regression 166–171, 284
  in significance test of mean 103, 104
  in two-group analysis of covariance 304,
    305
  in unpaired comparison of means (two-
    sample *t* test) 108–111, 207, 213
  related to variance ratio distribution 117,
    212, 228, 244, 284, 301, 321
  table 564, 565
Tables
  presentation of data in 7–9, 13, 551–553
  statistical 560–580
Tardive dyskinesia 275, 276, 385, 445
Test-based confidence limits 513, 517

Test of significance *see* Significance, test
Tetanus antitoxin 417–419
Ties in ranking 455–458
Time domain 376–378
Time series 5–7, 375–380, 555
  autoregressive 377, 378
  computer programs 555
  frequency domain 379, 380
  harmonic analysis 379
  moving-average 378
  seasonal trend 347, 379, 531
  spectral analysis 379, 380
  time domain 376–378
  trend removal 377
Titres
  antibody 3
  geometric mean 30, 31
Tolerance
  as collinearity measure 323
  in biological assay 547, 548
Tranquillizers 107, 108
Transformation 7, 214, 377
  and interactions 257
  in generalized linear model 422
  in multiple regression 327
  linear 386, 387
  logarithmic 292, 327, 387–391
  logit (logistic) 394, 424
  power 390
  probit 392–394, 424, 550
  purposes of 387
    linearizing 387, 389, 390
    normalizing 387, 389
    variance-stabilizing 387
  reciprocal 391
  square 391
  square-root 390, 391
Trend
  diagrammatic representation of 5–7
  direction of 154
  in counts 410, 411, 421, 422
  in large contingency table 408–410
  in population size 343–345
  in proportions 231
    chi-square test 404–406, 420, 421
    combination of subsets 420, 421
    exact test 404, 405, 557
    rank sum test 457, 458
  linear 154
  removal 377
  seasonal 347, 379, 531
Trial
  clinical *see* Clinical trials
  in random sequence 41

outcomes (events) 41
  independent 45
  mutually exclusive 44
Trimmed mean 401
Trypanosome counts 19
Tumours *see* Cancer
2×2 table 132–141, 146, 552
  chi-square (χ^2) test 132–137, 146
  combination 217, 218, 415–419, 511–513
  continuity correction 136, 137, 140, 141, 146
  exact test 137–141, 558
  mid-P test 140, 141, 557
  of means 135
Two-way table
  of frequencies *see* Contingency tables
  of measurements 237–245
    non-orthogonal 276–282, 427
    two rows or columns 279–282, 427
Type-I error 197
Type-II error 197

Unbiased estimator 86
Unimodal distribution 25
Uterine weights of rats 105

Vaccination
  trial 187
  yellow fever 3
Variable 15
  categorical 15
  continuous 16
  controlled 290
  dependent 310, 312, 313
  discrete 16
  dummy 84, 337, 340, 361, 362
  explanatory *see* Explanatory variables
  independent 310, 313
  indicator 337
  predictor 313
  prognostic 469, 483
  qualitative 15, 402
    nominal 15, 402
    ordinal 15, 402
  quantitative 15, 402
  random 48
Variance 35
  analysis of *see* Analysis of variance
  components of 172, 219–223, 272–275
  confidence limits for 114, 115
  difference between estimates (paired data) 117, 118, 171, 172
  estimated 36
    sampling distribution of 85–88

Variance (*continued*)
from frequency distribution   38–40
heterogeneity of, test for   234
inequality of, in comparison of
     means   111–114
inflation factor   323
of random variable   53, 54
ratio (F, VR)   115–117
   degrees of freedom for   115–117
   distribution   115–117, 121, 122
   in analysis of covariance   306
   in analysis of variance   212
   in comparison of slopes   299–301
   in multiple regression   318
      for deletion of variables   320, 321
   in regression   284, 285
   in test for linearity   285–287
   related to other distributions   117, 121,
      122, 212, 216, 228, 244, 284, 301,
      321, 514
   table   566–569
residual *see* Residual, variance
see also specific distribution entries
Variate   15
canonical   369–372
see also Variable
Variation
coefficient of   40, 91, 92, 389
measures of   26, 31–40
reduction in   189
Varimax method   353
Virus lesions (pocks)   17, 23, 113, 114, 217
Visual analogue scale   353

Visual display unit (VDU)   11
Vitamin
assay   287, 288, 540–543
supplementation   3, 503, 504

Wald test   429
Washout period   245
Weibull distribution   483
Weight gain
and birth weight   160–163, 167, 168,
     285
and protein content   110, 111
Weighting
by reciprocal of variance   215–219, 230,
     293, 294, 512, 515, 544
   in multiple regression   334, 335, 338
empirical   216, 424–428
Welch's test   112, 149
Wilcoxon
one-sample (signed rank sum)
      test   450–453
   table   577
two-sample (rank sum) test   407, 453–460,
     467, 468, 481
   table   578
Worm counts   213, 214

Yates's correction   136
Yeast cell counts   235, 236
Youden square   266
Youden's misclassification index   523, 524

z-value *see* Standardized, normal deviate